Radiographic Interpretation for the Small Animal Clinician

Second Edition

Radiographic Interpretation for the Small Animal Clinician

Second Edition

Jerry M. Owens, D.V.M.
Diplomate, American College of Veterinary Radiology
Bay Area Veterinary Specialists
San Leandro, California
Veterinary Radiology Services and Veterinary Telerad
San Rafael, California

Darryl N. Biery, D.V.M.
Diplomate, American College of Veterinary Radiology
Professor of Radiology
Department of Clinical Studies
University of Pennsylvania
School of Veterinary Medicine
Philadelphia, Pennsylvania

SANS TACHE

Williams & Wilkins
A WAVERLY COMPANY

BALTIMORE • PHILADELPHIA • LONDON • PARIS • BANGKOK
HONG KONG • MUNICH • SYDNEY • TOKYO • WROCLAW

Editor: Caroll C. Cann
Managing Editor: Leah Ann Kiehne Hayes
Marketing Manager: Diane Harnish
Production Editor: June Choe

351 West Camden Street
Baltimore, Maryland 21201-2436 USA

Rose Tree Corporate Center
1400 North Providence Road
Building II, Suite 5025
Media, Pennsylvania 19063-2043 USA

Printed in the United States of America

First Edition, 1992 by the Ralston Purina Company

Library of Congress Cataloging-in-Publication Data

Owens, Jerry M.
Radiographic interpretation for the small animal clinician / Jerry M. Owens, Darryl N. Biery. --2nd ed.
p. cm.
Includes bibliographical references (p.) and index.
ISBN 0-683-06684-6
1. Dogs—Diseases—Diagnosis. 2. Cats—Diseases—Diagnosis. 3. Veterinary radiography. I. Biery, Darryl N. II. Title.
SF991.094 1998
636.7'089607572—dc21 98-41669
CIP

99 00 01 02 03
1 2 3 4 5 6 7 8 9 10

Preface

We are very pleased to have created this second edition of *Radiographic Interpretation for the Small Animal Clinician.* The first edition, published in 1982, was generously supported and distributed by the Ralston Purina Company to veterinary students and veterinary practitioners throughout the United States. The book was also translated into Italian, German, and Japanese and has been used worldwide in teaching radiology. We are grateful for the relationship with Ralston Purina who made our vision for this book a reality, and for their continuing cooperation that has resulted in this new edition published by Williams & Wilkins.

The text has been significantly expanded, with five new chapters. The first chapter, on the scope of diagnostic imaging, includes the principles and applications of diagnostic radiology, ultrasound, computed tomography, magnetic resonance imaging, and scintigraphy. The second and third chapters on the principles of radiographic interpretation, contrast media, and radiographic contrast procedures have been increased in scope. Within the chapters of each anatomic region, many new disease entities, tables, and drawings have been added, increasing their depth and breadth. For each disease or condition, the discussion is in an outline consisting of clinical correlations, radiographic findings, and other recommended imaging procedures. It is anticipated that the reader will understand the concepts of radiographic interpretation resulting in the ability to recognize and diagnose many diseases in the dog and cat. As with the first edition, we envision this new book to be used in teaching radiology to veterinary students and to serve as a practical guide and resource for small animal practitioners.

Jerry M. Owens, Darryl N. Biery

Acknowledgments

We gratefully acknowledge many individuals who participated in this project. Carroll Cann and his staff at Williams & Wilkins have been very supportive and encouraging throughout the 3 years of creating this second edition. We are also thankful to our colleagues who helped edit and constructively criticize many of the chapters. The artistic talent of Rhonda Sharpe, who provided all of the new illustrations, is gratefully appreciated as the book would not have the same impact without them. We also thank our wives and families for allowing us the time to complete this second edition.

Contents

Preface v

1. The Scope of Diagnostic Imaging in Small Animal Practice 1

Philosophy of Imaging 1
Imaging Interpretation 1
Types of Imaging Procedures 1
Diagnostic Radiology 1
    Radiographic Technique 3
    Positioning 3
    Film Identification 3
Fluoroscopy 4
Diagnostic Ultrasound 4
Computed Tomography 6
Magnetic Resonance Imaging 7
Nuclear Medicine Imaging 8

2. Principles of Radiographic Interpretation 9

Introduction 9
Radiopacity 9
Basic Radiographic Opacities 10
    Bone Opacity 10
    Soft Tissue Opacity 10
    Fat Opacity 10
    Gas Opacity 10
Geometry of the Radiographic Image 10
Radiographic Interpretation 11
    Viewing Area 11
    Three-Dimensional Concept 11
    Process of Examining the Radiographs 11

3. Radiographic Contrast Procedures 15

Patient Preparation 15
Contrast Media 15
    Types of Contrast Media 15
    Ionic and Nonionic 15
    Barium Sulfate Contrast Media 16
    Adverse Effects of Barium Sulfate . . . 17
    Adverse Effects of Negative Contrast Media 17
Contrast Examination Techniques 17
    Intravenous Urography 17
    Cystography 18
    Double Contrast Cystography 18
    Positive Contrast Cystography 18
    Pneumocystography 18
    Urethrography 18
    Vaginography 18
    Esophagography 20
    Gastrography 20
    Upper Gastrointestinal Study 21
    Barium Enema 21
    Double Contrast Barium Enema 21
    Pneumocolon or Positive Contrast Colonic Examination 22
    Peritoneography 22
    Myelography 22
    Epidurography 23
    Discography 23
    Arthrography 23
    Angiography: Selective and Nonselective 23
    Venous Portography 24
    Pneumopericardiography 24
    Fistulography 24
    Tracheography and Bronchography . . 25
    Pleurography 25
    Sialography 25

Dacryocystorhinography 25
Otic Canalography 25
Rhinography 25
Lymphography 25

4. Extremities 27

Anatomy 27
Normal Bone Development and Growth 27
Accessory Ossification Centers and Sesamoid Bones 27
Variable Ossification Centers 28
Clinical and Radiographic Correlations 28
Radiographic Technique 29
Radiographic Interpretation 30
Definitions 34
Diseases/Disorders 36
Osteoporosis 36
Osteopetrosis 36
Ectrodactyly 36
Polydactyly 36
Syndactyly 37
Hemimelia 37
Chondrodysplasia 37
Pituitary Dwarfism 38
Congenital Hypothyroidism 38
Multiple Epiphyseal Dysplasia 38
Enchondrodystrophy 38
Dwarfism of Alaskan Malamutes 38
Dwarfism of Norwegian Elkhound . . . 39
Chondrodysplasia of Great Pyrenees 39
Skeletal-Retinal Dysplasia in Labrador Retrievers 39
Ocular-Skeletal Dwarfism in Samoyed 39
Metaphyseal Tibial Dysplasia 39
Mucopolysaccharidosis 40
Feline Osteodystrophy 40
Osteogenesis Imperfecta 40
Hypertrophic Osteodystrophy 40
Retained Enchondral Cartilage of the Distal Ulna 41
Rickets 42
Growth Arrest Line (Growth Retardation Line) 42
Hypertrophic Osteopathy 42
Panosteitis 43
Lead Poisoning 43
Bone Infarcts 43
Fractures 43
Fracture Healing 47
Radiographic Evaluation of Fracture Healing 47
Fracture Complications 48
Diseases/Disorders 48
Classification of Fracture Complications 48
Delayed Union 48
Nonunion 49
Malunion 49
Pseudoarthrosis 49
Premature Physeal Closure 49
Osteomyelitis: Bacterial and Mycotic 50
Protozoan Osteomyelitis 52
Neoplasia 53
Diseases/Disorders 53
Primary Benign Bone Tumors and Cysts 53
Primary Malignant Bone Neoplasia 54
Metastatic Malignant Bone Neoplasia 54
Musculocutaneous Soft Tissue Diseases . . . 56
Diseases/Disorders 56
Soft Tissue Swelling 56
Musculocutaneous Soft Tissue Masses 56
Musculocutaneous Emphysema 56
Soft Tissue Mineralization 57
Foreign Bodies 58
Arteriovenous Fistula 58
Lymphadenopathy 58
Lymphedema 58

5. Joints 59

Anatomy 59
Synovial Joints (Diarthroses) 59
Fibrous Joints (Synarthroses) 59
Cartilage Joints (Synchondroses) 59
Radiographic Technique 60
Projections 60
Radiographic Interpretation 60
Clinical and Radiographic Correlations 61
Diseases/Disorders 61
Congenital Malformations 61
Conformational Deformities 62
Osteochondrosis and Osteochondritis Dissecans 62
Trauma 62
Physeal Injury 63
Osteoarthritis 63
Infectious Arthritis 63
Bacterial Arthritis 63
Mycoplasma and L-Forms of Bacterial Arthritis 64
Rickettsial Arthritis 64
Spirochetal Arthritis 64
Viral Arthritis 64
Fungal Arthritis 64

Noninfectious Arthritis 64
Idiopathic Polyarthritis 65
Systemic Lupus Erythematosus 65
Polyarthritis/Polymyositis Complex 65
Polyarthritis/Meningitis Syndrome 65
Sjogren Syndrome 65
Familial Renal Amyloidosis 65
Heritable Polyarthritis 66
Polyarteritis Nodosa 66
Erosive Arthritis 66
Rheumatoid Arthritis 66
Reiter Disease 67
Feline Polyarthritis 67
Polyarthritis of the Greyhound 67
Synovial Cell Sarcoma 67
Primary Bone Sarcoma 67
Metastatic Neoplasia 68
Synovial Osteochondromatosis 68
Villonodular Synovitis 68
SHOULDER 68
Radiographic Technique 68
Disease/Disorders 68
Luxation 68
Fracture 69
Osteochondrosis/Osteochondritis Dissecans 69
Biceps Tendinopathy 70
Supraspinatus and Infraspinatus Tendinopathy 70
Shoulder Dysplasia 72
Osteoarthritis 73
ELBOW 73
Radiographic Technique 73
Diseases/Disorders 74
Elbow Dysplasia 74
Osteochondrosis/Osteochondritis of Humeral Condyle 74
Ununited Anconeal Process 76
Fragmented Medial Coronoid Process . 76
Distractio Cubiti 78
Incomplete Ossification of Humeral Condyle 79
Luxation 79
Subluxation 79
Medial Epicondylar Spur 79
CARPUS 80
Radiographic Technique 80
Diseases/Disorders 80
Luxation/Subluxation 80
Fracture 80
DIGITS—Metacarpus/Metatarsus/Phalanges 80
Radiographic Technique 80
Radiographic Anatomy 81
Diseases/Disorders 81
Fracture/Luxation 81
Sesamoid Bone Fractures 82
Digital Neoplasia 82
COXOFEMORAL JOINTS AND PELVIS 82
Radiographic Technique 82
Radiographic Anatomy 83
Diseases/Disorders 83
Coxofemoral Luxation 83
Fractures of the Pelvis 83
Sacroiliac Luxation 84
Femoral Head/Neck Fractures . . 84
Ischemic Necrosis of Femoral Head 85
Hip Dysplasia 86
Hip Dysplasia Control Programs . 89
STIFLE 92
Radiographic Technique 92
Diseases/Disorders 92
Cranial Cruciate Ligament Injury 92
Caudal Cruciate Ligament Injury 93
Osteochondrosis/Osteochondritis Dissecans 93
Luxation 94
Avulsion of the Tendon of Origin of the Long Digital Extensor . . . 94
Avulsion of the Origin of the Popliteal Muscle 94
Intraarticular Ossification 94
Avulsion of the Tibial Tuberosity 94
Patellar Luxation/Subluxation . . 95
Ruptured Patellar Tendon 99
TARSUS 102
Radiographic Technique 102
Diseases/Disorders 102
Luxation/Subluxation 102
Calcanean Tendon Injury 103
Osteochondrosis/Osteochondritis Dissecans 103

6. Skull 105

Radiographic Technique 105
Other Imaging 108
Radiographic Anatomy 108
Radiographic Interpretation 110
CRANIAL VAULT (CALVARIUM) . . . 110
Radiographic Anatomy 110
Diseases/Disorders 110
Hydrocephalus 110
Occipital Dysplasia 111
Fractures 112
Temporomandibular Subluxation or Luxation 112
Infection 112

Craniomandibular Osteopathy 112
Lesions of the External, Middle, and Inner Ear 113
Neoplasms 114
NASAL CAVITY AND PARANASAL SINUSES 116
Radiographic Anatomy 116
Diseases/Disorders 116
Fractures of the Face and Frontal Area 116
Infections 116
Neoplasms Involving the Nasal Cavity 117
TEETH 118
Radiographic Anatomy 118
Effect of Age 119
Radiographic Examination 120
Diseases/Disorders 120
Dental Anomalies 120
Dental Calculus 120
Dental Decay (Caries) 120
Tooth Resorption 120
Periodontal Disease 121
Apical Infection 121
Fractures of Tooth 122
Metabolic Diseases 122
Neoplasms of the Teeth and the Oral Cavity 123
SALIVARY GLANDS 124
Radiographic Anatomy 124
Diseases/Disorders 124
Sialolithiasis 124
Sialocoele 124
Salivary Duct Fistula 124
Neoplasms 124
Nasolacrimal Duct Abnormalities 125

7. Spine 127

Vertebral Development 127
Vertebral Anatomy 127
Radiographic Technique 127
Other Imaging 127
Radiographic Interpretation 128
Myelography 129
Interpretation 129
Diseases/Disorders 131
Spinal Bifida 131
Block Vertebra 132
Hemivertebra 132
Transitional Vertebrae 133
Sacrococcygeal Dysgenesis 134
Spinal Curvature Deformities 134
Osteoporosis 134
Hypervitaminosis A in the Cat 135
Mucopolysaccharidosis 135
Atlantoaxial Subluxation 136
Cervical Spondylopathy 137
Lumbosacral Instability 137
Osteochondrosis 138
Calcinosis Circumscripta 138
Spinal Trauma 139
Intervertebral Disk Disease 140
Schmorl's Nodes 142
Dural Ossification 142
Spondylosis Deformans 142
Disseminated Idiopathic Skeletal Hyperostosis 143
Osteoarthritis of the Articular Facets 143
Spondylitis 143
Diskospondylitis 144
Osteochondromatosis 144
Neoplasia 145

8. Thorax (Noncardiac) ... 147

Radiographic Technique 147
Standard Projections 147
Supplemental Projections 147
Radiographic Anatomy 147
Radiographic Interpretation: Systematic Evaluation 150
LARYNX AND HYOID BONES 150
Radiographic Interpretation 150
Diseases/Disorders 151
Laryngeal Hypoplasia 151
Laryngeal Paralysis 151
Laryngeal Neoplasia 151
The Hyoid Bones 152
TRACHEA AND MAJOR AIRWAYS 152
Radiographic Interpretation 152
Diseases/Disorders 153
Hypoplastic Trachea 153
Tracheal Stenosis 153
Trachea Collapse 153
Endotracheal Masses 153
Tracheal Rupture 154
Tracheal Foreign Body 154
Tracheitis 154
Bronchial Collapse 154
Bronchitis 154
Bronchiectasis 155
Bronchial Obstruction 155
Lower Airway Disease 156
LUNG 156
Radiographic Interpretation 156
Patterns of Lung Disease 158
Alveolar Pattern 158
Interstitial Pattern 158

Bronchial Pattern 158
Vascular Pattern 158
Diseases/Disorders 160
Pulmonary Edema 160
Pulmonary Hemorrhage 162
Pulmonary Hematomas and Pneumatoceles 162
Pneumonia 162
Interstitial Pneumonia 163
Aspiration Pneumonia 163
Eosinophilic Pneumonia 164
Pulmonary Abscess 164
Atelectasis 165
Emphysema 165
Pulmonary Cysts, Bullae and Blebs, and Other Cavitating Lung Lesions 165
Chronic Obstructive Pulmonary Disease 165
Lung Torsion 166
Pulmonary Thrombosis and Thromboembolism 166
Adult Respiratory Distress Syndrome 167
Parasitic Pneumonia 167
Toxoplasmosis 167
Paragonimus 167
Aeleurostrongylus 168
Mycotic Pneumonia 168
Histoplasmosis 168
Blastomycosis 168
Coccidioidomycosis 169
Nocardiosis 169
Cryptococcosis 169
Pneumocystis 169
Pulmonary Neoplasia 169
Primary Pulmonary Neoplasia . 169
Metastatic Pulmonary Neoplasia 170
MEDIASTINUM 171
Radiographic Anatomy 171
Diseases/Disorders 171
Mediastinal Shift 171
Pneumomediastinum 172
Mediastinal Mass 172
Diffuse Mediastinal Enlargement 173
Focal Mediastinal Enlargement . 174
PLEURA AND PLEURAL SPACE . . . 174
Normal Anatomy 174
Radiographic Anatomy 174
Diseases /Disorders 175
Pleural Effusion 175
Pleural Thickening 176
Pleural Neoplasms 177
Other Pleural Masses 178
Pneumothorax 178
THORACIC WALL 179
Diseases/Disorders 179
Soft Tissue Abnormalities 179
Congenital Anomalies of the Chest Wall 180
Pectus Excavatum 180
Pectus Carinatum 180
Sternal Dysraphism 180
Fractures of the Sternum and Ribs 181
Masses of the Thoracic Wall . . 181
DIAPHRAGM 182
Radiographic Anatomy 182
Radiographic Interpretation 182
Bilateral Displacement of the Diaphragm 182
Unilateral Displacement of the Diaphragm 182
Diseases/Disorders 183
Diaphragmatic Hernia 183
Diaphragmatic Tumors 183
Diaphragmatic Abscess 184

9. Heart 185

Radiographic Technique 185
Exposure Technique and Film Quality 185
Standard Projections 185
Supplemental Projections 185
Contrast Radiography 185
Other Imaging 186
Radiographic Anatomy of Normal Canine and Feline Heart 186
Lateral Projection 186
Dorsoventral Projection 188
Radiographic Interpretation 189
Normal Heart Size and Shape 189
Normal Variables for Heart Size and Shape 190
Evaluation of Heart Chamber Enlargement 192
Right Atrial Enlargement 192
Right Ventricular Enlargement 192
Left Atrial Enlargement 193
Left Ventricular Enlargement 193
Generalized Heart Enlargement 194
Evaluation of Major Vessels 194
Aortic Arch and Aorta 194
Pulmonary Artery Segment Enlargement 194
Caudal Vena Cava 195
Evaluation of the Pulmonary Circulation 195
Hypovascularity 195
Hypervascularity 195
Diseases/Disorders 195
Congestive Heart Failure 195

Microcardia 196
Congenital Heart Disease 197
Patent Ductus Arteriosus (Left to Right Shunt) 198
Reverse Patent Ductus Arteriosus (Right to Left Shunt) 199
Pulmonic Stenosis 199
Aortic Stenosis 200
Ventricular Septal Defect 201
Tetralogy of Fallot 201
Atrioventricular Valve Malformation and Dysplasia 201
Vascular Ring Anomalies 202
Situs Inversus 202
Acquired Heart Disease 203
Chronic Valvular Disease 203
Mitral Valvular Insufficiency 203
Tricuspid Valvular Insufficiency 204
Infectious Endocarditis 205
Dirofilariasis 205
Canine Heartworm Disease 206
Feline Heartworm Disease 206
Cardiomyopathy 207
Canine Dilated Cardiomyopathy 207
Doberman Pinscher Cardiomyopathy 208
Boxer Cardiomyopathy 208
English Cocker Spaniel Cardiomyopathy 209
Canine Hypertrophic Cardiomyopathy 209
Feline Hypertrophic Cardiomyopathy 209
Feline Restrictive Cardiomyopathy 210
Feline Congestive Cardiomyopathy 211
Intermediate (Indeterminate) Cardiomyopathy 211
Hyperthyroid Myocardial Disease 212
Systemic Hypertension 212
Myocardial Neoplasia 212
Heart Base Tumors 212
Aortic Thromboembolism 213
Pericardial Diseases 213
Anatomy and Physiology 213
Peritoneopericardial Diaphragmatic Hernia 214
Pericardial Cysts 214
Pericardial Effusion 214
Constrictive Pericarditis 215
Pericardial Masses 216

10. Abdomen: Peritoneal and Retroperitoneal Cavities 217

Anatomy 217
Radiographic Interpretation 217
Diseases/Disorders 217
Loss of Abdominal Detail 217
Intraabdominal Gas Accumulation 219
Intraabdominal Focal Opacities 220
Abdominal Lymph Nodes 221
Peritoneal Hernias 221

11. Gastrointestinal System 223

Radiographic Anatomy 223
Diseases/Disorders 223
Pharyngeal Inflammation 223
Pharyngeal and Retropharyngeal Masses 223
Dysphagia and Cricopharyngeal Achalasia 224
ESOPHAGUS 225
Radiographic Anatomy 225
Contrast Radiography 226
Diseases/Disorders 227
Esophagitis 227
Esophageal Foreign Bodies 227
Vascular Ring Anomalies 227
Esophageal Stricture 228
Esophageal Neoplasia 229
Esophageal Diverticuli 229
Megaesophagus 230
Gastroesophageal Intussusception 230
LIVER 231
Radiographic Anatomy 231
Normal Radiographic Appearance 231
Diseases/Disorders 233
Liver Enlargement 233
Decreased Liver Size 234
GALL BLADDER 235
Anatomy 235
Radiographic Anatomy 235
Diseases/Disorders 235
Cholecystitis 235
Cholelithiasis 236
Parasitic Disease of the Gall Bladder and/or Bile Ducts 236
SPLEEN 237
Radiographic Anatomy 237
Radiographic Interpretation 237
Diseases/Disorders 237
Splenomegaly 237
Splenic Torsion 238
Splenic Neoplasia 238
Splenic Abscess 238
Splenic Rupture 239
PANCREAS 239
Radiographic Anatomy 239
Diseases/Disorders 239
Pancreatitis 239
Pancreatic Masses 240
STOMACH 240

Radiographic Anatomy 240
Radiographic Interpretation 241
Diseases/Disorders 242
Gastric Enlargement 242
Gastric Wall Abnormalities . . . 244
Gastric Emptying 244
Acute Gastritis 244
Chronic Gastritis 245
Gastric Ulcers 245
Gastric Neoplasia 246
Gastric Foreign Bodies 247
Gastric Dilation and Volvulus . 247
Pyloric Outflow Obstruction . . 248
SMALL BOWEL 249
Radiographic Anatomy 250
Radiographic Interpretation 250
Contrast Radiographs 250
Contrast Media 251
Diseases/Disorders 251
Enteritis and Inflammatory Bowel Disease 251
Intestinal Obstruction 251
Linear Foreign Bodies 253
Intussusception 253
Small Bowel Neoplasia 254
Mesenteric Volvulus 254
Mesenteric Thrombosis 254
Intestinal Perforation 255
LARGE BOWEL 255
Radiographic Anatomy 255
Radiographic Findings 255
Contrast Radiographs 257
Diseases/Disorders 258
Acute Colitis 258
Chronic Colitis 258
Cecal Inversion 259
Neoplasia 259
Perineal Hernia and Perineal Diverticuli/Rectal Diverticuli 260
Imperforate Anus 260

12. Urinary System and Adrenal Glands 261

Radiographic Technique 261
KIDNEYS AND URETERS 261
Radiographic Anatomy 261
Radiographic Interpretation 262
Survey Radiographs 262
Causes of Observed Variations . 262
Contrast Radiographs 264
Intravenous Urography 264
Indications for Intravenous Urography 264
Interpretation of the Intravenous Urogram 265
Diseases/Disorders 265
Congenital Renal Disease 265
Ectopic Ureter 266
Nephritis and Pyelonephritis . . 266
Renal Cysts 267
Feline Perirenal Cysts 267
Renal and Ureteral Calculi . . . 268
Hydronephrosis 268
Renal Neoplasia 269
Renal and Ureteral Rupture . . . 269
URINARY BLADDER AND URETHRA 270
Radiographic Anatomy 270
Radiographic Interpretation 270
Survey Radiographs 270
Contrast Radiographs 271
Diseases/Disorders 272
Cystitis 272
Cystic Calculi 272
Ruptured Bladder 273
Emphysematous Cystitis 273
Neoplasms of the Urinary Bladder 273
URETHRA 274
Anatomy 274
Radiographic Interpretations 274
Contrast Radiographs 274
Diseases/Disorders 275
Urethritis 275
Urethral Calculi 275
Ruptured Urethra 275
Urethral Neoplasia 276
Urethrorectal Fistula 276
ADRENAL GLANDS 276
Radiographic Anatomy 276
Radiographic Interpretation 276
Diseases/Disorders 276
Adrenal Gland Enlargement . . 277
Adrenal Gland Mineralization . 277
Hypoadrenocorticism (Addison's Disease) 277
Pheochromocytoma 277
Hyperadrenocorticism (Cushing's Syndrome) 277

13. Genital System 279

Male 279
PROSTATE GLAND 279
Anatomy 279
Radiographic Anatomy 279
Radiographic Findings 279
Diseases/Disorders 279
Benign Prostatic Hypertrophy . 279
Prostatitis, Prostatic Abscess . . 281
Prostatic Calculi/Prostatic Mineralization 282

Paraprostatic Cyst 282
Prostatic Neoplasia 282
TESTICLE 283
Radiographic Interpretation 283
Diseases/Disorders 283
Cryptorchidism 283
Orchitis/Epididymitis 283
Testicular Torsion 283
Testicular Neoplasia 284
Infections and Tumors of the Penis 284
Fractures of the Os Penis 284
Female 284
Radiographic Anatomy 284
Radiographic Findings 284
Contrast Radiographs 285
OVARIES AND UTERUS 285
Diseases/Disorders 285
Ovarian Masses 285
Uterine Masses 285
The Gravid Uterus 286
Dystocia and Fetal Death 287
Cystic Endometrial Hyperplasia/Pyometra Complex 287
Cervical Masses 288
Diseases of the Vagina 288
Hermaphroditism 289

Suggested Readings . . . 291

Glossary 293

Index 299

chapter one

1

The Scope of Diagnostic Imaging in Small Animal Practice

Diagnostic imaging is important in small animal practice. It enables the visual evaluation of normal and abnormal anatomy and the recognition and diagnosis of many diseases. Most practices use radiology as their major diagnostic imaging modality, although other modalities, such as ultrasound and endoscopy, are increasingly being used by many practitioners. All imaging modalities have enhanced the practitioner's level of diagnostic accuracy, and provide methods to more closely monitor therapy. As noninvasive studies, they provide excellent alternatives to more invasive procedures, such as surgical exploration.

Other imaging modalities, such as fluoroscopy, computed tomography (CT), magnetic resonance imaging (MRI), and scintigraphy (nuclear medicine) of dogs and cats, have also enabled veterinarians to diagnose more diseases. These more sophisticated and expensive modalities are available to veterinary practitioners, often at referral specialty practices, veterinary teaching hospitals, and human imaging medical centers.

PHILOSOPHY OF IMAGING

The small animal clinician usually chooses an imaging modality that is cost-effective, readily available, easily performed, and accurately interpreted in a timely manner. Financial constraints are often imposed by the animal owner, and this may affect the choice of procedure and/or the extent of diagnostic imaging performed.

Survey radiographs are part of a complete clinical workup, as in lameness, cardiopulmonary, gastrointestinal or genitourinary tract disease; assessment of body trauma; dental examinations; metastatic survey before surgical removal of a malignant tumor; or in a search for polyostotic or multiple organ diseases. Radiographic studies are also used to follow a disease process and to monitor the effectiveness of therapy, as in animals with orthopedic, cardiac, pulmonary, or oncologic disease.

After assessment of the initial survey radiographs (coupled with the clinical assessment and review of the animal's data base), additional radiographs and/or other imaging studies may be needed for a diagnosis. The small animal clinician needs to decide the most appropriate order of imaging modalities, whether that be additional radiographs (such as oblique or stress views), radiographic contrast procedure, or another imaging modality (such as ultrasound, fluoroscopy, endoscopy, CT, magnetic resonance, or scintigraphy).

IMAGING INTERPRETATION

Every generated image should be interpreted and a written report of the interpretation should be included as part of the patient's record. Many practitioners have their images reviewed by a veterinary radiologist. The radiologist provides an expert's opinion in interpreting the images and may provide guidance for additional imaging examinations that could be helpful in diagnosis and treatment. Diplomates of the American College of Veterinary Radiology (board certified veterinary radiologists) in private practice and in veterinary teaching hospitals provide consultation services to the practitioner.

TYPES OF IMAGING PROCEDURES

DIAGNOSTIC RADIOLOGY

Diagnostic radiology utilizes an x-ray machine that produces ionizing radiation in the form of electromagnetic energy.

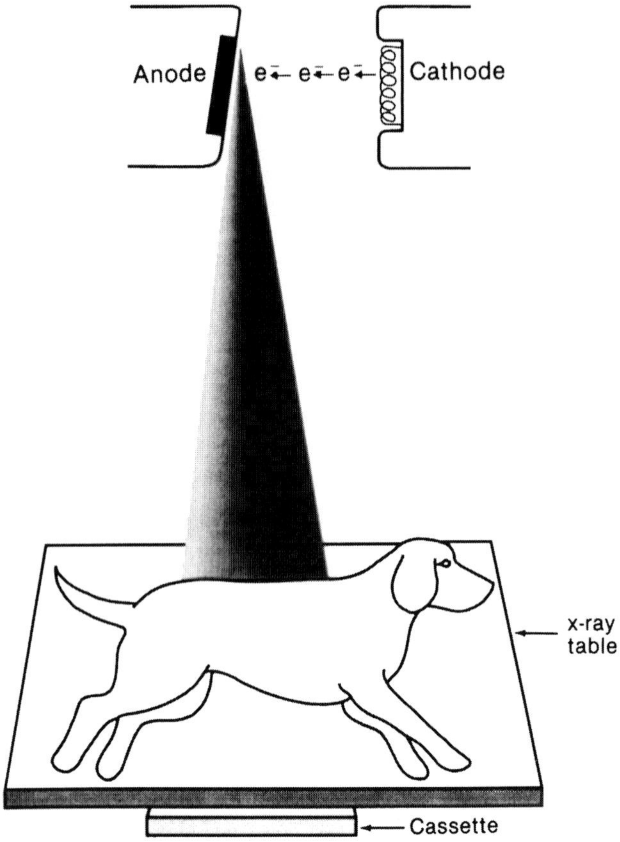

Figure 1.1. Schematic drawing of x-ray production showing collimation of x-ray beam and positioning of dog for a right-left lateral recumbent radiographic projection of the abdomen. (From Perry RL. Principles of conventional radiography and fluoroscopy. In: The Veterinary Clinics of North America [Small Animal Practice] [Diagnostic Imaging], 1993;23(2):237. Reprinted with permission of W.B. Saunders, Philadelphia.)

An x-ray machine consists of an x-ray tube, high voltage generator, and a control panel. Within the x-ray tube, the cathode contains a heated filament that produces electrons that are accelerated across a high voltage potential to strike a tungsten target at the anode. X-rays, as a form of electromagnetic energy, are emitted from this target and directed out of the x-ray tube through a glass window. The quality of the x-ray beam (wavelength) is controlled by the kilovoltage (kVp) and the quantity by the milliamperage-seconds (mAs). The x-ray beam is then restricted by collimation and directed to the animal (Figure 1.1).

The wavelength energy characteristics of x-rays enable them to penetrate and be attenuated by the different density and volume of body tissues. This results in five basic radiographic opacities: air, fat, soft tissue/fluid, bone, and metal (Figure 1.2). Air attenuates little of the x-ray beam, allowing nearly the full x-ray beam to expose and blacken the x-ray film. Conversely, bone and metal will attenuate a larger proportion of the x-ray beam than air, fat, or soft tissues (muscle, blood, urine, and other fluids), and as a result bones appear more radiopaque (whiter) on the film, even when superimposed on other tissues. Thick structures attenuate more x-rays than thin structures of the same tissue composition. Anatomic structures are seen on radiographs when they are outlined (contrasted) in whole or in part by tissues of different density. For example, pulmonary vessels are visible because of air in the lung. Fat in the abdomen enables visualization of the margins of the liver, spleen, and kidneys, which are of soft tissue opacity.

The image on an x-ray film is produced by a photochemical reaction when the x-rays pass through the body to the film. The film is usually placed within a cassette containing intensifying screens that emit light when exposed to x-rays. This light exposes the film. When the exposed film is processed, the visible image is apparent on the x-ray film as a radiograph.

The primary purpose of intensifying screens is to reduce radiation exposure by using the shortest exposure time possible. Less than 5% of the film density on the radiograph results from the direct effect of the x-rays and more than 95% of the density is caused by the effect of light emitted from the rare earth phosphors or calcium tungstate phosphors of the intensifying screen. Because film and screen systems vary in speed, detail, contrast, and latitude, the choice depends on the veterinarian's preference. In general, rare earth speed film/screen systems with a speed of 400 are recommended for most anatomic regions in the dog and cat. Slower speed systems

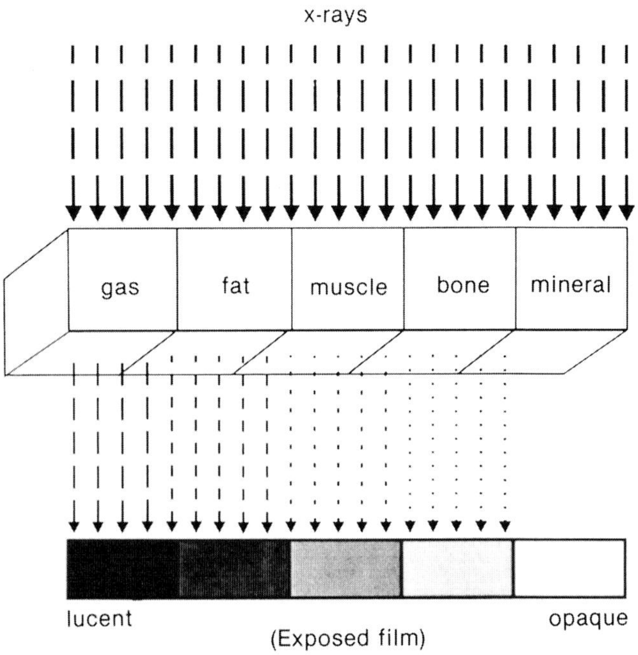

Figure 1.2. X-ray attenuation by tissue that results in five basic radiographic opacities. (From Perry RL. Principles of conventional radiography and fluoroscopy. In: The Veterinary Clinics of North America [Small Animal Practice] [Diagnostic Imaging], 1993;23(2):249. Reprinted with permission of W.B. Saunders, Philadelphia.)

will provide more detail, but require more exposure with the possibility of more motion artifact.

X-ray film is composed of a clear plastic base covered by an emulsion containing silver halides. Light or x-rays cause a physicochemical alteration in the silver, which then blackens when developed in processing chemicals. The degree of film blackening is related to the intensity of the x-ray beam and to the time and temperature of the developing process. The type of x-ray film used must be compatible with the intensifying screen. The type of film and screen selected should be based on the amount of detail and contrast required to obtain the best diagnostic quality radiograph for a specific body region.

Radiographic Technique

1. High-quality diagnostic radiographic images are necessary to provide accurate interpretation and assessment of the image. The quality radiograph should have optimal radiographic density, adequate contrast, minimal patient motion, and proper patient positioning.
2. Motion artifact is frequently encountered, but is usually can be eliminated by using short exposure times (1/60 or 1/120 second), fast film screen systems, and effective patient restraint. Whenever possible, chemical and/or mechanical restraint devices (sandbags, foam cushions, tape, rope) should be used to position the animal for the radiographic examination to decrease or eliminate unnecessary ionizing radiation exposure to personnel.
3. A reliable radiographic exposure technique chart is essential to the production of consistently high-quality diagnostic radiographs. A separate exposure technique chart for each anatomic region should be designed for the x-ray machine using a standardized focal-film distance, grid and nongrid techniques, speed of film-screen system, and processing technique. Most technique charts are based on centimeter thickness of the anatomic region. However, even when using an accurate technique chart, there are some situations in which technique adjustments of kVp and mAs are necessary to optimize the radiographic quality. Examples include obese or thin patients, and disease conditions such as pleural effusion, pneumothorax, ascites, and contrast studies.

Positioning

The veterinary technician and veterinarian need to participate in the decision-making process regarding the most appropriate radiographic projections and the selection of exposure factors that would most likely yield the best quality diagnostic image. Most radiographic projections are described by the direction that the x-ray beam enters and exits the animal (Figure 1.3). Thus a ventrodorsal projection of the thorax is one in which the x-ray beam passes through the thorax by entering the ventral surface of the thorax and exiting through the dorsal surface of the thorax. A right-left lateral recumbent projection of the thorax or abdomen is one in which the x-ray beam passes from the right to the left side of the body. A right lateral decubital projection of the chest or abdomen is one made with the animal in right lateral recumbency using a horizontal x-ray beam.

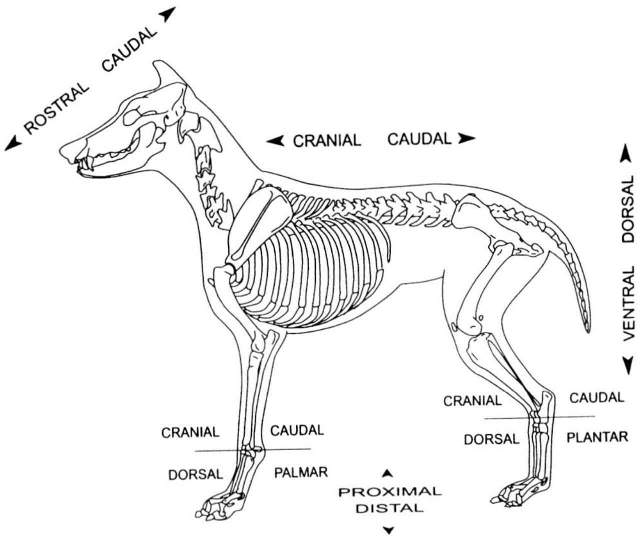

Figure 1.3. Drawing illustrating the anatomic nomenclature that is used to describe the direction of the x-ray beam for radiographic projections. (Reprinted with permission from Morgan JP. Techniques of Veterinary Radiography, 5th ed. Iowa State University Press; 1993:113.)

Film Identification

Every radiograph should be labeled in some manner to identify the animal and date of the examination. It is preferable to identify the film permanently within the emulsion by using devices, such as lead markers and photo "flashing." The radiograph is a medical legal record, and the identification needed may vary depending on the requirements of a state's practice act, or requirements of a specific organization. It is suggested that the following information permanently be included on each film.

1. Name of veterinarian or veterinary hospital
2. Name of client and animal
3. Date
4. Radiographic projection and body markers (e.g., VD, DV, R, L)

Other information may also be included:

1. Age, sex, and breed of animal
2. Address and telephone number of veterinary hospital
3. Breed registry number
4. Radiographic projection
5. Anatomic region
6. Other projection or body markers (e.g., oblique, horizontal)
7. Time of day

FLUOROSCOPY

Fluoroscopy uses an x-ray tube and a fluoroscopic screen with an image intensifier. The technique provides for real time radiographic viewing of moving anatomic structures. It can provide assessment of motility and function of the pharynx, esophagus, stomach, and bowel; evaluate respiratory function, such as tracheal or bronchial collapse; and observe diaphragmatic movement. It is also useful in interventional studies, such as directed aspirates or biopsies of internal organs or structures, and in placement of angiographic and other catheters.

An image-intensified fluoroscopic system consists of a fluoroscopic x-ray tube, an image intensifier tube, and either a mirror imaging or television viewing system. Most fluoroscopic systems have the fluoroscopic tube located under the table. X-rays are generated from the tube and pass through the animal to enter an image intensifier tube, which has an input fluorescent screen. Within the image intensifier tube, the x-rays are converted into visible light photons, then into photoelectrons that are accelerated across the tube and focused by electrostatic lenses toward the anode. When these electrons collide with the output fluorescent screen, light is produced. The fluoroscopist sees the image either directly through a series of lenses and mirrors or indirectly through a closed circuit television system. Options in the imaging recording system allow the images to be stored on x-ray film, photographic film, videotape, or on hard disk (Figure 1.4).

Radiation exposure to personnel is the major disadvantage of doing fluoroscopy in animals. Therefore, fluoroscopic studies should be done using an image intensifier tube and used only when specifically indicated. The fluoroscopy should be performed by a veterinary radiologist or similarly trained person who is knowledgeable about radiation protection and the equipment.

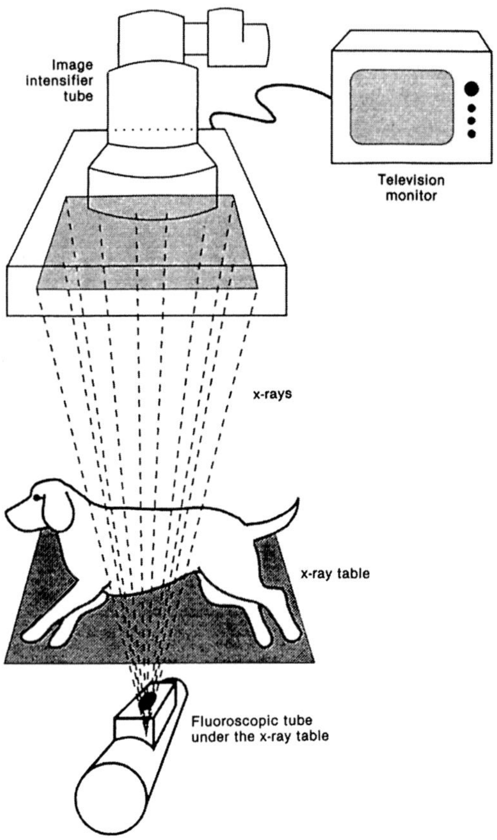

Figure 1.4. Illustration of imaging a dog using an image-intensifier tube in a fluoroscopic system. X-rays pass through the animal and enter the image-intensifier tube where a fluoroscopic image is formed. The image is observed on a television monitor. (From Perry RL. Principles of conventional radiography and fluoroscopy. In: The Veterinary Clinics of North America [Small Animal Practice] [Diagnostic Imaging], 1993;23(2):251. Reprinted with permission of W.B. Saunders, Philadelphia.)

DIAGNOSTIC ULTRASOUND

Ultrasound has greatly expanded the diagnostic imaging capabilities for dogs and cats. It provides a safe, economical, and noninvasive imaging modality in defining soft tissue architecture (of organs and structures) and the assessment of organ function (gastric and intestinal motility, echocardiography, and fetal viability). Ultrasound has reduced the need for many contrast radiographic examinations. It aids in guiding diagnostic or therapeutic needle aspirations and biopsies of organs or lesions for cytologic, bacteriologic, or histopathologic preparations. No ionizing radiation hazard or other known safety consideration is present with ultrasound.

However, ultrasound is highly ultrasonographer and ultrasonologist dependent. The production of quality diagnostic images requires patience, skill, and experience by those performing the ultrasound examination. There are many sources of error in imaging and interpretation, and numerous artifacts and pitfalls must be recognized to prevent misdiagnosis.

The ultrasound transducer converts electrical energy into a brief pulse of high frequency sound waves that are then transmitted into the animal's tissues. The transducer then functions as a receiver, detecting echoes of sound energy reflected from the tissues. Sound is transmitted less than 1% of the time, thus more than 99% of the time, the transducer is waiting for the returning echoes. The depth of a structure producing an echo is determined by the amount of "round trip" time of the transmitted pulse and the returning echo, assuming an average speed of sound through tissues of 1540 m/second. An image, representing the organs and tissues in the field of view, is produced by computer analysis of the time delay and amplitude (multiple closely spaced ultrasound pulses) of the returning echo. Images are updated approximately 30 times/second and provide real time assessment of cardiac movement, vascular pulsations, and gastrointestinal peristalsis (Figure 1.5 A, B).

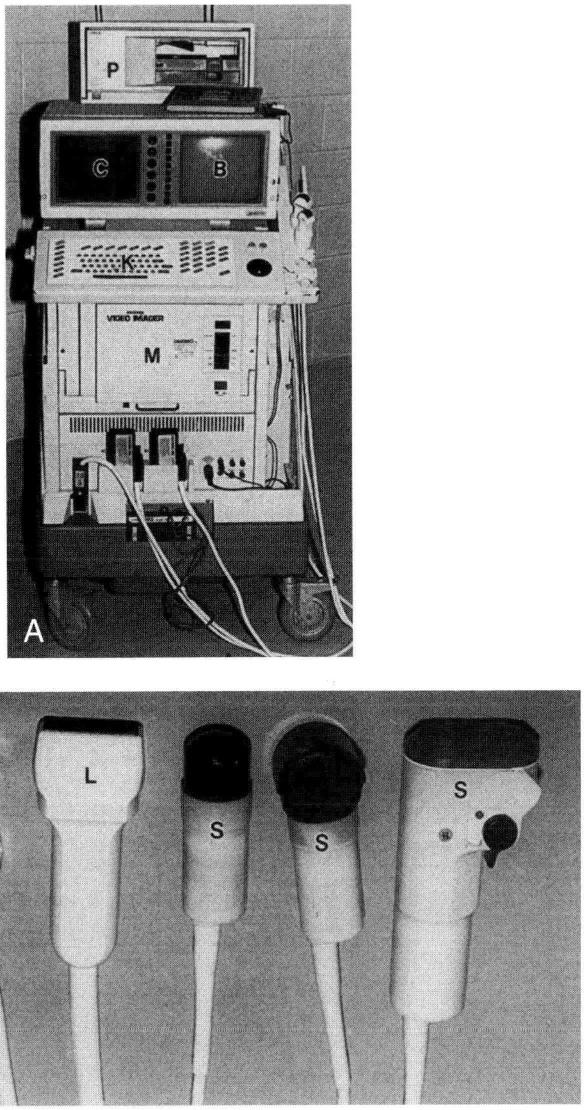

Figure 1.5. **A)** Example of an ultrasound machine. P, printer; C, color monitor; B, black and white monitor; K, keyboard controls; M, camera. (From Cartee RE. Instruments and their operation. In: Cartee RE, Selcer JA, Hudson ST, et al. Practical Veterinary Ultrasound. Lea & Febiger; 1995:12. With permission of Williams & Wilkins, Baltimore.) **B)** Examples of different kinds and sizes of ultrasound transducers. Types include linear array (L), Mechanical Sector (S), curved linear (CL). (From Cartee RE. Instruments and their operation. In: Cartee RE, Selcer JA, Hudson ST, et al. Practical Veterinary Ultrasound. Lea & Febiger; 1995:10. With permission of Williams & Wilkins, Baltimore.)

Transducers produce ultrasound at various frequencies. Higher frequency emitting transducers (e.g., 7.5–10 MHz) provide better spatial resolution, but cannot image deep tissues. Lower frequency emitting transducers (e.g., 2.5–5 MHz) can image deeper tissues, but produce images with less resolution. Images may be produced in any anatomic plane by adjusting the orientation and angulation of the transducer and patient position.

Ultrasound image quality is influenced by the type of transducer (frequency), gain settings, focal zone location, and patient preparation. Patient preparation should include clipping the hair over the region of interest, wetting the skin with water or alcohol, and liberal application of acoustic gel to ensure good contact, thereby allowing sound transmission from the transducer to the animal's tissues. Air and bone reflect a large percentage of the ultrasound beam and produce image artifacts. An ultrasound "window" (avoiding gas or bone) should be selected to image deeper tissues.

Doppler ultrasound is an important adjunct to real time gray-scale ultrasound imaging. The Doppler effect is a shift in the frequency of the returning echoes, as compared to the transmitted pulse, caused by the reflection of the sound waves from moving objects. The moving objects are usually red blood cells in flowing blood. If the blood flow is away from the transducer, the echo frequency shift is lower; if blood flow is toward the transducer, the echo frequency shift is higher. The amount of frequency shift is proportional to the relative red blood cell velocity. Therefore, Doppler ultrasound can detect the presence of blood flow, determine flow direction and flow velocity. The Doppler frequency information can be displayed in a variety of image modes; as a time-velocity waveform (spectral Doppler) or with the colors assigned to the frequency shifts superimposed on the gray-scale image (color Doppler).

Interpretation of ultrasound images is best done by the radiologist or clinician who, with transducer in hand, personally examined the patient. When done by a skilled person, the ultrasound examination is a dynamic extension of the physical examination. During the ultrasound examination, many suspected masses or lesions can be palpated, artifacts can be differentiated from true lesions, and three-dimensional anatomic relationships can be assessed.

Ultrasound examinations are usually recorded on videotape. Individual frame images also can be captured on thermal or photographic paper or on x-ray film by using a multiformat camera. These images can be reviewed by others, bearing in mind that the hard copy recorded images serve only to document the dynamic, real time examination. Questions regarding interpretation are often best answered by the individual performing the examination.

COMPUTED TOMOGRAPHY (CT)

Computed tomography is valuable in imaging many diseases in the dog and cat. CT imaging has most commonly been used for diagnosing diseases of the brain, nasal and sinus cavities, orbit, mediastinum, lung, liver, adrenal gland, elbow joint, and spine. Although CT is a noninvasive imaging technique, ionizing radiation from the x-ray tube is produced.

Computed tomography uses a computer to mathematically reconstruct a cross-sectional image of a body area from measurements of x-ray transmission through thin slices of patient tissue (Figure 1.6). In the machine, a narrow, collimated beam of x-rays is generated on one side of the patient. Sensitive detectors on the opposite side of the patient measure the amount of x-ray transmission through a tissue slice of the patient. Most CT units can provide slice thicknesses from 1 to 10 mm and usually take 1 to 3 seconds to acquire data from an individual slice. These measurements are repeated many times from different directions as the x-ray tube rotates around the patient (Figure 1.7).

The resulting image is made up of a matrix of picture elements (pixels), each of which represents a volume element (voxel) of patient tissue (Figure 1.8). To produce an image, shades of gray (CT numbers) are assigned to ranges of pixel values. Using variable "window settings" the degree of contrast and latitude can be altered to best produce an image for bone, air filled lung, and soft tissues.

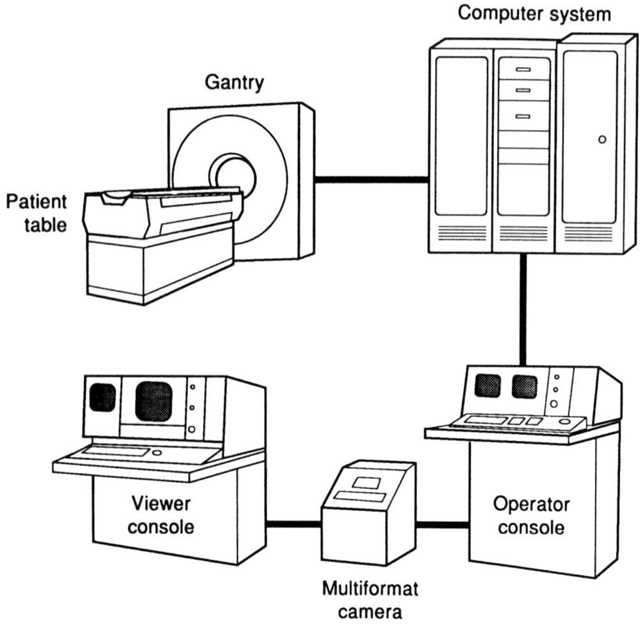

Figure 1.6. Components of a computerized tomography unit. (From Hathcock JT, Stickle RL. Principles and concepts of computed tomography. In: The Veterinary Clinics of North America [Small Animal Practice] [Diagnostic Imaging], 1993;23(2):401. Reprinted with permission of W.B. Saunders, Philadelphia.)

Superior osseous and soft tissue differentiation enables the production of images without superimposition of overlying structures.

Intravenous iodinated contrast media is often administered in CT to enhance the density differences between lesions and surrounding parenchyma, to demonstrate vascular anatomy and vessel patency, and to characterize lesions by their patterns of contrast enhancement. Defects in the blood-brain barrier associated with tumors, infection, hemorrhage, or other lesions allow contrast media to accumulate within abnormal tissues for improved visibility on the CT image. In other tissues, the contrast diffuses into the extravascular spaces enhancing the lesions on the CT image. In addition to giving iodinated contrast media intravenously, contrast media can be administered orally or rectally to enhance CT imaging of the esophagus, stomach, and bowel.

MAGNETIC RESONANCE IMAGING (MRI)

Magnetic resonance imaging is a technique that provides a noninvasive digitized anatomic image by means of magnetic fields and radio waves (Figure 1.9). MRI is based

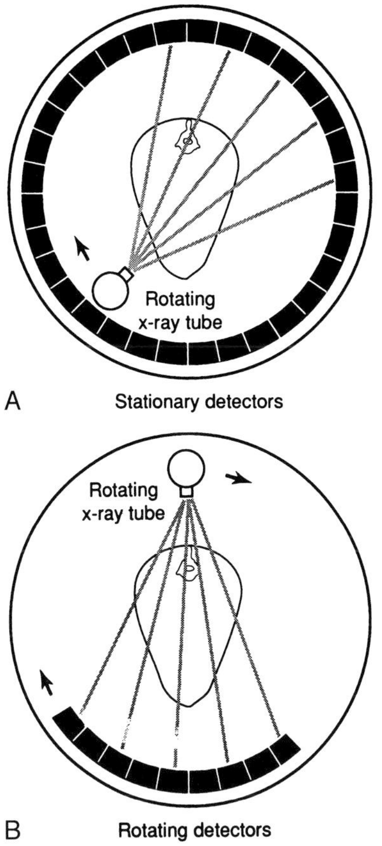

Figure 1.7. Illustrations of the rotation of the x-ray tube in a CT unit around the patient. The detectors may be stationary **(A)** or rotate with the x-ray tube **(B)**. (From Hathcock JT, Stickle RL. Principles and concepts of computed tomography. In: The Veterinary Clinics of North America [Small Animal Practice] [Diagnostic Imaging], 1993;23(2):410. Reprinted with permission of W.B. Saunders, Philadelphia.)

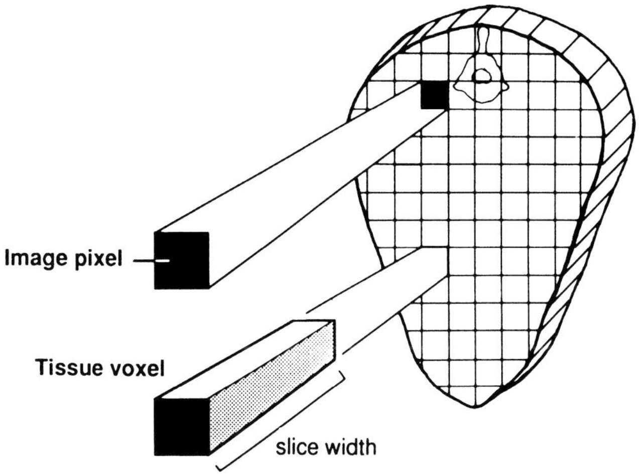

Figure 1.8. The CT image is composed of a matrix of tiny squares called pixels. The pixels of the CT image are two-dimensional representations of a three-dimensional block of tissue (voxel) from the body slice. (From Hathcock JT, Stickle RL. Principles and concepts of computed tomography. In: The Veterinary Clinics of North America [Small Animal Practice] [Diagnostic Imaging], 1993;23(2):400. Reprinted with permission of W.B. Saunders, Philadelphia.)

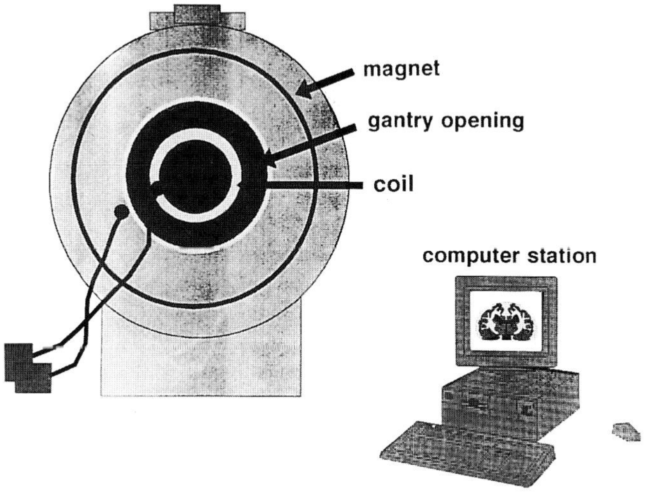

Figure 1.9. Components of a magnetic resonance imaging unit (MR). (From Shores A. Magnetic resonance imaging. In: The Veterinary Clinics of North America [Small Animal Practice] [Diagnostic Imaging], 1993;23(2):438. Reprinted with permission W.B. Saunders, Philadelphia.)

on the ability of a few protons within the body to absorb and emit radiowave energy when the body is placed within a strong magnetic field. Different tissues absorb and release radiowave energy at different, detectable, and characteristic rates. MRI uses a static low (<0.1 tesla) to high (>1 tesla) magnetic field, a coil for detection of the radio frequency signals, and a computer. The changes in cellular orientation within the body are detected, analyzed, and reconstructed as images by a computer. Water is the major source of the higher MR signals in tissues other than fat. Bone and collagenous tissues are low in water content and produce a low MR signal. The computer also enables one to set parameters for the image study, formulates and transmits instructions for the production of a radiofrequency pulse sequence that is directed at the region of interest, and analyzes the sampled data to produce the image. Specific contrast media (nonferrous) can also be used with MRI.

The image produced with MRI provides outstanding soft-tissue contrast. Superior differentiation within the soft tissues of the body enable visualization of cartilage, tendon, muscle, and ligaments as well as differentiating differences within the soft tissues of all internal organs, including the spinal cord, heart, lung, abdominal viscera, and the white and gray matter of the brain.

There is no ionizing radiation risk, but there are safety considerations for patients and operators who have ferromagnetic implants, foreign bodies, or metallic devices such as a pacemaker. Metallic objects (i.e., bullets, shrapnel, vascular slips, skin staples, pocket pens) may move and cause additional injury or become projectiles within the magnetic field.

NUCLEAR MEDICINE IMAGING (SCINTIGRAPHY)

Nuclear imaging is a modality that provides diagnostic information on the functional status of an organ or body part. Radiopharmaceutical drugs that emit radioactive gamma rays are administered into the patient, and after the radionuclide has been deposited in the organ or tissue of interest, a gamma scintillation camera is used to detect ionizing gamma rays emitted from the animal's body. The radionuclide distribution is usually recorded as an image on x-ray film. While CT, MRI, and ultrasound provide images that are high in spatial resolution and primarily anatomic, most scintigraphic images are more sensitive, but less specific.

Nuclear imaging procedures use the concept of the tracer principle. A radioactive element (radionuclide) by itself or adhered to another molecule is administered into the body and is used by the body without interfering with normal physiologic mechanisms. When imaging of the tracer is performed, the image reflects the biodistribution of the tracer, modified by physiologic, anatomic, and pathologic processes.

A radiopharmaceutical drug is a compound to which a radionuclide has been attached. The compound dictates the biodistribution of the radiopharmaceutical. Many radiopharmaceuticals act like analogs of natural biologic compounds. For example, ^{99m}Tectinetium sodium (^{99m}Tc) pertechnetate is analogous to the iodine molecule and readily distributes to the thyroid, salivary glands, stomach, and kidneys. ^{99m}Tc sulfur colloid acts like a colloid particle of approximately 1 μm in size and distributes throughout the reticuloendothelial system of the liver, spleen, and bone marrow. ^{99m}Tc methylene diphosphonate (MDP) acts like phosphate and is adsorbed onto bone crystals and is useful in bone imaging. ^{99m}Tc macroaggregated albumin (MAA) causes capillary blockade and is useful in the diagnosis of pulmonary thromboembolism.

Examples of scintigraphic studies in dogs and cats are:

1. Thyroid scintigraphy, using either radioiodine or ^{99m}Tc, is useful for assessing thyroid hyperactivity, determining whether one or both thyroid lobes are involved, detecting the presence of ectopic thyroid tissue, and estimating the size and relative activity of the thyroid gland.
2. Brain scintigraphy uses various ^{99m}Tc compounds. Brain lesions that disrupt the blood-brain barrier allow accumulation of the radiopharmaceutical in the local extracellular space and are visualized as a "hot spot" on the image. Experience has shown that this procedure is a good screening technique for brain tumors, but less sensitive than CT and MR in the detection of degenerative and inflammatory brain lesions.
3. Bone scintigraphy, usually with ^{99m}Tc diphosphonate compounds, is primarily used in the dog and cat to evaluate for metastatic bone disease and as an aid to localization of lameness. However, bone scintigraphy can also be used to detect for occult stress fracture, avascular necrosis, osteomyelitis, osteoarthritis, and for postoperative assessment of bone grafts and prostheses.
4. Scintigraphy to assess portosystemic shunts can be done by infusing ^{99m}Tc pertechnetate into the colon. The radiopharmaceutical is rapidly absorbed through the colon into the venous system. In normal dogs, the radioactivity is observed first in the liver, before it is detected in the heart. In animals with portosystemic shunts, some of the radioactivity can be detected in the heart before or at the same time as detection in the liver. The severity of the shunt can be estimated by use of computer analysis calculations on how much of the shunt fraction represents the percentage of portal blood flow that bypasses the liver and joins the systemic circulation.
5. Scintigraphic imaging also can be used to observe and evaluate gastric emptying, renal function, pulmonary perfusion, and for pulmonary ventilation studies.

chapter two

2

Principles of Radiographic Interpretation

INTRODUCTION

The interpretation of radiographs is based on the recognition and analysis of structures with different relative radiopacities on a radiograph. These different radiopacities are formed by the following basic principles of radiography.

1. X-rays, also known as photons, are a form of radiant energy having short wavelengths capable of penetrating tissue.
2. X-ray photons will, in part, be absorbed or attenuated by the tissue, and in part will pass through the tissue to interact with and expose the x-ray film.
3. Absorption of x-rays within tissue is a function of the atomic number and thickness of the tissues:
   a. Tissue and objects with a higher atomic number will absorb more radiation than will structures with a lower atomic number.
   b. Thicker tissue and objects will absorb more radiation than thinner structures of similar composition.
   c. The greater the amount of tissue absorption, the fewer the number of x-rays that expose the film and the more radiopaque the image on the film.
4. The radiograph (exposed and developed x-ray film) will display a range of radiopacities from white to black; radiopaque densities will appear more white and radiolucent densities will appear more black.
5. The resultant radiographic image is recognizable as an anatomic form that can be interpreted and used as a valuable clinical diagnostic aid.

RADIOPACITY

The relative difference in radiopacities (from radiolucent to radiopaque) of various objects and tissues makes their differentiation possible. The degree of radiopacity is a function of:

1. The atomic number of the substance
   a. The higher the atomic number, the more radiopaque is the tissue or object;
   b. Certain materials have an absolute atomic number.

Example	*Atomic Number*
Lead	82
Barium	56
Iodine	51

   c. The basic body tissues are a composite of many molecules and thereby have an atomic value that is termed an effective atomic number.

Example	*Approximate Effective Atomic Number*
Air/gas	1.8
Fat	6.5
Water	7.5
Muscle	7.6
Bone	12.3

2. The thickness of the tissue; the thicker the tissue or object, the more radiopaque it will appear on the radiograph.
3. Composite opacities; superimposed types and thicknesses of tissue and structures assume an additive or summation radiopacity on the radiograph. Examples of these include:
   a. A pulmonary vessel seen superimposed on the more radiolucent lung will appear less radiopaque than a similar vessel seen superimposed on the heart.
   b. The area where the caudal pole of the right kidney is superimposed over the cranial pole of the left

kidney will appear more radiopaque than the individual kidney.

BASIC RADIOGRAPHIC OPACITIES

The basic radiographic opacities are a spectrum from radiopaque (white) to radiolucent (black). The order of most radiopaque to most radiolucent is: metal, bone, soft tissue/fluid, fat, and gas. For example, fat is more radiolucent than soft tissue and bone, but more radiopaque than gas.

Bone Opacity

1. Bone is primarily composed of calcium and phosphorous.
2. A normal variation in bone radiopacity exists within the same bone and between separate bones because of:
   a. Different ratios of compact bone to spongy bone
   b. Different ratios of trabecular bone to intertrabecular spaces
   c. Different ratios of cortex to medullary canal
3. Bone is assessed radiographically as being more or less radiopaque than normal.
   a. Sclerotic bone is more radiopaque (less radiolucent) than normal.
   b. Porotic bone is less radiopaque (more radiolucent) than normal.

Soft Tissue Opacity

1. Is also referred to as water opacity.
2. Includes the radiographic opacities of normal soft tissue such as muscle, and solid and/or fluid-filled organs such as heart, liver, spleen, kidneys, and urinary bladder.
3. Variations in volume, thickness, and degree of compactness of soft tissue radiopacities create a spectrum of varying summation opacities on the radiograph.

Fat Opacity

1. Fat is more radiolucent than bone and soft tissue, but less radiolucent (more radiopaque) than gas/air.
2. Fat produces radiographic contrast for differentiation and visualization of the edges for many organs and structures:
   Examples include:
   a. The fat-containing falciform ligament located between the ventral liver margin and the abdominal wall enables visualization of the ventral liver border and the peritoneal surface of the adjacent abdominal wall.
   b. The omentum, between the stomach and the spleen, enables differentiation of the gastric wall from the spleen.
   c. Fascial planes contain fat and occasionally enable visualization of muscle groups.
   d. Fat within the retroperitoneal space enables visualization of the kidneys and other retroperitoneal structures such as aorta, caudal venal cava, and occasionally a portion of the circumflex artery.
3. In an immature or emaciated animal, the type of fat or lack of sufficient fat for radiographic contrast prevents the visualization of many organs and structures.

Gas Opacity

1. Gas or air is the most radiolucent opacity within the body and is easily recognized. Gas provides good contrast between other radiographic opacities.
2. The radiolucency of air provides contrast to visualize the more radiopaque structures:
   a. In the chest, structures of soft tissue opacity, such as the heart, aorta, and pulmonary vessels, are visible because the contrast is provided by the air-filled alveoli and airways of the lung.
   b. In the intestine, the bowel wall (of water opacity) is visible because of the gas within its lumen and the mesenteric fat adjacent to the outer wall.
3. In some contrast radiographic procedures, certain gases are introduced into structures/organs to enhance radiographic contrast (e.g., urinary bladder, peritoneal cavity).

GEOMETRY OF THE RADIOGRAPHIC IMAGE

The appearance of a radiographic image depends on the following factors:

1. *Size of the x-ray tube focal spot;* the smaller the focal spot, the greater the definition and detail of the image. Focal spot size of 0.6 to 1.0 mm produces less penumbra for better detail than 2 mm, but x-ray tube loading capacity is more.
2. *Distance of the object from the x-ray tube focal spot (focal spot-object distance);* the larger the distance between the object and the focal spot, the less magnification and the better the detail. The focal-spot film distance should be as large as is practical (90–100 cm is recommended for most small animal radiographic units).
3. *Distance of the object from the film (object-film distance);* the closer the object is to the film, the sharper the image and detail and the less the distortion and magnification. The body part of interest should be as close to the film as possible. If the body part is thin enough to use a nongrid technique, a tabletop technique is preferred to putting the cassette in the tray beneath the tabletop.
4. *Alignment;* The more perpendicular the object is to the central x-ray beam and film, the less distorted the image. Structures on the margins of a radiograph are distorted more than those in the middle of the radiograph.
5. *Heel effect and patient positioning;* the thicker part of the patient's body part should be placed toward the

cathode side of the x-ray tube where the x-ray beam has more intensity. Usually, this is significant only if using low techniques and in radiographing large dogs (e.g., pelvis, thorax, and abdomen).

RADIOGRAPHIC INTERPRETATION

Viewing Area

The environment in which the radiographs are viewed and interpreted is important and should consist of:

1. A quiet area
2. An area that can be adequately darkened to allow good illumination of radiographs
3. Adequate number of viewboxes (at least two) with appropriate bulbs
4. Bright light illuminator with rheostat (e.g., 60–100 W bulb)
5. Preferably, radiographic interpretation should be done when full attention can be given to the interpretation.

Three-Dimensional Concept

1. When viewing radiographs, one must mentally create a three-dimensional image from a radiograph that has only two dimensions.
2. A minimum of two radiographic projections, made at right angles to one another, is necessary to create a three-dimensional perspective.
3. Anatomy and radiology textbooks and skeletons are helpful as aids in radiographic interpretation.
4. To recognize an abnormality, one must first look for it. To see it, one must know about it.

Process of Examining the Radiographs

1. Determine that the radiograph is that of the patient being evaluated.
2. Have at least two projections (made at right angles to each other) available for evaluation.
3. Determine the position of the patient during the x-ray exposure and that the body is correctly identified (e.g., right or left side).
4. Verify that the radiographs are of good diagnostic quality and have adequte detail and contrast, proper centering, collimation, and processing.
5. Examine the entire radiograph systematically and thoroughly.
   a. All organs or structures on the radiograph should be examined in a deliberate order, concentrating on the anatomy of each structure.
   b. Even though an abnormality may be obvious, all structures should be evaluated before focusing on the obvious abnormality.
6. Describe all the radiographic abnormalities including:
   a. Changes in position of an organ or structure (Table 2.1)
   b. Variations in size (Table 2.2)
   c. Variations in contour or shape (Table 2.3)
   d. Variations in number (Table 2.4)
   e. Alterations in radiopacity (Tables 2.5 and 2.6)
   f. Alterations in the architectural pattern (Table 2.7)
   g. Changes in function (Table 2.8)
7. Integrate the radiographic findings with clinical data.
   a. Requires knowledge of disease patterns and pathogenesis.
   b. Requires knowledge of the statistical incidence of disease relative to age, sex, and breed predisposition.
8. Formulate list of differential diagnoses with the possibilities listed in order of the most likely diagnosis.
9. Include a written interpretation of the radiographic findings and differential diagnosis (or only the diagnosis) in the animal's record.

TABLE 2.1

Changes in Position of an Organ or Structure

1. The organ may be either pushed, pulled or displaced away from its normal position.
2. The organ may become twisted or rotated on its axis.
3. The organ may have an ectopic position.

TABLE 2.2

Variations in Size of an Organ or Structure

1. An organ may increase in size because of:
   a. Hypertrophy
   b. Hyperplasia
   c. Inflammation
   d. Neoplasia
   e. Edema
   f. Congestion
2. An organ may decrease in size because of:
   a. Atrophy
   b. Hypoplasia
   c. Congenital anomaly

TABLE 2.3

Variation in Contour or Shape of an Organ or Structure

1. Maldevelopment
2. Trauma
3. Hypertrophy or hyperplasia
4. Neoplasia
5. Localized atrophy
6. Necrosis
7. Localized loss of tissue turgor (e.g., bowel ileus)
8. Ulceration

TABLE 2.4

Variations in Number of Organs or Structures

1. Accessory ossification centers
2. Supernumerary digits or teeth
3. Absence or anomaly in the number or pairs of ribs
4. Absent kidney
5. Ureteral duplication

TABLE 2.5

Increased Radiopacity in an Organ or Structure

1. Increased radiopacity within an air-containing space (e.g., fluid-filled tympanic bulla, pulmonary mass)
2. Soft tissue mineralization (e.g., dystrophic mineralization)
   a. Calcified hematoma
   b. Chronic inflammation associated with abscess, tumor, or granuloma
   c. Chronic pancreatitis
   d. Fat saponification
3. Metastatic mineralization in normal tissue caused by a calcium phosphorus disturbance.
   a. May occur in the following:
      1) Primary hyperparathyroidism
      2) Secondary renal or nutritional hyperparathyroidism
      3) Pseudohyperparathyroidism
      4) Hyperadrenocorticism
   b. Common sites of metastatic mineralization include:
      1) Renal parenchyma (nephrocalcinosis)
      2) Arterial vessels (e.g., aorta, celiac, mesenteric, iliac)
      3) Gastric rugae
4. Metaplasia or osteoblastic activity
   a. Bone tumor (e.g., osteosarcoma)
   b. Heterotopic bone formation in lung (pulmonary osteomas)
5. Precipitated calcium deposition
   a. Gallbladder (cholelithiasis)
   b. Kidney (nephrolithiasis)
   c. Urinary bladder (cyctic calculi)
   d. Salivary gland (sialolithiasis)
   e. Prostate gland (prostatic calculi)

TABLE 2.6

Increased Radiolucency of an Organ or Structure

1. The presence of gas in abnormal sites such as:
   a. Subcutaneous emphysema
   b. Mediastinal emphysema (pneumomediastinum)
   c. Cavitation of an abscess or tumor
   d. Gas forming infection in a hollow viscus:
      1) Emphysematous cystitis
      2) Emphysematous cholecystitis
      3) Emphysematous metritis
2. Bone that is more radiolucent than normal, as may occur in:
   a. Osteoporosis or osteomalacia
   b. Osteomyelitis
   c. Neoplasia

TABLE 2.7

Alterations in the Architectural Pattern of an Organ or Structure

1. Changes in the bronchovascular pattern of the lungs
2. Changes in the trabecular pattern or cortical thickness of bone
3. Changes in the thickness of the wall of the urinary bladder or bowel
4. Changes in the integrity of the abdominal wall (e.g., hernia)

TABLE 2.8

Alterations in Function of an Organ or Structure

1. Changes in excretion (e.g., cholecystography, urography)
2. Changes in functional transit time (e.g., gastrointestinal and vascular contrast studies)

chapter three

3

Radiographic Contrast Procedures

Radiographic contrast procedures use positive and/or negative contrast media to enhance the visualization of individual organs and/or structures that are inadequately seen on the survey radiographs. Survey radiographs are always made before a contrast study, to ascertain that a contrast study is needed and to provide a baseline from which to evaluate the contrast study.

Indication

Special studies provide additional information, morphologic and/or functional, which is helpful to:

1. Make a definitive diagnosis.
2. Evaluate the character of a suspected lesion seen on survey radiographs.
   a. Identify an organ's size, shape, position, and contour.
   b. Evaluate the mucosal surface of a viscus or its luminal contents.
   c. Evaluate the wall of a viscus for a mural or extramural lesion.
   d. Provide assessment of organ function.
3. Aid in determining appropriate therapy (e.g., surgery).

PATIENT PREPARATION

Patient preparation is important for every contrast study. The amount of preparation done varies for each type of contrast study (e.g., cleaning and drying the animal's hair, and cleansing the gastrointestinal [GI] tract). Preparation should also include being prepared for possible medical emergencies that could be associated with a contrast reaction.

CONTRAST MEDIA

Types of Contrast Media

1. Positive contrast media absorb x-rays efficiently and are more radiopaque than the soft tissues. The most common types of positive contrast media used are barium and iodinated compounds.
2. Negative contrast media do not absorb x-rays and thus are more radiolucent than soft tissue and fat. The more common types of negative contrast media include room air and carbon dioxide. Infrequently, oxygen and nitrous oxide are used.

Ionic and Nonionic

1. Most ionic-iodinated contrast media are tri-iodinated derivatives of benzoic acid. These compounds form salts in solution with the anion (iodine) and the cation (sodium, meglumine, or iothalamate), which provide biologic stabilization.
2. Most ionic-iodinated media are hyperosmolar, have low protein binding capacity, and are excreted through the kidneys by glomerular filtration.
3. Some ionic-iodinated media are available with higher protein binding and are excreted through the biliary system.
4. Newer nonionic compounds are water soluble, do not dissociate into ions in solution, and thus have a lower osmolarity and lower incidence of adverse reactions.
5. Nonionic media (e.g., iopamidol and iohexol) are used primarily for myelography in the dog and cat, but they also are used for urography and angiography. In the GI tract, the nonionic media have all the advantages of ionic water-soluble iodides and none of their disadvantages. Advantages include: safety, rapid transit time, good radiographic opacification of the GI tract, and no residue coating to interfere with endoscopy or surgery.
6. Nonionic contrast media are more expensive than ionic iodinated agents. Although the cost may be prohibitive in medium and larger dogs (approximately 10 times the cost), it is cost-effective in cats and small dogs.
7. Examples of iodinated contrast agents commonly available for use in dogs and cats are:

Brand Name	Iodinated Form	Manufacturer
Conray & Conray 43	Ionic	Mallinckrodt
Optiray 240, 320 & 350	Nonionic	Mallinckrodt
Hypaque 76	Ionic	Nycomed
Renovist & Renografin 76	Ionic	Squibb
Isovue (iopamidol)	Nonionic	Squibb
Omnipaque (iohexol)	Nonionic	Nycomed
Visipaque (iodixanol)	Nonionic	Nycomed

Excretion of iodinated ionic and nonionic contrast media

1. Ionic and nonionic contrast agents share common biologic characteristics of low molecular weight, low lipid solubility, and rapid glomerular filtration.
2. Maximum plasma levels occur immediately after injection. Renal glomerular filtration without tubular reabsorption occurs rapidly and is the primary route of excretion from the body.
3. Alternative routes of excretion (<2%) are through the biliary system and the small bowel mucosa.
4. Contrast clearance occurs more slowly in the brain than in other organs. Clearance mechanisms may include: crossing the blood-brain barrier back into the capillary bed, diffusion from the cerebrospinal fluid into the venous circulation, and active transport from the choroid plexus.

Side effects of iodinated contrast media

1. Incidence of adverse reactions relates to many factors including: type, concentration, and volume of contrast media; type of contrast procedure performed, speed of infusion, and the history of prior contrast reactions. Reactions are less frequent with nonionic iodinated contrast media.
2. It is thought that the physiologic reactions result from an increase in hemic viscosity, endothelial damage, hypervolemia, vasodilatation, edema with neurotoxicity, depressed myocardial contractility, and/or systemic toxicity.
3. Although rarely reported in the dog and cat, contrast-induced reactions include acute renal failure, transient pulmonary edema, and vomiting. Proposed mechanisms of toxicity include direct tubular toxicity, renal ischemia, intratubular obstruction, hypotension, or possibly some immune complex reaction. Acute renal failure is recognized on the radiographs by seeing an immediate nephrogram and an absence of pelvic or ureteral opacification. The nephrogram becomes more radiopaque with time.
4. Contrast media reactions can be minimized by using minimum effective doses, maintaining adequate patient hydration, using general anesthesia to prevent vomiting, and being prepared for possible medical emergencies. Contrast-induced reactions in humans (<1% incidence), such as renal failure, are associated primarily with intravenous or intraarterial contrast administration in patients with preexisting renal disease, diabetes mellitus, multiple myeloma, proteinuria, dehydration, and hypertension.
5. Orally administered contrast media can cause osmotic diarrhea and dehydration. This is less of a problem with nonionic preparations.
6. If pulmonary aspiration or inadvertent tracheal injection occurs, pulmonary edema and atelectasis may result. Nonionic contrast media are less reactive in the lung than the iodinated contrast media (Table 3.1).

TABLE 3.1

Types of Contrast Reactions

1. Most common
   a. Nausea and vomiting
   b. Skin erythema
   c. Facial swelling
   d. Pulmonary edema
   e. Osmotic diuresis
   f. Hypotension
   g. Local irritation at injection site
2. Less common
   a. Laryngeal edema
   b. Vascular collapse
   c. Cerebral edema and seizures
   d. Arrhythmias
   e. Renal failure
   f. Death

Treatment of contrast reactions

1. Most reactions are mild and transient and require no specific therapy.
2. More severe reactions may require specific treatment depending on the clinical signs present. Intravenous fluid therapy, oxygen, corticosteroids, atropine, epinephrine, valium, or antihistamines are administered according to standard therapeutic protocols.

Barium Sulfate Contrast Media

1. Barium sulfate preparations are safely used for contrast visualization of the wall and lumen of esophagus, stomach, small and large bowel, and occasionally, for bronchography and rhinography.
2. Barium is biologically inert and not hypertonic, metabolized or absorbed by the GI tract.
3. The efficacy of barium as a contrast agent is caused, in part, by its high degree of radiopacity and its adherence to suspending agents, such as carboxymethyl cellulose, for coating mucosal surfaces. When micropulv-

erized and suspended, it efficiently coats the bowel and provides an excellent medium for assessing the mucosa of bowel and patency of GI tract.

4. Barium Sulfate USP ($BaSO_4$ United States pharmacopeia) is not recommended for contrast radiography. It does not suspend well when mixed with water, and rapidly precipitates and provides an overall inferior study when compared to other barium mixtures that are premixed suspensions of micropulverized barium.
5. Examples of barium sulfate contrast media for use in dogs and cats are:

Brand Name	Form	Manufacturer
Microtrast	$BaSO_4$ paste	Picker
Esophotrast	$BaSO_4$ paste	Rhone-Poulenc Rorer
E-Z Paste	$BaSO_4$ paste	E-Z-EM
Novopaque	$BaSO_4$ suspension	Picker
Barotrast	$BaSO_4$ suspension	Rhone-Poulenc Rorer
Polibar	$BaSO_4$ suspension	E-Z-EM

Adverse Effects of Barium Sulfate

1. Barium sulfate preparations have few direct adverse effects unless deposited outside the GI tract. If extravasated into the peritoneal cavity, mediastinum, or pleural cavity because of esophageal or GI perforation, barium may cause a granuloma with or without inflammatory disease, and may cause adhesions.
2. Barium in the trachea or lung usually results from patient aspiration when administering barium for a GI contrast study. Other causes include esophageal fistula or the incorrect placement of an oro or nasal gastric tube when administering the barium.
3. If large amounts of barium are present in the major airways of the lung, the clinical effect is airway obstruction and hypoxia. Clinically, if severe respiratory distress is present, it is recommended that the barium be removed by endotracheal suction. Barium that becomes alveolarized does not constitute a major problem if the volume is minor. With time, most will be cleared through the ciliary system of the bronchioles or through alveolar macrophages and will ultimately migrate and localize in the draining tracheobronchial lymph nodes. Barium may also stay within the alveolic or terminal bronchioles.
4. Barium is thought to have some therapeutic effects on the GI tract related to the protective coating action and the binding of bile acids, toxins, bacteria, and gas.

Adverse Effects of Negative Contrast Media

1. The major adverse effect is gas embolism and death if gas inadvertently gains access to the vascular system during or after completion of the procedure. This has occurred in pneumocystography (especially in the cat) when room air is used and hematuria is present, or there is overdistension of the bladder during the contrast study.
2. It is advised that a more soluble gas, such as carbon dioxide or nitrous oxide, be used for both pneumoperitoneography and pneumocystography.
3. Nonfatal embolization usually requires symptomatic support and time allowing for absorption of the intravascular gas. It is recommended that the animal be positioned in left lateral recumbency to trap the gas in the right ventricle and to prevent embolization of the pulmonary outflow tract.

CONTRAST EXAMINATION TECHNIQUES

The following technical methodology for contrast radiography is provided as a guideline. Variations depend on the specific reasons for the study, available equipment, status of the patient, and the veterinarian's experience.

It is important that the radiographic studies be conducted in a systematic manner using a predetermined technique (e.g., patient preparation, type and volume of contrast media, patient positioning, filming intervals). Following in a progressive manner over several minutes or hours, modifications of technique, such as additional radiographic views or changes in filming sequence, may be necessary depending on radiographic findings and status of the patient. Survey radiographs made immediately before the contrast study help determine the correct radiographic exposure factors and serve as a comparative baseline for subsequent contrast radiographs.

Intravenous Urography (IVU), Excretory Urography (EU), Intravenous Pyelography (IVP)

A progressive radiographic study is done after intravenous injection of iodinated contrast media to visualize the kidneys, ureters, and urinary bladder. Sequential radiographs show contrast enhancement of the renal vasculature (vascular phase), parenchyma (nephrogram phase), renal collecting system, and ureters (pyelogram phase) as contrast media is excreted by the kidneys and passes through the renal collecting system, ureters, and into urinary bladder.

Indications

1. Evaluate the size, shape, and position of the kidneys, ureters, and bladder.
2. Investigate the cause and source of hematuria, pyuria, dysuria, suspected calculi or masses, and urinary incontinence.
3. Determine the effect of retroperitoneal or intraabdominal masses on the structure, position, and function of the urinary tract.

4. Evaluate the result of trauma to the urinary tract.
5. Qualitative assessment of renal function and patency of the urinary tract.
6. Postoperative assessment of the urinary tract.

Contraindications

1. Anuria
2. Severe dehydration
3. Severe uremia is a contraindication because of the expectant poor contrast opacification of the urinary tract as a result of decreased glomerular filtration.
4. Prior contrast reaction.

Technique

1. Obtain and evaluate survey abdominal radiographs.
2. Animal preparation includes 24-hour fast and appropriate cleansing enemas to evacuate the GI tract.
3. The animal should be well hydrated.
4. Sedation or anesthesia is commonly helpful for animal positioning and application of compression.
5. Rapid intravenous infusion of iodinated contrast media at a contrast dose of 180 mg iodine/kg body weight when normal renal function is present. If the creatinine is greater than 2.0, an increased dose of contrast of 360 mg iodine/kg body weight is recommended. Maximum dose of 90 mL of contrast media in the dog and 15 mL in the cat has been recommended.
6. Radiographic sequence:
   a. Zero time: ventrodorsal and lateral projections
   b. 3 to 5 minutes: ventrodorsal or ventrodorsal and lateral projections
   c. 10 to 15 minutes: ventrodorsal and lateral projections
   d. Additional radiographs made at 30 minutes to 2 hours may be needed if urinary excretion is delayed.
   e. Ventrodorsal oblique projections of the caudal abdomen at 5 to 15 minutes may be helpful in evaluating the distal ureters and ureterovesicular junctions.
7. Abdominal compression
   a. Compression of urinary bladder can provide better visualization of the renal collecting system and proximal ureters by delaying drainage of the contrast.
      1) May be inappropriate if there is a caudal abdominal mass.
      2) Usually requires sedation or anesthesia for proper application of compression.
   b. If the renal pelves and proximal ureters are adequately visualized at 5 to 10 minutes, release the compression and take immediate radiographs of the distal ureters and urinary bladder.
8. If an ectopic ureter is suspected, pneumocystography, done in conjunction with an intravenous urogram, may better visualize the distal ureters and ureterovesicular junctions.

Cystography

Cystography is a contrast evaluation of the urinary bladder using negative contrast (pneumocystogram), positive contrast (cystogram), or both (double contrast cystogram). These studies are used to morphologically evaluate the urinary bladder position, integrity, distensibility, wall thickness, and for intraluminal or intramural lesions such as tumors, diverticula, or calculi.

Indications

1. Investigate causes of dysuria, hematuria, urinary infections, incontinence, or the abnormal appearance of the urinary bladder as seen in the survey radiographs.
2. Evaluate for bladder integrity (e.g., traumatic rupture) or location (e.g., abdominal or perineal hernia).

Selection of appropriate contrast study

1. Positive contrast cystography is the procedure of choice to evaluate for bladder wall integrity and bladder position. Mural masses may be seen if projections are made tangential to the lesion. However, iodinated contrast media can obscure intraluminal abnormalities such as calculi.
2. Double contrast cystography provides the best mucosal detail and is optimal to assess for calculi and mural masses.
3. Pneumocystography is least preferred for most situations. There is increased risk of air embolism, especially if severe hematuria is present. Bladder wall thickness, most calculi, and mural lesions may be seen. A pneumocystogram is insensitive for identifying the size or location of a bladder wall tear.

Technique

1. Preparation of the animal includes a 24-hour fast and cleansing enemas to evacuate the colon and rectum.
2. Sedation or anesthesia is preferred.
3. Obtain and review survey abdominal radiographs.

Double Contrast Cystography

1. Catheterize and empty the urinary bladder using aseptic technique.
2. Flush and remove blood clots if present.
3. Infuse gas sufficient to distend the bladder:
   a. "Rule of thumb" dose is 2 to 4 mL/kg body weight.
   b. Palpate bladder to prevent overdistension.
   c. Room air can be used; however, more soluble gases are preferred (e.g., carbon dioxide, nitrous oxide).
4. Inject small volume of iodinated contrast media into bladder lumen.
   a. 1 to 2 mL for a cat or small dog
   b. 2 to 10 mL for larger dogs
5. Roll the animal 360° to coat the mucosa with contrast.
6. Obtain lateral and ventrodorsal oblique projections.
7. Inject additional air if further distension of bladder is required and then obtain additional projections.

Positive Contrast Cystography

1. Catheterize and empty the urinary bladder using aseptic technique.
2. Flush and remove blood clots if present.
3. Infuse diluted contrast media (dilute 1 part contrast to 3 parts water) at a dose sufficient to distend the bladder.
   a. Rule of thumb dose is 2 to 4 mL/kg body weight, but more or less may be required (e.g., thickened fibrotic bladder or bladder atony).
   b. Palpate the bladder to prevent overdistension.
4. Obtain lateral and ventrodorsal oblique projections.
5. Inject additional contrast media if further distension of bladder is required and then obtain additional projections.

Pneumocystography

1. Catheterize and empty the urinary bladder using aseptic technique.
2. Flush and remove blood clots if present.
3. Infuse gas sufficient to distend the bladder.
   a. Rule to thumb dose is 2 to 4 mL/kg body weight, but more or less may be required (e.g., thickened fibrotic bladder or bladder atony).
   b. Palpate bladder to prevent overdistension.
   c. Room air may be used; however, more soluble gases are preferred (e.g., carbon dioxide, nitrous oxide).
4. Obtain lateral and ventrodorsal projections.
5. Inject additional air if further distension of bladder is required and repeat radiographic projections.

Urethrography

A contrast study of the urethra usually is made using positive contrast media to evaluate the location and morphology of urethra. Most often used to evaluate for stricture, rupture, neoplasia, calculi, or the prostatic urethra.

Indications

1. Investigate causes of stranguria, hematuria, or dysuria.
2. Evaluate for abnormal position of the urethra or urinary bladder (e.g., abdominal or perineal hernia).
3. Use as a supplemental contrast study of the urinary tract before or after a cystogram.
4. Aid in the diagnosis of a congenital anomaly (e.g., ectopic ureter).

Technique

1. Preparation of the animal with a cleansing enema to evacuate the colon and rectum.
2. Sedation or anesthesia is preferred.
3. Survey radiographs of ventrodorsal and lateral projections. In a male dog an additional lateral view is obtained of the perineal and penile regions with the rear legs pulled cranially.
4. Male dog:
   a. Place balloon tip catheter (e.g., Foley) in the distal urethra, prefilled with iodinated contrast media to prevent the injection of air bubbles, thereby avoiding erroneous diagnosis of calculi or other filling defects.
   b. For prostatic assessment, the catheter is placed into distal pelvic urethra at the level of the ischial arch.
   c. Infuse undiluted contrast media retrograde at a dose of 5 to 15 mL (sufficient to fill the urethra).
   d. Obtain a lateral projection (including the perineal area), the end of infusion when the urethra is distended maximally.
   e. Repeat the infusion for each additional projection that may be clinically indicated (e.g., ventrodorsal or oblique projections).
   f. Procedure can be performed after a cystogram by moving the catheter caudally to the level of the ischial arch.
5. Female dog:
   a. A voiding urethrogram can be performed after a cystogram by applying pressure to the urinary bladder with a radiolucent paddle or wooden spoon.
   b. A retrograde urethrogram can be performed by either of the following techniques:
      1) After a positive contrast cystogram has been performed, inject undiluted contrast through the catheter while pulling the catheter caudally and obtain a lateral radiograph during contrast infusion.
      2) Using a balloon tip catheter (e.g., Swan Ganz, Foley), place the catheter into the distal urethra, inflate the balloon, and make an injection of 5 to 10 mL of contrast media, making a lateral radiograph during the end of active infusion. Repeat the retrograde infusion for ventrodorsal or obliquc projcctions.
6. Male or female cats:
   a. Retrograde urethrography is difficult to perform because of the small urethral size.
   b. Swan Ganz catheters may be used as described above for the dog.
   c. Process can be performed as a voiding study by filling the bladder with contrast and obtaining lateral and/or oblique projections while expressing the bladder during abdominal compression.

Vaginography

Radiographic study using a retrograde infusion of positive contrast media for a morphologic evaluation of the vagina, cervix, and urethra. Negative contrast media may also be used, but is generally less satisfactory, especially for visualization of the urethra.

Indications

1. Evaluate for vaginal masses (extraluminal, intramural, and intraluminal), strictures or fistulae.
2. Evaluate for ectopic ureter.

Technique

1. A balloon tip catheter (e.g., Foley) is inflated inside the vestibule.
2. Undiluted iodinated contrast media is infused at a dose of 5 to 30 mL to adequately fill the vagina.
3. Obtain a lateral projection of the pelvis and caudal abdomen while the vagina is distended with contrast media.

Esophagography

Radiographic study is done using positive contrast media to evaluate esophageal location and morphology. Fluoroscopy is the optimum technique for the assessment of esophageal motility and function.

Indications

1. Assessing an animal with suspected esophageal disease based on clinical signs of regurgitation, gagging, or dysphagia.
2. Evaluating an animal with a foreign body, stricture, or trauma to the esophagus.
3. Evaluating the esophagus for abnormal position in an animal with a cervical or mediastinal mass.
4. Assessment of esophageal motility.

Contrast media

1. For mucosal assessment, use barium sulfate paste or thick liquid barium at a concentration of 80 to 100% w/v.
2. If esophageal perforation is suspected, use iodinated contrast media first. Occasionally, a perforation is better demonstrated with barium than with iodinated contrast media.
3. If megaesophagus is present, use barium sulfate at 30% w/v.
4. If a stricture is suspected, feed varying sizes of barium-filled gelatin capsules or barium-injected marshmallows or mix thick barium with food.
5. A bolus of barium can also be infused cranial to a suspected esophageal lesion through an oro or naso esophageal tube.
6. Barium-soaked kibble can be fed to evaluate the passage of a large bulky food bolus from the oropharynx into the stomach.

Patient preparation

1. Survey radiographs of the cervical region and thorax.
2. Sedation and anesthesia are not recommended because esophageal motility will be altered.

Technique

1. Administer barium contrast media by syringe into the buccal pouch at a dose of 5 to 20 mL and allow the animal to swallow two to three times to ensure coating of the esophagus. If iodinated contrast is used, a recommended dose is 5 to 10 mL.
2. Obtain right lateral and right ventrodorsal oblique projections.
3. Additional swallows of contrast can be administered if additional radiographs are required to verify suspected lesions.

Gastrography

Gastrography is a radiographic contrast study of the stomach using negative, positive, or double contrast techniques for evaluation of gastric morphology and function. Morphologic lesions can be intraluminal, mural, or extramural. A double contrast study, especially if done with fluoroscopy, is the most sensitive contrast study for detecting a gastric lesion.

Indications

1. Assessment of an animal with clinical signs suggestive of gastric disease including vomiting, hematemesis, cranial abdominal pain, anorexia, or a cranial abdominal mass.
2. Evaluate for a suspected mural or intraluminal gastric lesion based on survey radiographs or endoscopy.
3. Evaluate for gastric displacement (e.g., diaphragmatic hernia, volvulus, or adjacent abdominal mass).
4. Evaluate for suspected pyloric outflow obstructive disease.

Technique

1. Obtain and review survey abdominal radiographs.
2. Ideally, no sedation or anesthesia should be given for a functional study. If necessary, acepromazine should be used because it is reported to have the least effect on altering motility.
3. General anesthesia or sedation can be used for morphologic evaluation of the stomach.
4. For pneumogastrogram:
   a. Pass an orogastric tube into the stomach.
   b. Infuse sufficient gas to make the stomach tympanic.
      1) Rule of thumb dose is 40 to 60 mL in a cat.
      2) Rule of thumb dose is 50 to 300 mL in a dog.
   c. Obtain right lateral, left lateral, dorsoventral, and ventrodorsal projections.
5. For positive contrast gastrogram:
   a. Pass an orogastric tube into the stomach.
   b. Infuse barium sulfate 30% w/v
      1) Rule of thumb dose is 0.5 to 3 mL/kg body weight in a cat.
      2) Rule of thumb dose is 2 to 3 mL/kg body weight in a dog.
   c. Obtain right lateral, left lateral, dorsoventral, and ventrodorsal projections.
6. For double contrast gastrogram:
   a. Pass an orogastric tube into the stomach.
   b. Infuse barium sulfate 30 to 50% w/v, 0.5 to 1.0 mL/kg body weight. In addition, glucagon, 0.10 to 0.35 mg/kg body weight, also may be administered intra-

venously to facilitate the distention of the stomach and delay gastric emptying.
c. Infuse sufficient gas to make the stomach tympanic.
d. Carefully roll the animal 360°.
e. Obtain right lateral, left lateral, dorsoventral, and ventrodorsal projections.
f. The stomach may need to be redistended with more air (because of loss by regurgitation) for additional radiographs.
g. Fluoroscopic observation with concurrent radiographic filming is helpful for detecting lesions.

Upper Gastrointestinal Study (UGI)

Upper gastrointestinal study is a radiographic study using positive contrast media to provide functional and morphologic evaluation of the small intestine.

Indications:

1. Assessment of the size, shape, and position of the small intestine
2. Clinical signs of small bowel disease such as vomiting, anorexia, or abdominal pain
3. Diagnose partial or complete small bowel obstruction (mechanical ileus) caused by foreign body, tumor, intussusception, hernia, or adhesions.

Technique

1. Obtain and review survey abdominal radiographs.
2. If chemical restraint is necessary, acepromazine sedation in the dog (0.1 mg/kg body weight) or ketamine anesthesia in the cat (10–20 mg IV) may be used.
3. Pass orogastric tube and infuse contrast media.
4. For a barium examination:
   a. Use barium sulfate 30% w/v;
      1) Rule of thumb dose is 2.5 to 3 mL/kg body weight in a cat.
      2) Rule of thumb dose is 1.8 to 2.7 mL/kg body weight in a dog.
   b. Obtain sequential radiographs.
      1) For a dog, usually obtain lateral and ventrodorsal projections at 5 minutes, 30 minutes, and hourly thereafter, until the contrast is seen in the large intestine.
      2) For a cat, usually obtain lateral and ventrodorsal projections at 5 minutes, 15 minutes, 30 minutes, and every 30 minutes thereafter, until the contrast is seen in the large intestine.
5. For iodinated contrast examination:
   a. Use oral ionic or nonionic iodinated contrast media (e.g., Oral Hypaque, Iohexol)
      1) Dose is 0.5 to 1.0 mL/kg body weight in a cat.
      2) Dose is 0.25 to 0.50 mL/kg body weight in a dog.
   b. Obtain sequential radiographs. A more rapid transit time than with barium should be expected, and lateral and ventrodorsal projections should be made more frequently (usually every 10 to 30 minutes) until the contrast is seen in the large intestine.

Barium Enema (BE)

Barium enema is a radiographic study made with retrograde infusion of negative contrast, positive contrast, or both (double contrast) for the morphologic assessment of the large bowel. The large bowel cannot be properly evaluated after oral administration of contrast medium because the colon will not be sufficiently distended and artifactual filling defects will be present as a result of mixture of barium and the luminal contents. The rectum and anal canal cannot be evaluated with a barium enema.

Indications

1. Assess the size, shape, and position of the large bowel.
2. Assess the position of the colon caused by a caudal abdominal or pelvic mass.
3. Determine whether gas or fluid-filled bowel loops are of small bowel or large bowel origin.
4. Clinical conditions and signs in which a barium enema would be helpful in making diagnosis:
   a. Ileocolic intussusception or cecal inversion
   b. Mechanical or functional large bowel obstruction
   c. Mucosal lesion of the colon (colitis, tumor)
   d. A mass extrinsic to the large bowel
   e. Diarrhea often with red blood or mucus
   f. Tenesmus or dyschezia
   g. Abnormally shaped feces (e.g., small diameter)
5. Complications are rare. Perforation may occur secondary to either disease of the bowel wall or as a result of faulty contrast technique. Inadvertent filling of the distal small bowel may obscure visualization of the colon and cecum.
6. Endoscopy is a more accurate technique for the assessment of the colon.

Double Contrast Barium Enema

Technique

1. Thoroughly clean the large bowel with oral laxatives and warm water enemas.
2. Obtain and review survey abdominal radiographs.
3. General anesthesia is required.
4. Instillation of a balloon catheter (cranial to the anal sphincter) that completely occludes the anal canal.
   a. With the animal in left lateral recumbency, slowly infuse a dilute barium sulfate mixture (10–20% w/v) into the large bowel with an adequate volume to completely fill the large bowel and cecum. Rule of thumb dose is 1.0 to 2.5 mL/kg body weight.
   b. Obtain ventrodorsal and lateral abdominal radiographs. If the large bowel is insufficiently distended, additional contrast should be administered and the radiographs repeated.
   c. Evacuate the barium and, with the animal in right lateral recumbency, infuse air to redistend the colon.

d. Obtain ventrodorsal and lateral abdominal radiographs.
e. Deflate and remove balloon catheter.

Pneumocolon or Positive Contrast Colonic Examination

Technique

1. Obtain and review survey abdominal radiographs.
2. Cleansing enema is optional because this study is usually done to verify the position of the large bowel.
3. Anesthesia or sedation usually is unnecessary, unless a balloon catheter is used.
4. Insert a soft catheter or dose syringe rectally and inject gas or positive contrast media sufficient to fill the large bowel.
5. Obtain lateral and ventrodorsal radiographs.

Peritoneography: Celiography

Peritoneography is a radiographic contrast study of the peritoneal cavity using negative or positive contrast media to outline the peritoneal surface of the diaphragm, abdominal wall, and serosal surfaces of the abdominal viscera.

Indication

Assess the integrity of the diaphragm or abdominal wall for congenital or acquired hernias.

Technique

1. Obtain and review survey abdominal radiographs after the urinary bladder is emptied.
2. Anesthesia or sedation is preferred.
3. A needle or catheter is placed into the peritoneal cavity lateral to midline and caudal to the umbilicus.
4. For a positive contrast study:
   a. After a test aspiration to insure that neither a viscus nor vessel has been punctured, iodinated contrast media is infused (Rule of thumb dose of 0.1 to 0.25 mL/kg body weight mixed with an equal volume of sterile saline). Nonionic contrast is recommended.
   b. The animal is carefully rolled 360° to insure that the contrast is distributed throughout the peritoneal cavity.
   c. Radiographs are obtained, including right and left lateral, ventrodorsal, and dorsoventral projections.
5. For a negative contrast study:
   a. After a test aspiration to insure that neither a viscus nor vessel has been punctured, infuse gas at a sufficient dose to make the abdomen tympanic. Nitrous oxide or carbon dioxide is preferred over oxygen or room air because of increased solubility.
   b. It is recommended that initially the animal be in a left lateral recumbent position, so that, should embolization occur, the gas is trapped in the right atrium and the chance of air embolization and possible death is minimized.
   c. Radiographs are obtained including right and left lateral, ventrodorsal, and dorsoventral projections.
   d. Nitrous oxide and carbon dioxide are rapidly absorbed and do not require removal. However, room air, if used, should be removed.

Myelography

Myelography is a radiographic contrast examination of the spinal cord using nonionic contrast media injected into the subarachnoid space.

Indications

1. Aid is diagnosis of an animal with myelopathy and clinical signs of pain, paresis, or paralysis.
2. Assess the spinal cord relative to its size and position within the spinal canal.
3. Determine sites of cord compression related to extradural, intradural, or intramedullary disease.
4. Not of value for diagnosing disseminated myelopathies, meningopathies, or nerve root lesions.

Technique

1. Obtain and review survey spinal radiographs with the animal under general anesthesia.
2. Perform aseptic spinal puncture of the subarachnoid space at either the cisterna magna or an interarcuate space of caudal lumbar spine (usually L5–L6) using a 20 to 22 gauge spinal needle.
3. It is preferable (but not essential) to remove cerebral spinal fluid at a volume equal to the amount of contrast media that will be injected.
4. Slowly inject nonionic contrast media (e.g., iohexol, iopamidol) at a dose sufficient to fill the subarachnoid space (dose range of 0.03–0.07 mL/kg body weight).
5. After the contrast has been injected, a radiograph can be obtained with the needle still in place or the needle can be removed. Obtain ventrodorsal and lateral radiographs of the spine. Supplemental projections (e.g., dorsoventral, oblique, extended and flexed lateral) should be made as needed.
6. Depending on the flow of the contrast media, the body may be tilted to aid in moving the contrast and for better filling of subarachnoid space at a specific site.

Epidurography

Epidurography is a radiographic contrast study of the epidural space using positive contrast to assess the cauda equina and proximal portions of the nerve roots.

Indications

1. Aid in assessing the cauda equina for compression or displacement as a result of a constricting lesion, tumor, or disk protrusion or extrusion.

2. Difficult study to perform because the epidural space may not be clearly defined and contrast media may not flow freely.

Technique
1. Obtain and review survey spinal radiographs with the animal under general anesthesia.
2. With the animal in sternal or lateral recumbency, place a spinal needle aseptically into the floor of the spinal canal through the lumbosacral or coccygeal interarcuate space.
3. Inject nonionic contrast media at a dose sufficient to fill the epidural space (rule of thumb dose is 2–10 mL).
4. Remove the needle and obtain radiographs including lateral, flexed lateral, extended lateral, and ventrodorsal or dorsoventral projections.

Discography
Discography ia a radiographic study for visualizing the central portion of an intravertebral disk.

Indications
1. Evaluate the size and shape of the central cavity of the disk.
2. Determine the amount and position of herniated nuclear disk material or annular rupture.
3. More commonly done in animals with cauda equina syndrome because the needle can be more accurately positioned in this region of the spine. In other spinal regions, fluoroscopy is usually needed for accurate positioning of the needle.

Technique
1. Obtain and review survey radiographs of the spinal region with the animal under general anesthesia. First, evaluate for congenital anomalies or degenerative disease, which may affect the placement of the needle into the disk.
2. With the animal in lateral recumbency, place the spinal needle aseptically through interarcurate ligament and spinal canal into the disk.
3. Inject nonionic contrast media into the disk. A rule of thumb dose is 0.25 to 3.0 mL, varying with the size of the disk and the amount of observable degeneration. If resistance is encountered during injection, reposition the needle tip.
4. Obtain radiographs including neutral lateral, hyperflexed lateral, hyperextended lateral, and dorsoventral or ventrodorsal projections.

Arthrography
Arthrography is a radiographic contrast study of a joint using positive or negative contrast media to outline the margins of the joint and to assess the articular cartilage, intraarticular ligaments, tendons, meniscal cartilage, and joint capsule.

Indications
1. Evaluate for osteochondrosis (e.g., shoulder, elbow, stifle) and diseases of tendons and ligaments.
2. Supplemental procedure when a diagnosis cannot be made from survey radiographs, or to determine whether an articular cartilage flap is attached or detached.
3. Assessment for the presence of free bodies within the joint.
4. Positive contrast arthrography provides more information than negative contrast arthrography.
5. Double contrast arthrography is not recommended because of problems with numerous artifacts created by air mixing with the positive contrast media.

Technique
1. General anesthesia is usually necessary.
2. Obtain and review survey radiographs of the joint, including lateral and caudocranial projections.
3. Perform an aseptic articular puncture.
4. Remove as much joint fluid as possible (analysis of synovial fluid is recommended.)
5. Inject contrast media.
   a) For a positive contrast study, nonionic contrast media is preferred.
      1) Dilute contrast (1 part contrast, 2 parts water).
      2) Rule of thumb dose of 1 to 6 mL is used for the shoulder and stifle joints, depending on the animal's size.
   b) For a negative contrast study, air is used.
6. Remove the needle and manipulate the joint to insure uniform filling of the joint.
7. Obtain radiographs including lateral, caudocranial, and lateral oblique projections as required to adequately visualize the joint and the articular surfaces.

Angiography: Selective and Nonselective
Angiography is a radiographic contrast study made using iodinated contrast media and a sequence of radiographs to visualize the circulation (heart, arteries, and veins). Selective angiography is the placement of a catheter, as near to the suspected lesion as possible, for delivery of positive contrast media.

Selective angiography requires specialized equipment (e.g., special catheters, contrast media injector, rapid film recording device, fluoroscopy). Nonselective angiography is limited to certain cardiac and vascular diseases and is less accurate in demonstrating lesions than selective angiography. Nonselective angiography, however, can be adequately performed with routine radiographic equipment.

Indications
1. Evaluate the size and shape of the cardiac chambers.
2. Aid in differentiating some types of feline cardiomyopathy.

3. Detect right to left shunts.
4. Identify cardiac masses or intracardiac thrombi.
5. Diagnose a large pericardial effusion.
6. Evaluate the aorta, main pulmonary arteries, and cranial or caudal vena cava for displacement or occlusion by thrombosis, embolus, mass, or stricture.

Technique

1. General anesthesia is required for selective angiography. Sedation may be acceptable for nonselective angiography, depending on the status of the animal and indication for study.
2. Method for nonselective cranial vena cava and cardiac angiography:
   a. Obtain and review survey thoracic radiographs.
   b. Place indwelling 14 to 18 gauge catheter into the cephalic or jugular vein.
   c. Make a bolus injection of iodinated contrast media (dose of 0.1–0.25 mg/kg body weight) with a total injection time of 1 to 3 seconds.
   d. Obtain a radiograph at the end of the injection, and additional radiographs every 1 to 3 seconds to follow the contrast through the heart. Use of a rapid film changer or cassette tunnel allows multiple radiographs over a short period of time.
   e. Additional injections of contrast can be made (total dose received of 1.0 mL/kg body weight if additional radiographs are needed to complete the study.
3. Method for nonselective caudal vena cava venography:
   a. Obtain and review survey abdominal radiographs.
   b. Catheterize a peripheral vein (e.g., saphenous or recurrent lateral metatarsal).
   c. With the animal in lateral recumbency, inject iodinated contrast media at a dose of 0.10 to 0.25 mL/kg body weight at a rate of approximately 1 to 2 mL/second.
   d. Near the end of the injection, obtain a lateral radiograph of the abdomen.
   e. Reposition the animal into dorsal recumbency and reinject an additional bolus of contrast media and obtain a ventrodorsal projection.

Venous Portography

Venous portography is a radiographic contrast study of the portal venous system using positive contrast media injected into the spleen or mesenteric vein.

Indications

1. Assessment of the portal venous system for a suspected portosystemic shunt.
2. Aid in differentiating whether a portosystemic shunt is intrahepatic or extrahepatic.
3. Splenoportography is less accurate than mesenteric venography for the detection and characterization of a venous shunt.

Technique

1. Obtain and review survey abdominal radiographs.
2. Administer contrast media with catheter placed in the jejenal vein at laparotomy or into the spleen by percutaneous puncture.
3. Rule of thumb dose of iodinated contrast media is 0.1 to 0.25 mL/kg body weight.
4. Lateral projections of the abdomen are obtained during and after infusion. The timing and number of radiographic exposures needed may vary with the size and location of the shunt.
5. If needed, the animal is repositioned in dorsal recumbency with another injection of contrast media and additional sequential radiographs.

Pneumopericardiography

Pneumopericardiography is a radiographic contrast study using negative contrast media to visualize the pericardial sac and epicardium of the heart.

Indications

1. Usually performed in animals with pericardial effusion, after pericardiocentesis.
2. Diagnose epicardial, pericardial, and heart base masses.
3. Rarely needed, if ultrasound is available.

Technique

1. Place an indwelling catheter into the pericardial sac at the right fifth or sixth intercostal space.
2. Remove as much pericardial fluid as possible.
3. Infuse air or carbon dioxide at a volume approximately 75% of the fluid volume that was removed.
4. Obtain right lateral, left lateral, dorsoventral, and ventrodorsal projections.

Fistulography

Fistulography is a radiographic contrast study using positive, negative, or double contrast media to visualize the character, depth, and origin of fistulous tracts and draining wounds.

Indications

1. Assess location and extent of draining wound that has not responded to medical or surgical therapy when surgical intervention is being considered.
2. Detect the presence of a foreign body or a sequestra associated with osteomyelitis.

Technique

1. Obtain and review survey radiographs of the region.
2. Insert a catheter into the sinus or fistula. A balloon tip catheter may be useful to prevent leakage at the cutaneous margin.

3. Inject ionic or nonionic iodinated contrast media at a dose sufficient to fill the cavity and, if possible, leave the catheter in place.
4. Obtain radiographs, including lateral and orthogonal projections.

Tracheography and Bronchography

Tracheography and bronchography are radiographic contrast studies using positive contrast media to visualize the luminal anatomy of the trachea and bronchi.

Indications

1. Assess partial or complete airway obstruction by tumor, foreign body, or stricture.
2. Demonstrate tracheal or bronchial fistulas, abscesses, cysts, and other mural or intraluminal lesions.
3. Diagnose and evaluate the extent of bronchiectasis.

Technique

1. Obtain and review survey radiographs of thorax.
2. The animal must be anesthetized and intubated.
3. Selectively place a catheter through the endotracheal tube (using fluoroscopy or endoscopy) to the site of the suspected lesion in the trachea or specific bronchus. It is advisable to study no more than one lung at a time.
4. With the suspected lesion site placed in a dependent position, infuse positive contrast media to effect (usually 1 to 4 mL, if the lesion is limited to one lung lobe).
5. Sterile barium sulfate suspension is the contrast media of choice (50–60% w/v).
   a. Barium is relatively inert as a bronchographic media. (It may cause a mild reaction that readily and quickly subsides, usually within a few days.)
   b. Most is eliminated by the ciliary-mucous transport system, but some may become alveolarized and ultimately collect in the regional lymph nodes.
6. Keeping the lobe or lesion site dependent, obtain lateral, ventrodorsal, and when needed, oblique radiographic projections. Radiographs obtained during inspiration and expiration may be helpful.

Pleurography

Pleurography is a radiographic contrast study using negative or positive contrast media to visualize the parietal and visceral pleural surfaces.

Indications

1. Delineate pleural or extrapleural masses from pulmonary masses.
2. Delineate a mass lesion in the mediastinum.
3. Diagnose pleural adhesions.

Technique

1. Obtain and review survey radiographs of thorax.
2. General anesthesia is recommended.
3. Inject iodinated contrast media or gas into pleural cavity with aseptic technique, preferably with an indwelling catheter. Stop injection if respiratory distress develops.
4. For a positive contrast pleurogram:
   a. Mix sterile ionic or nonionic contrast media with lidocaine hydrochloride (1 part lidocaine, 9 parts contrast).
   b. Rule of thumb for contrast dose is 0.25 mL/kg body weight.
5. For a negative contrast pleurogram:
   a. Inject room air at volume of 50 mL for a small dog or cat, 100 mL for a medium dog, and 200 mL for a large dog.
6. Obtain left lateral, right lateral, ventrodorsal, and dorsoventral projections.

Sialography

Sialography is a radiographic contrast study using positive contrast media to visualize the salivary ducts and glands (i.e., parotid, sublingual, submandibular).

Indications

1. Need to evaluate a salivary mucocoele.
2. Confirm or exclude a salivary gland or duct rupture.
3. Confirm salivary duct obstruction, stricture, mass, or other lesion.

Technique

1. Obtain and review survey radiographs of skull and neck with the animal under anesthesia.
2. Cannulate the salivary duct using a 23 to 27 gauge lacrimal needle.
3. Inject 0.1 to 0.3 mL of iodinated contrast media.
4. Obtain lateral and ventrodorsal radiographic projections.

Dacryocystorhinography

Dacryocystorhinography is a radiographic contrast study using positive contrast media to visualize the nasolacrimal duct.

Indications

1. Assess for causes of chronic, recurring, or intractable conjunctivitis and dacryocystitis.
2. Diagnose stricture, obstruction, and alterations in lumen size and course of nasolacrimal duct.

Technique

1. General anesthesia is required.
2. Obtain and review survey radiographs of the nasal region including lateral and ventrodorsal projections.
3. Cannulate the superior or inferior lacrimal puncta with a 23 to 27 gauge lacrimal needle.
4. Inject iodinated contrast media until several drops are seen in the external nares.

5. Placing the nose slightly dependent will prevent the contrast media from flowing retrograde into the nasal cavity.
6. Obtain lateral and ventrodorsal radiographic projections.

Otic Canalography

Otic canalography is a radiographic contrast study using positive contrast media to visualize the external auditory canal.

Indication

1. Detect rupture of the tympanic membrane.
2. Helpful when tympanic membrane cannot be seen directly.

Technique

1. Obtain and review radiographs of skull with ventrodorsal and rostrocaudal open mouth projections.
2. Infuse 2 to 5 mL of iodinated contrast media into the ear canal.
3. Obtain ventrodorsal and rostrocaudal open mouth projections.

Rhinography

Rhinography is a contrast study of the nasal cavity using positive contrast media.

Indications

1. Assess for obstruction of the nasal cavity or nasopharynx.
2. Common clinical signs include nasal discharge, reverse sneezing, pharyngeal discharge, or upper airway obstruction.
3. Indicated if nasal radiographs and endoscopy are inconclusive.

Technique

1. Obtain and review radiographs of the nasal cavity and nasopharyngeal region (lateral and open mouth ventrodorsal projections).
2. Under general anesthesia, infuse 2 to 10 mL of positive contrast (either iodinated media or 20–30% barium sulfate) into the ventral nasal meatus.
3. With the infused side dependent, elevate the nose approximately 15° to encourage caudal gravitational flow of contrast media.
4. Obtain lateral and open mouth ventrodorsal projections.

Lymphography/Lymphangiography

Lymphography or lymphangiography is a radiographic contrast study of the lymphatic vessels and the lymph nodes. The contrast evaluation of the lymph system is restricted to those areas that are connected to peripherally accessible lymphatics or lymph nodes such as lymphatics of the extremities, the head, the lumbar cistern, and the thoracic duct.

Indications

1. To assess the peripheral lymphatic circulation in animals with congenital or acquired edema of the extremities.
2. To assist in the evaluation of the thoracic duct in chylothorax to differentiate traumatic rupture from obstruction or lymphangiectasia and to assess the effectiveness of surgical ligation.

Technique

1. Obtain and review survey radiographs of the affected limb.
2. Inject 0.5 to 1.5 mL of a dilute vegetable dye into the interdigital space. The dyes patent blue (2–3%) or Evan's blue (2–3%) are most often used.
3. Surgically expose the dorsal metatarsal or metacarpal region and isolate a blue stained lymphatic vessel.
4. Cannulate the lymphatic vessel with a 25 to 27 gauge needle and infuse 2 to 20 mL of iodinated contrast media by hand or through an infusion pump.
5. To evaluate the cisterna chyli and thoracic duct, an alternate approach is to cannulate a mesenteric lymphatic vessel or the cisterna directly.
6. Obtain radiographs of the limb and draining regions (e.g., abdomen, pelvis, cranial thorax).

chapter four

4

Extremities

ANATOMY

Normal Bone Development and Growth

1. Most bones of the skeleton develop by endochondral ossification through ossification in preexisting cartilage. The bones of the face and the cranium are formed by intramembranous ossification.
2. In endochondral ossification, a typical long bone (Figure 4.1A) develops from a primary center of ossification, usually the diaphysis, and from secondary centers of ossification, known as epiphyses. The ends of the diaphysis, called the metaphyses, are separated from the epiphysis by the physis in the immature animal.
3. Other secondary ossification centers, called apophyses, also contribute to the overall shape of the bone and serve for attachment of tendons. They do not contribute to the overall length of the bone (e.g., greater trochanter of femur).
4. The growth in bone length occurs at the physis (or epiphyseal cartilage), an area composed of active growing cartilage. When growth ceases, the physis cartilage stops growing. It undergoes closure with ossification and no further length is possible. Closure of that physis of various bones takes place at different, but predictable times. Ranges in the dog and cat are established. (See Table 4.1 on Canine Physis Closure and Table 4.2 on Feline Physis Closure.) (Figure 4.1B).

TABLE 4.1

Canine Physis Closures in Days[a]

Bone	Days Average	Days Range	Bone	Days Average	Days Range
Scapula			*Os coxae*		
Tuber scapulae	186	117–210	Ilium	112	
Humerus			Ischium	112	
Proximal epiphysis	375	273–465	Pubis	112	
Medial condyle	187		Os acetabulum	112	
Lateral condyle	187		Tuber ischii	292	
Medial epicondyle	216	187–240	*Femur*		
Radius			Femoral head	320	129–540
Proximal epiphysis	258	136–330	Trochanter major	320	129–540
Distal epiphysis	318	136–510	Trochanter minor	269	129–360
Ulna			Distal epiphysis	330	136–392
Proximal epiphysis	258	161–450	*Tibia*		
Distal epiphysis	308	217–450	Condylea	322	143–413
Carpus			Tibial tuberosity	249	143–435
Intermediate	101		Distal epiphysis	313	136–495
Radial	101		Medial malleolus	138	138
Central	110		*Fibula*		
Epiphysis of accessory	135	113–180	Proximal epiphysis	297	136–360
Metacarpus			Distal epiphysis	288	136–495
Proximal epiphysis of I	145		*Tarsus*		
Distal epiphysis of II–V	203	165–240	Fibular tarsal	159	
Phalanx			Three and four	101	
Proximal			*Metatarsal*		
Proximal epiphysis of I		141	Distal epiphysis II–V	217	165–270
Proximal epiphysis of II–V	186	131–224	*Phalanx*		
Middle			*Proximal*		
Proximal epiphysis of II–V	183	131–224	Proximal epiphysis II–V	187	161–210
			Middle		
			Proximal epiphysis II–V	187	161–210

[a]Adapted from Newton/Nunamaker. Textbook of Small Animal Orthopedics. Philadelphia: J. B. Lippincott; 1985:1110–1111 (table C-2).

TABLE 4.2

Feline Epiphyseal Plate Closures in Days[a]

Bone	Days	Bone	Days
Scapula		*Sesamoids*	140
Tuber & coronoid process	112	*Femur*	
Humerus		Femoral head	210–280
Proximal epiphysis	547–730	Greater trochanter	196–252
Medial condyle	98	Lesser trochanter	238–308
Lateral condyle	98	Distal epiphysis	378–532
Medial epicondyle	112–126	*Tibia*	
Radius		Proximal epiphysis	350–532
Proximal	196	Tibial tuberosity	350–532
Distal	406–616	Distal epiphysis	280–364
Ulna		*Fibula*	
Proximal (tuberosity of olecranon)	266–364	Proximal epiphysis	378–504
Distal epiphysis	406–700	Distal epiphysis	280–392
Carpus		*Tarsus*	
Accessory carpal bone epiphysis	112–126	Fibular tarsal	210–364
Metacarpus		*Metatarsal*	
Distal epiphysis II–V	203–280	Distal epiphysis II–V	224–308
Phalanges		*Phalanx*	
Proximal		Proximal II–V	126–168
Proximal epiphysis II–V	126–154	Middle II–V	126–154
Middle		*Sesamoid*	
Proximal epiphysis	112–140	Metatarsophalangeal	70–112
		Lateral sesamoid in gastrocnemius muscle	70–112
		Medial sesamoid in gastrocnemius muscle	154
		Popliteal muscle in sesamoid	112–140

[a]Breed, unknown; number, 37.
(Smith RN: Fusion of ossification centres in the cat. J Small Anim Pract 1969;10:523.)
From Newton/Nunamaker. Textbook of Small Animal Orthopedics. Philadelphia: J. B. Lippincott; 1985:1110–1111 (table C-2).

Accessory Ossification Centers and Sesamoid Bones

Accessory ossification centers include the normal sesamoid bones and other focal areas of ossification that occur near joints. Knowledge of these centers of ossification is important because they must be differentiated radiographically from traumatic chip fractures and osteophytes.

Sesamoid bones are formed in tendons or ligamentous tissue over which tendons pass. They are located near freely moving joints.

1. Stifle. Four sesamoid bones are normally present in the stifle joint of the dog and cat. These include: the patella, two proximal fabellar sesamoid bones (within the medial and lateral tendons of the heads of the gastrocnemius muscle), and the popliteal fabellar sesamoid bone (in the tendon of the popliteal muscle).
   a. The popliteal fabella is sometimes absent in the cat and smaller dogs.
   b. The fabellae may have more than one center of ossification (i.e., be multipartite), which must be distinguished from fractures of these bones.
2. There is a sesamoid bone in the elbow joint of some dogs (usually the larger breeds). The sesamoid bone is within the tendon of origin of the supinator muscle located adjacent to the craniolateral aspect of the radial head. When present, it is usually bilateral (Figure 4.2).
3. A sesamoid bone is often present in the carpus in the tendon of the insertion of the abductor pollicis longus muscle, and located medial to the carpal-metacarpal joint (Figure 4.3).
4. In the tarsus of some dogs, there are two plantar sesamoid bones located in the tarsometatarsal fibrocartilage. A lateral plantar sesamoid bone is present in approximately 50% of dogs and a medial tarsometatarsal sesamoid bone is present in approximately 30% of dogs (Figure 4.4).
5. There are sesamoid bones in the second, third, fourth, and fifth digits of the front and rear feet. Each metacarpophalangeal and metatarsophalangeal joint has three sesamoid bones, including a singular dorsal sesamoid bone and two palmar (or plantar) sesamoid bones. The sesamoid bones of the digits normally ossify from one center of ossification. In the dog, however, multipartite sesamoid bones are commonly seen and must be differentiated from fractures of these bones. Multipartite sesamoid bones of the digits have been most commonly reported in dogs (e.g., 2nd and 7th palmar sesamoid bones of digits 2 and 5), and usually have no associated clinical signs (Figure 4.5 A, B).
6. Accessory ossification centers or ossicles can occur in many locations, usually adjacent to joints and embedded within the joint capsule. These ossicles need to be clinically and radiographically differentiated from chip fractures. (See Figures 4.6 through 4.10 and Table 4.3 on Accessory Ossification Centers.)

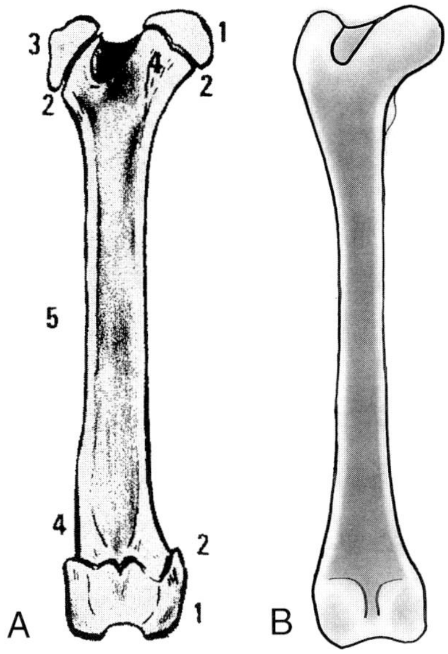

Figure 4.1. **A)** Normal femur (immature long bone). **1**) epiphysis, **2**) physis, **3**) apophysis, **4**) metaphysis, and **5**) diaphysis. **B)** Normal femur (mature long bone). Physes are closed.

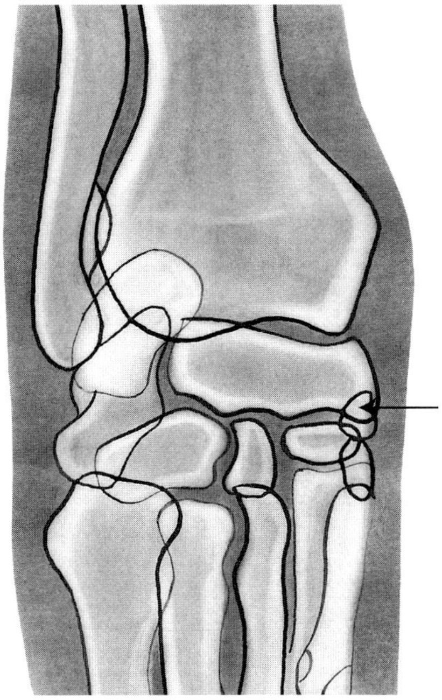

Figure 4.3. Normal canine carpus (dorsopalmar projection). Sesamoid bone (arrow) in the tendon of insertion of the abductor pollicis longus muscle on medial side of carpus.

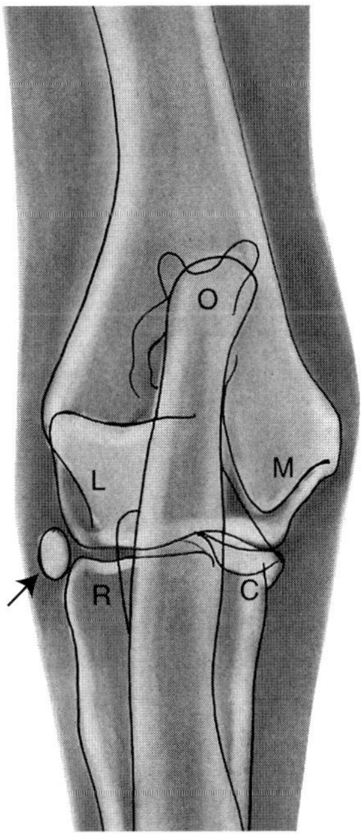

Figure 4.2. Normal canine elbow (craniocaudal projection). Sesamoid bone (arrow) in tendon of supinator muscle on craniolateral side of elbow. Other landmarks include radial head (**R**), coronoid process of ulna (**C**), the medial humeral condyle (**M**), the lateral humeral condyle (**L**), and olecranon (**O**).

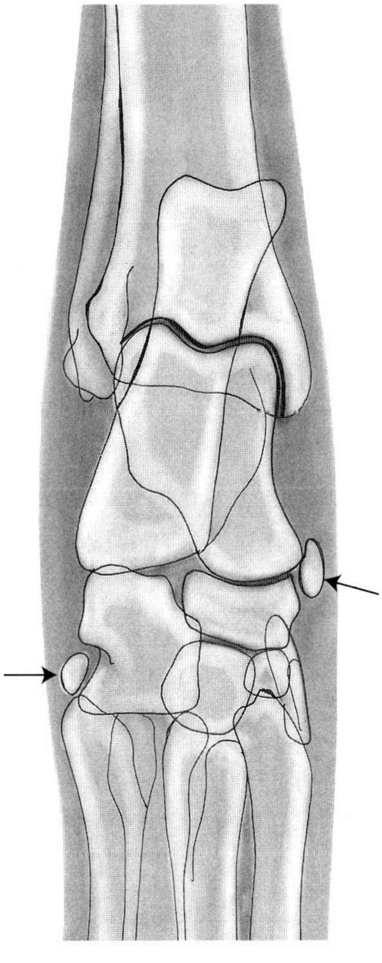

Figure 4.4. Sesamoid bones of canine tarsus (dorsoplantar projection). Lateral plantar sesamoid bone (straight arrow) and medial tarsometatarsal sesamoid bone (curved arrow).

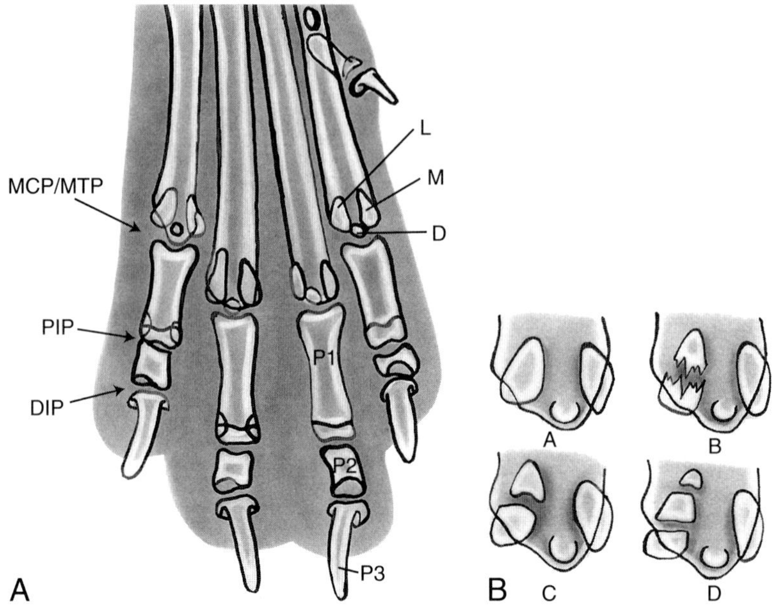

Figure 4.5. **A)** Dorsopalmar or dorsoplantar projection of normal fore and rear digits. Note the medial (**M**) and lateral (**L**) palmar sesamoid bones and dorsal sesamoid bone (**D**) at each metacarpophalangeal joint. Other landmarks are metacarpal-phalangeal and corresponding metatarsal-phalangeal joints **(MCP/MTP)**, proximal interphalangeal joints (**PIP**), and distal interphalangeal joints (**DIP**). There are two palmar (plantar) sesamoid bones (**L&M**) and a singular dorsal sesamoid bone (**D**) immediately proximal to the MCP and MTP joints. **B)** Normal paired palmar (plantar) sesamoid bones are depicted in (**A**) a fracture of a sesamoid bone (**B**) and congenital bipartite (**C**) and tripartite sesamoid (**D**) bones.

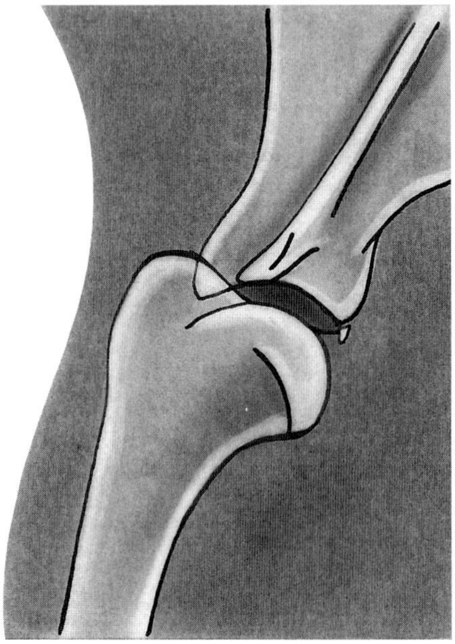

Figure 4.6. Ossicle on the caudal margin of the glenoid. These are usually bilateral and most often present in medium to large breed dogs.

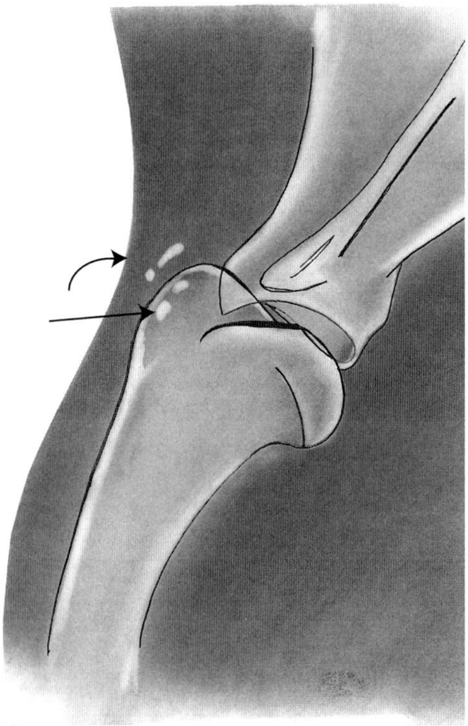

Figure 4.7. Sesamoid bones adjacent to humerus. Sesamoid in the tendon of the infraspinatus muscle (straight arrow) and sesamoid in the tendon of the supraspinatus muscle (curved arrow).

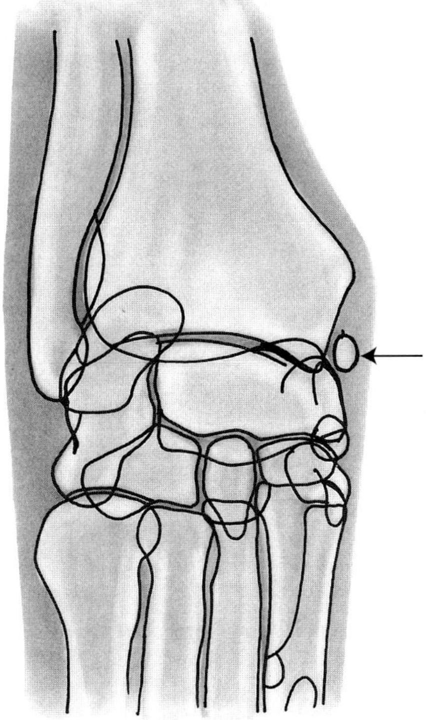

Figure 4.8. Sesamoid bone in the medial radiocarpal ligament in the canine carpus (arrow).

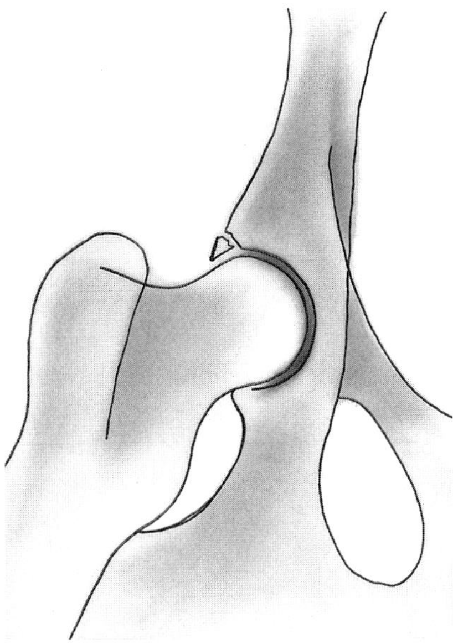

Figure 4.9. Ossicle on the dorsal acetabular rim of canine pelvis. These are usually seen on the ventrodorsal view of the pelvis and in medium to large breed dogs.

Variable Ossification Centers

1. The anconeal process is a normal secondary center of ossification present in medium and large breed dogs. It develops at approximately 11 weeks of age and usually fuses with the ulna by 16 to 20 weeks of age. In smaller dogs and cats, the anconeal process develops as an extension of the proximal ulnar metaphysis. In one form of elbow dysplasia, the anconeal process fails to unite (united anconeal process) (Figure 4.11).

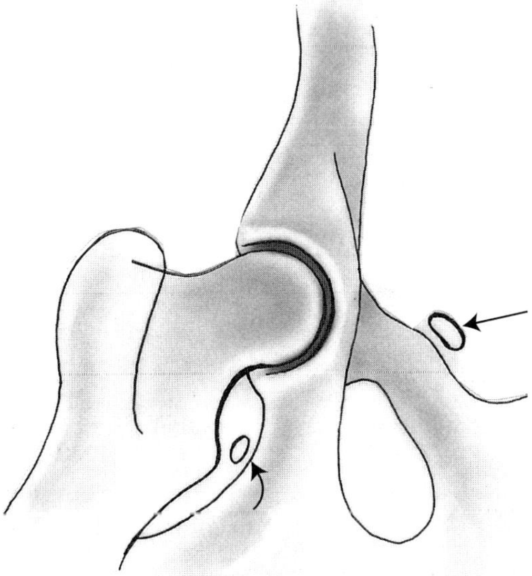

Figure 4.10. Accessory ossification in the pelvis. Sesamoid bone in the tendon of the iliopsoas muscle (curved arrow) and sesamoid bone in the tendon of the psoas minor adjacent to the iliopectineal eminence (straight arrow).

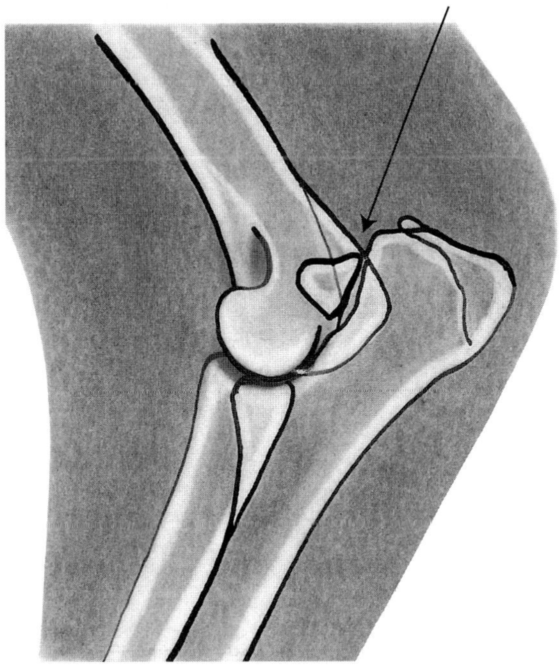

Figure 4.11. Ununited anconeal process of ulna. A radiolucent cleavage line (arrow) at the base of the anconeal process.

TABLE 4.3

Accessory Ossification Centers

1. Ossicle on the caudal margin of the glenoid (Figure 4.6).
2. Sesamoid bone in the tendon of the deltoid muscle adjacent to the acromion process of the scapula.
3. Sesamoid bone in the tendon of the infraspinatus muscle adjacent to the greater tubercle of the humerus (Figure 4.7).
4. Sesamoid bone in the tendon of the supraspinatus muscle adjacent to the greater tubercle of the humerus (Figure 4.7).
5. Sesamoid bone in the tendon of supinator muscle of the elbow (Figure 4.2).
6. Sesamoid bone in the medial radiocarpal ligament of carpus (Figure 4.8).
7. Ossicle on the dorsal acetabular margin of pelvis (Figure 4.9).
8. Sesamoid bone in the tendon of the iliopsoas muscle adjacent to the lesser trochanter of the proximal femur (Figure 4.10).
9. Sesamoid bone in the tendon of the psoas minor muscle adjacent to the iliopectinal eminence (Figure 4.10).

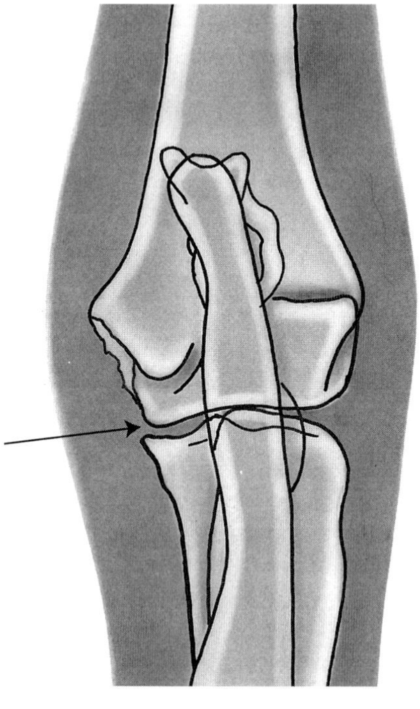

Figure 4.12. Craniocaudal view of elbow. Degenerative joint disease is present secondary to ununited medial coronoid process. Osteophytes are present on the medial humeral condyle adjacent to an irregular medial coronoid process (arrow).

2. The medial coronoid process of the ulna develops as an accessory ossification center in some dogs. If this process becomes fragmented, fractured, or fails to unite with the ulna, elbow dysplasia results (Figure 4.12).
3. The os penis bone normally ossifies from one center of ossification. However, it may ossify from two or more centers. Incomplete ossification also may occur, usually on the proximal end, and mimic a fracture.

CLINICAL AND RADIOGRAPHIC CORRELATIONS

1. The radiographic changes of bone are a reflection of the underlying disease process. Radiographic changes include alterations of size, shape, contour, and radiopacity.
2. When making a differential diagnosis, it is helpful to categorize the radiographic findings of a bone lesion as having an aggressive or nonaggressive pattern. Benign lesions, such as a healing fracture, usually have a nonaggressive pattern. Conversely, malignant bone tumors usually appear aggressive.
3. In general, bone lesions take time to develop, and with many disorders, the early radiographic lesions may be nonspecific. Follow-up radiographs are often helpful in establishing a diagnosis. For example, in septic arthritis, erosive and/or proliferative changes may be undetectable for 10 to 14 days.
4. Preexisting radiographic lesions may obscure abnormalities associated with a second disease process. For example, periarticular osteophytes and subchondral sclerosis associated with degenerative joint disease may obscure the bony changes associated with infection or neoplasia.
5. Diagnosis of some bone diseases can be based on a characteristic radiographic appearance, the animal's clinical signs and history. In other instances, however, different diseases have similar radiographic abnormalities.
6. Radiographic abnormalities commonly lag behind clinical signs, laboratory results, and other parameters. Follow-up radiographs may be necessary for further and more definitive assessment.
7. Correlation of clinical parameters, radiographic findings, and pathologic findings are essential for an accurate diagnosis. When the radiographic diagnosis is in conflict with other clinical findings, further investigation is indicated.
8. In some bone diseases, there may be a poor correlation between clinical signs and radiographic findings. It is also true that the severity of the clinical signs cannot be predicted with certainty from the radiographic findings.
9. The results of the initial radiographic examination may suggest the need for other additional radiographic projections, other imaging studies, clinical tests, biopsy, or other diagnostic procedures.

RADIOGRAPHIC TECHNIQUE

1. Standard projections
   a. At least two radiographs, which are made perpendicular to each other (e.g., craniocaudal and lateral projections).
   b. The joints (proximal and distal to the bones radiographed) should be included.
2. Supplementary radiographic projections
   a. Comparison projections of the contralateral limb
   b. Special projections (e.g., oblique, stress/compression, tangential/tunnel)
   c. A skeletal survey consisting of lateral projections of all four extremities, spine, and skull may be indicated (e.g., systemic or multifocal diseases such as metastatic bone neoplasia).

RADIOGRAPHIC INTERPRETATION

1. Bone lesions can be caused by developmental, metabolic, nutritional, infectious, traumatic, and neoplastic causes. Radiographically, the bone can react to these disease processes in a limited number of ways. Bone changes can include:
   a. Increased radiopacity (osteoblastic or osteosclerosis)
   b. Decreased radiopacity (osteolysis or osteoporosis)
   c. Presence of a periosteal reaction (e.g., solid, amorphous, laminar, sun-burst)
2. Soft tissue alterations observed on a radiograph can be helpful in interpreting a bone lesion. Soft tissue changes can include:
   a. Swelling or mass
   b. Atrophy
   c. Displacement or obliteration of normal structures, such as fascial planes
   d. Mineralization
   e. Presence of a radiopaque foreign body
   f. Emphysema as a result of infection, fistulous tract, or puncture wound
3. The following should be noted when a bone lesion is observed.
   a. Location of lesion (See Figure 4.1)
      1) Periosteum
      2) Cortex
      3) Medullary canal
      4) Epiphysis, physis, metaphysis, or diaphysis
      5) Joint
      6) Monostotic or polyostotic
      7) Focal, multifocal, or generalized
   b. Type of bone production or bone destruction and the margination (aggressive or nonaggressive pattern)
   c. Involvement of the cortex and/or subchondral bone including thickening, thinning, lysis, or sclerotic changes.
      1) Thickened cortex (e.g., healed fracture, chronic osteomyelitis)
      2) Thinned cortex (e.g., disuse bone atrophy, osteoporosis, bone cyst)
      3) Broken cortex (e.g., traumatic fracture, pathologic fracture)
4. Type of periosteal reaction: listed from least aggressive to most aggressive type pattern (Figure 4.13).
   a. Smooth (nonaggressive)

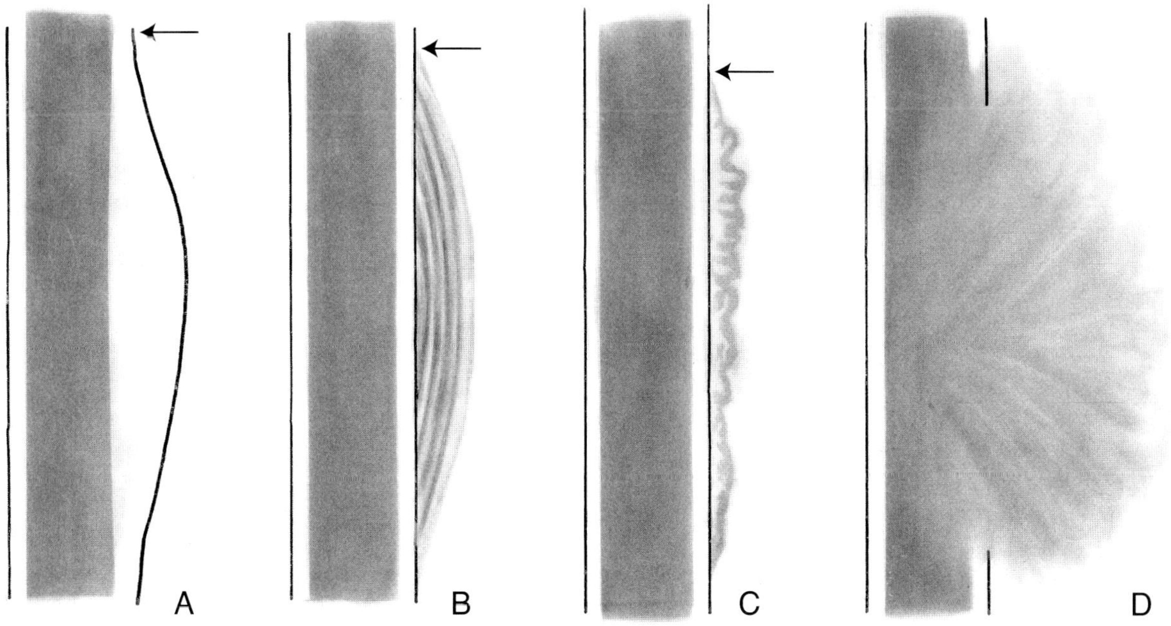

Figure 4.13. Types of periosteal reaction and Codman's triangle (arrows): **A)** Smooth, **B)** Laminar, **C)** Amorphous/lacy, and **D)** Sunburst.

1) Periosteal reaction is smooth and homogenous with a well-defined margin
2) Differential diagnosis:
   a) Trauma to periosteum and cortex
   b) Healing or healed fracture

b. Amorphous to lacy
1) Periosteal new bone usually has sharp margins with smooth irregular enlargements.
2) Differential diagnosis:
   a) Osteomyelitis
   b) Hypertrophic osteopathy
   c) Tumor

c. Laminar or onion skin
1) The periosteal new bone is laid down in layers along the diaphysis of the bone.
2) Differential diagnosis:
   a) Trauma
   b) Osteomyelitis
   c) Tumor (uncommon)
   d) Hypertrophic osteopathy

d. Sunburst or spiculated (aggressive)
1) Periosteal new bone is poorly demarcated and radiates from the cortex.
2) Differential diagnosis:
   a) Malignant tumor
   b) Healing fracture with motion present
   c) Active osteomyelitis

e. Codman's triangle (Figure 4.13)
1) The angle at which the elevated periosteum meets the cortex.
2) Not helpful in the differential diagnosis of a benign versus malignant lesion.
3) Differential diagnosis:
   a) Subperiosteal hemorrhage
   b) Osteomyelitis
   c) Tumor

Definitions (Table 4.4)

1. *Nonaggressive and aggressive patterns.* An estimation is made of activity (or rate of change) of a bone lesion. This is done by characterizing the radiographic pattern of the bony change (i.e., type of osteolysis, sclerosis, periosteal reaction). In many lesions, there is a continuum or admixture of aggressive and nonaggressive findings.

a. Nonaggressive pattern
1) Inactive or slowly progressive lesion that is usually associated with benign diseases.
2) Characterized radiographically by:
   a) Sharp and well-defined lesion margin, usually with a smooth contour
   b) Short transition zone between lesion and normal bone
   c) Smooth and homogenous periosteal reaction
   d) Organized trabecular bone
3) Differential diagnosis:
   a) Healed fracture
   b) Traumatic periostitis
   c) Chronic osteomyelitis
   d) Bone cyst
   e) Benign tumor (Osteoma, Enchondroma, and Osteochondroma)

b. Aggressive pattern
1) Active or rapidly progressive lesion that is commonly associated with malignant diseases.
2) Characterized radiographically by:
   a) Poorly defined or indistinct lesion margin
   b) Thick, hazy, and/or poorly defined transition zone between lesion and normal bone
   c) Moth eaten and/or permeative lysis
   d) Active periosteal reaction, usually laminar or sun-burst pattern
3) Differential diagnosis:
   a) Malignant bone tumor (primary and metastatic)
   b) Osteomyelitis (mycotic and bacterial)

2. *Bone Radiopacity:* the apparent radiopacity or radiolucency of bone representing a summation of calcium ions in bone that relates to the amount of x-ray photon absorption. A wide range of mineral (from 20 to 70%) may be removed before the loss is observed radiographically as a loss of bone opacity. Discrete lesions with mineral loss are often more easily visible.
3. *Osteoporosis*: decrease in radiopacity of one or more bones as a result of decreased bone mass. Also referred to as osteopenia or bone atrophy. Causes include disuse, senility, and hormonal, metabolic, and nutritional imbalance.
4. *Osteolysis*: a localized area of bone loss caused by removal or loss of bone calcium. Bones appear more radiolucent than normal. Causes include bone tumor, bone cyst, and osteomyelitis.
5. *Osteomalacia*: a softening of the bones and decreased bone mass because of faulty mineralization of osteoid. Bones appear more radiolucent than normal and may mimic the radiographic appearance of osteolysis. Most

TABLE 4.4

Radiographic Definitions

1. Nonaggressive and aggressive patterns
2. Bone radiopacity
3. Osteoporosis
4. Osteolysis
5. Osteomalacia
6. Osteosclerosis
7. Myelosclerosis
8. Osteopetrosis

diseases with osteomalacia have concurrent osteoporosis. Causes include hypertrophic osteodystrophy, rickets, osteogenesis imperfecta, calcium/phosphorus imbalance, protein deficiency, and renal tubular diseases such as Fanconi syndrome.
6. *Osteosclerosis*: an increased radiopacity of bone affecting compact and cancellous bone, also known as eburnation. Causes include degenerative joint disease (osteoarthritis) and osteomyelitis.
7. *Myelosclerosis*: an increased radiopacity of cancellous bone with normal appearing cortical bone. Causes include panosteitis, renal osteodystrophia fibrosa, marrow tumor, bone infarcts, and feline leukovirus infection.
8. *Osteopetrosis*: an increased bone radiopacity usually resulting from prenatal bone that has not converted to cancellous bone. Causes include congenital osteopetrosis, hypervitaminosis D, and some types of myelofibrosis.

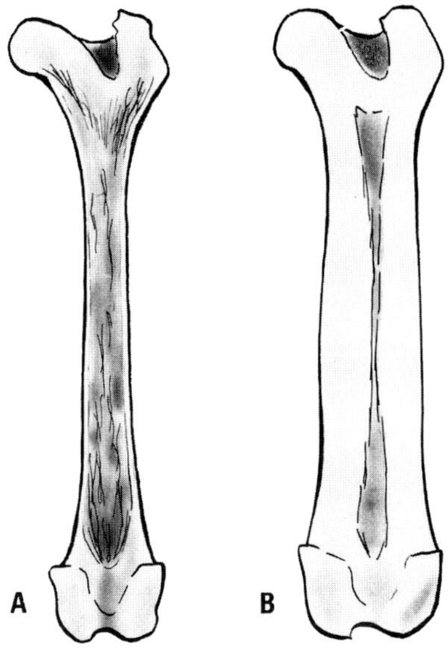

Figure 4.14. Metabolic bone disease. **(A)** Osteoporosis and **(B)** Osteopetrosis.

DISEASES/DISORDERS

Osteoporosis

Clinical correlations:

1. Also known as osteopenia or bone atrophy.
2. Common causes include:
   a. Disuse
   b. Senile
   c. Hormonal imbalance
   d. Metabolic imbalance
   e. Secondary hyperparathyroidism (nutritional and renal)
   f. Hyperadrenocorticism
   g. Steroid therapy
3. Less common causes:
   a. Myeloma
   b. Lymphosarcoma
   c. Primary hyperparathyroidism
   d. Pseudohyperparathyroidism
4. Growth deformities and pathologic fractures may occur if osteoporosis affects the immature animal.

Radiographic findings (Figure 4.14A)

1. Decrease in bone radiopacity (more radiolucent than normal)
2. Cortical thinning
3. Double cortical line (intracortical resorption of bone)
4. Prominent and coarse trabeculae
5. May be localized or generalized
   a. Localized in disuse atrophy (e.g., immobilized leg)
   b. Generalized in systemic disease
6. Pathologic fractures and/or bone deformities are most common in secondary renal or nutritional hyperparathyroidism, if osteoporosis is severe.

Osteopetrosis

Clinical correlations

1. Also is known as marble bone.
2. Condition is rare in dogs and cats.
3. Causes include:
   a. Hypervitaminosis D
   b. Idiopathic
   c. Some forms of myelofibrosis
4. May cause anemia if the medullary canal is significantly compromised.

Radiographic findings (Figure 4.14B):

1. Thickened cortex of all axial and appendicular bones.
2. Chalky opaque appearance to the affected bones.

Ectrodactyly

Clinical correlations:

1. Also known as split hand deformity.
2. A variety of congenital malformations in bones of the limb (most commonly affecting the longitudinal axis of the metatarsal or metacarpal bones).
3. No noted predisposition by breed or sex in cats and dogs.
4. Usually unilateral.

Radiographic findings (Figure 4.15):

1. Variable manifestations observed with separation of metacarpal and/or metatarsal bones.
2. Associated anomalies such as digit aplasia, metacarpal and/or metatarsal metahypoplasia and fusion, and elbow subluxation/luxation.

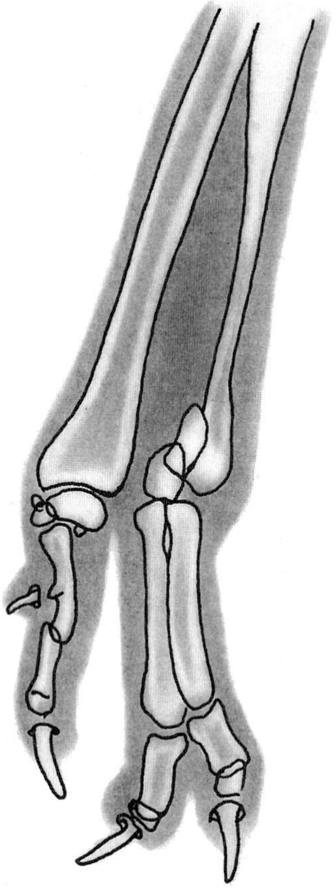

Figure 4.15. Ectrodactyly. Abnormal limb development with separation of the metacarpal bones and digits with digit aplasia.

Polydactyly

Clinical correlations

1. Presence of one or more extra digits.
2. An extra digit adjacent to the first digit is common in dogs and cats.
3. Is inherited as an autosomal dominant trait with a variety of expressions.
4. No apparent clinical significance, other than propensity for traumatic injury of the supernumerary digit.

Radiographic finding:

1. One or more extra digits present.
2. Digit development varies from partial to complete.

Syndactyly

Clinical correlations

1. Bony or soft tissue union of two or more digits.
2. Varying modes of inheritance have been described.
3. Minimal to no clinical significance.

Radiographic finding

1. Bony fusion of one or more digits.

Hemimelia

Clinical correlations

1. Congenital anomaly in which one normally paired bone is partially or completely absent.
2. Commonly affects the radius/ulna and tibia/fibula.
3. A moderate gait abnormality is usually present because of the deformity.

Radiographic findings

1. Either the radius (or ulna) or the tibia (or fibula) is partially or completely absent.
2. The existing bone of the affected pair is usually larger than normal in diameter.
3. The joints, proximal or distal to the site of hemimelia, is often subluxated or luxated.

Chondrodysplasia (Table 4.5)

Clinical correlations

1. May be either proportionate or disproportionate dwarfism.
2. Chondrodysplasia (including achondroplasia and endochondrodystrophy) are inherited deformities of the bony skeleton resulting from abnormal cartilage development. Affected animals are stunted and have lateral bowing of the forelimbs, lateral deviation of the paws, carpal enlargement, and forward slanting of the body.
3. The basic bone development (ossification centers and physis closure times) is similar to that in nonchondrodystrophic animals.
4. Many breeds have been selectively bred for the desired chondrodysplasia characteristics. These phenotypic characteristics, which result in proportional and disproportional dwarfs, are considered normal for the breed.

TABLE 4.5

Types of Chondrodysplasia

1. Proportionate dwarfism
2. Disproportionate dwarfism
3. Pituitary dwarfism
4. Congenital hypothyroidism
5. Multiple epiphyseal dysplasia
6. Enchondrodystrophy
7. Dwarfism of Alaskan Malamutes
8. Dwarfism of Norwegian Elkhound
9. Chondrodysplasia of Great Pyrenees
10. Skeletal/Retinal Dysplasia in Labrador Retriever
11. Ocular/Skeletal Dwarfism in Samoyed

a. Examples of proportionate chondrodystrophoid breeds include many of the miniature breeds such as Toy Poodle, Miniature Poodle, and Miniature Schnauzer.
b. Examples of disproportionate chondrodystrophoid breeds include: Dachshund, Basset Hound, Bulldog, Pug, Beagle, Pekinese, Lhasa Apso, Welsh Corgi, Scottish Terrier, Cairn Terrier, and Munchkin cats.
c. The disproportionate chondrodystrophoid breeds commonly have conformational anomalies that include stunted limbs, bowed limbs, and deviated paws.
d. Some animals also have one or more bone and other anomalies such as hemivertebra, elbow and patella luxation, stenotic nares, and elongated soft palates.

5. When chondrodysplasia is abnormal for the breed, it is commonly referred to as dwarfism.
   a. Many of dwarfism traits are reported to be recessively inherited in dogs and cats.
   b. Some breeds have a higher reported frequency than others (i.e.. Alaskan Malamute, Norwegian Elkhound, Great Pyrenees, Labrador Retrievers, Samoyed).

Radiographic findings
Variety of changes depending on the breed and type of proportionate or disproportionate dwarfism (e.g., curved and short bones).

Pituitary Dwarfism
Clinical correlations
1. Results from inadequate growth hormone.
2. Is a proportionate dwarfism with diminutive stature, slow growth and delayed retention of juvenile hair coat. Symmetrical alopecia and hyperpigmentation often develop later.
3. May have other anomalies (e.g., patent ductus arteriosus, megaesophagus).
4. Most commonly reported in the German Shepherd.

Radiographic findings:
1. Delayed centers of ossification
2. Normal to delayed closure of epiphyseal growth plates (physes).
3. Disordered or incomplete ossification of epiphyses

Congenital Hypothyroidism
Clinical correlations
1. Also called cretinism
2. A disproportionate dwarfism caused by arrested development of the thyroid gland, defective thyroid hormone synthesis, or iodine deficiency.
3. May have myxedematous features, lethargy, juvenile hair coat, anemia, hypercholesterolemia, and/or hydrocephalus.
4. Lethargy and constipation are prominent clinical features.
5. Causes reduced bone formation and remodeling, which result in short limbs, kyphosis, a broad and short skull, and delayed dental eruption.
6. If hypothyroidism occurs after cessation of bone growth, no dwarfism or radiographic changes are present.

Radiographic findings
1. Delayed closure of fontanelles and shortened facial bones.
2. Ossification of epiphyses is delayed.
3. Epiphyseal stippling observed and delayed physeal closure.
4. Cortical thickening of long bones.
5. Abnormal shaped vertebra often "hook shaped" with kyphosis.

Multiple Epiphyseal Dysplasia
Clinical correlations
1. Reported in Beagles and Miniature Poodles.
2. Presents as disproportionate dwarf with short limbs, spinal kyphosis, and enlarged joints.
3. May have hind limb dysfunction at birth. Usually by 2 to 3 weeks of age, poor growth and retardation in standing and walking can be recognized.

Radiographic findings
1. Deformed and mottled epiphyses are most commonly seen affecting the carpal and tarsal joints, but can also affect the vertebrae and long bones. Is difficult to recognize after 4 months of age when the mottled epiphyses become incorporated within the ossified bone.
2. Can mimic early changes of ischemic necrosis in the femoral heads.
3. Secondary degenerative joint disease commonly occurs as a sequel.

Enchondrodystrophy
Clinical correlations
1. Reported in English Pointers.
2. Dwarfism, with lateral bowing of forelimbs, is usually observed by 10 weeks of age.
3. Affected dogs have a bunny-hopping gait and abnormal locomotion.

Radiographic findings
1. The extremities are shortened, often most prominently affecting the radius and ulna.
2. The physes are widened and irregular, and the metaphyses are flared.
3. Mandibular prognathism may be present.

4. With maturity, the physeal and metaphyseal abnormalities often regress; however, the bone deformities persist.
5. Degenerative joint disease often develops as a sequel.

Dwarfism of Alaskan Malamutes

Clinical correlations

1. Is a disproportionate dwarfism resulting from abnormal endochondral bone formation.
2. Is transmitted as a simple autosomal recessive trait.
3. The body length and skull size are normal.
4. The limbs are shortened, exhibiting a lateral bowing of the forelimbs, enlargement of both distal radii and ulnas, and lateral deviation of the feet as a result of asynchronous growth of the radius and ulna.
5. Anemia and stunted growth may be present.

Radiographic findings

1. The changes are most obvious in the carpal region and are best recognized at 5 to 12 weeks of age, but are present as early as 7 to 10 days of age.
2. The distal ulnar metaphysis and physis are abnormally shaped. Other physes may also be irregular, and enlarged with an abnormal flared shape.
3. The bony trabeculae of the metaphyses appear coarse and disorganized.
4. The ossification of the epiphyseal ossification centers are delayed.

Dwarfism of Norwegian Elkhound

Clinical correlations

1. Is a disproportional dwarfism caused by generalized disturbance of endochondral ossification.
2. The mode of inheritance is not fully known.
3. The skull is of normal size, the body tends to be shortened and the legs are disproportionately shortened.
4. The forelimbs are bowed and relatively shorter than the hind limbs.

Radiographic findings

1. The radii and ulnas are bowed, with increased width and flaring of the distal radial and ulnar metaphyses.
2. There is a delayed ossification of the carpal bones.
3. There is reduction in the length of vertebral bodies.

Chondrodysplasia of Great Pyrenees

Clinical correlations

1. Disturbance of endochondral ossification
2. Probable mode of inheritance is a simple autosomal recessive trait.
3. Shortened body length with normal skull size
4. Forelimbs are shortened and bowed.

Radiographic findings

1. The changes are usually visible by 8 weeks of age.
2. Flaring and flattening of the metaphyses
3. There is increased opacity at the junction of the primary and secondary spongiosa.
4. Usually, there is underdevelopment of the epiphyses and carpal bones.
5. Often, the vertebrae are abnormally shaped and incompletely developed with poorly ossified vertebral endplates.

Skeletal-Retinal Dysplasia in Labrador Retrievers

Clinical correlations

1. Is a disproportionate dwarfism with skeletal and ocular defects.
2. Associated ocular abnormalities include impaired vision with retinal dysplasia, retinal detachment, and cataract formation.
3. Is probably an autosomal recessive trait.
4. Normal body length but shortened limbs are the result of retarded growth of the radii, ulnas, femurs, and tibias.
5. Valgus deformity of carpi and straight, hyperextended hind legs

Radiographic findings

1. The long bones are shorter than normal (i.e., radii, ulnas, femurs, tibias and fibulas)
2. Delayed ossification of the epiphyses usually can be detected at 8 weeks of age
3. There are irregularities of the distal ulnar physis and retained enchondral cartilage may be present in the metaphysis.
4. Delayed development of the coronoid process, the medial humeral condyle and the anconeal process. The anconeal process may be hypoplastic or ununited.
5. Degenerative joint disease of the hips and stifles commonly occurs.

Ocular-Skeletal Dwarfism in Samoyed

Clinical correlations

1. Is a disproportionate dwarfism with shortened limbs and ocular defects (e.g., retinal detachment and cataracts).
2. An autosomal recessive mode of inheritance
3. A small stature with the pelvic girdle higher than the thoracic girdle is characteristic.
4. There is a varus deformity of elbows and valgus deviation of the distal forelimbs.
5. Doming of the forehead is prominent.

Radiographic findings

1. The long bones of the limbs are shorter than normal.
2. Flaring of some metaphyses may be present.
3. There is asynchronous growth of the radius and ulna with valgus deviation of the feet.

Metaphyseal Tibial Dysplasia

Clinical correlations

1. Abnormal development of the distal tibial metaphysis leading to pes varus.
2. Reported in Dachshunds as an autosomal recessive defect.
3. May be unilateral or bilateral with abnormal curvature of the tibia.
4. Lameness in affected leg may be observed from 2 to 6 months of age.

Radiographic findings

1. The tibia is shortened and curved.
2. The deformity of tibia and fibula is most prominent at the distal end with a beak-shaped exostosis on the medial metaphysis of distal tibia.
3. The lateral groove of trochlea of tibia is shallow with incongruity of the talocrural joint.
4. Secondary degenerative disease of talocrural joint commonly occurs as a sequel.

Mucopolysaccharidosis

Clinical correlations

1. Is a genetic inborn error of metabolism that results in connective tissue abnormalities and affects the musculoskeletal, ocular, neurologic, and circulatory systems.
2. Inherited as an autosomal recessive trait.
3. Different types have been described in dogs and cats.
   a. Type I occurs in Plott hound dogs and domestic cats and is attributable to alpha-L-iduronidase deficiency with excessive urinary excretion of dermatan and heparan sulfates.
   b. Type VI has been recognized in cats of Siamese ancestry and in dogs (Miniature Pinscher and Welsh Corgi). In cats, it is caused by a deficiency of arylsulfatase B; in dogs it is the result of excessive dermatan sulfate. Dogs have an excessive amount of dermatan, heparan, and chondroitin sulfates in the urine.
   c. Type VII has been recognized in dogs and cats and result from deficiency of beta glucuronidase.
4. Common clinical signs are:
   a. Facial dysmorphia including large head, depressed nasal bridge, hypertelorism, micrognathism, short neck, and stubby malformed teeth.
   b. The cornea is clouded.
   c. Generalized skeletal deformities are present, including severe dysostosis multiplex with swollen and stiff joints.
   d. The body size is smaller than normal.
   e. May have cardiac anomalies and hydrocephalus.
   f. Approximately 25% of Type VI cats have caudal paresis secondary to spinal cord compression.

Radiographic findings (Figure 4.16 A, B)

1. Changes are usually least severe in Type I and most severe in Type VII.

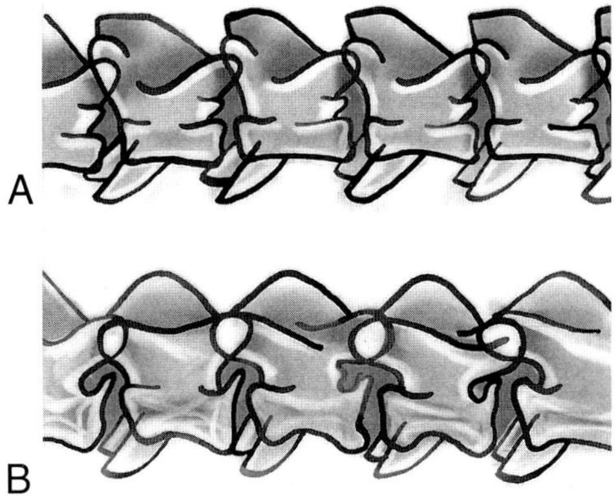

Figure 4.16. Mucopolysaccharidosis (MPS). Feline lumbar spine. **A)** Normal and **B)** Mucopolysaccharidosis. Notice the shortened and deformed vertebral bodies.

2. Epiphyseal dysplasia, dysgenesis, and deformity of most appendicular joints, including delayed ossification of the epiphyses and metaphyseal flaring.
3. Midfacial bones are shortened.
4. Pectus excavatum is often present.
5. Diaphyseal enlargement of the long bones
6. The clavicle may be widened and the ribs are often oar-shaped.
7. The vertebral abnormalities include epiphyseal dysplasia, end plate sclerosis, hypoplasia of the odontoid process, and widening and fusion of the vertebrae.
8. Coxofemoral luxation
9. Mild to severe osteoporosis
10. Degenerative joint disease and spondylosis

Feline Osteodystrophy

Clinical correlations

1. An autosomal-dominant inherited disease in fold ear cats (e.g., Scottish Fold cats).
2. Developmental derangement of the epiphyseal cartilage.
3. Affected cats may have lameness, deformed limbs, thickened tail base with short and inflexible tail, overgrowth of nails, and partial deafness.

Radiographic findings

1. Shortening and thickening of the metacarpal, metatarsal, and the phalangeal bones
2. Exostoses are most commonly seen on the plantar aspect of the tarsal and metatarsal bones.
3. Coccygeal vertebrae are thickened and shortened.
4. Degenerative joint disease and bony ankylosis of the carpus and tarsus.

Osteogenesis Imperfecta

Clinical correlations

1. A generalized condition resulting from a defect in collagen production, which causes fragile bones.

2. Is an autosomal-recessive inherited disease with several different forms.
3. Deformed limbs, blue sclera, thin skin, teeth discoloration, and occasional deafness are characteristics of the disorder.
4. Pathologic fractures are common.

Radiographic findings

1. Osteoporosis with pathologic fractures
2. Deformed limbs secondary to various stages of fracture healing, frequently with malunion fractures
3. The rib cage is small with compromised thoracic viscera.

Hypertrophic Osteodystrophy (HOD)

Clinical correlations

1. Most commonly seen in rapidly growing large and giant breed dogs from 3 to 6 months of age.
2. Is an osteomalacia disease of unknown etiology, although numerous etiologies have been proposed. Among these are:
   a. Nutritional over supplementation, imbalance of dietary calcium and phosphorus
   b. Vitamin C deficiency
   c. Infection with link to respiratory disease, including distemper
3. Primarily affects the metaphyses of the long bones. The metaphyses are frequently swollen, warm, and painful. It can also cause changes in the mandible, the cranium, and the ribs.
4. Severely affected dogs may have systemic illness with fever, depression, anorexia, and are reluctant to stand or walk.
5. Prognosis is good for most affected dogs because the disease is usually self-limiting. Severely affected dogs may have the sequel of retarded bone growth and limb deformities, including enlarged metaphyses and pes valgus.
6. Some dogs die of concurrent septicemia.

Radiographic findings (Figure 4.17)

1. Affects all long bone metaphyses. Changes are usually bilaterally symmetrical and most severe in the distal radius and ulnar metaphyseal regions.
2. Abnormal radiolucent lines are visible within the metaphyses.
3. Metaphyseal flaring and sclerosis may occur.
4. Paraperiosteal new bone formation may develop later in the long bone metaphyses. The flaring and irregularity are symmetrical and are most obvious in the distal ulnar and radial metaphyses. Although rare, periosteal changes may progress to involve the entire diaphysis and occur in other bones (i.e., mandible).
5. Forelimb deformity resulting from asynchronous growth of the radius and ulna is occasionally a sequel.
6. Cranial hyperostosis, a disease in the Bullmastiff, may also cause similar appendicular changes, plus hyperostosis and a periosteal reaction in the calvarium and sinus frontalis regions.
7. Need to differentiate from the normal, irregular and opaque metaphyses in rapidly growing, large breed dogs.

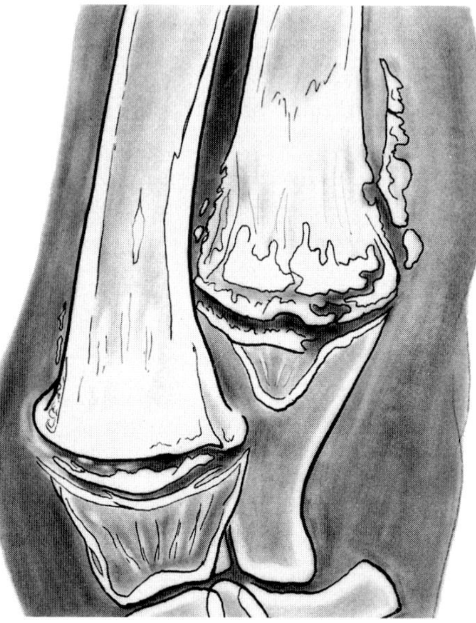

Figure 4.17. Hypertrophic osteodystrophy (HOD). There are radiolucent zones of bone in the metaphyses of distal radius and ulna and paraperiosteal new bone formation. The physes are normal.

Retained Enchondral Cartilage of the Distal Ulna

Clinical correlations

1. Results from a temporary or permanent retention of enchondral cartilage in the distal ulnar metaphysis.
2. Usually is self-limiting and is usually an incidental finding with no clinical significance. If it persists long enough, however, it can retard the growth of the ulna resulting in a bowing deformity (radius curvus) and pes valgus deformity.
3. Is more common in large and giant breed dogs that are growing rapidly (e.g., Great Danes, Saint Bernard, and Setters).
4. May occur concurrently with other diseases (e.g., hypertrophic osteodystrophy).

Radiographic findings (Figure 4.18)

1. Triangular or cone-shaped radiolucent defect that extends from the distal ulnar physis into the distal metaphysis.
2. Is usually bilaterally symmetrical.

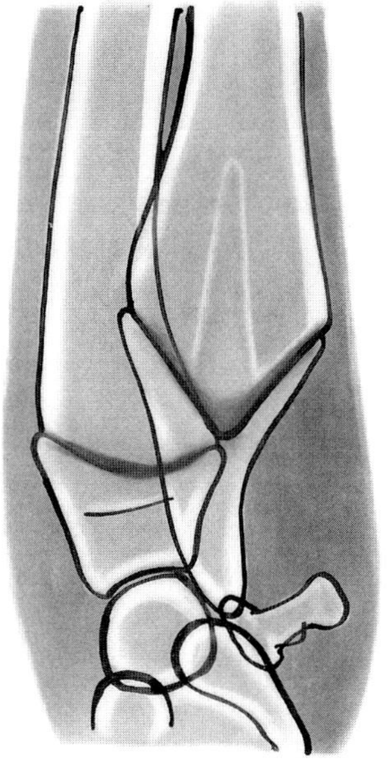

Figure 4.18. Retained enchondral cartilage of the distal ulna. The ulnar metaphysis contains a well-defined triangular radiolucent cartilage core. Soft tissue swelling is also present. The physes and epiphyses are normal.

Rickets

Clinical correlations

1. Rickets is a rare disease in dogs and cats.
2. Results from a deficiency of vitamin D.

Radiographic findings

1. Affects all physes.
2. Widening and delayed ossification of the physis.
3. Flaring of the metaphyses.
4. May result in severe deformity of the affected bones.

Growth Arrest Line (Growth Retardation Line)

Clinical correlations

1. No known clinical significance.
2. Is reported to represent periods when rate of bone formation has changed, either increasing or decreasing. Is often secondary to dietary changes or systemic illness.

Radiographic findings (Figure 4.19)

1. Radiopaque thin horizontal lines usually in the diaphysis of the long limb bones, most commonly in the femurs.
2. The lines tend to be bilaterally symmetrical.

Hypertrophic Osteopathy (HO)

Clinical correlations

1. Also known as hypertrophic pulmonary osteopathy, hypertrophic pulmonary osteoarthropathy (HPOA), pulmonary osteoarthropathy, and Marie's disease.

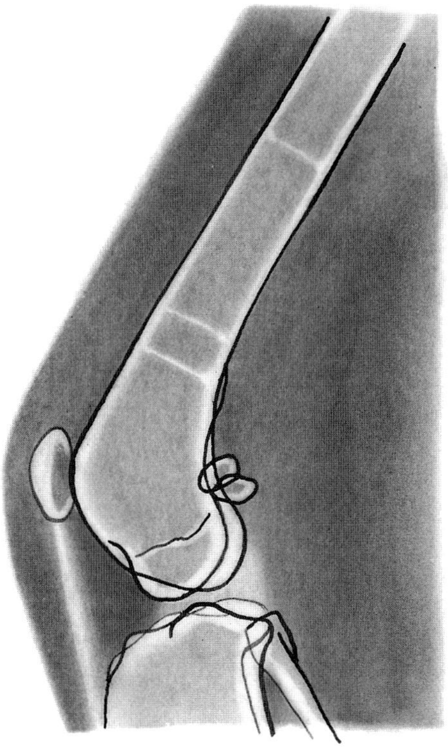

Figure 4.19. Growth arrest lines.

2. Causes soft tissue swelling of the extremities, which are bilaterally symmetrical, especially involving the distal portions of the limbs.
3. Lameness and pain on palpation are usually present.
4. Unknown cause, though usually associated with primary or metastatic pulmonary neoplasia, but can also occur with other thoracic diseases (e.g., bronchopneumonia, *Spiroceoca lupi*, congestive heart failure).
5. May occur secondary to abdominal disease (e.g., hepatic or urinary bladder neoplasia, cystic calculi).
6. If the primary lesion is removed, the bone lesions usually gradually resolve.

Radiographic findings (Figure 4.20)

1. Periosteal proliferations along the diaphyses of the affected bones with adjacent soft tissue swelling. Periosteal pattern is usually smooth, lacy, and/or palisading, but also variable, depending on the severity and chronicity of the thoracic or abdominal lesion.
2. Radiographic changes are usually bilaterally symmetrical and present in both fore and rear limbs.
3. The earliest changes are usually seen in the metacarpal and metatarsal bones, progressing to involve the long bones of all four legs, and less commonly, the carpal and the tarsal bones.
4. The joints are unaffected.
5. Occasionally, the periosteal changes also involve other bones (i.e., vertebra, pelvis).

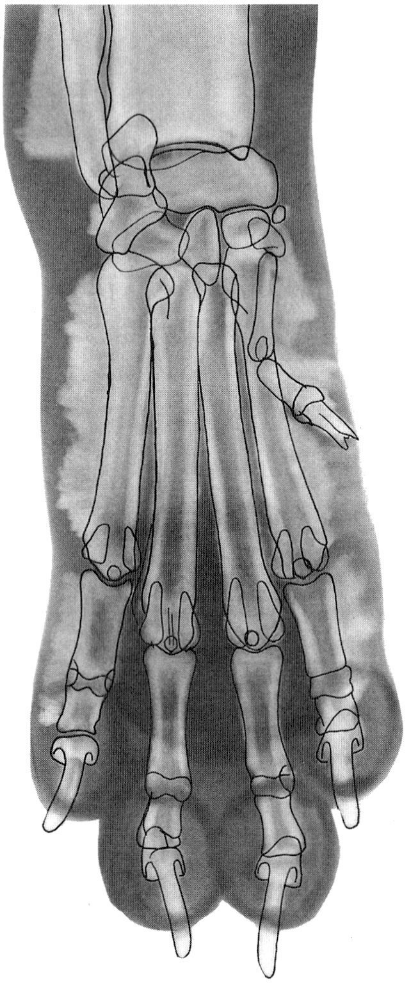

Figure 4.20. Hypertrophic osteopathy (HO). Palisading periosteal reactions are present on the metacarpal bones and phalanges.

Panosteitis

Clinical correlations

1. Also known as enostosis and eosinophilic panosteitis.
2. A self-limiting disease with unknown etiology. There may be some hereditary predisposition, and or association with viral, bacterial, or transient vascular causes.
3. Occurs most commonly in large and giant dogs, especially the German Shepherd. Usually occurs in dogs that weigh greater than 40 lb, and in the Basset Hound.
4. Most commonly affects dogs from 4 to 12 months of age, but is occasionally seen in older dogs.
5. Shifting leg lameness with pain, usually affecting a single limb is characteristic, but several limbs may be affected simultaneously or sequentially.
6. Disease affects long tubular bones of the appendicular skeleton (i.e., femur, tibia, humerus, radius, and ulna), but can also affect metacarpal and metatarsal bones.

Radiographic findings (Figure 4.21 A and B)

1. Increased intramedullary radiopacity is the most common change and is characterized by:
   a. Blurring and accentuation of the trabecular bone pattern
   b. Hazy and diminished contrast seen between the medulla and the cortex.
   c. Abnormal areas may be small or large. Coalescing lesions may occupy most of the diaphyseal medullary cavity.
   d. The lesions are usually most prominent near the nutrient canal of the affected bone.
2. Endosteal bone is thickened and/or roughened.
3. Periosteal new bone is usually smooth or laminar.
4. One or more of the above radiographic abnormalities may be present simultaneously.

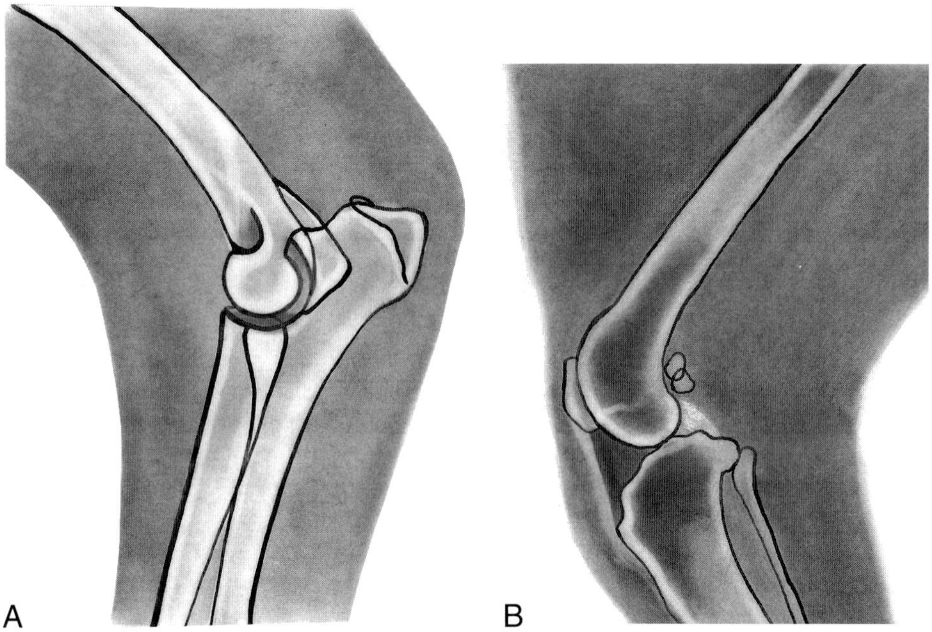

A B

Figure 4.21. **A)** Panosteitis. Myelosclerosis in the distal humerus and mid radius and ulna. **B)** Myelosclerosis in femur and tibia with a smooth periosteal reaction.

Lead Poisoning

Clinical correlations

1. Condition is rare.
2. Results from acute or chronic ingestion of lead containing substances.
3. In acute lead poisoning, common clinical signs include vomiting, diarrhea, abdominal pain, and seizures and/or dementia.
4. In chronic lead poisoning (plumbism), vague gastrointestinal signs, weight loss, dementia, or anemia may be observed.

Radiographic findings

1. If lead ingestion is recent, metallic foreign material may be seen in the GI tract.
2. In most clinical cases the radiographic examination is normal.
3. Thin sclerotic bands may be seen in the metaphyses of immature animals, usually most apparent in the distal radius and ulna.

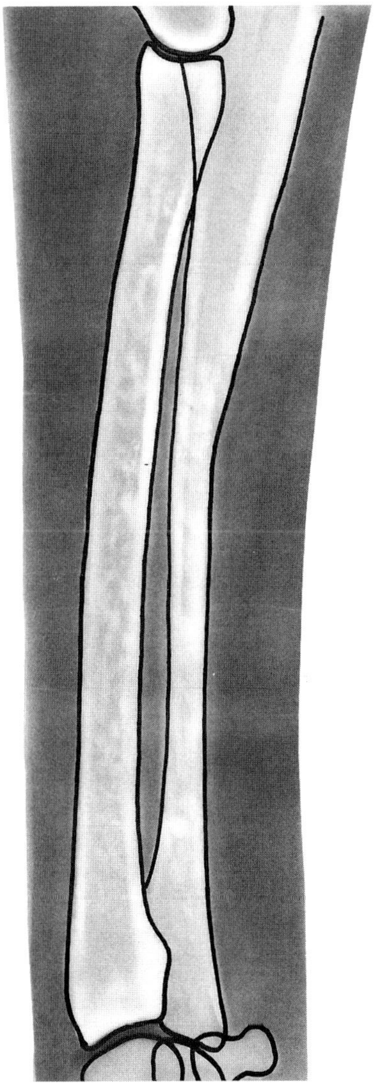

Figure 4.22. Bone infarcts. Irregular foci of increased radiopacity within the medullary cavity of the radius and ulna.

Bone Infarcts

Clinical Correlation

1. Caused by necrosis within the medullary cavity of one or more bones.
2. Commonly associated with a concurrent, primary bone sarcoma that is located at another site. Has been reported most often in Schnauzers, but can occur in any breed.
3. May be secondary to other causes such as vasculitis and emboli.
4. Usually no clinical signs are associated with the bone infarcts.

Radiographic findings (Figure 4.22)

1. Irregular or distinctly increased radiopacity seen in the medullary cavity of one or more bones (i.e., long bones of limbs, diploe of cranium).
2. Narrowed medullary cavity width.
3. A portion of medullary cavity has radiopacity similar to the cortical bone.
4. Must differentiate from other diseases that may cause generalized myelosclerotic changes in bone (i.e., feline leukemia virus infection in cats and erythrocyte pyruvate kinase deficiency in Basenjis).

FRACTURES

1. A fracture is defined as a break or discontinuity in a bone. On radiographs, fractures are usually seen as a radiolucent line. However, compacted fractures can create an increased opacity and microfractures are usually invisible.
2. Classification of fracture types (Table 4.6)
   a. Complete or incomplete (relative to the degree of bone continuity)

TABLE 4.6

Types of Fractures

1. Incomplete or complete fracture
2. Closed or open fracture
3. Compression fracture
4. Pathologic fracture
5. Stress fracture

1) Incomplete fracture: a fracture in which the bone has a broken cortex, but the bone is not in complete discontinuity (Figure 4.23 A, B).
   Types of incomplete fracture include:
   a) Greenstick fracture: The bone cortex is broken on the convex side.
   b) Torus fracture: The bone cortex is broken (buckles or folds) on the concave side.
2) Complete fracture: Fracture extends through the entire cortex. A simple fracture has one line while a mutiple fracture has two or more noncontinuous fracture lines.
   Types of fracture configuration (Figures 4.24 A, B and 4.25 A, B):
   a) Transverse
   b) Oblique
   c) Spiral
   d) Comminuted: three or more fragments
      (1) Butterfly fragment: a wedge-shaped bone fragment
      (2) Segmental fracture: a fracture with two fracture lines that isolates a segment of the long bone

b. Closed or Open:
   1) Closed fracture: overlying skin and soft tissue are intact.
   2) Open fracture: overlying skin and soft tissues are perforated.

c. Compression fracture: a fracture in which the end portions of bone fragments are impacted into each other, usually causing shortening or collapse of the bone. Often, no distinct fracture line is visible.

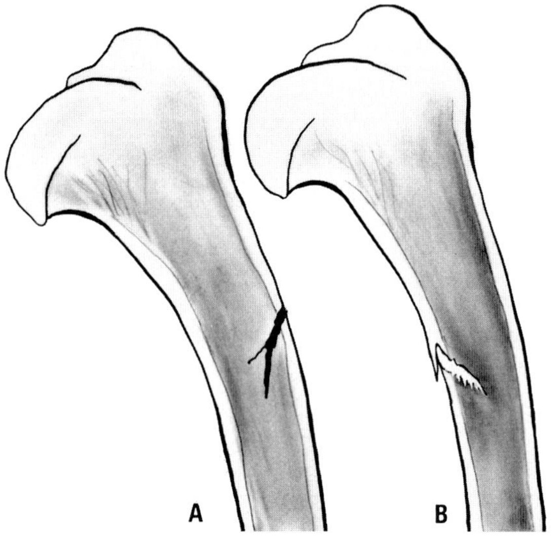

Figure 4.23. Incomplete fractures: **A)** Greenstick. **B)** Torus.

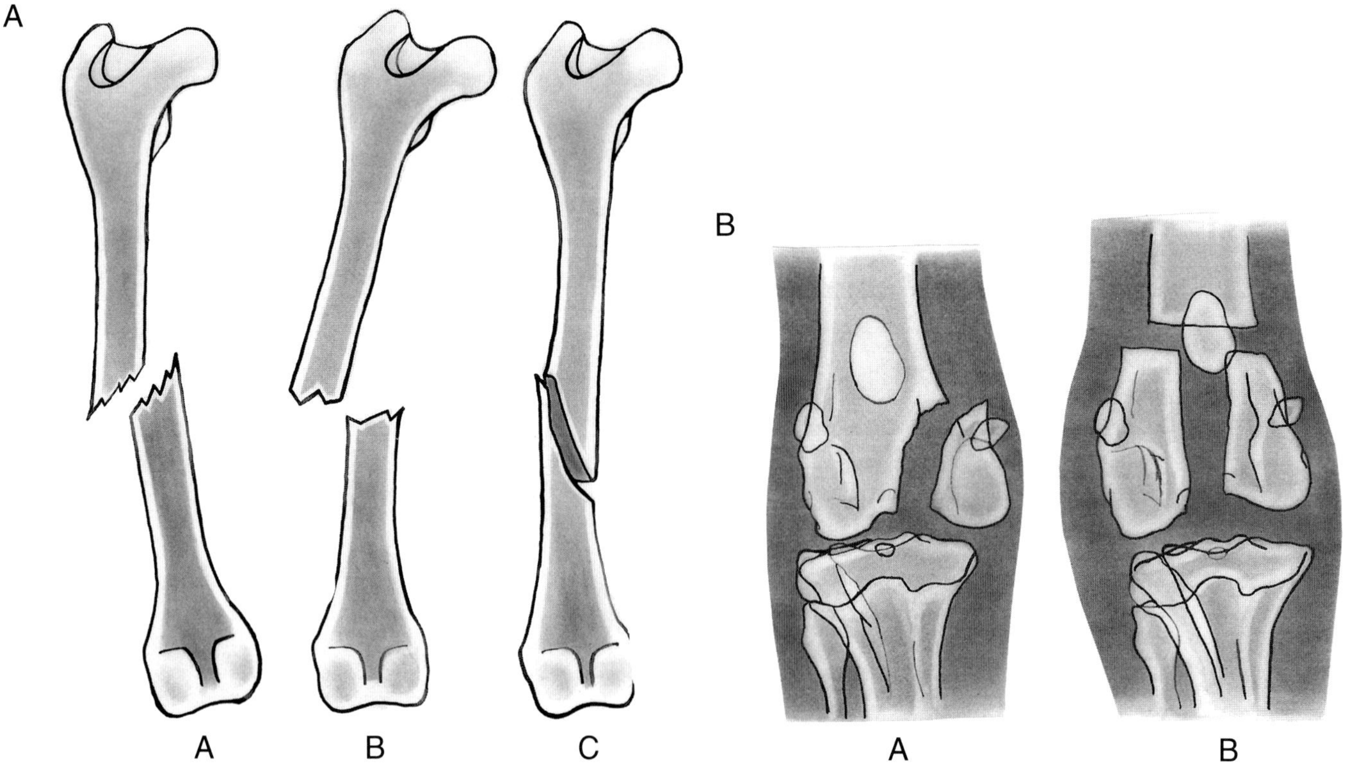

Figure 4.24. **A)** Types of complete fractures: (**A**) Oblique, (**B**) Transverse, and (**C**) Spiral. **B)** Types of condylar fractures: (**A**) Medial condylar fracture of femur and (**B**) Intercondylar and supracondylar fracture of femur ("Y" fracture).

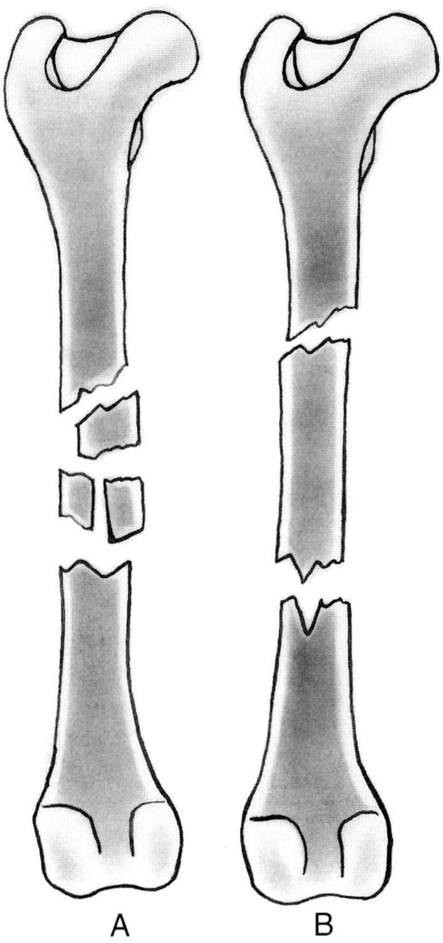

Figure 4.25. Comminuted fractures: **A)** Segmental with butterfly fragments. **B)** Segmental.

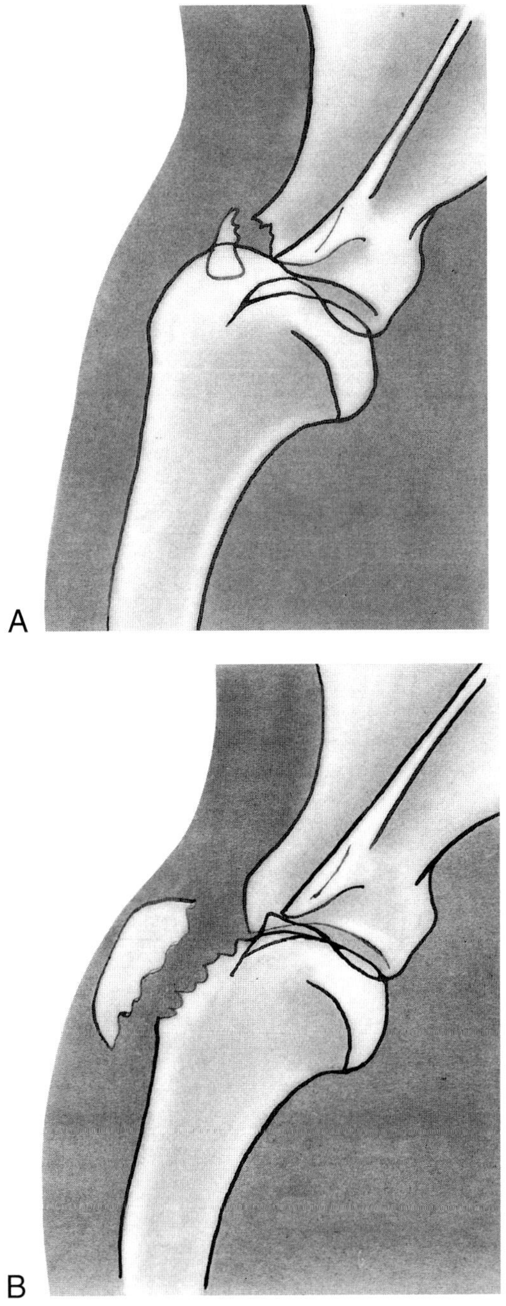

Figure 4.26. **A & B)** Avulsion fractures. (**A**) Avulsion of scapular tuberosity and (**B**) Avulsion of humeral tubercle.

d. Pathologic fracture: a fracture through bone that has been weakened by an underlying disease or developmental defect (e.g., tumor, hyperparathyroidism, bone cyst, fracture through incomplete ossification of humeral condyle in Spaniels).
e. Stress fracture (a fatigue fracture): fracture results when a repetitive stress causes interruption in the bone structure at a faster rate than can be offset by the bone's reparative process.
f. Fracture classification by location (Figures 4.26 A, B and 4.27)
   1) Avulsion fracture: a fracture that involves the bony insertion of a ligament or a tendon, usually involving an apophysis or sesamoid bone.
   2) Physis fracture: these fractures occur in immature animals and are classified according to the degree of involvement of the epiphysis, physis, and metaphysis. The Salter Harris fracture types (grades I to V) are correlated with the increasing probability of growth deformity occurring when a fracture heals.

3. Radiographic description of a fracture should include (Table 4.7):
   a. Location in bone
   b. Type of fracture
   c. Configuration/direction of fracture (spiral, transverse, oblique)
   d. Involvement of a joint, if present (articular or nonarticular)
   e. Apposition (none, partial, complete)
   f. Displacement and angulation (overlapping, distracted)

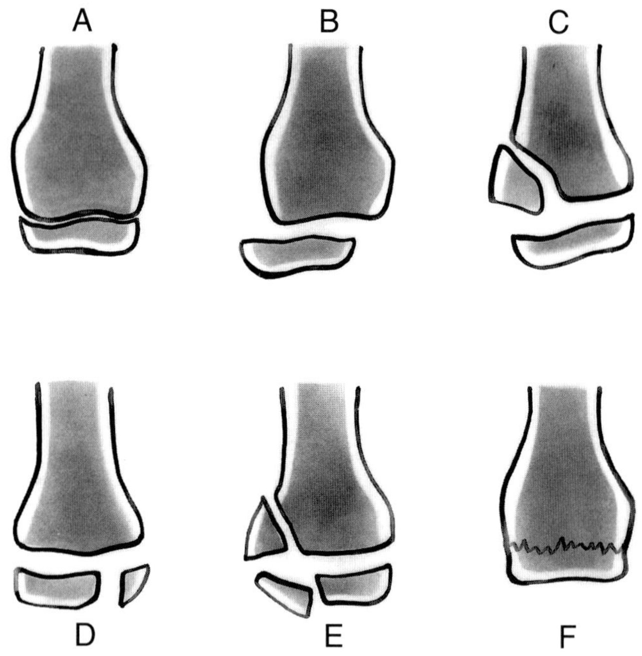

Figure 4.27. Salter Harris Classification: **A)** Normal; **B)** Type I (physis only); **C)** Type II (metaphyseal fragment); **D)** Type III (Epiphyseal fragment); **E)** Type IV (metaphyseal and epiphyseal fragments); **F)** Type V (compression or impaction of physis).

TABLE 4.7

Description of Fracture

1. Location in bone
2. Type of fracture
3. Configuration or direction of fracture
4. Articular or nonarticular
5. Degree of apposition of the fracture segments
6. Displacement and angulation

g. Rotation, displacement, and apposition can be altered by radiographic positioning. The position of the distal fragment is usually described in relationship to the proximal fragment and rotation by the amount of twisting about the bone's longitudinal axis.

FRACTURE HEALING (Table 4.8)

1. Fractures heal by the proliferation of periosteal and endosteal bone.
2. Stages of fracture healing include (Figure 4.28):
   a. Release of various factors (e.g., systemic mitogens and growth factors) at the site of a fracture to promote production and differentiation of specialized cells at that site.
   b. A blood clot leads to organization by granulation tissue between fragments.
   c. Production of callus: The amount of osteoclastic and osteoblastic activity at fracture site and the amount of periosteal and endosteal callus produced varies greatly with location, type of fracture, and age of animal.
      1) Callus is usually visible 10 to 14 days after fracture, but may be visible as early as 3 to 5 days, especially in young animals.
      2) Callus modeling involves the restitution of original bone contour and function.
      3) Callus remodeling involves the conversion to lamellar bone with periosteal and endosteal apposition.

TABLE 4.8

Factors Affecting Fracture Healing

1. Blood supply
2. Location of fracture in bone
3. Configuration of fracture
4. Method of reduction of fracture
5. Age of the animal
6. Other systemic illness or debilitating disease
7. Presence of concurrent infection
8. Presence of motion at fracture site

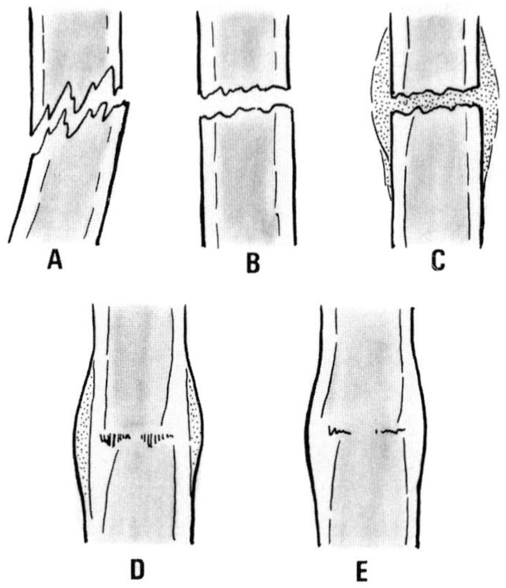

Figure 4.28. Stages of fracture healing.

4) Minimal callus formation occurs with the healing of membranous bone fractures.
3. Factors affecting speed of fracture repair.
   a. Local blood supply, which may be altered by reduction and/or removal of the hematoma
   b. Location of fracture
      1) Metaphyseal fractures tend to heal faster then diaphyseal fractures.
      2) Some locations tend to heal more slowly (e.g., distal radius and ulna, distal tibia).
   c. Configuration of fracture.
      1) Spiral and oblique fractures heal faster than transverse fractures.
      2) Comminuted fractures may have fragments of bone that lack a viable blood supply and this may delay their healing.
   d. Method of reduction of the fracture
      1) The more rigid the fixation of the fracture, the more likely primary union will occur.
      2) Intramedullary fixation, such as an intramedullary pin, may disrupt the medullary and endosteal blood supply, and result in a slowing of the healing process.
   e. Age of the patient affects the rate of healing with young animals healing faster than older animals. In adequately stabilized fractures, radiographic and clinical bone healing is usually observed from 6 to 8 weeks.
   f. Presence of a concurrent infection or other debilitating disease may delay bone healing.

RADIOGRAPHIC EVALUATION OF FRACTURE HEALING

1. A fracture can be considered healed if there is:
   a. Bone continuity of the cortex.
   b. A complete calcified and ossified bridging callus.
   c. No remaining visible fracture line.
2. After internal and external fracture reduction, follow-up radiographic evaluations are usually made at the following time sequence:
   a. Immediately after reduction for evaluation of:
      1) Alignment and degree of reduction of fractured bones
      2) Position of the fixation device (either internal or external)
   b. At 2 weeks, 4 weeks, and 6 weeks postoperatively for the evaluation of:
      1) Change in alignment and reduction of the fracture.
      2) Change in the position of the fixation devices.
      3) Evidence of infection.
      4) Progress of callus formation.
   c. If the fracture is not healing, additional radiographs are made at subsequent 4 week intervals or as needed, until complete fracture healing is apparent. Removal of the internal or external fixation device can be considered when the fracture is healed.

FRACTURE COMPLICATIONS

Radiographic findings indicating possible fracture healing complications include:

1. The absence of callus formation. (May be normal with rigid internal compression and excellent anatomic reduction.)
2. Exuberant callus formation around the fracture site.
   a. Sequel to periosteal stripping from original trauma or surgical intervention
   b. Incomplete stability or motion at the healing fracture site
   c. Infection
3. Change in angulation or rotation of the fracture fragments
   a. Inadequate surgical reduction and alignment
   b. Motion at the fracture site
   c. Change in fracture fixation device
4. Lysis at the fracture site and separation of the ends of the fracture fragments
   a. The presence of soft tissues between the fractured fragments (e.g., muscle).
   b. Motion at the fracture site
   c. Infection
5. Zone of radiolucency around the fixation devices (e.g., screws, intramedullary pins)
   a. Motion
   b. Infection
   c. Electrolysis
6. Soft tissue changes of swelling, atrophy, and/or dystrophic mineralization and joint contracture
7. Bone deformity caused by premature physis closure

DISEASES/DISORDERS

Classification of Fracture Complications (Figures 4.29 A, B and 4.30)

Delayed Union

Clinical correlations

1. The bones do not unite within the expected period of time (usually 6–8 weeks), but healing is gradual and will eventually occur (Figure 4.29A).
2. Common causes:
   a. Motion at the fracture site
   b. Infection at the fracture site
   c. Older patient
   d. Configuration/type and site of fracture
   e. Pathologic bone (e.g., neoplasia, osteoporosis)

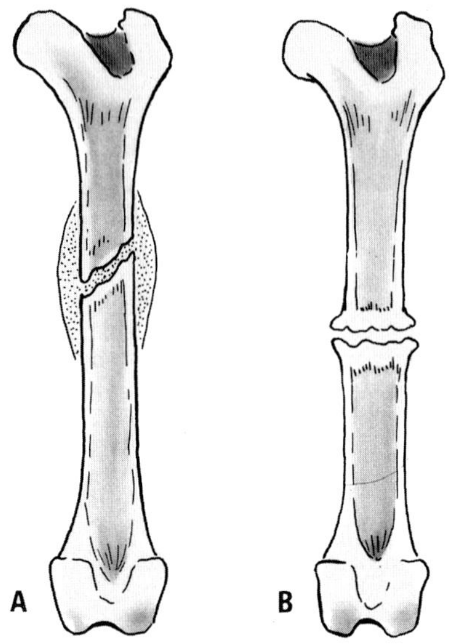

Figure 4.29. Fracture complications. **A)** Delayed union. **B)** Nonunion.

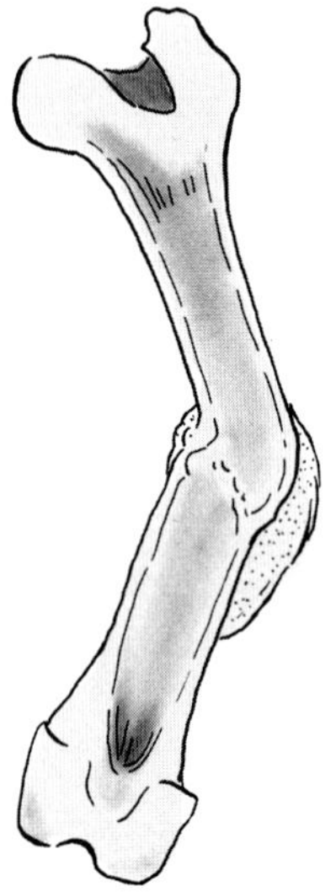

Figure 4.30. Malunion.

Radiographic findings

1. Persistent presence of a radiolucent fracture line.
2. Minimum periosteal reaction with incomplete bridging callus at the fracture site

Nonunion

Clinical correlations

1. Bone healing ceases before complete healing occurs (Figure 4.29B).
2. Common causes:
   a. Motion at the fracture site
   b. Avascularity at the fracture site
   c. The presence of infection or foreign material at the fracture site
   d. Interposed tissue (e.g., muscle, fat) at the fracture site

Radiographic findings

1. The ends of the fracture fragment become smooth, rounded, and sclerotic with no radiographic evidence of bridging callus. Bone may also atrophy.
2. The medullary canal (at the fracture site) is sealed with a sclerotic bony margin.
3. There may be a pseudoarthrosis (false joint) at the fracture site.

Malunion

Clinical correlations

1. The healed union of a fracture with angular or rotary deformity.
2. Normal function of the bone may be compromised (Figure 4.30).
3. Common causes
   a. Improper reduction
   b. Rotation, angulation, or collapse of the fracture fragments during the healing process

Radiographic findings

1. Bone appears healed with good callus formation, but is malaligned, rotated, or distracted.
2. Bone is shortened.
3. May cause adjacent joint to be more flexed or extended than normal.

Pseudoarthrosis

Clinical correlations

1. An inability to form normal callus in healing
2. Cause is unknown.

Radiographic findings

1. Discontinuity between bones at pseudoarthrosis site with no visible callus
2. Ends of bone may become tapered.
3. Osteoporosis of the bone if weight bearing

Premature Physeal Closure

Clinical correlations

1. Usually occurs as sequel to trauma.
2. May also be sequel to other conditions such as developmental anomalies (e.g., dwarfism), other trauma (internal fracture fixation), and other disorders.
3. Can affect any physis of a bone, but most clinical problems occur in the distal radius and ulna where premature closure causes disproportional growth of the two bones.
4. Amount of growth deformity will depend on the amount and severity of premature physis closure; more significant in young dogs of large and giant breeds.
5. Radiographs of the opposite limb should be made for comparison of the physes and lengths of the bones.

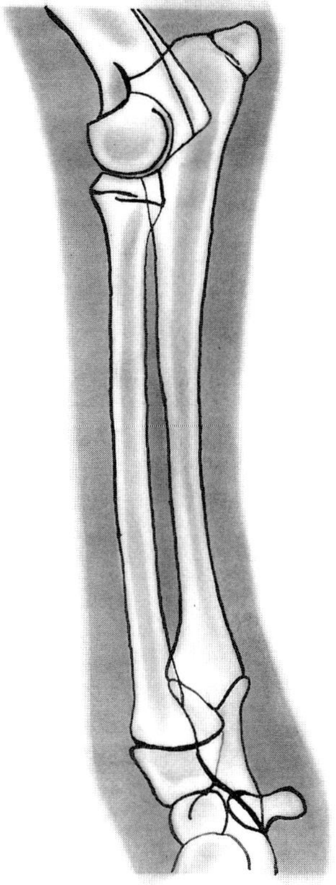

Figure 4.31. Premature physeal closure. **A)** Normal foreleg with open radial and ulnar physes. **B)** Premature closure of distal ulna physis with radius curvus and elbow subluxation.

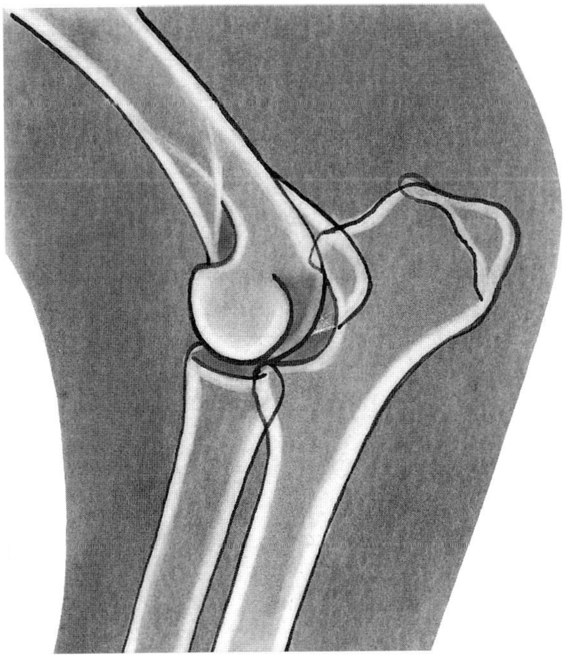

Figure 4.32. Close up lateral projection of elbow with humeroulnar subluxation from premature closure of the distal ulna physis.

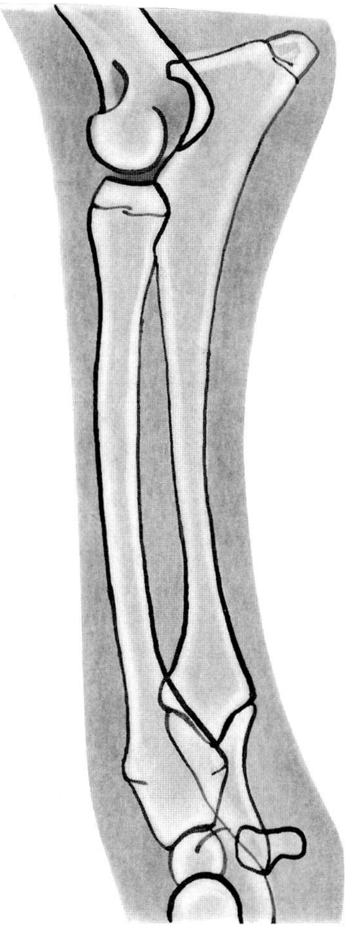

Figure 4.33. Premature physeal closure of the distal radius with a disproportionate shorter radius compared to ulna. Elbow subluxation is also present.

Radiographic findings (Figures 4.31 A, B through 4.34 A, B):

1. Premature closure of physis
2. Deformity of bone and limb

Premature closure of the distal ulna

1. Partial or complete closure (obliteration) of the distal ulnar physis
2. Cranial and medial bowing of the radius (radius curvus) with valgus pes deformity
3. Subluxation and/or degenerative joint disease of the radiocarpal joint as a sequel
4. Subluxation and/or degenerative joint disease of the humeroulnar joint as a sequel

Premature closure of the distal radius

1. Partial or complete closure (obliteration) of the distal radial physis
2. Subluxation and/or degenerative joint disease of the humeroulnar joint as a sequel

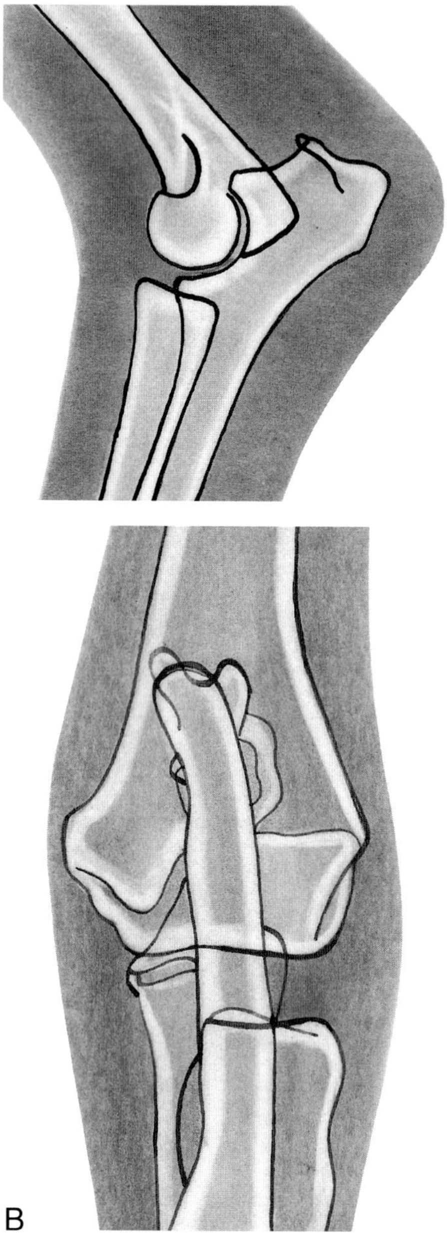

Figure 4.34. Close up lateral projection of humeroradial joint subluxation resulting from premature closure of the distal radial physis. **(A)** Lateral projection and **(B)** Craniocaudal projection.

3. Subluxation and/or degenerative joint disease of the humeroradial joint as a sequel
4. Distal displacement of the ulnar styloid process
5. Degenerative joint disease of the carpal joint as a sequel
6. Varus pes deformity

Premature symmetrical closure of the distal radial and the distal ulnar physes

1. Short radius and ulna
2. Subluxation and/or degenerative joint disease of the elbow and/or carpal joints as a sequel

Osteomyelitis: Bacterial and Mycotic

Clinical correlations

1. Bacterial osteomyelitis
   a. Routes of infection include:
      1) Open reduction and internal fixation of a closed fracture
      2) Open fracture and traumatic injury
      3) Previous surgery
      4) Extension to bone from soft tissue infection (e.g., bite wound, gunshot wound)
      5) Puncture wounds (e.g., bite wound)
      6) Hematogenous infection
         a) Localized infection
            (1) Periodontal disease
            (2) Rhinitis
            (3) Otitis media
            (4) Paronychia
   b. Fever, pain, swelling, and leukocytosis are usually present
   c. *Staphylococcus* spp. is present in 40 to 50% of monomicrobial infections.
      1) More than 40% of bone infections are polymicrobial with mixtures of gram positive and gram negative bacteria.
      2) Anaerobic infections occur in 15% or more cases, but are often difficult to isolate. A fistulous tract may be present in a chronic infection.
2. Mycotic osteomyelitis.
   a. Geographic distribution:
      1) *Coccidioides immitis*: most common in southwestern and western United States
      2) *Blastomyces dermatitidis*: most common in southwestern and midwestern United States
      3) *Histoplasma capsulatum*: most common in midwestern United States
      4) *Cryptococcus neoformans*: throughout United States
      5) *Aspergillosis spp*: throughout United States
   b. May be monostotic or polyostotic.
   c. May have other systemic illness such as pneumonia, lymphadenopathy, pericardial effusion, fever, and leukocytosis.

Radiographic findings (bacterial and mycotic osteomyelitis):

1. Acute osteomyelitis (Figure 4.35)
   a. Earliest stage has no bone abnormality, only soft tissue swelling
   b. Subsequently, (in 7–14 days) there is often a proliferative periosteal reaction
      1) Tends to extend along the shaft of the diaphysis.
      2) Rarely involves a joint.
   c. Radiolucent line between the periosteal new bone and the cortex

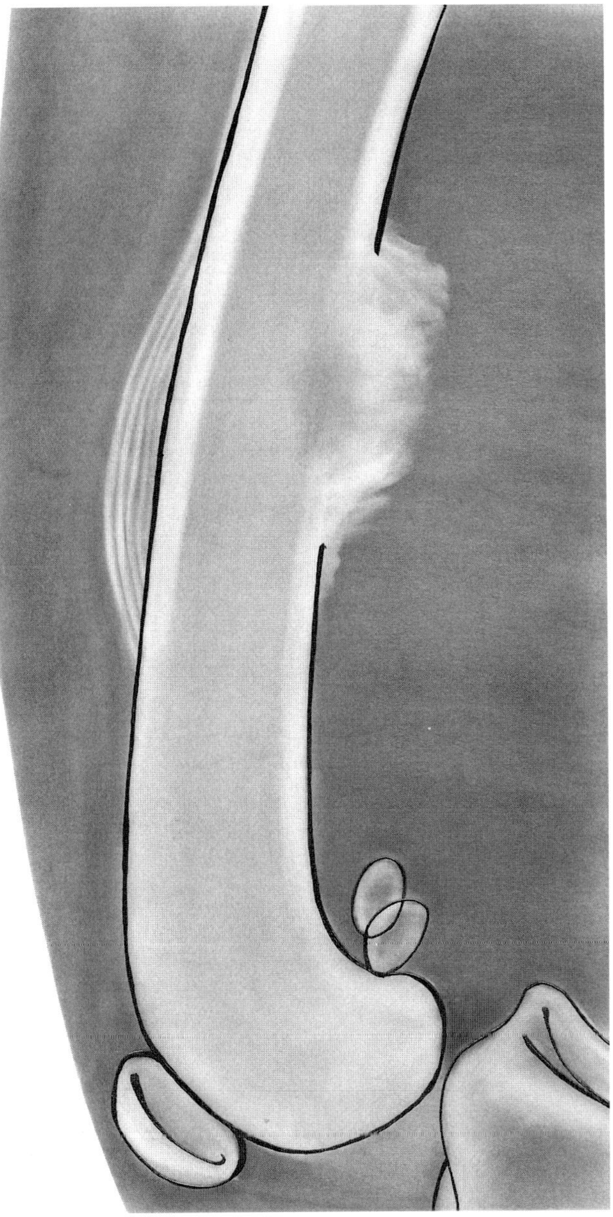

Figure 4.35. Chronic bacterial osteomyelitis. There is lysis within the medullary cavity of the mid femoral diaphysis with smooth and irregular periosteal reactions on the cranial and caudal cortex. Note radiolucent line between cortex and periosteal reaction.

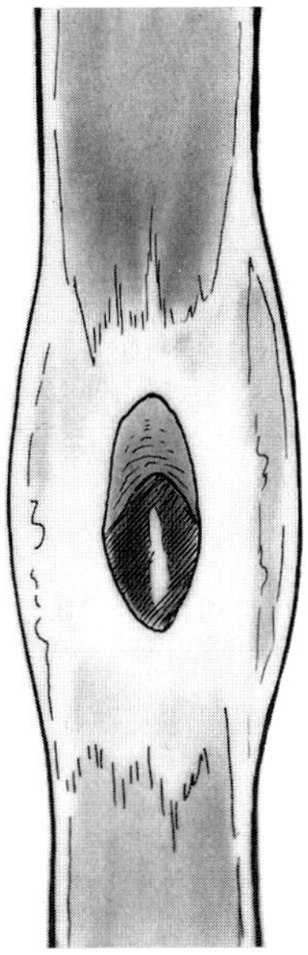

Figure 4.36. Chronic bacterial osteomyelitis. Notice the radiopaque sequestrum within the relatively more radiolucent involucrum.

   d. Lysis of cortical and medullary bone
   e. Bone abscess: (referred to as Brodie abscess if infection is a sharply delineated focus in a bone)
   f. Diffuse adjacent soft tissue swelling
2. Chronic osteomyelitis (Figures 4.36 and 4.37)
   a. Sclerotic margin around areas of lysis as a result of the bone's attempt to wall-off the infection
   b. Sequestrum formation (an avascular piece of bone)
   c. Periosteal proliferation may be present or absent.
   d. Adjacent soft tissue swelling

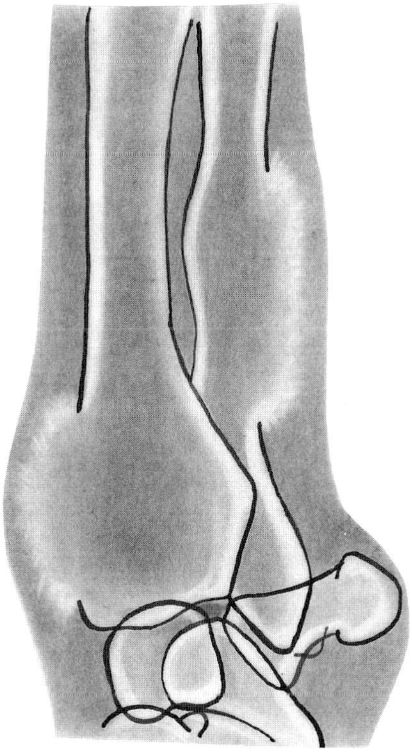

Figure 4.37. Mycotic osteomyelitis of distal radius and ulna with polyostotic expansile osteolytic and osteoblastic bony lesions. Active periosteal reactions and adjacent soft tissue swelling are also present.

e. Gas visible in fistulous tract or radiopaque foreign body may be present; contrast radiography may aid in delineating fistulous tract or foreign body.

Protozoan Osteomyelitis

Clinical correlations

1. Hepatozoon canis genus causes infection in many organs (e.g., bones, liver, spleen, muscles, bowel, myocardium). Protozoan-infected tick is ingested.
2. Uncommon in dogs and rare in cats.
3. More common in southern and southwestern United States.
4. May produce clinical signs of fever, inappetence, bloody diarrhea, lameness, and neurologic manifestations.

Radiographic findings

1. Periosteal proliferation of long bones of limb, pelvis, and/or vertebrae.

NEOPLASIA

DISEASES/DISORDERS

Primary Benign Bone Tumors and Cysts

Clinical correlations

1. Less common than malignant tumors.
2. Bone cyst and cartilaginous exotosis is usually seen in young dogs and cats.
3. Lesions do not usually cause lameness or other signs unless the tumor interferes with function of the limb or joint (i.e., compression of spinal cord, displaced ligaments or tendons, or if a pathologic fracture occurs).
4. Tumors are usually slow growing, but malignant transformation can occur.
5. May have phenotypic deformity at site of lesion (e.g., inherited multiple cartilaginous exostosis, enchondromatosis).
6. Feline osteochondromatosis usually occurs in flat or irregular bones (e.g., pelvis, vertebra) in mature cats. The tumor contains viral particles resembling feline leukemia virus FELV and feline sarcoma virus (FSV).
7. Osteochondroma is inherited in dogs, especially the polyostotic form.
   a. The lesion usually affects the long bones of young animals and the growth of the tumor ceases when the animal is skeletally mature.
   b. Most commonly reported in Great Danes, Saint Bernards, and Hounds.

Radiographic findings (Figures 4.38 through 4.40)

1. Osteoma
   a. There is an opaque cortical lesion of bone with a smooth periosteal reaction.
2. Enchondroma
   a. There is smooth enlargement of the cortical bone.
   b. The bone trabeculae may be seen within the tumor.
   c. Occasionally a radiolucent center is present within the tumor.
3. Bone cyst
   a. Is usually solitary (monostotic), but may be polyostotic.
   b. Is usually located in the diaphysis or metaphysis of a long bone.
   c. Expansile radiolucent lesion is sometimes seen, usually with septation and cortical thinning.
   d. Well-demarcated transition zone is present.
   e. Pathologic fracture may be a sequel.
4. Exostosis
   a. Smooth bony enlargement protruding outward from a bone.
   b. Commonly has a triangular shape and is located in epiphyseal or metaphyseal region (e.g., distal ulna).
5. Osteochondroma
   a. Also known as osteochondromatosis and multiple cartilaginous exotosis in dogs, and as feline osteochondromatosis in cats.

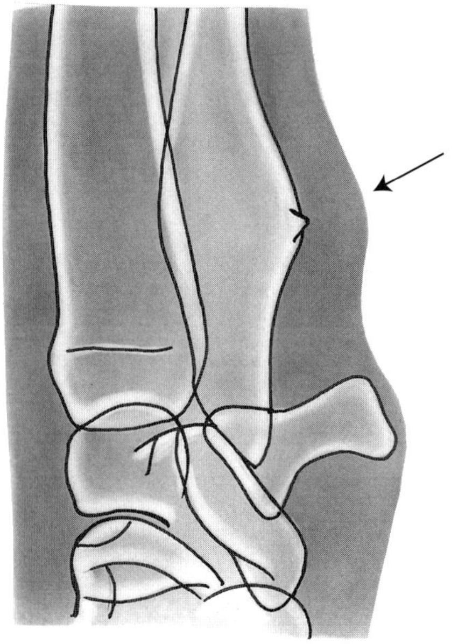

Figure 4.38. Exotosis. There is a smooth protuberance extending from the ulnar cortex with adjacent soft tissue swelling (arrow).

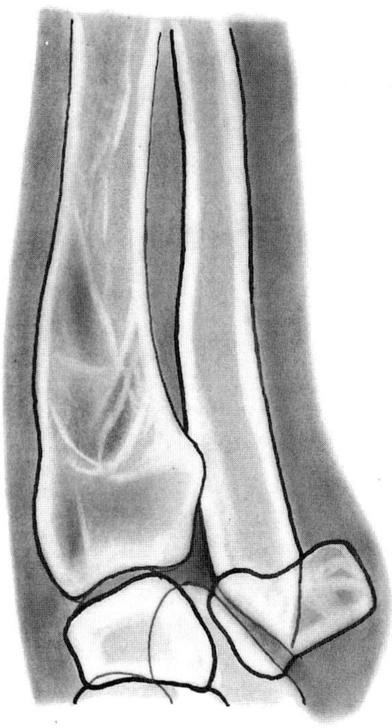

Figure 4.39. Bone cyst. Radiolucent septated benign cyst in distal metaphysis of the radius. Many bone cysts have a more demarcated margin between the cyst and normal bone.

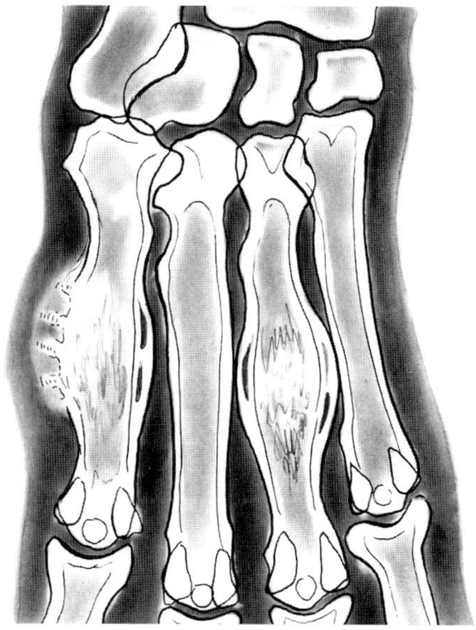

Figure 4.40. Osteochondroma. Expansile bony masses arising from two separate metacarpal bones.

   b. Amorphous and variable sized bony masses with irregular contours involving rib, long bone, digit, and/or vertebra.
   c. Commonly expansile in appearance, usually extending away from the bone.
   d. Lesion may be solitary (monostotic) or polyostotic.

Primary Malignant Bone Neoplasia

Clinical correlations

1. Usually occurs in large and giant breed dogs of middle to older age.
2. May have acute onset or progressive lameness of affected limb.
3. Osteosarcoma is the most common primary bone tumor in dogs and cats. Other primary tumors include fibrosarcoma, chondrosarcoma, hemangiosarcoma, malignant histiocytoma, lymphosarcoma, and myeloma.
4. Osteosarcoma occurs most commonly in the metaphysis of the long bones in the dog, with site predilections as follows.
   a. Proximal humerus
   b. Distal radius
   c. Distal and proximal ulna
   d. Proximal and distal femur
   e. Proximal and distal tibia
5. Malignant neoplasia may occur at the site of a previous fracture, or chronic osteomyelitis.
   a. Usually more than 5 years after the fracture occurred.
   b. Usually occurs in the diaphysis of long bones.
   c. More common in large breed dogs.
   d. Has been reported to be associated with metallic implants, most often when electrolysis has occurred with the use of two different kinds of metals.

Radiographic findings (Figures 4.41)

1. Usually is a solitary focal lesion in metaphysis of a bone. Rarely occurs in diaphysis or epiphysis.
2. Aggressive radiographic pattern is commonly present.
   a. The lesion has a poorly demarcated margin a wide transition zone between the normal and abnormal bone.
   b. Osteolytic and/or osteoblastic activity, commonly with cortical erosion. Approximately 5% of osteosarcomas have osteolysis only.
   c. There is active and aggressive periosteal reaction and approximately 33% of osteosarcoma cases have sun-burst periosteal reaction. Periosteal new bone may be tumor bone or reactive bone.
   d. Localized soft tissue swelling
   e. Usually does not involve joint or other bones.
   f. A pathologic fracture may be present.
3. Radiographic appearance of primary tumors is similar to metastatic tumors and mycotic osteomyelitis.

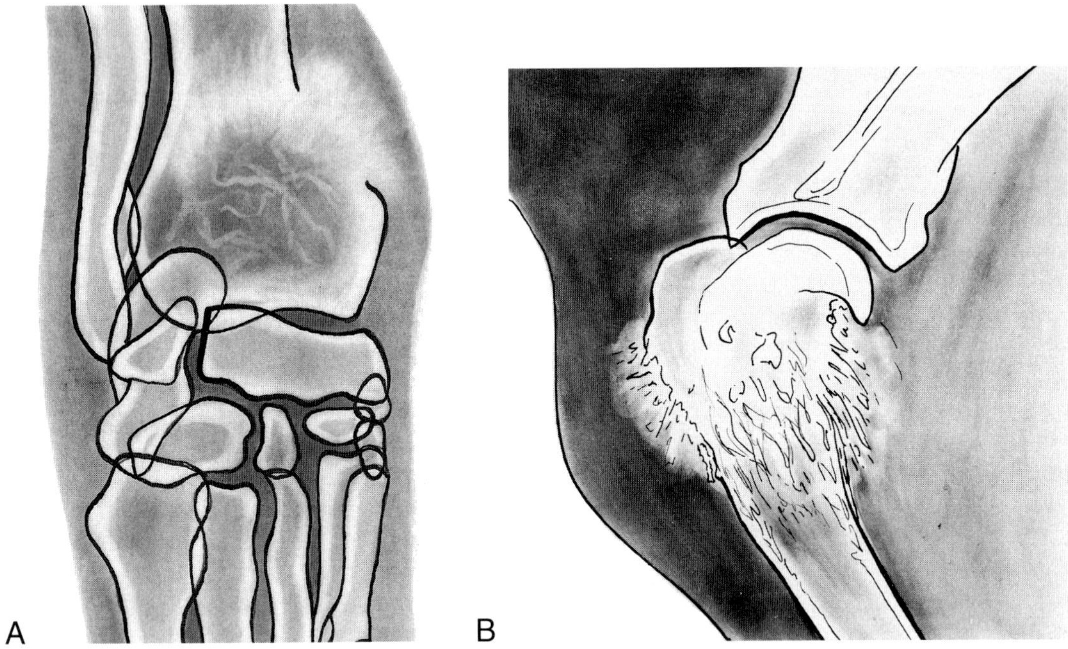

Figure 4.41. **A)** Primary malignant bone neoplasia. Aggressive expansile lytic and poorly demarcated tumor of the distal radius. Note aggressive sunburst periosteal reaction and cortical erosion. **B)** Primary malignant bone neoplasia of proximal humeral metaphysis. There is an osteoblastic lesion with cortical destruction, a sunburst periosteal reaction, and adjacent soft tissue swelling.

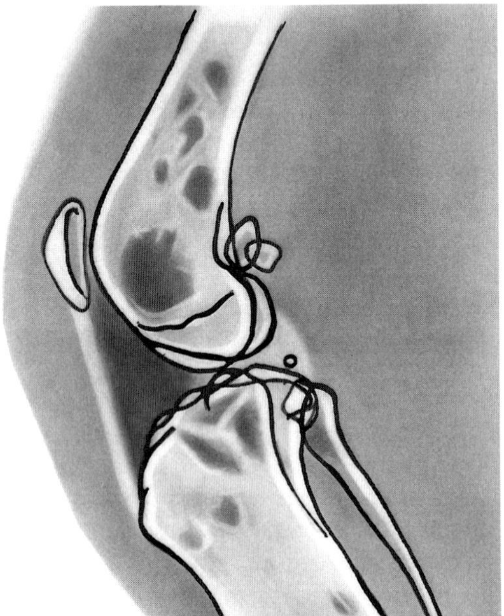

Figure 4.42. Metastatic malignant bone neoplasia of femur and tibia characterized by multiple aggressive appearing, poorly marginated lytic lesions.

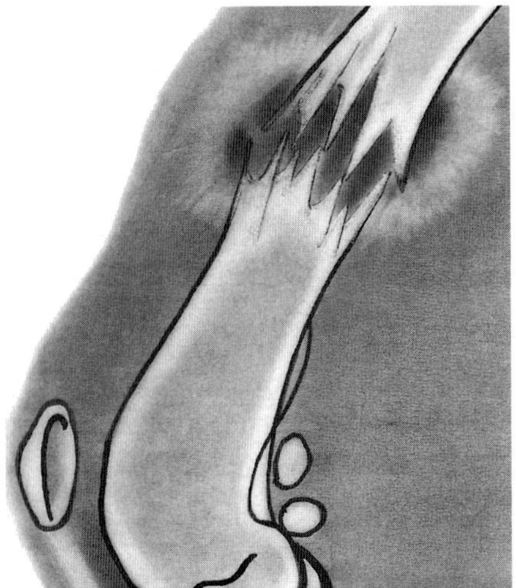

Figure 4.43. Metastatic malignant bone neoplasia characterized by an aggressive lytic lesion in mid femur with a pathologic fracture.

Metastatic Malignant Bone Neoplasia

Clinical correlations

1. Is usually seen in older animals, often in animals that have or are being treated for neoplastic disease.
2. There is no breed predilection.
3. Metastatic tumors of bone usually occur in the diaphysis, but can affect any location in any bone.
4. Often has concurrent pulmonary or other organ metastasis.
5. Any malignant tumor can metastasize to bone, but most frequently they are epithelial rather than mesenchymal. Mammary, pulmonary, prostate, and bone tumors are the most common to metastasize to bone.

Radiographic findings (Figures 4.42 and 4.43):

1. Usually involves more than one bone of the appendicular or axial skeleton.
2. When involving a long bone, it usually affects the diaphyseal and metaphyseal regions.
3. It usually has aggressive radiographic appearance with both osteolytic and osteoblastic changes.
4. Metastatic carcinomas of the bladder, urethra, or prostate can cause a smooth or irregular periosteal reaction on the ventral margins of vertebrae (lumbar, sacral, coccygeal), pelvis, and femur.

MUSCULOCUTANEOUS SOFT TISSUE DISEASES

1. Diseases of the skin, muscle, fibrous connective tissue, tendons, ligaments, joint capsule, cartilage, blood vessels, and lymphatic vessels can produce radiographic abnormalities.
2. The radiographic appearance of the soft tissues adds valuable information about a disease process. Radiographs of bone disease commonly include soft tissue alterations.
3. Soft tissue disease may represent a musculoskeletal lesion limited to only the soft tissues, or it may be the result of an underlying bone disease such as osteomyelitis in which soft tissue changes occur before bony changes.
4. A reduction in radiographic technique (e.g., soft tissue technique instead of bone technique) is helpful to better visualize the soft tissues.
5. Common radiographic abnormalities include: swelling, atrophy, displacement, or obliteration of normal structures such as fascial planes, mineralization, a radiopaque foreign body, abnormal radiopacity (e.g., lipoma), or emphysema.
6. When present, one or more of the soft tissue changes may imply possible cause or site of the disease process. For example, if the soft tissue swelling is poorly defined, the disease process is more likely to be an infiltrative lesion rather than an organized hematoma or abscess.
7. Comparison radiographs of the contralateral limb are commonly helpful when confirming lesions (e.g., atrophy, loss of fascial plane).

DISEASES/DISORDERS

Soft Tissue Swelling

Clinical correlations

1. Commonly caused by edema and hemorrhage associated with trauma (e.g., fracture) or infection.
2. May occur anywhere in limb.
3. May be localized or generalized.

Radiographic findings

1. Commonly is invisible radiographically, especially if within muscle.
2. The size (thickness) of the soft tissue structures is increased.
3. There is a diffuse increase in radiopacity, which is ill defined because fluid obliterates the normally distinct boundary between muscles and fat.
4. There is a loss of normal fascial planes. Subcutaneous spaces may have a fine striated or mottled soft-tissue radiopacity with the margins gradually fading into normal soft tissue opacity.
5. Subperiosteal hemorrhage is invisible, until the periosteum reacts to the irritation by depositing calcium, which usually takes 7 to 10 days after the onset of infection or a trauma. Mineralization develops more rapidly in immature animals than in aged animals.

Musculocutaneous Soft Tissue Masses

Clinical correlations

1. Localized masses can be associated with trauma, infection, or neoplasia and are best assessed by physical palpation and correlation with the clinical history.
2. Solid masses are often caused by peripheral lymphadenopathy, benign tumors, or malignant tumors.

Radiographic findings

1. Tumor types cannot be differentiated with radiography.
2. There may be a well-defined or an ill-defined soft tissue radiopacity.
3. Fatty masses (e.g., lipoma, liposarcoma) are more radiolucent than adjacent soft tissue and are commonly located within fascial planes.
4. Adjacent structures may be displaced.
5. Swelling may contain dystrophic mineralization, gas, or a radiopaque or radiolucent foreign body.

Musculocutaneous Emphysema

Clinical correlations

1. There is an abnormal presence of gas or air within the soft tissues. The gas may be subcutaneous, interfascial, or intramuscular.
2. Gas may result from a penetrating wound, gas forming infection (e.g., Clostridia), or surgery.
3. If the emphysema is severe, crepitus can be palpated. When infection is present, the local area may be warm and painful and the animal may be febrile.

Radiographic findings

1. There is localized or generalized gas accumulation in the soft tissues.
2. When localized infection is present, multiple bubbles of gas may be seen.

Soft Tissue Mineralization

Clinical correlations

1. Seen in enthesopathy, ossifying tendinitis, myositis ossificans, calcinosis circumscripta, calcinosis cutis, and vascular mineralization.
2. There is deposition of calcium salts in the soft tissues.
3. A histologic examination is required to differentiate different types of mineralization (e.g., ossification or calcification).
4. Clinical signs are rare, unless the location interferes with function.
5. Classifications of mineralization in soft tissues (Table 4.9)
   a. Dystrophic mineralization is the deposition of calcium in dead, degenerating, or damaged tissue (e.g., tumor, abscess, hematoma, trauma).
   b. Metastatic mineralization is a deposition of calcium in tissue that is not the disease site, often as a result of altered calcium metabolism (e.g., hyperparathyroidism, hyperadrenocorticism).
   c. Myositis ossificans is the deposition of calcium in muscle, and often is secondary to metaplasia of connective tissue cells within the traumatized muscle.
   d. Ossifying tendonitis (enthesopathy) is the deposition of calcium at the insertion sites of muscles (e.g., gluteal tendon attachment on the trochanter major of femur).
   e. Calcinosis cutis is the deposition of calcium in the skin (e.g., as seen in Cushingoid animals).
   f. Calcinosis circumscripta (tumoral calcinosis) is the deposition of amorphous calcium in the subcutaneous tissue and skin, usually on the limbs, under foot pads and over bony prominences.
      1) More common in dogs than cats.
      2) Approximately 50% of cases in dogs are in German Shepherds, usually younger than 2 years of age.
      3) Mass is usually hard, well-circumscribed, and nonpainful.
      4) Common locations are shoulder, elbow, and regions of the foot.
   g. Vascular mineralization is the deposition of calcium in the walls of vessels.
      1) Systemic diseases (e.g., hypothyroidism, hyperparathyroidism, hyperadrenocorticism).
      2) Idiopathic (e.g., thoracic aorta of aged cats, abdominal aorta, and its major branches in dogs).

Radiographic finding (Figures 4.44 and 4.45)

Appearance of mineralization ranges from disorganized to highly organized radiopaque calcific densities within soft tissue.

TABLE 4.9

Soft Tissue Mineralization

1. Dystrophic mineralization
2. Metastatic mineralization
3. Myositis ossificans
4. Ossifying tendonitis (enthesopathy)
5. Calcinosis cutis
6. Calcinosis circumscripta
7. Vascular mineralization

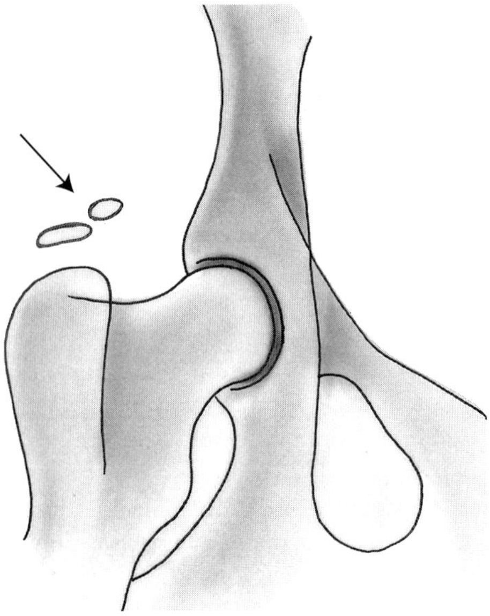

Figure 4.44. Mineralization in the tendon of the gluteal muscle.

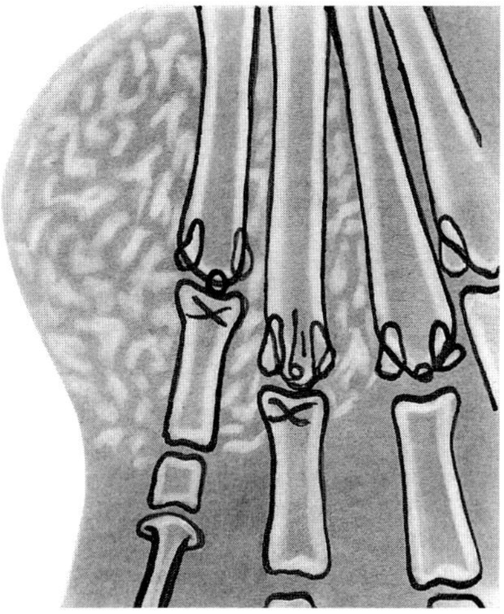

Figure 4.45. Calcinosis circumscripta. Amorphous mineralization is present within the soft tissues of the foot.

Foreign Bodies

Clinical correlations

1. Foreign bodies commonly found in soft tissues include needles, shrapnel, gravel, glass, wood, plastic, and plant material.
2. Depending on the type and location of the foreign body, clinical signs may vary from none to a draining tract.
3. May have other lesions (i.e., fracture with shrapnel).

Radiographic findings

1. Metallic foreign bodies (i.e,. bullet) are radiopaque and easily identified.
2. Gravel, glass, wood, and many plastic objects are of soft tissue radiopacity and often not visible.
3. At least two views (perpendicular to one another) are required to localize a foreign body.
4. Positive contrast fistulography may aid in determining the location and type of foreign body.
5. Other imaging
   a. Ultrasound
   b. Computed tomography (CT)
   c. Magnetic resonance imaging (MRI)

Arteriovenous Fistula

Clinical correlations

1. Is an abnormal communication between an artery and vein.
2. Most often is acquired lesion rather than congenital.
   a. History of soft tissue blunt trauma or surgery is most common.
   b. May be initiated by a traumatic vascular puncture or perivascular injection of irritating chemicals.
3. Depending on the site of the arteriovenous fistula and size, there may be a continuous bruit at the site.
4. Rarely is the fistula large enough to cause secondary congestive heart failure.
5. Most often reported in the limbs, but has also been reported in the ear, head, neck, and internal organs, (e.g., liver, lung, and bowel).
6. In the limb, the fistula site is usually a warm, nonpainful soft tissue swelling. Large fistulas can be painful and cause lameness.

Radiographic findings

1. There is localized soft tissue swelling at the site of the fistula.
2. Underlying osseous changes may be present, (e.g., periosteal reaction, cortical destruction).
3. Selective angiography is necessary to radiographically document the arteriovenous fistula.
4. Doppler ultrasound aids in determining the location, size, and direction of the blood flow through the fistula.

Lymphadenopathy

Clinical correlations

1. Is commonly associated with inflammatory or neoplastic diseases.
2. Peripheral lymph nodes are enlarged and palpable.

Radiographic findings

1. Normal peripheral lymph nodes may occasionally be visible because of radiolucency of the adjacent fat.
2. Enlarged peripheral lymph nodes are commonly visible and include the prescapular, popliteal, axillary, and inguinal nodes.
3. Lymphangiography may be helpful in assessing the size and structure of some lymph nodes.
4. Ultrasound is effective in evaluating the size and internal architecture of most lymph nodes.

Lymphedema

Clinical correlations

1. There is an abnormal accumulation of lymph fluid in the soft tissues, which most often occurs secondary to trauma, venous stasis, infection, or neoplasia.
2. In dogs with congenital lymphedema there is usually swelling of one or more limbs, which is usually attributable to hypoplastic (or absence) peripheral lymph nodes and deep lymphatic vessels.
   a. Edema is usually pitting and begins distally on the limbs.

b. It is noticeable at birth or within several months.
c. Pain and lameness are uncommon.
d. More commonly reported in the Bulldog and Poodle.
e. Differential considerations include neoplasia, cellulitis, vasculitis, and thrombosis.

Radiographic findings

1. Soft tissue swelling ranges from the distal portion to the entire limb and may affect one or more limbs.
2. Lymphangiography is necessary for a diagnosis.

chapter five

5 Joints

ANATOMY

A joint is formed when two or more bones are united by cartilaginous, fibrous, or elastic tissue. Joints are divided into three main groups based on the type of tissues that connect the bones. These are synovial joints (diarthrosis), fibrous joints (synarthrosis), and cartilaginous joints (synchondrosis). Some joints are also composed of more than one group (i.e., sacroiliac and tibiofibular joints are a combination of synovial and fibrous joints).

Synovial Joints (Diarthroses)

Synovial joints provide the greatest range of movement for mobility. Synovial joints enable the diverse movements of flexion, extension, adduction, abduction, circumduction, and rotation. All diarthrodial joints (e.g., ball and socket, hinge, condylar, pivot) have a joint cavity, joint capsule, synovial fluid, and articular cartilage. In some synovial joints, there may also be a meniscus and ligament (e.g., stifle joint). The joint capsule consists of a synovial membrane that lines the joint cavity and an outer fibrous capsule. The ends of the articulating surfaces are covered with articular cartilage, beneath which lies a thin plate of dense subchondral bone.

Examples: (Figure 5.1)

a. Joints of the extremities (e.g., shoulder, stifle, elbow, tarsus)
b. Articular facet joints of the vertebrae
c. Atlantoaxial joint
d. Articulations between the ribs and thoracic vertebrae (costovertebral joints) and between the costal cartilages and sternabra (sternocostal joints)
e. Temporomandibular joint

Fibrous Joints (Synarthroses)

Fibrous joints are the least movable and lack a joint cavity. Based on the type of tissue present within the joint surfaces, fibrous joints are classified as: syndesmosis, suture, and gomphosis unions. On survey radiographs, fibrous joints are usually seen as thin radiolucent lines. Commonly, they are not visible unless the central x-ray beam is perpendicular to the joint. In mature animals, many fibrous joints are no longer visible radiographically.

1. *Syndesmosis* fibrous joints have a considerable amount of intervening connective tissue.
   Examples:
   a. Attachment of the hyoid to petrous temporal bone
   b. Proximal and distal tibiofibular articulations (also have a small synovial joint)
   c. Interosseous ligament between the radius and ulna
2. *Suture* fibrous joints usually are confined to the flat bones of the skull and can be further subclassified according to shape of the opposed edges (i.e., serrated, squamous, foliate plane).
   Examples:
   a. Occipitoparietal suture
   b. Frontonasal suture
   c. Vomeromaxillary suture
3. *Gomphosis* fibrous joints are formed by the peridontal ligament, which attaches the cementum of each tooth to the alveolar bone of the socket. The peridontal ligament is not visible radiographically.

Cartilage Joints (Synchondroses)

Cartilage joints are formed by the union of two or more bones by hyaline cartilage, by fibrocartilage, or by a combination of the two. Cartilage joints are commonly classified into two types: hyaline cartilage and fibrocartilage. The radiographic appearance of joints changes with increasing age, varying between radiolucent to ossified (young to old).

1. Hyaline cartilage joints are usually temporary and represent persistent parts of the fetal skeleton or secondary cartilage of growing bones. Commonly, when adult status is reached, osseous fusion occurs and the joint no longer exists.

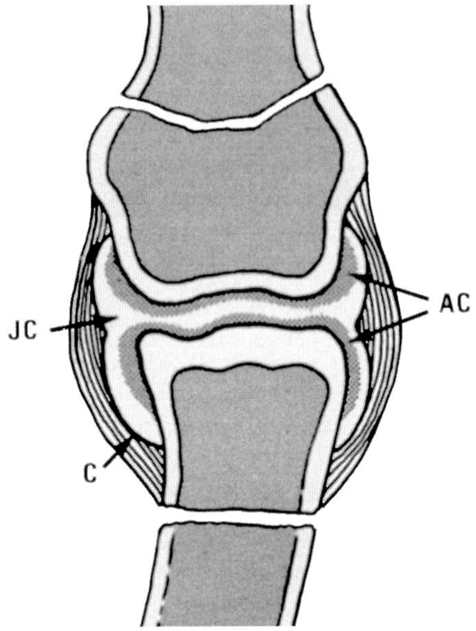

Figure 5.1. Typical synovial joint with articular cartilage (**AC**), a joint cavity (**JC**) containing synovial fluid, and an articular capsule (**C**).

Examples:
   a. Epiphyseal lines in bones (physes)
   b. Union of the femoral trochanter and humeral tubercles with the bone shafts
   c. Costochondral junctions (remain throughout life)
2. Fibrocartilage joints, also referred to as amphiarthroses, usually have an intervening plate of hyaline cartilage at each end and may occasionally ossify.
   Examples:
   a. Mandibular symphysis
   b. Pelvic symphysis
   c. Intervertebral discs
   d. Sternebrae

RADIOGRAPHIC TECHNIQUE

Projections

Standard projections: (should include the joint and portion of adjacent bones)
1. Craniocaudal or caudocranial projection
2. Lateral projection

Supplemental projections:
1. Medial and lateral oblique projections
2. Flexed or extended projections
3. Traction or torsion projections
4. Weight-bearing projections
5. Comparison views of contralateral joint

RADIOGRAPHIC INTERPRETATION

The interpretation of the images should include the following:
1. Examine the alignment of the bones.
   a. Excellent positioning is essential.
   b. Changes in alignment may indicate joint instability because of tearing or stretching of the supporting ligamentous structures.
2. Examine the soft tissues adjacent to the joint.
   a. Evaluate the contour and extent of soft tissue swelling or atrophy.
   b. Evaluate for changes in radiopacity within the soft tissues. These changes may indicate the presence of gas, mineralization, or foreign matter.
3. Evaluate the subjective width of the joint space.
   a. Weight-bearing radiographs (with the x-ray beam perpendicular to the joint) are essential for reliable assessment of joint space, but this projection is difficult to obtain in dogs and cats.
   b. Joint space narrowing may indicate destruction of the joint cartilage.
   c. Joint space widening may indicate joint effusion or ligamentous instability.
4. Evaluate for the presence of joint effusion. Joint capsule distension is usually associated with synovial effusion, but may also be caused by synovial membrane hypertrophy and hyperplasia, joint capsule fibrosis, or neoplasia.
   a. It is difficult to see radiographically, except in the tarsus and stifle.
      1) Observations on a lateral projection of the stifle joint:
         a) Cranial displacement or obliteration of the infrapatellar fat pad
         b) Caudal displacement of the joint capsule (seen by noting caudal displacement of the fat containing fascial planes)
         c) Cranial displacement of the patella (if effusion is severe)
      2) Observations on a lateral projection of the tibiotarsal joint:
         a) Cranial distension of the joint capsule (seen by noting cranial displacement of the periarticular fat)
         b) Caudal displacement of the joint capsule (seen between the distal caudal tibia and the fibular tarsal bone)
5. Examine the periarticular structures.
   a. Evaluate for degenerative osteophytes and enthesophytes at the articular margins.
   b. Evaluate for avulsion fractures involving the tendinous or ligamentous insertions.

Examples:
  1) Avulsion of the tibial tuberosity
  2) Avulsion of the supraglenoid tuberosity
  3) Avulsion of the round ligament in the hip

6. Examine the distribution of the joint lesions.
   a. Determine if monarticular (one joint) or polyarticular (two or more joints).
   b. Evaluate the extent and symmetry of the lesions.
7. Comparison radiographs of the contralateral limb frequently enable a better appreciation of an abnormality. Times when these comparisons are useful:
   a. Immature animals in which the physes are open and the epiphyses are incompletely ossified
   b. Traumatic conditions in which subtle joint lesions may be present

CLINICAL AND RADIOGRAPHIC CORRELATIONS

The causes of joint disease are many and include congenital, developmental, metabolic, degenerative, traumatic, inflammatory, and neoplastic diseases. An accurate clinical diagnosis is based on the clinical history, physical findings, laboratory data (including joint fluid analysis), and the evaluation of radiographic lesions. The radiographic changes are frequently nonspecific and vary depending on the length and severity of the underlying disorder. The types of abnormalities that may be seen radiographically include: (Figure 5.2)

1. Articular fracture and/or joint malalignment
2. Joint capsule distension (usually caused by effusion)
3. Decreased or increased joint space
4. Subchondral bone sclerosis
5. Subchondral erosion or cyst formation
6. Bone remodeling
7. Mineralization of periarticular or intraarticular soft tissues
8. Periarticular bone spurs (osteophytes and enthesophytes)

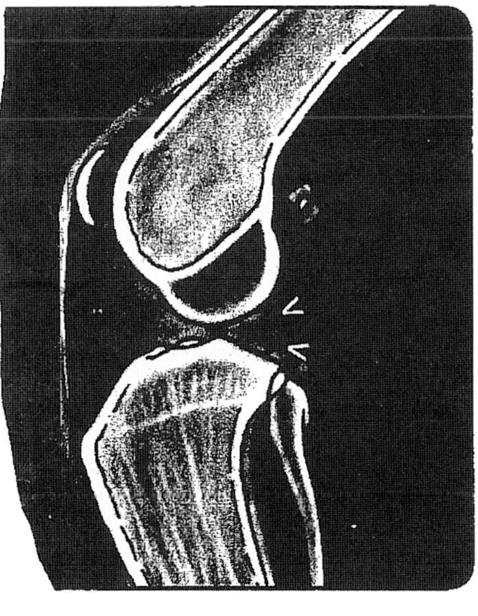

Figure 5.2. Joint effusion. Increased joint fluid in the stifle joint causes distension of the joint capsule (arrows) and partial obliteration of the infrapatellar fat pad.

A classification system, based on types of noninflammatory and inflammatory arthropathies, may aid the clinician in making a differential diagnosis or diagnoses. (See Table 5.1)

TABLE 5.1

Classification of Arthropathies

I. Noninflammatory:
  A. Degenerative joint disease
    1. Primary (e.g., storage diseases).
    2. Secondary (e.g., hip dysplasia, elbow dysplasia).
  B. Trauma (e.g., luxation, subluxation, articular fracture)
  C. Neoplastic (e.g., synovial cell sarcoma)

II. Inflammatory:
  A. Infectious (See Table 5.2)
    1. Hematogenous
      a. Umbilical infections in neonates
      b. Genitourinary infections
      c. Bacterial endocarditis
    2. Nonhematogenous
      a. Penetrating wounds
      b. Trauma, including postsurgical
      c. Bacterial endocarditis
      d. Nonsterile injections
    3. Direct extension from adjacent soft tissue
  B. Noninfectious
    1. Immunologic
      a. Erosive
        1) Rheumatoid arthritis
        2) Reiter disease
        3) Polyarthritis of the Greyhound
      b. Nonerosive (See Table 5.3)
        1) Idiopathic
        2) Systemic lupus erythematosus (SLE)
        3) Other

DISEASES/DISORDERS

Congenital Malformations

Clinical correlations

1. Congenital malformations of the bony skeleton and joints occasionally are seen. They rarely cause any clinical abnormality, unless the anomaly affects function of the joint.
2. Clinical lameness and gait disturbance may be present.

Radiographic findings

1. Findings depend on type and severity of the malformation.
2. Examples of radiographic findings are:
   a. Hypoplasia or aplasia of a developing epiphysis
   b. Congenital absence of a carpal or tarsal bone
   c. Hemivertebra

Conformational Deformities

Clinical correlations

1. Conformational deformities may be congenital or acquired. Acquired deformities are often secondary to trauma, nutritional imbalance, or metabolic disorders.
2. Trauma can cause joint subluxation, asymmetric physeal growth with angulation, and result in a malunion fracture.
3. Conformational defects in posture and limb development can result in abnormal angulation, which, with abnormal mechanical stresses, can lead to asymmetric joint pressure, epiphysiolysis, ligamentous degeneration, and secondary degenerative joint disease.

Radiographic findings

1. Findings vary with type and extent of conformational defects.
2. Examples include
   a. Valgus deformity of the forelimbs as seen in chondrodystrophoid dogs
   b. Functional hyperextension of the rear limbs, "cow" hocks, knock-knees (genu varum), and bow-legs (genu valgum).
   c. Ehler-Danlos syndrome—Joint hyperlaxity caused by increased connective tissue elasticity is seen as an inherited disorder. Degenerative joint disease also may be present.

Osteochondrosis (OC) and Osteochondritis Dissecans (OCD)

Clinical correlations

1. Osteochondrosis is a generalized disease of disturbed endochondral ossification. The thickened cartilage precursor fails to ossify, ossifies in an irregular manner, or is delayed in its ossification.
2. When osteochondrosis progresses and breaks through the articular cartilage and into the joint, the condition becomes osteochondritic dissecans.
3. In osteochondritic dissecans, a cartilage "flap" can then develop. This "flap" either remains attached or becomes free, and as a "free body" can become mineralized and grow in size as a "joint mouse."
4. Degenerative joint disease commonly occurs as a sequel.
5. Occurs most commonly in large and giant breed dogs that are less than 1 year of age.
6. Predisposing factors for development of osteochondrosis and osteochondritic dissecans include:
   a. Genetics
      1) Elbow osteochondritic dissecans has been shown to be inheritable in some dogs, notably the Labrador Retriever, the Golden Retriever, the Bernese Mountain dog, the Newfoundland, and other large and giant dog breeds.
   b. Metabolic
      1) Rapid growth and weight gain associated with nutrition, hormones, and genetic factors contribute to growth rate, weight gain, and cartilage/endochondral osteogenesis.
         a) It is twice as common in male dogs, which tend to grow more rapidly than females.
         b) Osteochondritic dissecans lesions can also occur in non–weight-bearing and nontraumatized sites, such as the distal ribs.
   c. Trauma
      1) Trauma plays a role in inciting or perpetuating cartilaginous changes at vulnerable sites.
      2) In the shoulder (during extension of the joint), the caudal margin of the glenoid may put added stress or pressure on the caudal humeral head, resulting in osteochondrosis.
6. Is most common in the shoulder, elbow, stifle, and tarsus of dogs.
   a. Shoulder (caudal aspect of humeral head) (See page 68)
   b. Elbow (humeral condyle, anconeal process, and coronoid process) (See page 73)
   c. Stifle (femoral condyles) (See page 92)
   d. Tarsus (trochlea of tibiotarsal bone) (See page 102)
7. Lesions are often self-limiting and may heal spontaneously, especially if small.

Radiographic findings (See following sections with Figures 5.14, 5.24, 5.59, and 5.73)

1. Osteochondrosis and osteochondritic dissecans appear similar with a flattened or radiolucent subchondral defect on the articular surface.
2. Osteochondritic dissecans may have:
   a. Flattened or radiolucent subchondral defect
   b. Joint effusion
   c. Mineralized cartilage flap
   d. Mineralized joint mouse
   e. Secondary degenerative joint disease (including bone spurs and subchondral sclerosis)

Trauma

Clinical correlations

1. Trauma can cause injury to the bones and cartilage as well as the supporting soft tissues of the joints including the ligaments, tendons, and the joint capsule.
2. Types of joint injuries:
   a. Sprain—implies an injury to the supporting ligaments of a joint. The degree of injury may range from partial to complete tearing of the ligamentous structures.
   b. Subluxation (partial dislocation)—implies a partial loss of contact between the articular surfaces of a joint.
   c. Luxation (dislocation)—implies a complete loss of contact between the articular surfaces of a joint.
   d. Fracture—implies a break in the articular cortex extending through the subchondral bone and articular cartilage into the joint.
   e. Congenital anomaly implies a predisposition that predisposes to fracture as seen in incomplete ossification of the humeral condyles in Cocker Spaniels and Brittany Spaniels.

Radiographic findings (See following sections with Figures 5.10, 5.32, 5.45, 5.63, and 5.72)

1. Visible abnormalities are based on alignment and appearance of bony structures.
2. Stress radiographs, such as hyperflexion and hyperextension projections, are often necessary to demonstrate subluxation of the carpus, tarsus, stifle, and hip.
3. Radiographic changes of osteoporosis, muscle atrophy, and bony remodeling may be observed with chronic joint subluxation or luxation.
4. Secondary degenerative joint disease with periarticular bone spurs, subchondral osteosclerosis, and bone remodeling usually occurs as a sequel.

Physeal Injury: (Epiphyseal growth plate injury)

Clinical correlations

1. Trauma may cause a delayed or premature closure of the long bone physes, which may result in shortening of the affected bone and secondary angular limb deformities.
2. Joint subluxation and malalignment often occur secondarily to asymmetric growth of adjacent bones (e.g., radius and ulna, tibia and fibula).
3. Clinical problems are often most significant in young, large and giant breed dogs, in which bone growth is faster and greater.
4. Asymmetric growth of the radius and ulna is common in chondrodystrophoid breeds (e.g., Bassett Hounds, Skye Terrier).

Radiographic findings (See Figures 4.31, 4.32, 4.33, and 4.34)

1. Variable joint deformities will be observed depending on the severity and length of time that the bone physis injury has been present.
2. Subluxation and degenerative joint disease are common sequelae.

Osteoarthritis (Table 5.1)

Clinical correlations

1. Osteoarthritis, also known as degenerative joint disease, is a noninflammatory disorder of synovial joints characterized by deterioration of the articular cartilage and formation of new bone at the periarticular margins and joint surfaces.
2. Involves a complex of interactive degradation and repair processes within the cartilage, bone, and synovium.
3. Osteoarthritis can be classified as primary or secondary.
   a. Primary osteoarthritis results from normal wear and tear with no known specific or predisposing cause.
   b. Secondary osteoarthritis results from a known specific or predisposing cause (i.e., previous trauma, OCD, elbow dysplasia, hip dysplasia).
4. Is the most common type of arthropathy in dogs and cats.

Radiographic findings (See Figure 4.12 and following sections with Figures 5.18, 5.27, 5.28, 5.52, 5.58, and 5.74)

1. Early in the disease, the joint appears normal.
2. Increased periarticular soft tissue swelling may be present as a result of joint effusion and/or thickening of the articular or periarticular soft tissues.
3. Narrowing or ablation of the joint space may be apparent.
4. Subchondral bone sclerosis is the result of the dual processes of attrition and new bone deposition. Occasionally in severe disease subchondral cyst formation develops.
5. Osteophyte formation (bone spurs) often form at the margins of the articular surface.
6. Enthesophytes develop at the bone tendon interface.
7. Mineralization of the intraarticular and periarticular soft tissues may occur.

INFECTIOUS ARTHRITIS (Table 5.2)

Bacterial Arthritis

Clinical correlations

1. Infectious arthritis is characterized by an inflammatory response in the synovial membrane and joint fluid.
2. Bacteria can gain entrance into a joint through the bloodstream, penetrating wounds, or as a postoperative complication.

TABLE 5.2

Infectious Arthritis

1. Bacterial arthritis
2. Mycoplasma and L form bacterial arthritis
3. Rickettsial arthritis
4. Spirochetal arthritis
5. Viral arthritis
6. Fungal arthritis

3. In puppies and kittens, umbilical infections (omphalophlebitis) are occasional sources of septic arthritis.
4. In older animals, bacteremia associated with infections of the teeth or oral cavity, lung, genitourinary tract, and the skin can be responsible for infectious arthritis. In cats, it often is associated with bite wounds.
5. Organisms commonly involved in joint infections include: *Streptococcus, Staphylococcus, Corynebacteria, Pasteurella, Salmonella, Brucella,* and fungal organisms.
6. Affected dogs and cats will show variable signs of illness including fever, lameness, anorexia, and lethargy.
7. In most instances, the arthritis is monarticular and most commonly involves the shoulder, carpus, elbow, stifle, or a cubital joint.
8. Predisposing conditions may include: immunosuppression, diabetes, and penetrating wounds.

Mycoplasma and L-Forms of Bacterial Arthritis

1. L-form bacteria (cell wall deficient bacteria) can have joint involvement in cats often secondary to a bite wound with fistulous subcutaneous infections.
2. Mycoplasma infections occurs most often in immunocompromised animals.

Rickettsial Arthritis

1. Rickettsia and rickettsial-like organisms infect dogs through tick bites and often cause a polyarthropathy as part of the systemic illness.
2. Rocky Mountain Spotted Fever (*R. rickettsii)* Ehrlichiosis (*E. canis, E. equi, E. risticii,* and *E. sennetsu*) are the most common organisms.

Spirochetal Arthritis

1. Lyme disease, a spirochetal infection, is caused by *Borrelia burgdorferi* and is transmitted by tick bites.
2. Infected animals may be asymptomatic.
3. Arthropathy can be monarticular or polyarticular.
4. The joint fluid is usually inflammatory with many polymorphonuclear neutrophils.

Viral Arthritis

1. Viral arthritis causes joint pain as a postviral infection.
2. Fever may be present.
3. Polyarthropathy with inflammatory joint fluid is common.
4. Is self-limiting without any residual joint disease.

Fungal Arthritis

1. May be an extension of osteomyelitis or as a primary granulomatous synovitis from a hematogenous infection.
2. Infectious agents include:
   a. *Coccidioidomycosis immitis*
   b. *Blastomyces dermatiditis*
   c. *Cryptococcus neoformans*
   d. *Sporotrichum schenckii*
   e. *Aspergillus terreus*

Radiographic findings

1. Usually normal, but may show mildly increased articular or periarticular soft tissue swelling and joint effusion.
2. Early signs of infectious arthritis include soft tissue swelling of the articular and periarticular structures.
3. There is increased joint effusion characterized by capsule distension and displacement of fascial planes (e.g., in the stifle, the effusion distorts or displaces the intrapatellar fat pad).
4. The joint space may appear widened because of increased joint fluid.
5. Later, subchondral bone destruction/erosion occurs, usually on both adjacent bony margins.
6. Chronically affected joints have subchondral bone sclerosis. The joint space is collapsed and there often is marked proliferative degenerative joint disease.

NONINFECTIOUS ARTHRITIS (Table 5.3)

Clinical correlations

1. The diagnosis is based on the history, clinical signs, laboratory tests, radiologic, and pathologic features. A tentative diagnosis can be made even when serologic abnormalities are absent or detected at insignificant levels, bacterial cultures are negative, and evidence of an underlying disease process is absent.
2. No clinical findings, test result, or radiographic findings are pathognomonic for any specific type of inflammatory joint disease. A specific diagnosis is substantiated most often by the elimination of other causes of polyarthritis.

Radiographic findings

1. Radiographs are usually normal.
2. Periarticular soft tissue swelling or joint effusion may be present.

TABLE 5.3

Noninfectious Arthritis

1. Idiopathic
   a. Type I: Uncomplicated idiopathic polyarthritis
   b. Type II: Idiopathic arthritis associated with infections remote from the joints
   c. Type III: Idiopathic arthritis associated with gastrointestinal disease
   d. Type IV: Idiopathic arthritis associated with neoplasia remote from the joints
2. Systemic lupus erythematosus (SLE)
3. Polyarthritis/polymyositis complex
4. Polyarthritis/meningitis syndrome
5. Sjogren syndrome
6. Familial renal amyloidosis of Chinese Shar Pei dogs
7. Heritable polyarthritis of the adolescent Akita
8. Polyarteritis Nodosa

---

3. In chronic cases, there may be proliferative degenerative joint disease and subchondral sclerosis.
4. Is indistinguishable from the many other causes of nonerosive degenerative joint disease.

Idiopathic Polyarthritis

1. Most common polyarthritis—cannot be classified into another subgroup of polyarthropathies.
2. There are four subcategories (Type I–Type IV).
   a. Type I—Uncomplicated Idiopathic Polyarthritis
      1) Most common form that is clinically recognized.
      2) Usually, affected dogs only have lameness.
      3) Other body systems may be involved including dermatitis, glomerulonephritis, uveitis, and retinitis.
      4) Production of immune complexes within the joints may initiate a type III hypersensitivity reaction.
      5) Can occur as side effect of sulfonamide therapy.
   b. Type II—Idiopathic arthritis associated with infections remote from the joints
      1) Affected animals usually have concurrent infections (tonsil, lung, oral cavity, urinary tract, uterus, eye, or skin).
      2) Affected animals may have major clinical signs related to lameness or infection.
      3) Treatment is directed at the infection.
      4) Lameness usually resolves spontaneously without need for corticosteroids.
   c. Type III—Idiopathic arthritis associated with gastrointestinal tract disease
      1) Major clinical signs are vomiting and diarrhea.
      2) May be caused by bacterial overgrowth in the bowel or associated with ulcerative colitis.
      3) It is believed that the increased permeability of the diseased bowel allows entry of potential antigens or toxins that in turn stimulate the production of immune complexes, which are then deposited in the joints or other tissues.
      4) Hepatopathic arthropathy can occur secondary to chronic active hepatitis and cirrhosis. The antigenic material (passing from the bowel) is probably inadequately phagocytized in the liver, thus allowing access to the general circulation.
   d. Type IV—Idiopathic polyarthritis associated with neoplasia remote from joints
      1) Lameness and the degree of polyarthritis usually are mild.
      2) Associated with a nonarticular neoplasm.

Systemic Lupus Erythematosus (SLE)

1. This disease involves the simultaneous or sequential development of autoimmune hemolytic anemia (AIHA), thrombocytopenia, leukopenia, glomerulonephritis, dermatitis, polymyositis, pleuritis, central nervous system (CNS) disease, and symmetric polyarthritis.
2. The etiology is obscure in dogs and cats; but may be caused by an underlying viral infection with some genetic predisposition.
3. Autoimmunity and immune complex hypersensitivity are characteristic of the disease.

Polyarthritis/Polymyositis Complex

1. Polyarthritis is complicated by polymyositis.
2. Most frequently seen in the spaniel breeds.

Polyarthritis/Meningitis Syndrome

1. Affected animals usually have neck pain, fever, and stiffness.
2. Cerebrospinal fluid (CSF) has increased protein and white blood cells.
3. The disease has been reported in the Weimaraner, German Shorthaired Pointer, Bernese Mountain Dog, Boxer, and Akita.

Sjogren Syndrome

1. Characteristics of Sjogren syndrome include keratoconjunctivitis sicca, xerostomia, and polyarthritis.
2. Polyarthritis may be erosive or nonerosive.

Familial Renal Amyloidosis in Chinese Shar Pei Dogs

1. Is characterized by episodic fever and swelling of one or both tibiotarsal joints; occasionally other joints are affected.

2. The period between episodes varies, usually 4 to 6 weeks.
3. Renal amyloidosis often leads to renal failure.

Heritable Polyarthritis of the Adolescent Akita

1. Affected dogs are usually less than 1 year of age.
2. The clinical signs consist of polyarthritis, peripheral lymphadenopathy, and systemic illness with fever, lethargy, and anorexia.

Polyarteritis Nodosa

1. Affected animals often have meningitis and polyarthritis.
2. Episodic clinical signs of fever, stiffness, and depression are often seen.
3. Prognosis is good; usually self-limiting with maturity.

EROSIVE ARTHRITIS

Rheumatoid Arthritis (Table 5.4)

Clinical correlations

1. Is an immune-mediated disease with circulating autoantibodies against IgG (positive RF factor).
2. Occurs most often in middle-aged, small to medium dogs.

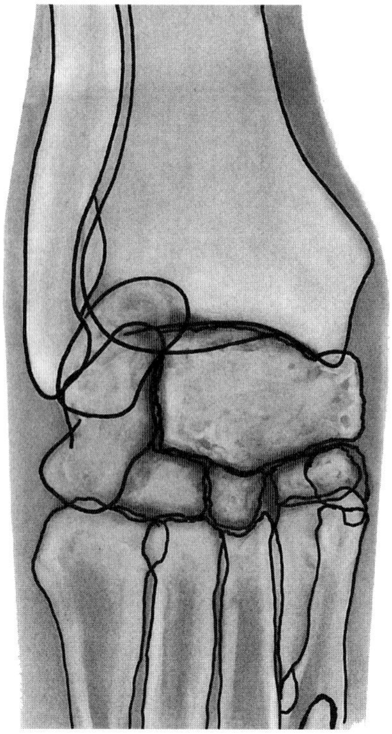

Figure 5.3. Erosive arthritis. Radiographic changes include marked subchondral bone erosion, loss of joint space, and periarticular soft tissue swelling.

TABLE 5.4

Criteria for the Diagnosis of Canine Rheumatoid Arthritis[a]

1. Stiffness after rest
2. Pain or tenderness in at least one joint
3. Swelling in at least one joint
4. Swelling of at least one other joint within 3 months
5. Symmetrical joint swelling
6. Subcutaneous nodules over bony prominences or extensor surfaces or in juxtaarticular regions
7. Destructive radiographic
8. Positive agglutination test for serum rheumatoid factor
9. Poor mucin precipitate from synovial fluid
10. Characteristic histopathologic changes in the synovial fluid
11. Definite rheumatoid arthritis is diagnosed when five of the criteria are satisfied. Arthritis criteria 1 to 5 must be present for at least 6 weeks.

[a]Data from the American Rheumatoid Association for the diagnosis of rheumatoid arthritis in humans.

3. There is variable degree of lameness and joint stiffness; symmetrical polyarthropathy usually is apparent.
4. The animal often has fever, lethargy, and inappetence.
5. The diagnosis is based on history, clinical signs, and radiographic findings and laboratory data.
6. The diagnosis may be based on serum rheumatoid factor (positive in approximately 75% of cases), synovial fluid analysis, and synovial biopsy.

Radiographic findings (Figure 5.3)

1. Periarticular soft tissue swelling and or distended joint capsule caused by joint effusion.
2. Decrease in width of joint space caused by cartilage destruction
3. Subchondral bone cysts and lytic changes in subchondral bone
4. Lytic changes at the attachment sites of ligaments in the juxtaarticular bone
5. Bone atrophy caused by disuse and hyperemic inflammation
6. Subluxation or luxation
7. Mineralization of the periarticular ligaments and/or joint capsule
8. Periarticular bony proliferation caused by periostitis and/or degenerative joint disease.

Reiter Disease

Clinical correlations

1. Has been reported in cats.
2. Is a progressive disease causing stiffness and lameness.

Radiographic findings

1. Marked periosteal new bone extending beyond the confines of the joint, usually most severe in the tarsal and carpal joints, but can also occur in the elbow and stifle joints.
2. Bone destruction and proliferation occurs at the attachment of the ligaments and tendons.

Feline Polyarthritis

Clinical correlations

1. Feline polyarthritis, also known as feline chronic progressive polyarthritis, occurs as a proliferative or deforming form of disease.
2. Inflammatory joint disease involving two or more joints and is characterized by inflammatory changes in the synovial membrane and systemic signs of illness (e.g., fever, malaise, anorexia).
3. Proliferative form occurs more commonly in young male cats and the erosive form in older male cats.
4. May be associated with infections of *Mycoplasma* species and L-form bacteria.
5. Secondary osteomyelitis may occur.
6. Arthritis usually is chronic and progressive.

Radiographic findings

1. Early changes are nonspecific, such as thickening and distension of the joint capsule and joint space widening caused by effusion.
2. Later radiographic changes may be erosive or nonerosive with periosteal changes on adjacent bones, pathologic fractures, and fibrous or bony ankylosis. In some cats, the lesions are only erosive and lack any periosteal reaction. Subluxation or luxation is common with the deforming form.
3. Cannot usually distinguish it from other arthritides, which have similar radiographic changes in the cat (e.g., Reiter disease).

Polyarthritis of the Greyhound

Clinical correlations

1. Usually affects young dogs, 3 to 30 months of age
2. Insidious onset with progressive lameness
3. Joint fluid indicates nonsuppurative polysynovitis
4. May be associated with *Mycoplasma spumans* infections

Radiographic findings

1. Polyarticular disease
2. Severe erosive disease with marked destruction of articular cartilage

Synovial Cell Sarcoma

Clinical correlations

1. More common in the larger appendicular joints (e.g., elbow, stifle).
2. Tumor can metastasize to the regional lymph nodes and lung.

Radiographic findings (Figure 5.4)

1. Early in the disease there is intraarticular and/or periarticular soft tissue swelling.
2. Later in the disease lytic lesions of multiple bones of a joint are commonly present and may be extensive.
3. Joint effusion or an intraarticular "mass" may be present. In the stifle, the patella may be displaced cranially.

Primary Bone Sarcoma

Clinical correlations

1. Primary bone sarcoma usually involve metaphyses of a long bone, and can occasionally extend into joint.
2. Osteosarcoma is the most common type. Other types of sarcomas include fibrosarcoma, chondrosarcoma, and hemangiosarcoma.
3. Prominent lameness and soft tissue swelling around the affected joint.

Radiographic findings

1. An admixture of aggressive osteolytic, osteoblastic lesions, and periosteal lesions are commonly present.
2. Radiographically, tumor types cannot be distinguished from one another.

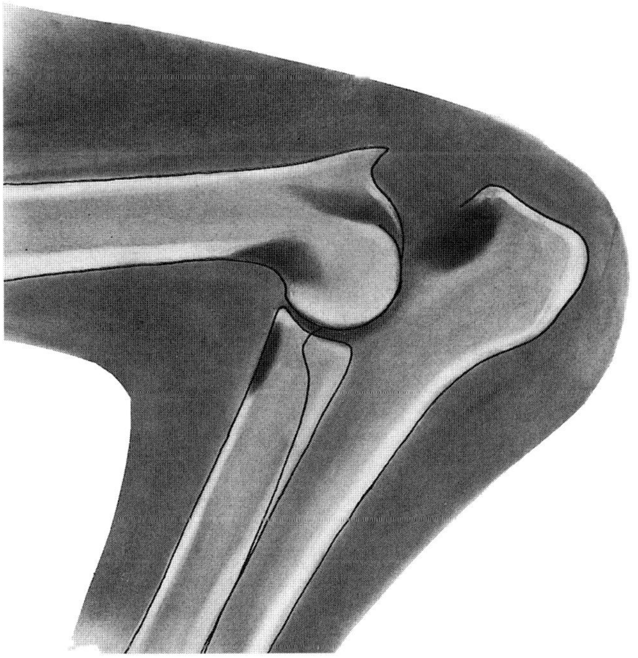

Figure 5.4. Synovial cell sarcoma in elbow causing lysis in humerus, ulna, and radius.

Metastatic Neoplasia
Clinical correlations
1. Metastatic tumors rarely involve the joints.
2. Feline lymphosarcoma can sometimes extend into synovial joints.

Radiographic findings
1. Soft tissue swelling is usually seen in periarticular or articular structures.
2. Subchondral lysis may be present.

Synovial Osteochondromatosis
Clinical correlations
1. Is a polyostotic joint disease, more common in cats than dogs.
2. Usually is bilateral and more often seen in mature cats.
3. In cats, most commonly seen in the stifle, elbow, shoulder, and digits.
4. In dogs, most commonly seen in the hip, stifle, and elbow.
5. Unknown cause, but it probably is attributable to metaplasia of synovial cells.
6. Usually, there is no lameness or other clinical signs, however affected joint may be stiff.

Radiographic findings (Figure 5.5 A, B)
1. Usually seen as bilateral symmetrical mineralization in a joint.
2. Mineralizations are often small.

Villonodular Synovitis
Clinical correlations
1. Rarely diagnosed in dogs and cats.
2. Thought to result from previous trauma or from chronic articular hemorrhage.
3. Joint fluid analysis indicative of mild inflammatory disease.
4. The diagnosis is based on synovial biopsy.

Radiographic findings
1. Subchondral cysts and/or lytic defects in the subchondral bone.
2. Radiographic signs can mimic synovial sarcoma.

SHOULDER

RADIOGRAPHIC TECHNIQUE
1. Heavy sedation (or, preferably, general anesthesia) is usually necessary for adequate positioning.
2. Standard projections:
   a. Lateral projection (Figures 5.6 and 5.7)
   b. Caudocranial projection (Figures 5.8 and 5.9)
3. Supplemental projections:
   a. Craniocaudal projection
   b. Lateral projections with pronation and supination
   c. Craniodistal-cranioproximal flexed projection

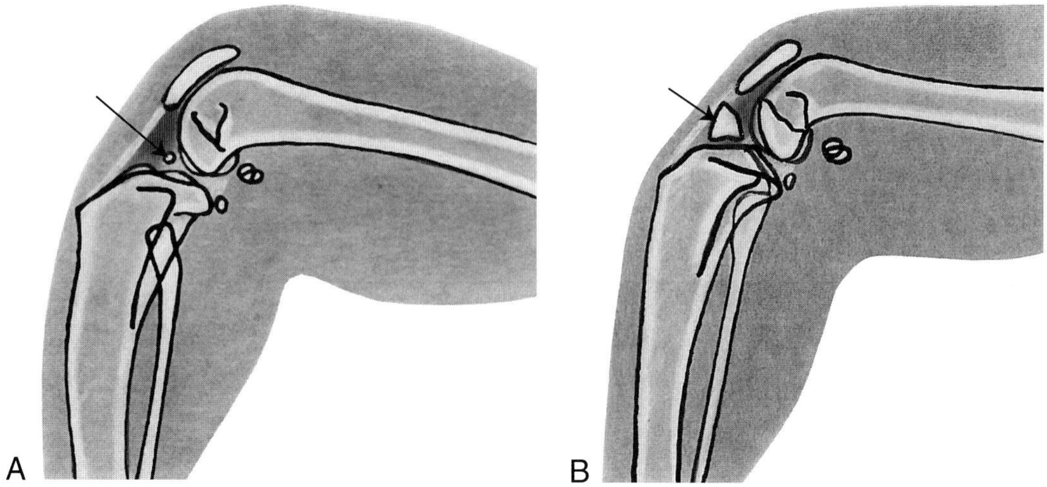

Figure 5.5. Synovial osteochondromatosis. Small **(A)** and larger **(B)** mineralized radiopacity within the cranial compartment of the stifle (arrow).

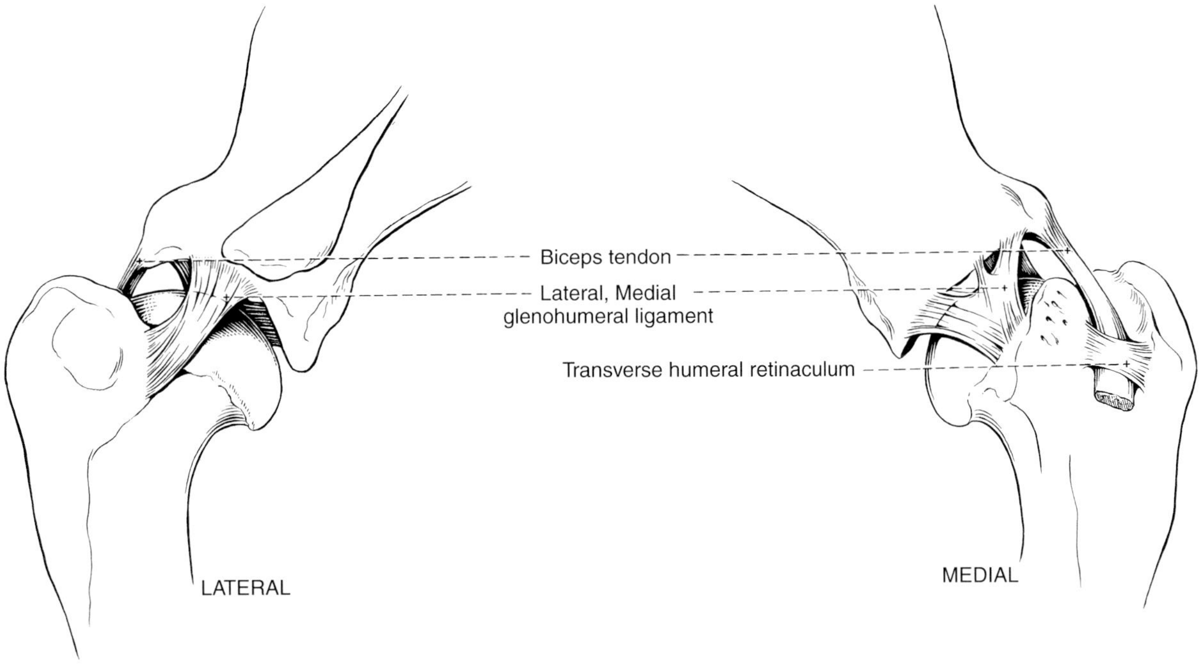

Figure 5.6. Left shoulder joint—lateral and medial views. (From Evans HE. Arthrology. In: Evans HE, ed. Miller's Anatomy of the Dog. 3rd ed. Philadelphia: W.B. Saunders; 1993:234. Courtesy of and with permission of Dr. Howard E. Evans.)

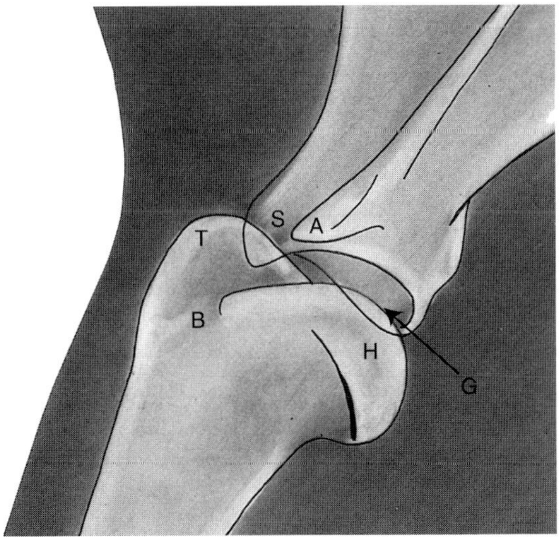

Figure 5.7. Normal canine shoulder (lateral projection). Major landmarks include humeral head **(H)**, greater tubercle **(T)**, bicipital groove **(B)**, scapular tuberosity **(S)**, and the glenoid cavity **(G)**. **(A)** is acromion.

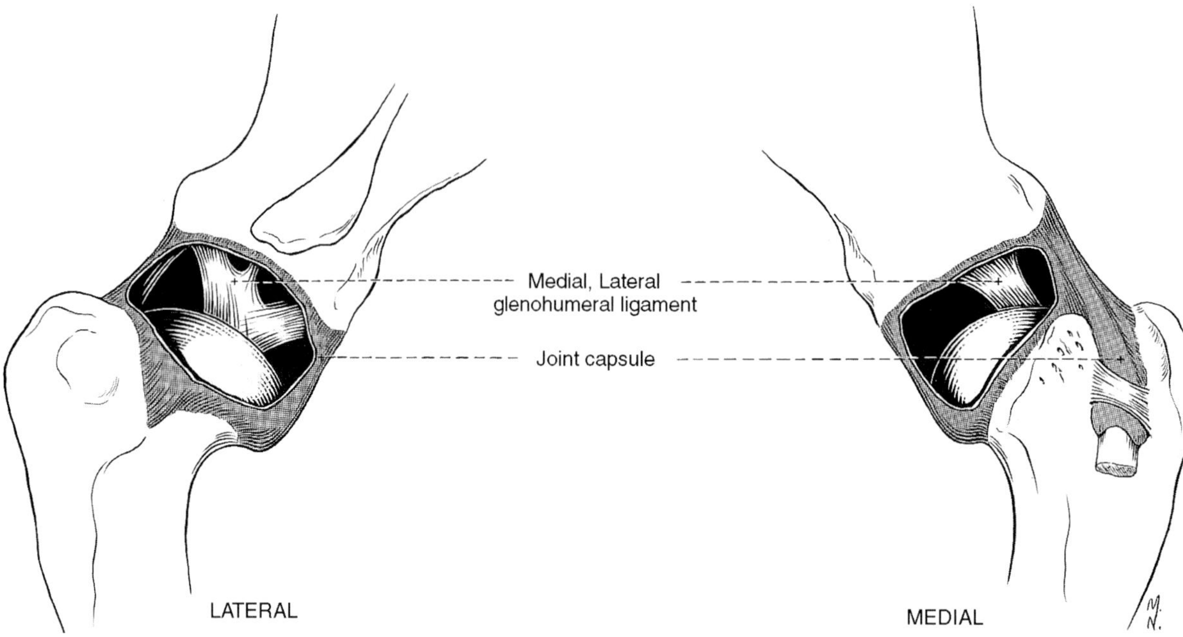

Figure 5.8. Capsule of left shoulder joint—lateral and medial views. (From Evans HE. Arthrology. In: Evans HE, ed. Miller's Anatomy of the Dog. 3rd ed. Philadelphia: W.B. Saunders; 1993:235. Courtesy of and with permission of Dr. Howard E. Evans.)

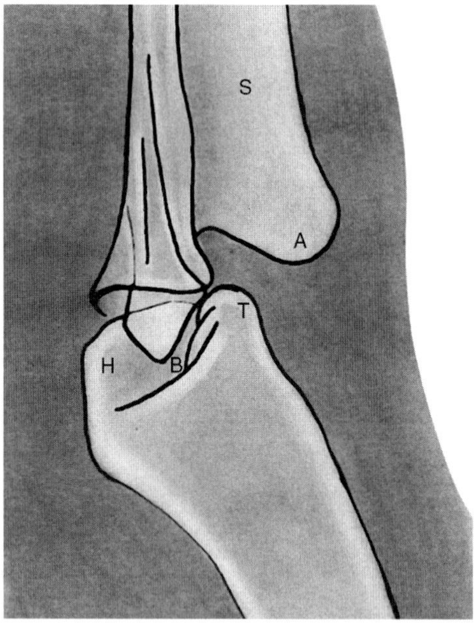

Figure 5.9. Normal canine shoulder (caudocranial projection). Major landmarks include humeral head **(H)**, greater tubercle **(T)**, bicipital groove **(B)**, acromion **(A)**, and spine of scapula **(S)**.

4. Contrast examinations:
   a. Positive contrast arthrogram
   b. Negative contrast arthrogram

DISEASES/DISORDERS

Luxation

Clinical correlations

1. Traumatic luxation of the shoulder can be cranial, lateral, or medial and is associated with tearing of the infraspinatus tendon, joint capsule, and glenohumeral ligament.
2. Medial luxations are more common in small breed dogs. Lateral luxations are more common in large breed dogs.
3. Congenital medial luxation (often bilateral), is seen most commonly in small dog breeds. It occurs because of laxity of the medial joint capsule and under development of the medial labrum of the glenoid. Most often it is recognized in the Chihuahua, Yorkshire Terrier, Miniature Poodle, Miniature Schnauzer, Japanese Spitz, and Pomeranian breeds.
4. On physical examination, the affected shoulder joint usually is painful on palpation, often with palpable crepitus.

Radiographic findings (Figure 5.10)

1. On the lateral view, an abnormal joint space (between the glenoid and humeral head) usually is identified.
2. Medial or lateral luxation is best diagnosed on the caudocranial projection.

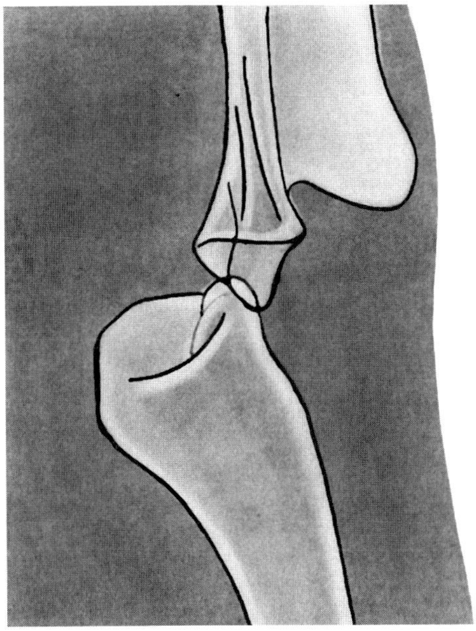

Figure 5.10. Luxation of shoulder. Humeral head is displaced medially.

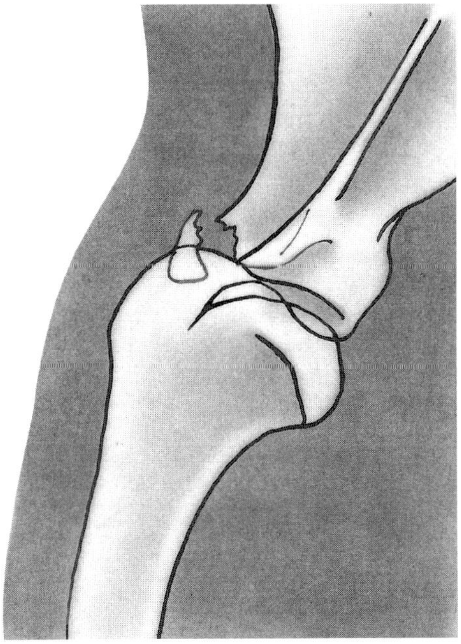

Figure 5.11. Avulsion of scapular tuberosity.

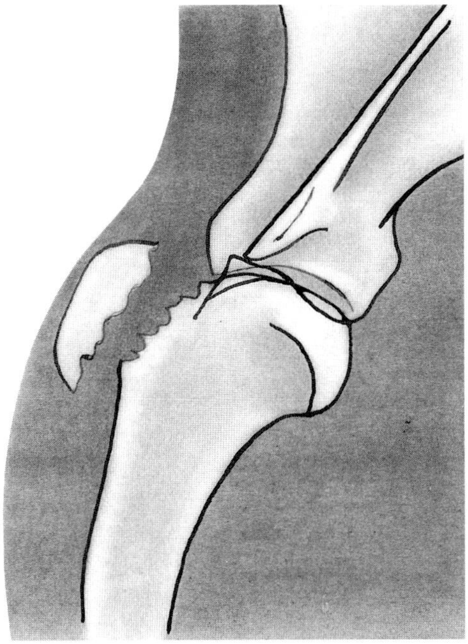

Figure 5.12. Avulsion of greater humeral tubercle.

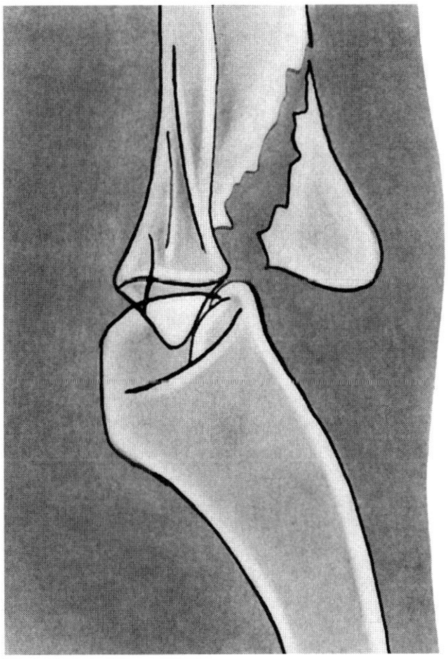

Figure 5.13. Avulsion of acromion and spine of scapula.

3. When positioning the shoulder for the radiographic examination, some luxations may spontaneously reduce.

Fracture

Clinical correlations

1. Fracture results from trauma and commonly involves a physes in immature animals.
2. There is an acute onset of non–weight-bearing lameness.

Radiographic findings

1. Common types of fractures include avulsion of:
   a. Scapular tuberosity (Figure 5.11)
   b. Greater tubercle of humerus (Figure 5.12)
   c. Acromion (Figure 5.13)

Osteochondrosis/Osteochondritis Dissecans (also see pages 74 and 93)

Clinical correlations

1. Lameness occurs when subchondral bone and cartilage degeneration cause an articular flap and involve the synovial joint.
2. Lameness usually is noticed in dogs 4 to 10 months of age, though some dogs are 12 months of age or older.
3. Is most common in large and giant breed dogs, but has been reported in more than 25 breeds.
4. More common in males
5. Lameness usually is unilateral, but lesions are present bilaterally in approximately 50% of the dogs.
6. An affected dog usually holds its leg slightly abducted and is reluctant to extend the shoulder.

Radiographic findings (Figures 5.14 and 5.15)

1. The most common finding is subchondral flattening or a radiolucent defect on the caudal articular surface of the humeral head. The radiolucent defect may represent either osteochondrosis or osteochondritis dissecans.
2. Osteochondritis dissecans may have:
   a. Mineralized cartilage flap
   b. Subchondral sclerosis
   c. Ossified free bodies, known as joint mice or osteochondromas, when present are usually in the caudal joint compartment or bicipital bursa. Need to differentiate free bodies from an ossicle sesamoid bone, or osteophyte on caudal glenoid margin (See Figure 4.6A).
   d. Degenerative joint disease is a common sequel.
3. Pronated and supinated lateral projections of the shoulder may be needed to identify the lesion.
4. Occasionally, a gas bubble may be visible within the joint. This is known as the vacuum phenomenon, and is created by a negative pressure within the joint allowing gas to enter the joint from the surrounding extracellular fluid. The vacuum phenomenon is not a radiographic finding of joint disease but is related to the technique of stress radiography.
5. Arthrography will delineate the articular cartilage, and usually will demonstrate a cartilage flap (if present) and the presence of free bodies as filling defects within the articular space.

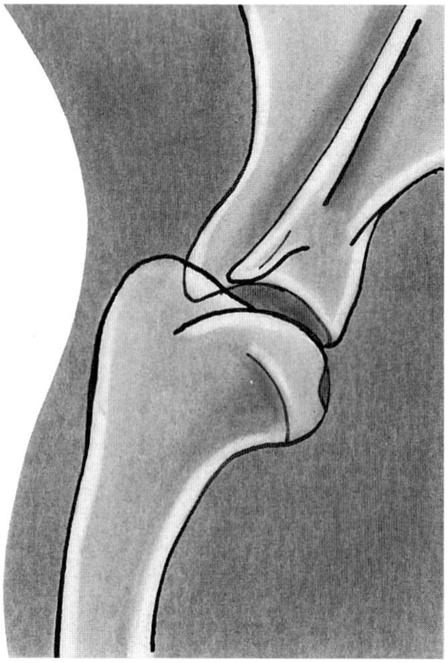

Figure 5.14. Osteochondrosis/osteochondritis dissecans. Flattened subchondral defect on caudal margin of humeral head.

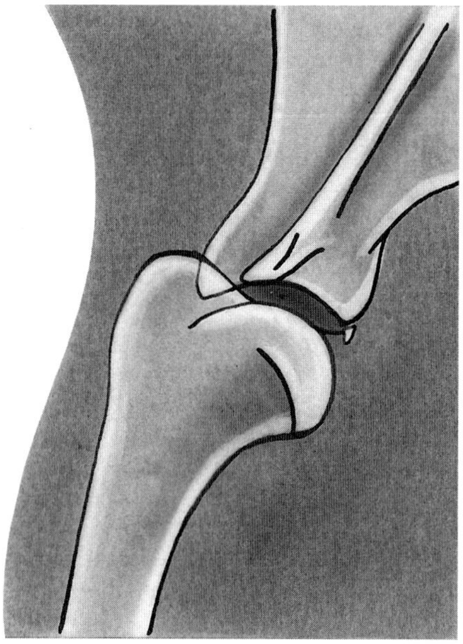

Figure 5.15. Normal accessory ossicle on caudal glenoid.

Biceps Tendinopathy

Clinical correlations

1. May be secondary to acute or chronic trauma or associated with chronic low grade inflammation (tenosynovitis).
2. The severity of injury ranges from incomplete separation of the tendon, often at the musculotendinous junction, to complete rupture of the tendon.
3. Clinical examination may reveal pain on palpation of the biceps muscle proximal to elbow or on flexion and palpation of the shoulder.

Radiographic findings (Figures 5.16 and 5.17)

1. Initially, the radiographs are normal, unless there is an avulsion fracture fragment of the tuber scapula.

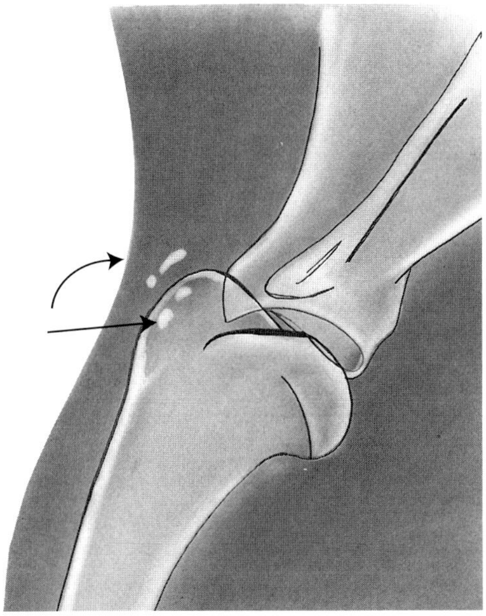

Figure 5.16. Mineralized opacities in the tendon of the infraspinatus muscle (straight arrow) and in the tendon of the supraspinatus muscle (curved arrow). These may represent sesamoid bones or foci of dystrophic calcification secondary to trauma.

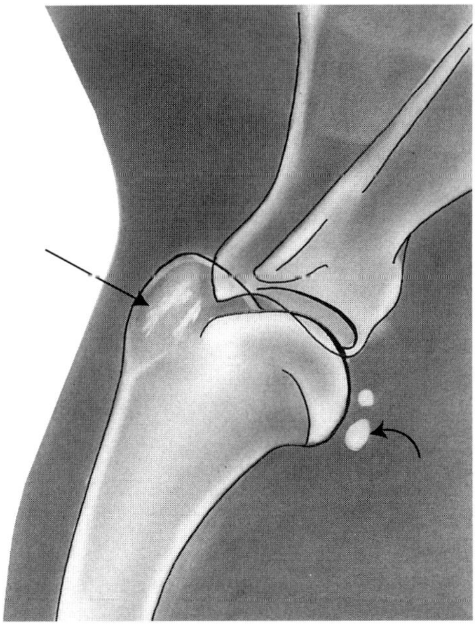

Figure 5.17. Bicipital tendinopathy (straight arrow) and joint mice (curved arrow).

2. With chronicity, mineralization may be visible within the tendon or within the intertubercular groove (e.g., on the lateral and craniodistal-cranioproximal flexed projections).
3. Secondary degenerative joint disease also may be present.
4. The observer must differentiate osteophytes from intraarticular free bodies as may occur in osteochondritis dissecans.
5. Arthrography can demonstrate abnormalities of the biceps tendon and the bursa.
   a. Incomplete filling of the bursa because of fibrosis or synovial hyperplasia of the joint capsule or tendon sheath.
   b. Irregularity of the tendon border
   c. Visualization of free bodies (as filling defects) within the contrast medium

Other imaging

1. Ultrasound
2. CT
3. MRI

Supraspinatus and Infraspinatus Tendinopathy

Clinical correlations

1. Most often seen in large breed dogs.
2. Presumably secondary to previous trauma.
3. Degree of lameness is variable.

Radiographic findings (Figure 5.16)

1. The lesion may be visualized on a lateral, caudocranial, or craniodistal-cranioproximal flexed projections.
2. In the supraspinatus tendon, mineralized opacities are often seen adjacent to the proximal aspect of the greater humeral tubercle.
3. In the infraspinatus tendon, mineralized opacities when present are seen superimposed over the greater tubercle, proximal to the bicipital bursa.
4. Difficult to differentiate from normal sesamoid bones.
5. Must differentiate from mineralization within the bicipital groove or bicipital tendon.

Shoulder Dysplasia

Clinical correlations

1. Is reported most often in Dachshunds.
2. Variable degree of lameness.

Radiographic findings

1. The humeral head is flattened, smaller than normal and sloped caudoventrally.
2. Malformation of the supraglenoid tubercle and glenoid cavity develops as a result of abnormal ossification.

Osteoarthritis

Clinical correlation

1. Is a degenerative joint disease, most often secondary to previous trauma, OCD, infection, or the result of immune mediated joint disease.

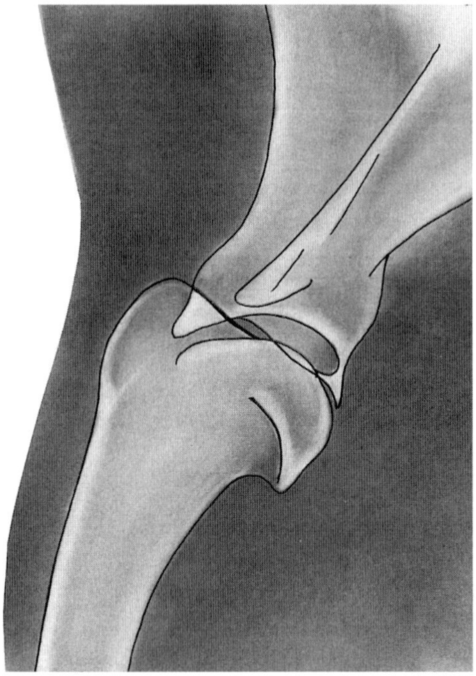

Figure 5.18. Degenerative joint disease. Proliferative bony changes are present on articular margins of humeral head and glenoid of scapula.

Radiographic finding (Figure 5.18)

1. Osteophytes commonly are seen on the caudal periarticular aspect of the humeral head and glenoid cavity (as seen on the lateral projection) and on the medial periarticular margins (as seen on the caudocranial projection).

ELBOW

RADIOGRAPHIC TECHNIQUE

1. Standard projections: (Figures 5.19 through 5.23)
   a. Lateral projections (neutral and flexed)
   b. Craniocaudal projection
2. Supplemental projections:
   a. Craniolateral-caudomedial oblique projection
   b. Cranial 10° caudomedial oblique projection
   c. Extreme flexed lateral projection
3. Contrast examination
   a. Arthrogram

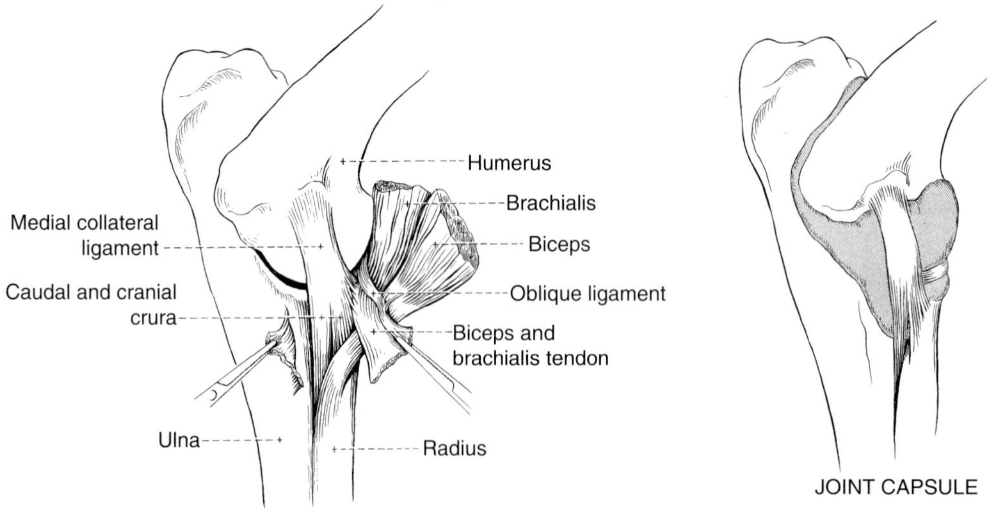

Figure 5.19. Left elbow joint, medial aspect. (From Evans HE. Arthrology. In: Evans HE, ed. Miller's Anatomy of the Dog. 3rd ed. Philadelphia: W.B. Saunders; 1993:236. Courtesy of and with permission of Dr. Howard E. Evans.)

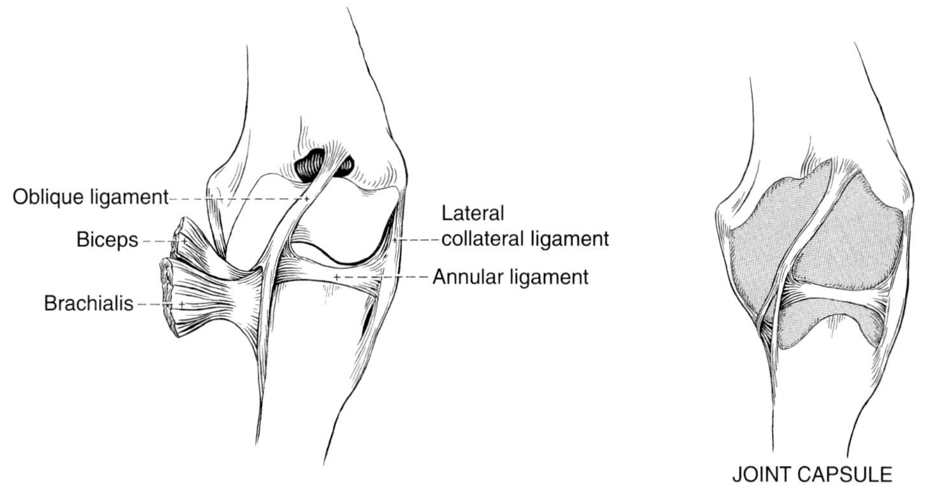

Figure 5.20. Left elbow joint, cranial aspect. (From Evans HE. Arthrology. In: Evans HE, ed. Miller's Anatomy of the Dog. 3rd ed. Philadelphia: W.B. Saunders; 1993:237. Courtesy of and with permission of Dr. Howard E. Evans.)

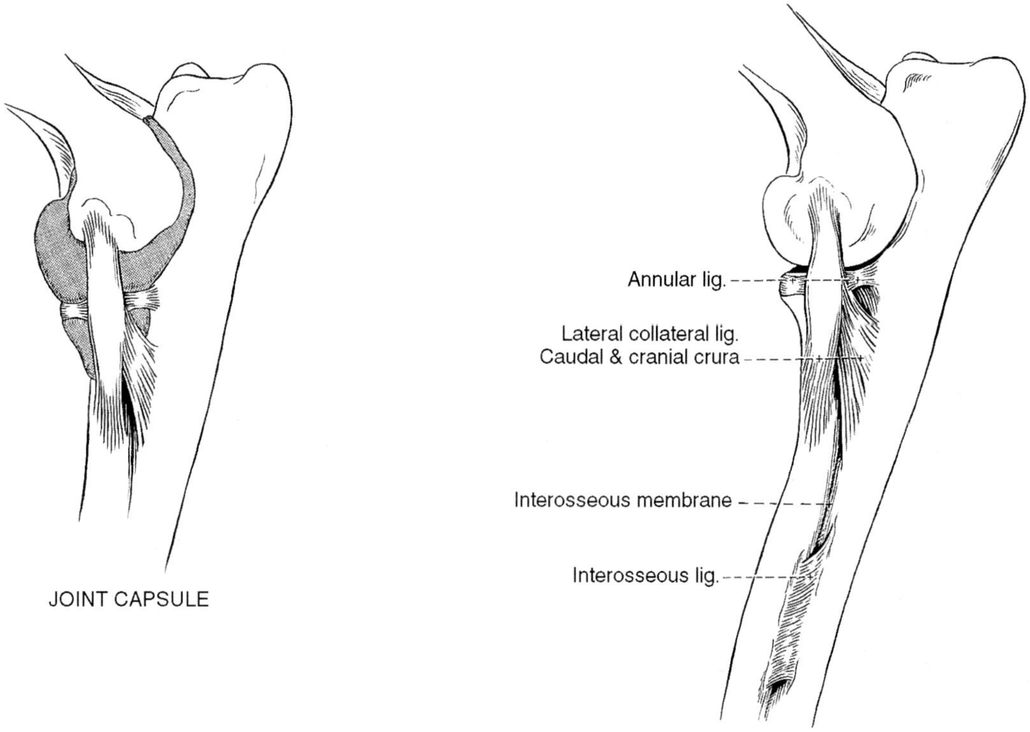

Figure 5.21. Left elbow joint, lateral aspect. (From Evans HE. Arthrology. In: Evans HE, ed. Miller's Anatomy of the Dog. 3rd ed. Philadelphia: W.B. Saunders; 1993:237. Courtesy of and with permission of Dr. Howard E. Evans.)

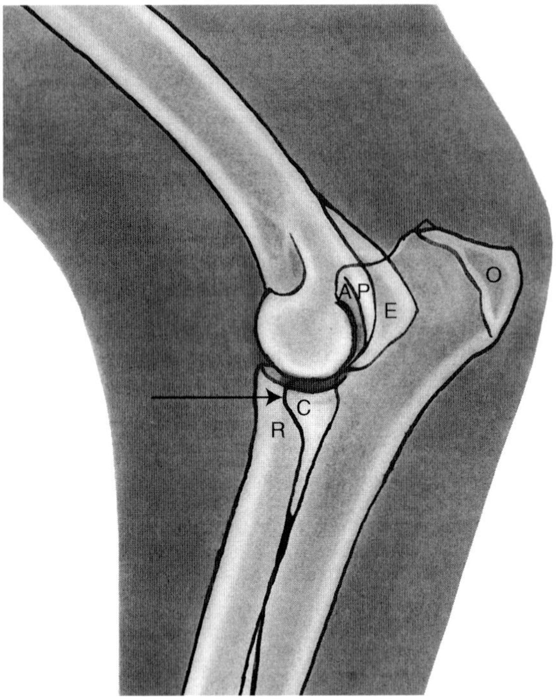

Figure 5.22. Normal canine elbow (lateral projection). Major landmarks are radial head **(R)**, olecranon **(O)**, anconeal process **(AP)**, medial humeral epicondyle **(E)**, and medial coronoid process **(C)** (arrow).

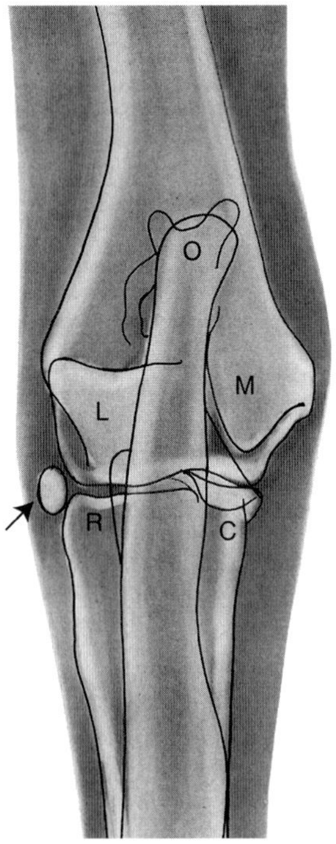

Figure 5.23. Normal canine elbow (craniocaudal Projection). Major landmarks are radial head **(R)**, olecranon **(O)**, medial humeral condyle **(M)**, lateral humeral condyle **(L)**, and medial coronoid process **(C)**. Note sesamoid bone in the tendon of the supinator muscle (arrow), a variant of normal.

DISEASES/DISORDERS

Elbow Dysplasia

Clinical correlations

1. A developmental abnormality that leads to malformation and degenerative disease of the elbow joint.
2. Subclassification of elbow dysplasias includes:
   a. Osteochondritis dissecans
   b. Fragmented medial coronoid process (FMCP)
   c. Ununited anconeal process (UAP)
   d. Distractio cubiti (elbow incongruity)
3. Is inheritable in many breeds of dogs, usually large breed dogs.
4. Affected dogs often exhibit lameness from 4 to 18 months of age; however, many affected dogs have no lameness.
5. Affected dogs may have one or more forms of elbow dysplasia, and the lesions are commonly bilateral.
6. Fragmented medial coronoid process (FMCP), ununited anconeal process (UAP), and OC of the humeral condyle are each considered to be a form of OC.

Radiographic findings

1. The International Elbow Working Group (IEWG) recommends that screening registries use the following radiographic criteria for the diagnosis of elbow dysplasia:
   a. Arthrosis—The degree of arthrosis is based on the osteophyte thickness on the proximal nonarticular margin of the anconeal process.
      1) Mild—less than 2 mm
      2) Moderate—from 2 mm to 5 mm
      3) Severe—more than 5 mm
   b. Malformed or fragmented medial coronoid process
   c. Ununited anconeal process
   d. Osteochondrosis of the humeral condyle
   e. Incongruity of the articular surface
   f. Mineralization in the deep tendon, caudal to the medial condyle
2. Other imaging
   a. CT
   b. MRI

Osteochondrosis/Osteochondritis of Humeral Condyle

Radiographic findings (Figure 5.24)

1. Is seen as a subchondral radiolucent bone defect on the medial humeral articular surface, usually best seen on the craniocaudal and oblique projections.
2. Degenerative joint disease, characterized by periarticular osteophytes and subchondral sclerosis, is commonly present.

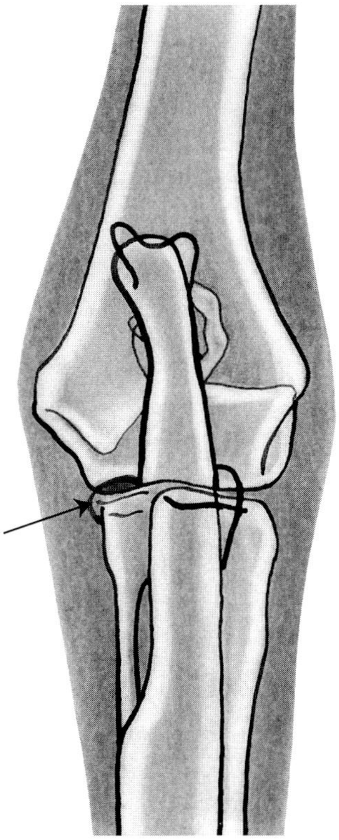

Figure 5.24. Osteochondrosis/osteochondritis dissecans. Subchondral defect on the medial humeral condyle (arrow).

Ununited Anconeal Process

Radiographic findings (Figure 5.25)

1. A radiolucent cleavage line is observed between the anconeal process and proximal ulna. This is seen best on the flexed lateral projection. (The anconeal process is a separate ossification center in most medium and large breed dogs, and normally ossifies and unites to the proximal ulna before 20 weeks of age.)
2. Degenerative joint disease, characterized by periarticular osteophytes and subchondral sclerosis, is commonly present and usually progressive.
3. Must differentiate UAP from fracture of the anconeal process, which results from trauma or disproportionate growth of radius/ulna.

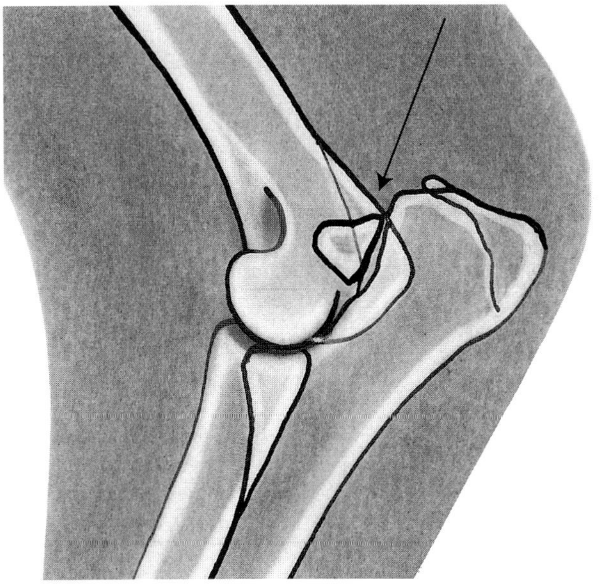

Figure 5.25. Ununited anconeal process (arrow).

Fragmented Medial Coronoid Process (FMCP)

Radiographic findings (Figures 5.26, 5.27, and 5.28)

1. Fragmented medial coronoid process is seldom visualized on radiographs.
2. Diagnosis is commonly presumptive and based on the radiographic presence of degenerative joint disease.
3. Degenerative joint disease is commonly characterized by osteophyte formation on the proximal nonarticular margin of the anconeal process, medial epicondyle, and the cranial margin of the radial head. Changes on the proximal margin of the anconeal process are best seen on an extreme flexed lateral projection.
4. Sclerosis of the coronoid process and trochlear notch, and/or a "step-like" subluxation between the articular surface of the radial head and the proximal ulna is commonly present.
5. Additional changes, associated with a concurrent me-

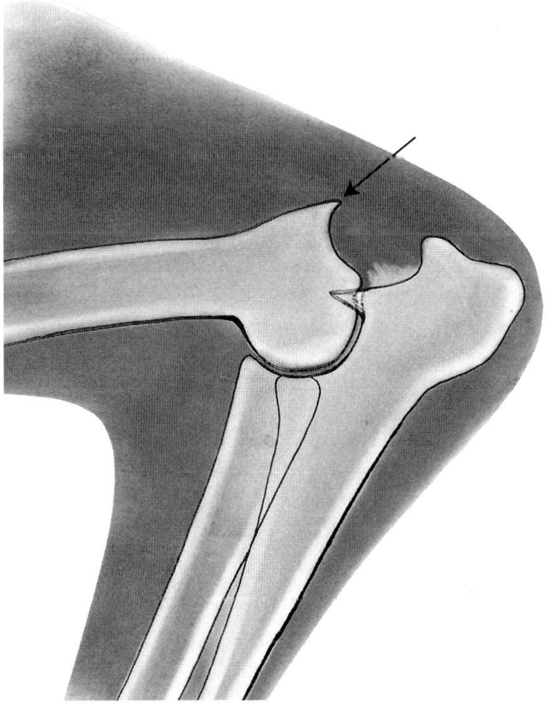

Figure 5.26. Elbow dysplasia (flexed lateral projection). Periosteal bone is present on proximal margin of the anconeal process. Also note spur on medical epicondyle (arrow).

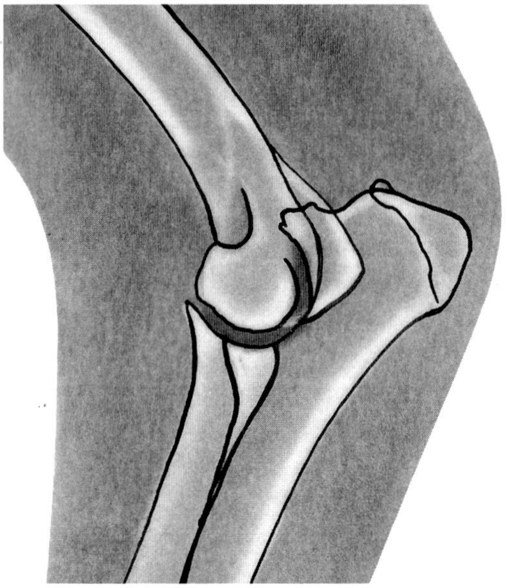

Figure 5.27. Degenerative joint disease. Osteophytes are present on the articular margins.

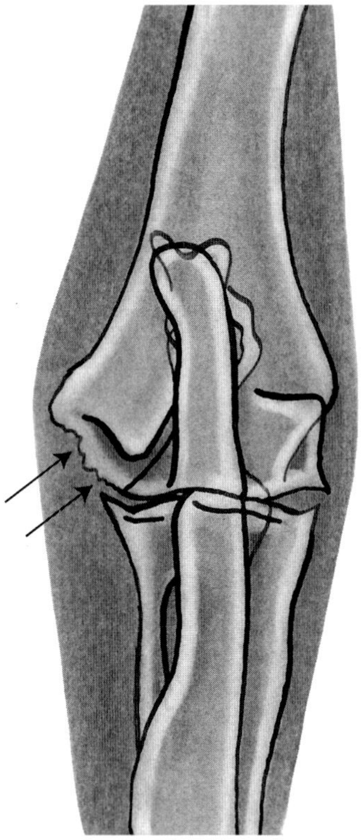

Figure 5.28. Degenerative joint disease of elbow secondary to elbow dysplasia. Osteophytes are prominent on the medial condyle and epicondyle (arrows).

dial fragmented coronoid process and/or ununited anconeal process, may be present.

Other imaging

1. CT
2. MRI

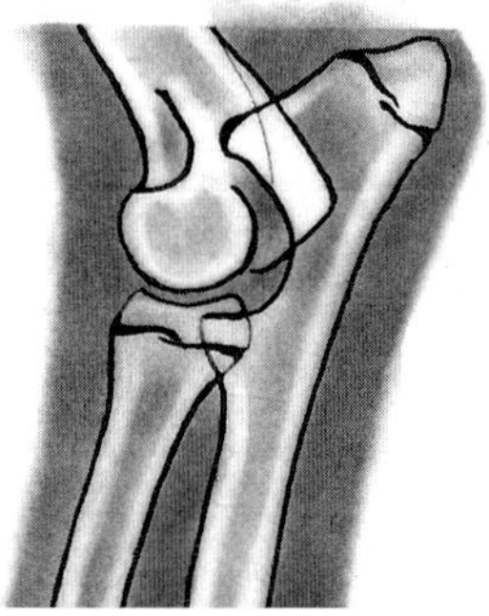

Figure 5.29. Distractio cubiti. Humeroulnar subluxation is secondary to disproportionately shorter ulna compared to radius.

Distractio Cubiti

Radiographic findings (Figure 5.29)

1. Distractio cubiti is also known as elbow incongruity.
2. Subluxation of humeroulnar joint results from asynchronous growth of the radius and ulna, and is usually best identified on the lateral projection.
   a. Is often bilateral.
   b. Chondrodystrophoid breeds are most commonly affected (i.e., Basset Hound, Dachshund, Welsh Corgi).
3. Degenerative joint disease, characterized by periarticular osteophytes and subchondral sclerosis, is commonly present and often progressive.
4. Must differentiate from other causes of elbow subluxation and asynchronous growth of radius and ulna (e.g., premature closure of distal ulna physis, retained enchondral cartilage of the distal ulna).

Incomplete Ossification of Humeral Condyle

Clinical correlations

1. There is incomplete ossification of distal humeral condyle where normal fusion occurs between the medial and lateral centers of ossification; is usually bilateral.
2. Ossification defect predisposes to fracture through the condyles with involvement of elbow joint.
3. Inheritance in Spaniels is probably recessive, with most reported in the Cocker Spaniel and Brittany Spaniel.
4. Affected dog usually develops an acute lameness caused by fracture through the intercondylar defect.

Radiographic findings (Figure 5.30 A, B)

1. Curvilinear radiolucent line is seen between the humeral condyles, with other long bone physes closed.
2. A displaced fracture of the distal humerus through the site of incomplete ossification may be identified.
3. Concurrent elbow arthrosis may also be present.

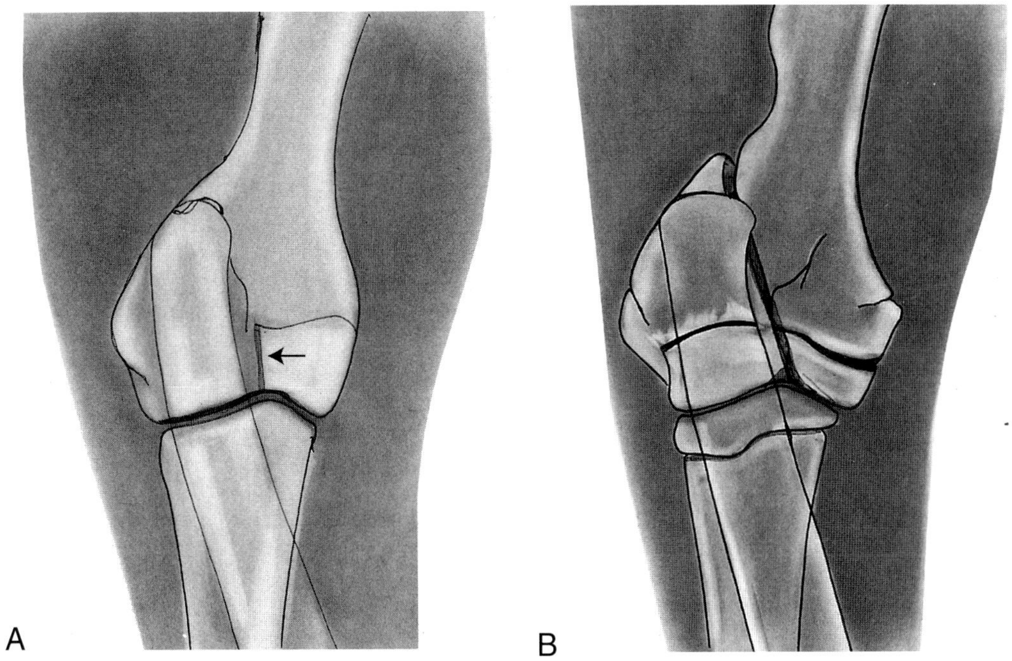

Figure 5.30. **A)** Incomplete ossification between medial and lateral humeral condyle (arrow). **B)** Fractured humeral condyle as sequel to trauma in incomplete ossification of the humeral condyle.

Luxation

Clinical correlations

1. Is usually caused by trauma.
2. Concurrent medial and lateral collateral ligament injury usually is present.

Radiographic findings

1. May have a small avulsion fracture associated with ligament injury.
2. Humeroradial joint luxation is often associated with a concurrent fracture of ulna (Figure 5.31).

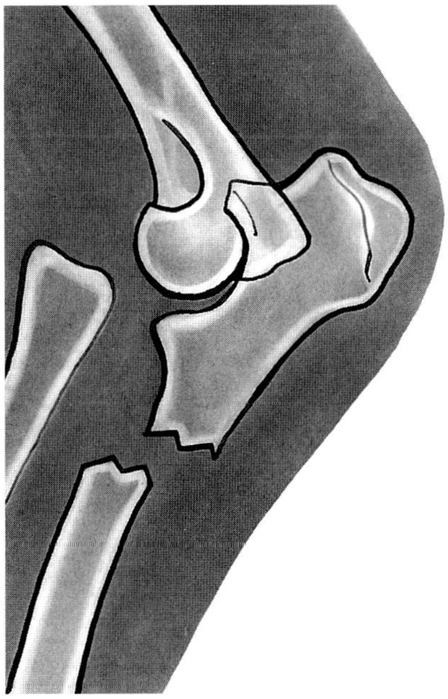

Figure 5.31. Monteggia fracture—ulnar fracture with humeroradial joint luxation.

Subluxation

Clinical correlations

1. Is usually secondary to growth plate (physis) injuries.
2. Premature closure of the distal ulna, causes shortening and distal subluxation of the humeroulnar joint, and may cause fracture of the anconeal process.
3. Premature closure of the distal radius may cause proximal subluxation of the humeroulnar joint and fracture of the medial coronoid process of the ulna.
4. Differentiate from distractio cubiti

Radiographic findings (Figure 5.32)

1. An abnormal joint space, affecting the humeroulnar or humeroradial joints
2. Comparison radiographs with the contralateral limb help to visualize the presence and degree of subluxation.

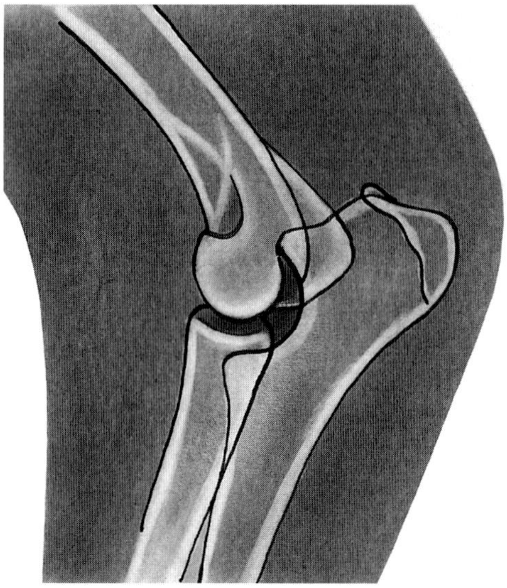

Figure 5.32. Humeroulnar joint subluxation secondary to growth deformity.

Medial Epicondylar Spur

Clinical correlations

1. Medial epicondylar spur is also known as flexor enthesopathy.
2. Is usually seen in large breed dogs.
3. There is variable degree of lameness, which often resolves with time.
4. May be traumatic or associated with osteochondrosis.

Radiographic findings (Figure 5.33)

1. On the lateral projection, an irregular spur or bony proliferation is seen extending caudally from the medial epicondylar ridge.
2. On the craniocaudal projection, focal mineralization is seen in the deep tendon medial and distal to the medial epicondyle.

CARPUS

RADIOGRAPHIC TECHNIQUE

1. Standard projections: (Figure 5.34 A, B)
   a. Craniocaudal projection
   b. Lateral projection
2. Supplemental projections:
   a. Medial and lateral oblique projections
   b. Flexed lateral projection
   c. Extended lateral projection
   d. Standing lateral projection (weight bearing)

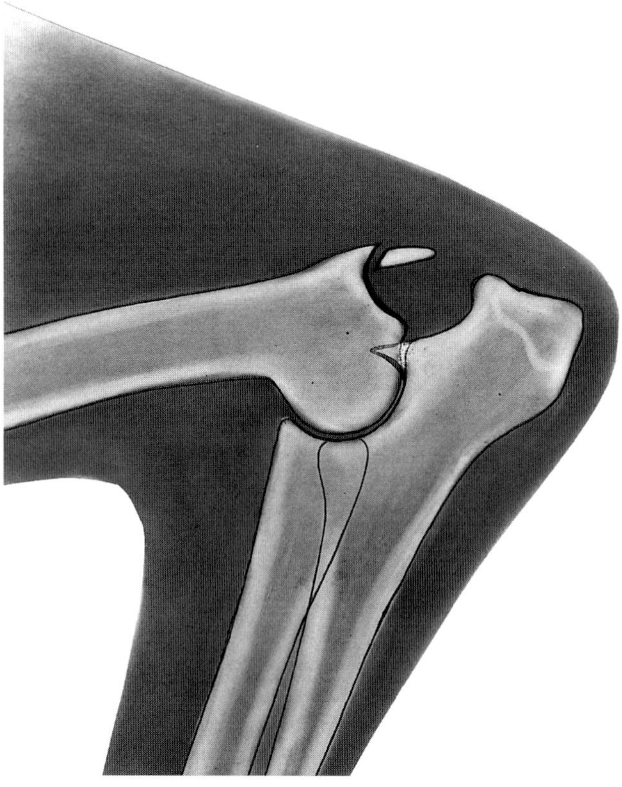

Figure 5.33. Medial humeral epicondylar spur and mineralization within the deep tendon.

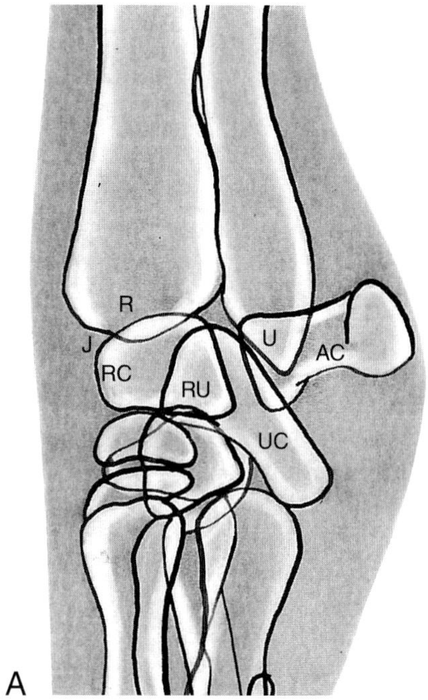

Figure 5.34. **A)** Normal canine carpus (lateral projection). Major landmarks are ulnar styloid **(U)**, distal radius **(R)**, radiocarpal joint **(J)**, radiocarpal bone **(RC)**, ulnar carpal bone **(UC)**, accessory carpal bone **(AC)**, superimposition of radiocarpal and ulnarcarpal bones **(RU)**.

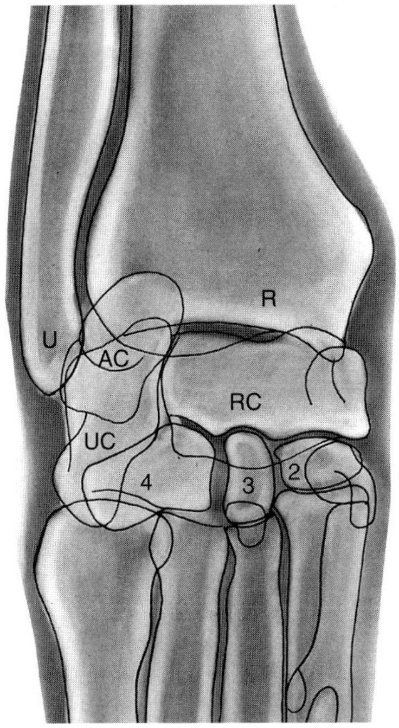

Figure 5.34. ***(continued)* B)** Normal canine carpus (craniocaudal projection). The major landmarks include the ulnar styloid **(U)**, the distal radius **(R)**, the carpal bones including accessory carpal **(AC)** radiocarpal **(RC)**, ulnar carpal bone **(UC)**, and carpal bones 2, 3, and 4 labeled accordingly.

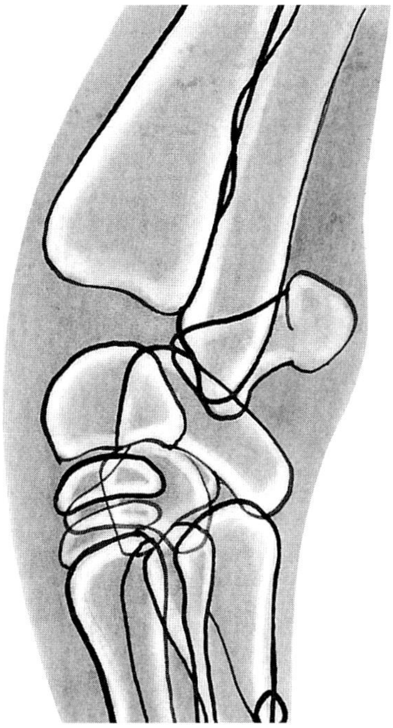

Figure 5.35. Radiocarpal joint subluxation.

DISEASES/DISORDERS

Luxation/Subluxation

Clinical correlations

1. Most often is seen in aged, overweight, or large breed dogs, resulting from repeated low-grade trauma with variable hyperextension of the carpus.
2. Acute hyperextension injury causes tearing of the palmar ligaments of the antebrachiocarpal, intercarpal, and carpometacarpal joints. It also tears the accessory carpal ligament, which anatomically extends from the distal border of the accessory carpal bone to the proximal caudal aspect of the 5th metacarpal bone.
3. Medial and lateral carpal instability usually is caused by injury to the radial or ulnar collateral ligaments.
4. Subluxation is more common than luxation.
5. Is often associated with avulsion, compression, or chip fractures of the carpal and proximal metacarpal bones.

Radiographic findings (Figure 5.35)

1. There may be an increased joint space or joint malalignment.
2. Articular or periarticular fractures may be present.
3. With chronic injury (or reinjury), periarticular osteophytes and periosteal reaction is usually present.
4. Optimally, radiographs should include oblique and stress projections to best demonstrate joint instability. Comparison radiographs of contralateral limb are frequently helpful.

Fracture

Clinical correlations

1. Often is associated with other injuries (e.g., strains, joint subluxation/luxation).
2. Fractures of the carpus are commonly chip, slab, or avulsion types.
3. Avulsion fractures of the distal radius and/or ulna is usually indicative of carpal instability.

Radiographic findings (Figure 5.36)

1. Identification of many of the fractures often necessitates oblique radiographic projections or other supplemental projections (e.g., stress radiographs with flexion, extension, and rotation).

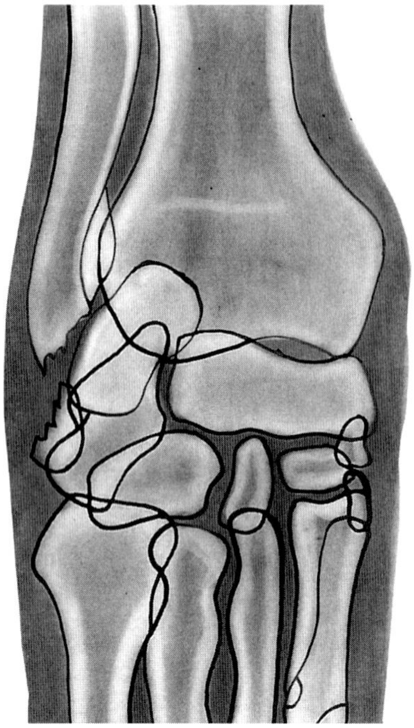

Figure 5.36. Fracture of ulnar styloid.

DIGITS — METACARPUS/ METATARSUS/ PHALANGES

RADIOGRAPHIC TECHNIQUE

1. Standard projections:
   a. Dorsopalmar/dorsoplantar projection.
   b. Lateral projection.
2. Supplemental projection:
   a. Oblique lateral projection

RADIOGRAPHIC ANATOMY (Figures 5.37 through 5.40)

1. Most dogs and cats have four metacarpal and four metatarsal bones with five digits.
2. Each metacarpal and metatarsal bones has two ossification centers: diaphysis and distal epiphysis.

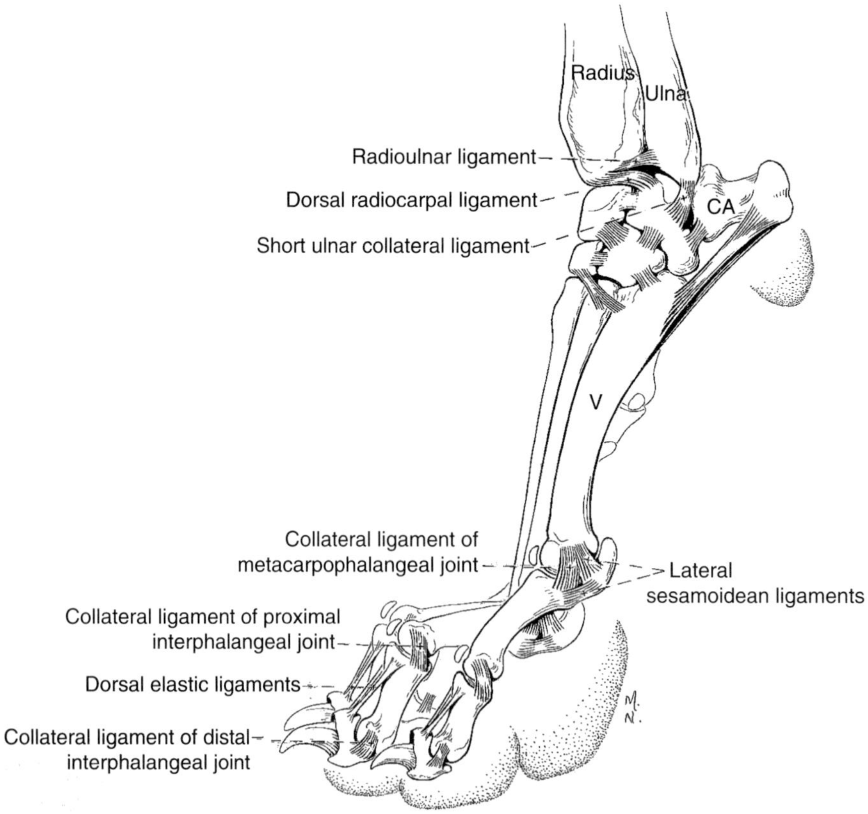

Figure 5.37. Ligaments of the left forepaw, lateral aspect. (From Evans HE. Arthrology. In: Evans HE, ed. Miller's Anatomy of the Dog. 3rd ed. Philadelphia: W.B. Saunders; 1993:242. Courtesy of and with permission of Dr. Howard E. Evans.)

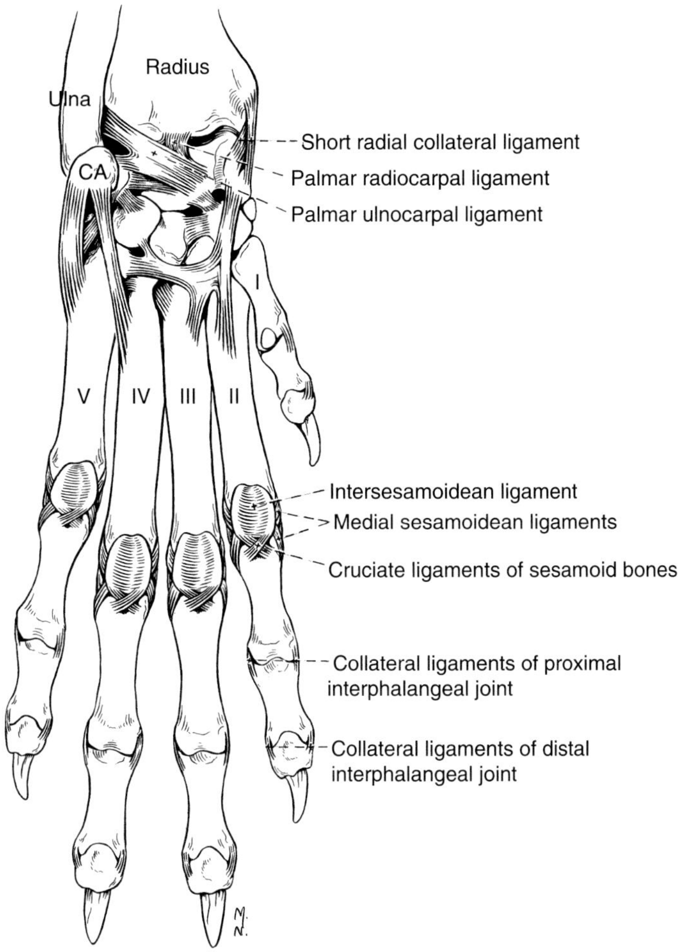

Figure 5.38. Deep ligaments of left forepaw, palmar aspect. (From Evans HE. Arthrology. In: Evans HE, ed. Miller's Anatomy of the Dog. 3rd ed. Philadelphia: W.B. Saunders; 1993:240. Courtesy of and with permission of Dr. Howard E. Evans.)

3. On each digit, numbered from medial to lateral (as 2 through 5), there are three phalanges. The first digit (dewclaw) is variably developed and commonly has only two phalanges.
4. Each phalanx has a single ossification center.
5. Normally, there are three sesamoid bones present in each metacarpophalangeal and metatarsophalangeal joint.
   a. Single dorsal sesamoid
   b. Paired palmar and plantar sesamoids
      1) Numbered from medial to lateral as 1 through 8.
      2) One or more palmar and plantar sesamoids may be multipartite, commonly on digits 2 and 5 in dogs.

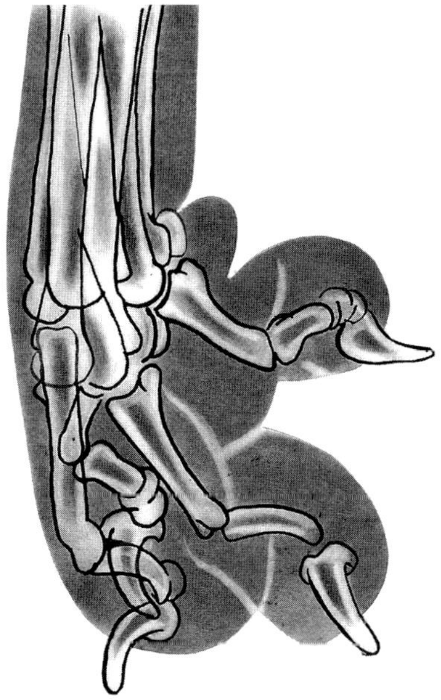

Figure 5.39. Normal canine foot (lateral projection).

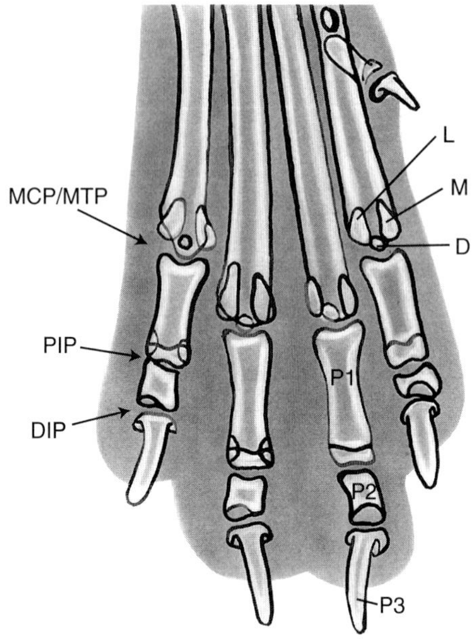

Figure 5.40. Normal canine foot (dorsopalmar/dorsoplantar projection). Major landmarks are metacarpal-phalangeal and corresponding metatarsal-phalangeal joints (MCP/MTP), proximal interphalangeal joints (PIP), and distal interphalangeal joints (DIP). There are two palmar (plantar) sesamoid bones (L&M) and a singular dorsal sesamoid bone (D) immediately proximal to the MCP and MTP joints.

DISEASES/DISORDERS

Fracture/Luxation

Clinical correlations

1. Digits are subject to trauma including luxation, subluxation, and fracture.
2. Fractures may be articular

Radiographic findings

1. Usually, fractures are readily identified.
2. Luxations may require two views to adequately assess.
3. If digits are not seen in profile, a normal digit can mimic the appearance of being subluxated.
4. Soft tissue swelling usually is visible.

Sesamoid Bone Fractures

Clinical correlations

1. Fractures are associated with hyperextension injury to digits, and most often affect the palmar sesamoids 2 and 7.
2. They are seen most often in heavy, large breed dogs.
3. Often seen in racing greyhounds, in the right front foot.

Radiographic findings

1. One or more fracture lines is seen with osteonecrosis and/or displacement of the fracture fragments.
2. Soft tissue swelling is variably present.
3. It is often difficult to differentiate fracture of a palmar or plantar sesamoid bone from a multipartite sesamoid anomaly (Figure 5.41).

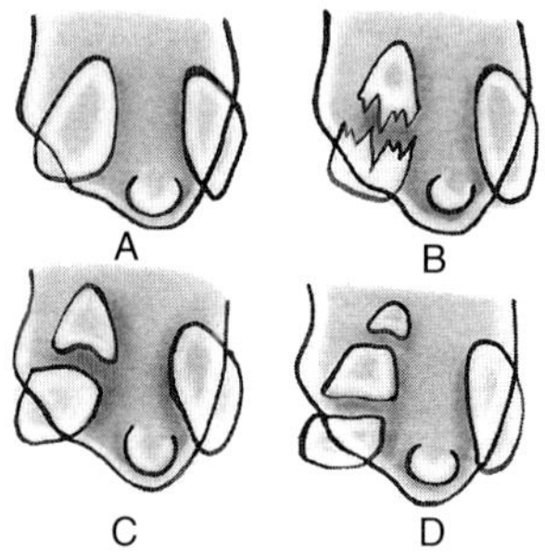

Figure 5.41. Phalangeal sesamoid bones. Normal paired palmar (plantar) sesamoid bones are depicted in **(A)**, a fracture of a sesamoid bone **(B)**, congenital bipartite **(C)** and tripartite sesamoid **(D)** bones.

Digital Neoplasia

Clinical correlations

1. Usually occurs in older dogs and cats.
2. One digit is affected with soft tissue swelling and pain. Occasionally, multiple digits on one or more feet can be involved.
3. Squamous cell carcinoma and malignant melanoma are the most common tumors.
4. Surgical biopsy often is necessary to differentiate from benign conditions (i.e., bone cyst, chronic osteomyelitis, or nail bed infection).

Radiographic findings (Figure 5.42)

1. Variable amounts of osteolysis of the third phalanx

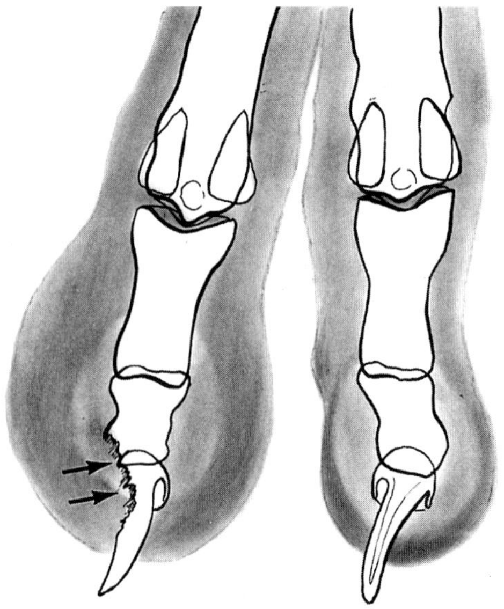

Figure 5.42. Soft tissue tumor of digit. Localized soft tissue swelling and bone lysis of second and third phalanges are seen.

2. Minimal or no periosteal reaction, unless complicated by infection
3. Nonspecific soft tissue swelling or mass
4. Differential diagnosis:
   a. Osteomyelitis—usually has periosteal reaction and extends proximally to involve the second phalanx—often with erosive arthritis of the distal interphalangeal joint (DIP)
   b. Intraosseous, epidermoid bone cyst—usually has focal lysis in the ungual process

THE COXOFEMORAL JOINTS AND PELVIS

RADIOGRAPHIC TECHNIQUE

1. Standard projections:
   a. Lateral projection
   b. Ventrodorsal hip extended projection
2. Supplemental projections:
   a. Frog-legged ventrodorsal projection
   b. Oblique lateral projection
   c. Dorsal acetabular rim projection (DAR)
   d. PennHIP (Synbiotics Corporation, San Diego, CA) distraction/compression projections

RADIOGRAPHIC ANATOMY (Figures 5.43 A, B and 5.44)

1. The acetabulum is formed by the union of the ilium, ischium, pubis and acetabular bone. These bones fuse at approximately 4 months of age.
2. An accessory ossification center is sometimes present at the craniodorsal acetabular rim (See Figure 4.10).
3. The proximal femur includes the head, neck, and three trochanters (greater, lesser, and third).
4. The hip includes the femoral head and acetabulum.

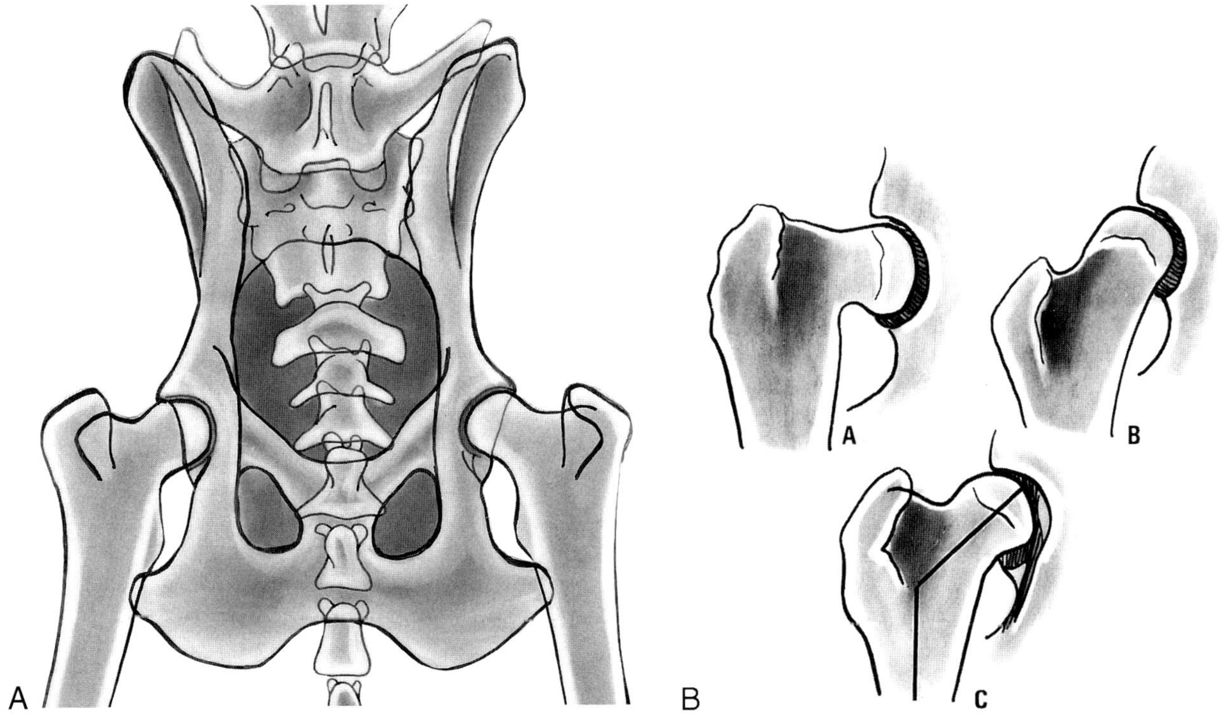

Figure 5.43. **A)** Normal canine pelvis and hips (ventrodorsal projection). **B)** Angle of the femoral neck. Coxofemoral joint conformation is in part determined by the angle between the femoral neck and femoral diaphysis. Coxa vara **(A)** and coxa valga **(B)** are compared with the normal angle **(C)**, which is approximately 130°.

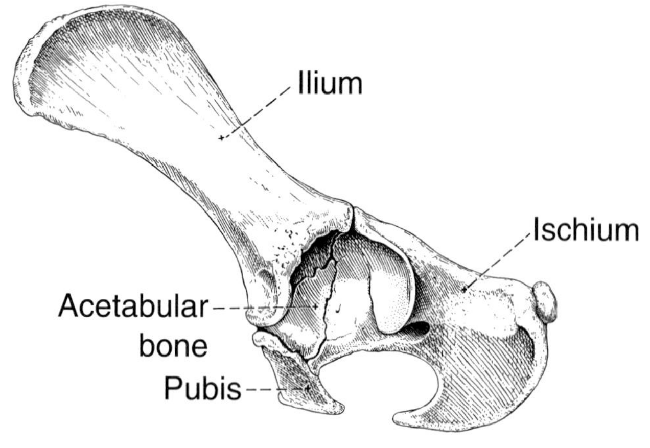

Figure 5.44. Left os coxae of young dog (lateral aspect). (From Evans HE. The Skeleton. In: Evans HE, ed. Miller's Anatomy of the Dog. 3rd ed. Philadelphia: W.B. Saunders; 1993:199. Courtesy of and with permission of Dr. Howard E. Evans.)

DISEASES/DISORDERS

Coxofemoral Luxation (other than associated with hip dysplasia)

Clinical correlations

1. Is the most commonly luxated joint in dogs and cats.
2. Is usually associated with blunt trauma.
3. Lameness usually is non–weight-bearing.
4. Limb usually is held adducted with some external rotation.
5. Commonly, other injuries also are present (i.e., soft tissue injuries of the urethra, bladder and rectum, ruptured urinary bladder, or diaphragmatic hernia).

Radiographic findings (Figure 5.45)

1. Most luxations are craniodorsal.
2. Caudoventral and medial luxations are less common.
3. Medial luxation is associated with acetabular fracture.
4. Lateral and ventrodorsal projections may be necessary for a diagnosis. Supplemental oblique lateral, or frog-legged ventrodorsal projections, may also be necessary, especially to evaluate for fractures of the acetabulum and other bony structures.
5. Common types of avulsion fractures:
   a. Insertion of round ligament (fovea capitus)
   b. Greater trochanter of femur

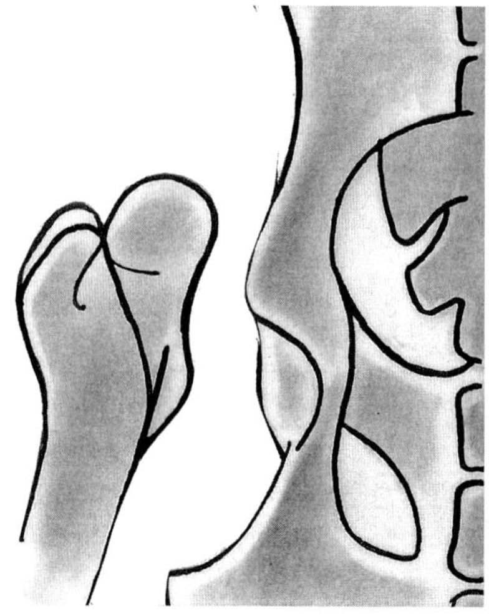

Figure 5.45. Coxofemoral luxation with craniolateral luxation of femoral head.

Fractures of the Pelvis

Clinical correlations

1. Fracture usually involves more than one bone of the pelvis.
2. If only one bone is fractured, a concurrent sacroiliac luxation is usually present.
3. The trauma may cause soft tissue injuries to urethra, bladder, rectum, and nerves (sciatic and pelvic).
4. Clinical problems with defecation and parturition may occur as a sequel to a narrowed pelvic canal and displaced pelvic fracture fragment.

Radiographic findings (Figure 5.46)

1. In addition to the standard lateral and ventrodorsal radiographic projections, oblique views may be necessary to identify all fractures adequately.
2. Fractures usually become displaced and are easily identified.
3. Commonly, other lesions are present (e.g., sacroiliac luxation, coccygeal fracture, retroperitoneal hematoma).
4. In patients with hematuria or a peritoneal effusion, consider urethrocystography and/or intravenous urography to evaluate urinary tract integrity.

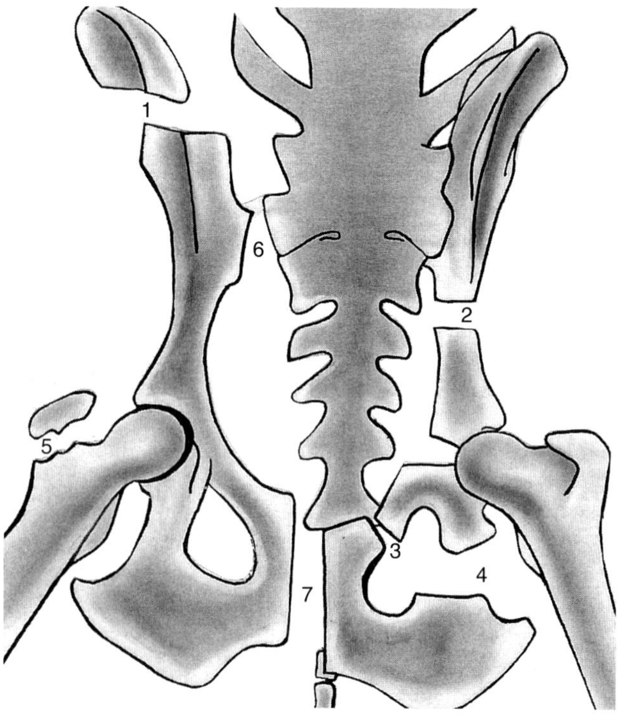

Figure 5.46. Pelvic fractures. Some of common pelvic fractures are depicted. These include wing of ilium **(1)**, shaft of ilium **(2)**, cranial ramus of pubic bone **(3)**, shaft of ischium **(4)**, greater trochanter of femur **(5)**, sacroiliac subluxation **(6)** and pubic symphyseal separation **(7)**.

Sacroiliac Luxation

Clinical correlations

1. Is commonly associated with other pelvic fractures.
2. May be unilateral or bilateral.

Radiographic findings (See Figure 5.46)

1. Is best diagnosed from a ventrodorsal projection of the pelvis.
2. Cranial displacement of the ilium, relative to the sacrum.
3. The smooth contour between the medial margin of the shaft of the ilium and the caudal margin of the sacrum is lost, resulting in a "step."

Femoral Head/Neck Fractures

Clinical correlations

1. Fracture has a traumatic etiology.
2. Types of fracture of the femoral head:
   a. Capital epiphysis
   b. Intracapsular femoral neck
   c. Extracapsular femoral neck
   d. Acetabulum

Radiographic findings (Figure 5.47)

1. Some fractures, such as those of the capital epiphysis, may appear reduced on one projection and distracted on another.
2. A ventrodorsal frog-legged projection may be helpful if the fracture is inadequately visualized on the ventrodorsal and oblique lateral projections.

Ischemic Necrosis of Femoral Head

Clinical correlations

1. Ischemic necrosis of the femoral head is also known as Legg-Calves Perthes disease.
2. Spontaneous necrosis of the femoral head is most often seen in immature toy and small-breed dogs.
   a. Is most common in Yorkshire Terrier, Toy Poodle, Pomeranian, Chihuahua, Jack Russell Terrier, West Highland White Terrier, Cairn Terrier, Manchester Terrier, Pug, and Dachshund.
   b. Is inherited as an autosomal recessive trait in the Toy Poodle, Yorkshire Terrier, and West Highland White Terrier.
   c. Necrosis may be unilateral or bilateral, and the lesion is usually self-limiting.
   d. Affected dogs are often lame, usually beginning at 4 to 10 months of age.
   e. If lameness is severe or chronic, disuse muscle atrophy is common.
3. Osteonecrosis can occur secondary to other causes of vascular insult, including an intracapsular femoral head and neck fracture.
4. As the osteonecrosis heals, there is remodeling of the femoral head and acetabulum with secondary degenerative joint disease.

Radiographic findings (Figure 5.48)

1. The initial change is a subtle radiolucency of the femoral capital epiphysis.

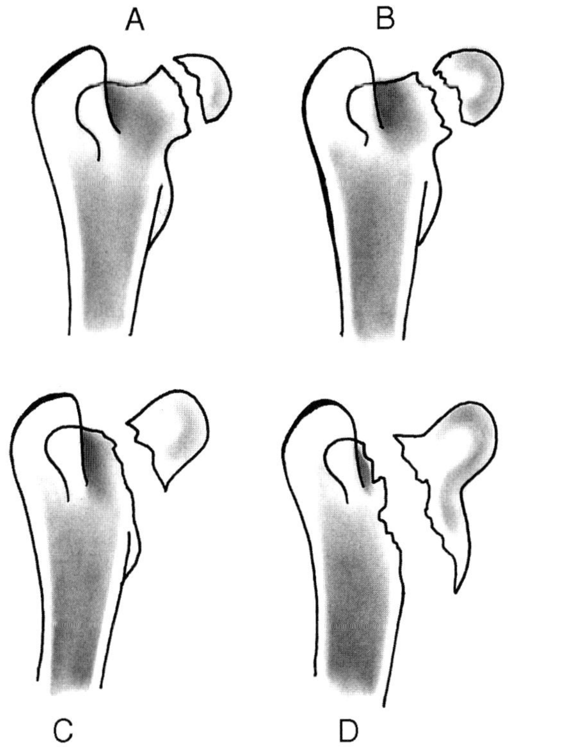

Figure 5.47. Femoral head and neck fractures. Fracture types include capital epiphysis (**A**), high cervical intracapsular (**B**), midcervical extracapsular (**C**), and low cervical extracapsular (**D**).

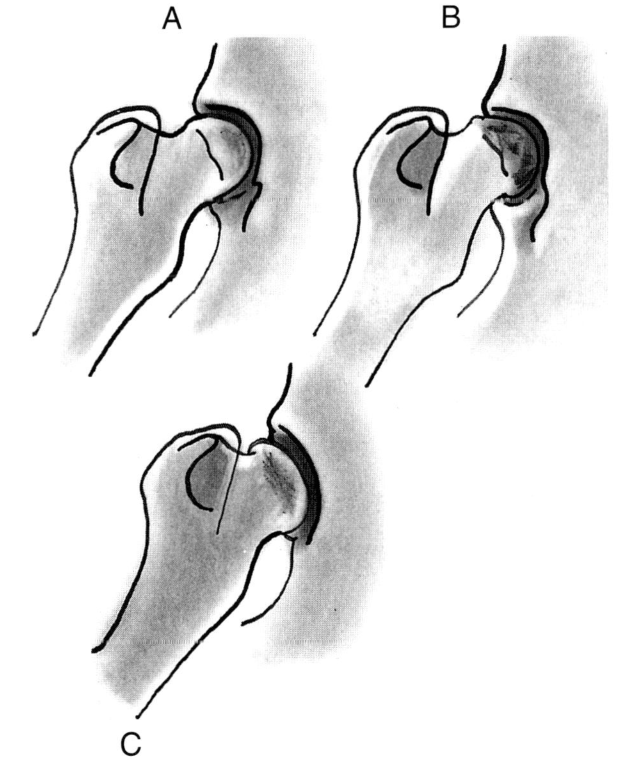

Figure 5.48. Ischemic necrosis of the femoral head. Early lytic changes in capital epiphysis (**A**) may be followed by greater lysis (**B**) with resultant remodeling of femoral head and degenerative changes (**C**).

2. With progression of necrosis, a widened joint space is seen with lysis and collapse of the femoral epiphysis, and occasionally, osteosclerosis is present in the femoral metaphysis.
3. Fractures of the epiphysis may occur.
4. Remodeling of the femoral head and neck results in an abnormally shaped head and acetabulum with secondary, proliferative, degenerative joint disease of the coxofemoral joint.

Hip Dysplasia

1. Hip dysplasia in dogs and cats is characterized by abnormal development of the hip joint.
   a. Varying amounts of laxity in the hip joint are thought to permit subluxation during early life; giving rise to varying degrees of shallow acetabuli, small and flattened femoral heads, and subsequent degenerative joint disease.
2. A genetic basis, that is polygenetic and multifactorial, has been reported.
   a. The estimates of heritability range from 0.2 to 0.6 in different dog breeds.
   b. Other factors affecting development of canine hip dysplasia include: growth rate and size, hypernutrition, level of dietary anion gap, in utero endocrine influences, and muscle mass.
3. All breeds of dogs are affected, but highest incidence is in large and giant breeds.
   a. Prevalence is estimated to range from 10 to 70% in many of the popular dog breeds.
4. It also affects purebred and domestic cats, short and long hair breeds.
5. The clinical signs vary in effect from mild to severe. Typically, dogs with the severe dysplasia exhibit lameness starting at 5 to 12 months of age. Dogs with milder dysplasia may be clinically normal.
   a. Common clinical signs include: abnormal gait, pain, low exercise tolerance, reluctance to rise or climb stairs, and muscle atrophy.
   b. Subtle pain and stiffness, mildly restricted range of joint motion, and crepitus may be present.
   c. Many dogs with hip dysplasia have minimal or no clinical signs.
6. Tentative diagnosis is based on history, clinical signs, and palpation. Definitive diagnosis is based on the radiographic findings of hip dysplasia.
7. Hip dysplasia is usually bilateral; however, unilateral dysplasia commonly occurs.
8. Radiographic technique is important for assessment of the hips.
   a. Hip extended ventrodorsal projection (Figure 5.49)
      1) Include caudal two lumbar vertebra, sacrum, pelvis, femurs, and stifle joints.
      2) Pelvis and femurs must be symmetrically positioned.
         a) Equal width of the wings of both ilia
         b) Equal size of the obturator foramina

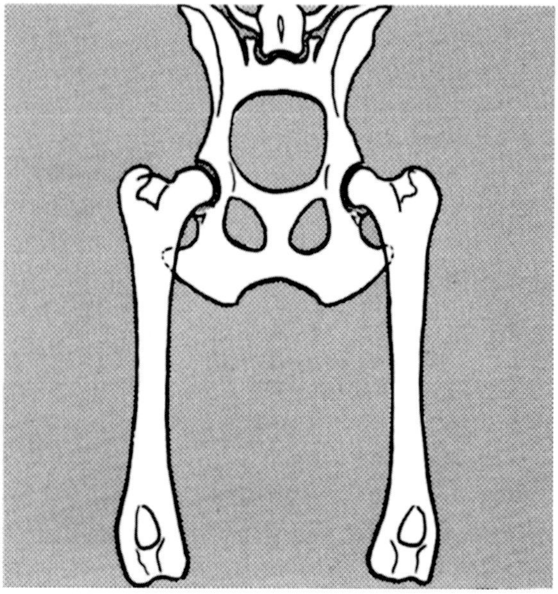

Figure 5.49. Normal canine hips (ventrodorsal hip extended projection). Proper positioning of the pelvis and femurs is denoted by symmetry of the pelvis, parallel femurs, and the patellae positioned on the midline of the distal femurs.

         c) Femurs extended and parallel. The patellas should be superimposed on the midline of the distal femurs.
      3) Congruity of the hip joint and the presence or absence of degenerative joint disease can be evaluated with this ventrodorsal projection.
      4) Criteria for radiographic diagnosis of hip dysplasia include:
         a) Femoral head subluxation or luxation
         b) Shallow acetabula
         c) Remodeling of the femoral head and neck
         d) Secondary degenerative joint disease of head, neck, and/or acetabulum
      5) The Norberg angle can also be measured (Figure 5.50). This angle is a numerical measurement of joint laxity or subluxation on the hip extended projection.
         a) The Norberg angle is defined by a line connecting the centers of the femoral heads and secondary lines from the centers of the femoral heads to the cranial acetabular rims.
         b) Norberg angle scores:
            1) An included angle of 105° and greater is considered normal.
            2) An included angle less than 90° is considered abnormal.
            3) An included angle from 90 to 105° is considered borderline.

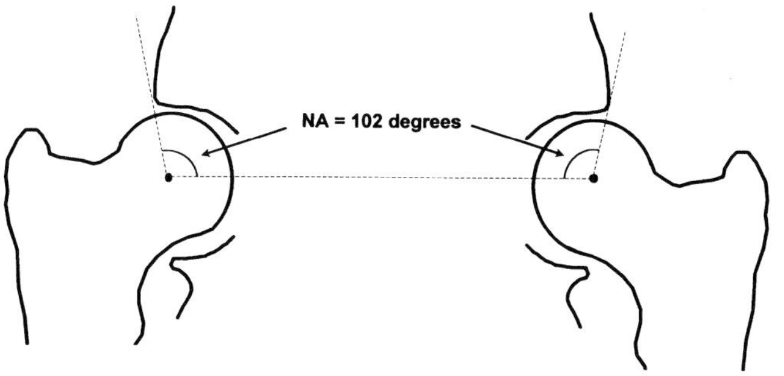

Figure 5.50. Norberg angle measurement of hips. On a ventrodorsal projection, it is the angle between a line connecting the femoral head center and a line from the center of the femoral head to the craniodorsal acetabular rim. (Courtesy of Dr. Gail K. Smith from "Diagnosis of Canine Hip Dysplasia" Canine Hip Dysplasia Symposium Western States Conference, 1995. As adapted from Smith GK. Current Concepts in the Diagnosis of Canine Hip Dysplasia. In: Bonagura JD, ed. Kirk's Current Veterinary Therapy, XII: Small Animal Practice. Philadelphia: W.B. Saunders; 1995. Used with permission.)

b. Distraction/Compression Projections (Figure 5.51 A, B)
   1) This specific, stress radiographic view (PennHIP) provides a quantitative measurement of passive hip laxity. The amount of passive hip laxity has been shown to relate directly to the probability of the hip developing degenerative joint disease.
   2) With the animal in dorsal recumbency, the femurs are positioned between 10° of flexion and 30° of extension, between 10 and 30° of abduction and between 0 and 10° of external rotation; approximately the neutral stance-phase of coxofemoral orientation.
   3) The compression projection is made with the femoral heads fully seated in the acetabula.
   4) The distraction projection is made by placing and levering a custom-designed device between the rear legs at the level of the ventral pelvis to create

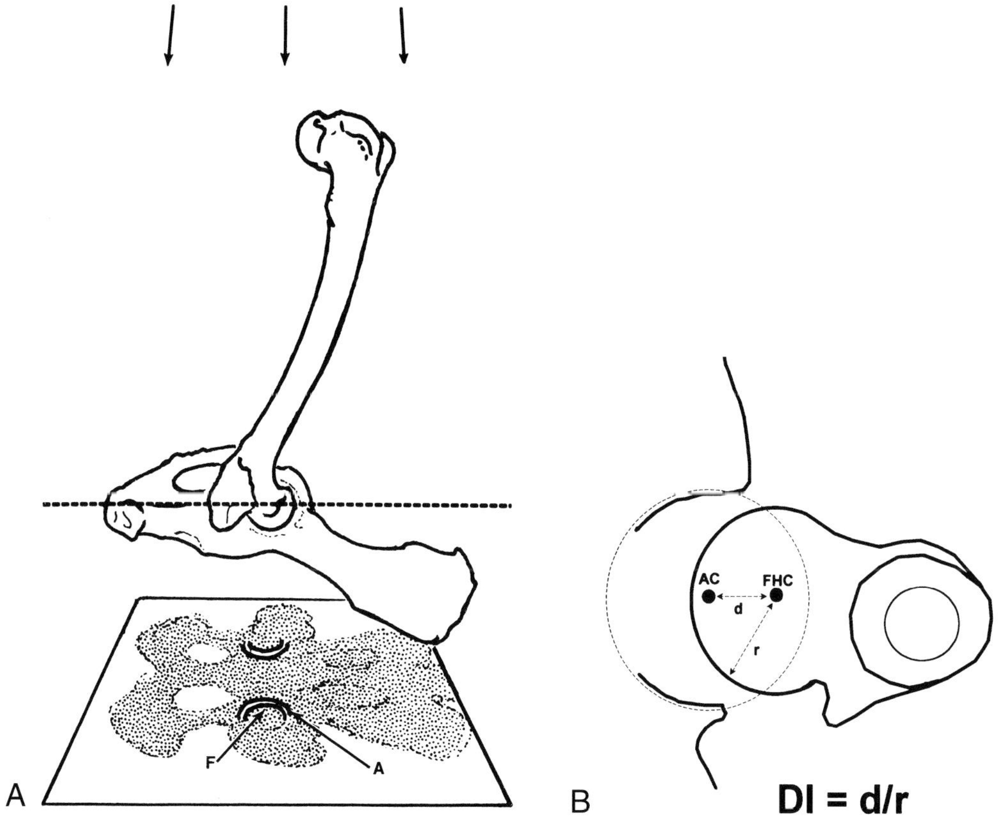

Figure 5.51. A) Schematic diagram of positioning for PennHIP distraction/compression projections. The dog is supine with the rear legs held in a neutral orientation for application of a lateral distractive load to the hips. The acetabulum **(A)** and femoral head **(F)** are imaged. (From Smith GK, Biery DN, Gregor TP. New concepts of coxofemoral joint stability and the development of a clinical stress-radiographic method for quantitating him joint laxity in the dog. JAVMA 1990;196(1):59–70. Used with permission of AVMA.) **B)** PennHIP (Synbiotics Corporation, San Diego, CA) distraction index (PennHIP DI) is determined by measuring separation distance **(d)** of the femoral head center **(FHC)** from acetabular center **(AC)** and dividing by the radius **(r)** of the femoral head. (Courtesy of Dr. Gail K. Smith from "Diagnosis of Canine Hip Dysplasia" Canine Hip Dysplasia Symposium Western States Conference, 1995. As adapted from Smith GK. Current concepts in the diagnosis of canine hip dysplasia. In: Bonagura JD, ed. Kirk's Current Veterinary Therapy, XII: Small Animal Practice. Philadelphia: W.B. Saunders; 1995. Used with permission.)

maximal lateral displacement of the femoral heads.

c. Dorsal Acetabular Rim Projection
   1) This radiographic projection provides a cross-sectional view of the dorsal acetabular rim.
   2) The animal is positioned in sternal recumbency with the tarsi positioned cranially and elevated 5 cm from the table. The x-ray beam passes through the long axis of the pelvis from cranial to caudal.
   3) The normal appearance for the acetabular rim is pointed and its slope is horizontal. If abnormal, the femoral head is displaced lateral to the dorsal acetabular rim.

Radiographic findings

1. The hip extended ventrodorsal projection shows: (Figure 5.52)
   a. Femoral head subluxation or luxation
   b. Shallow acetabula
   c. Remodeling of femoral head and neck
   d. Secondary degenerative joint disease (characterized by remodeling, bone spurs, and subchondral sclerosis of head, neck, and/or acetabulum)
2. Compression/Distraction—PennHIP (See Figure 5.51B)
   a. The Distraction Index (range, 0.0 to 1) is a quantitative measurement for the amount of passive hip laxity present. Distraction index measures the amount of laxity between compression and distraction of the femoral heads.

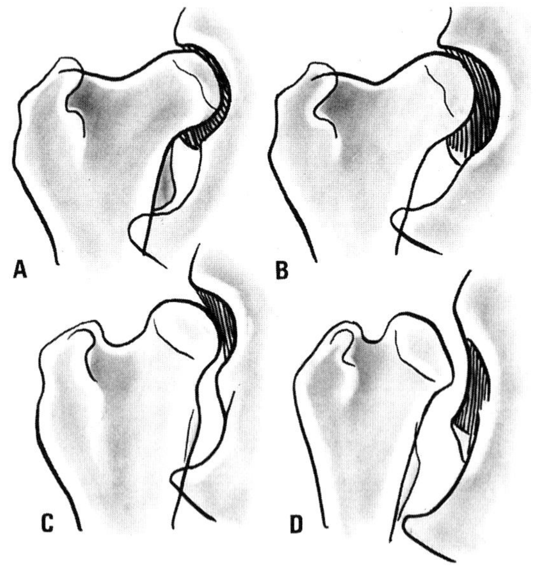

Figure 5.52. Canine hip dysplasia. Normal hip **(A)**, femoral head subluxation **(B)**, femoral head subluxation with shallow acetabulum and thickened femoral neck **(C)**, and femoral head luxation with shallow acetabulum and degenerative joint disease **(D)**.

   b. The lower the distraction index, the tighter the hip.
   c. The higher the distraction index, the greater the probability for developing degenerative joint disease associated with hip dysplasia
   d. The evaluation can be done in puppies as early as 16 weeks of age.

Hip Dysplasia Control Programs

In most countries of the world, there is some form of radiographic evaluation and registry to assist dog owners and breeders with the selection of dogs (e.g., no phenotypic evidence of joint disease).

In the United States, this is commonly done by practicing veterinarians, veterinary radiologists, veterinary surgeons, and several national organizations. The three most common organizations in the United States that provide services for the selection of phenotypically normal dogs are the following.

Orthopedic Foundation for Animals (OFA)

1. The OFA was established in the 1960s as a hip registry for dogs. A normal canine hip is based on a normal radiographic appearance to the hips when the dog is at least 24 months of age.
2. It is a closed registry, in which recorded information is available only to the animal's owner.
3. Each submitted radiograph is reviewed by three independent veterinary radiologists. A consensus opinion is provided to the owner and the referring veterinarian.
4. The grading system uses seven scoring categories:
   a. Excellent: normal hip conformation for dog's age and breed
   b. Good: normal hip conformation for dog's age and breed
   c. Fair: normal hip conformation for dog's age and breed
   d. Borderline hip conformation for dog's age and breed (follow-up radiographic examination is advised in 6 to 8 months)
   e. Mild hip dysplasia for dog's age and breed
   f. Moderate hip dysplasia for dog's age and breed
   g. Severe hip dysplasia for dog's age and breed
5. The accuracy of a radiographic diagnosis depends on the dog's age. For the German Shepherd, the published reliability of the hip extended ventrodorsal projection for diagnosis of hip dysplasia is:

   16% at 6 months of age
   69% at 12 months of age
   83% at 18 months
   95% at 24 months of age
6. The reliability reported for other breeds is approximately 85 to 90% at 24 months of age (i.e., Rottweiler, Golden Retriever, Shar Pei).

7. The OFA also provides radiographic assessment and a registry for other orthopedic diseases (elbow dysplasia, shoulder osteochondrosis, patella luxation) and some medical conditions.

Institute for Genetic Disease Control in Animals (GDC)

1. GDC developed a registry in the 1990s to evaluate and register dogs for hip dysplasia, elbow dysplasia, ostrochondrosis of extremity joints (shoulder, elbow, stifle, tarsus), and other genetically transmitted diseases.
2. This is an open registry in which information is accessible by breeders and others interested in identifying normal and affected individuals within the various dog breeds.
3. Submitted radiographs are evaluated by one to three radiologists with a consensus opinion provided.
4. Animals are evaluated at 12 months of age or older. The grading system for the hips includes three categories as follows:
   a. unaffected (excellent, good, or acceptable)
   b. indeterminate
   c. abnormal

PennHIP

1. PennHIP developed a method in the 1980s to more accurately evaluate individual dogs for joint laxity, which has been shown to be the major factor in the pathogenesis of canine hip dysplasia.
2. A hip-extended ventrodorsal projection is required plus distraction (D) and compression (C) projections. A specially designed device is used to obtain the D/C projections, and objective measurements are made to separate a normal dog with tight hips from a dog with increased joint laxity.
3. Veterinary practitioners are trained in the use of the distraction device, and radiographic technique for successful acquisition of radiographs for hip laxity assessment.
4. The radiographs obtained with this method are then quantitatively evaluated for degree of hip laxity and presence of degenerative joint disease.
   a. The amount of hip laxity is a valid predictor for the future development of degenerative joint disease associated with hip dysplasia. The less hip laxity (tighter), the better the hip.
5. The laxity index provides a ranking of a dog's hip tightness relative to other members of the same breed. Dogs with the tighter hips are less likely to develop hip dysplasia and pass the genetic tendency on to future generations.

STIFLE

RADIOGRAPHIC TECHNIQUE (Figures 5.53 through 5.56)

1. Standard projections:
   a. Lateral projection
   b. Caudocranial projection

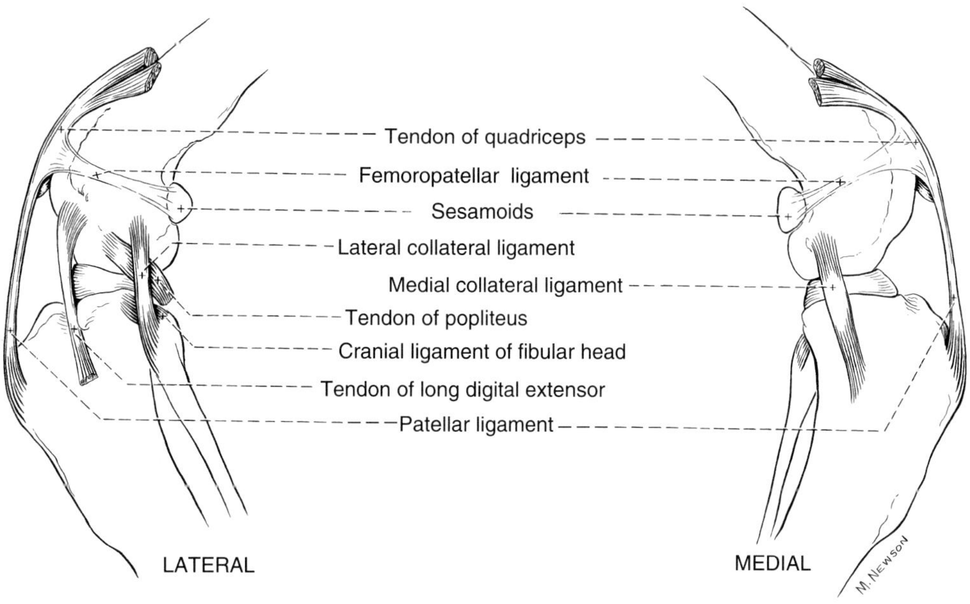

Figure 5.53. Ligaments of the canine stifle joint—lateral and medial views. (From Evans HE. Arthrology. In: Evans HE, ed. Miller's Anatomy of the Dog. 3rd ed. Philadelphia: W.B. Saunders; 1993:248. Courtesy of and with permission of Dr. Howard E. Evans.)

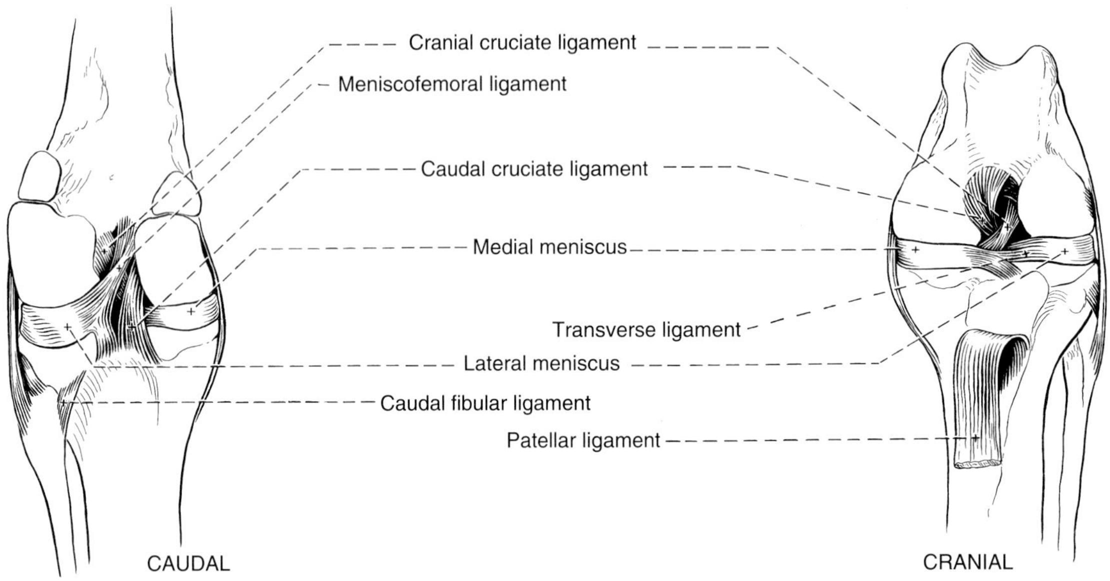

Figure 5.54. Ligaments of the canine stifle joint—cranial and caudal views. (From Evans HE. Arthrology. In: Evans HE, ed. Miller's Anatomy of the Dog. 3rd ed. Philadelphia: W.B. Saunders; 1993:246. Courtesy of and with permission of Dr. Howard E. Evans.)

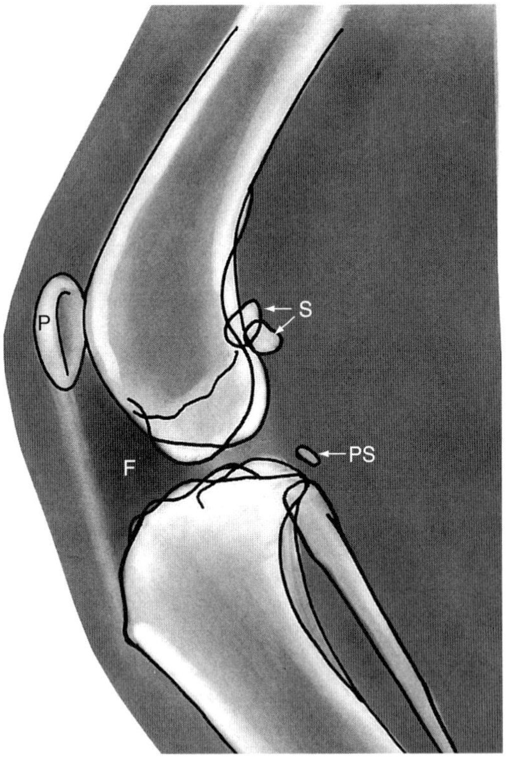

Figure 5.55. Normal canine stifle (lateral projection). Major landmarks include patella **(P)**, proximal sesamoid bones **(S)**, popliteal sesamoid bone **(PS)**, and infrapatellar fat pad **(F)**.

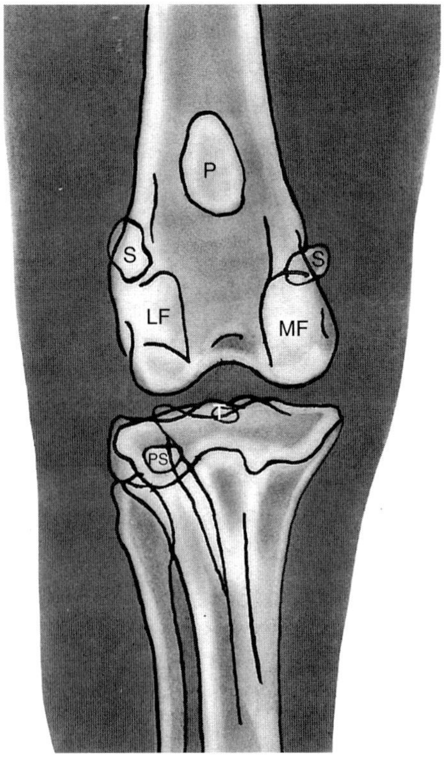

Figure 5.56. Normal canine stifle (caudocranial projection). Major landmarks include the patella **(P)**, medial femoral condyle **(MF)**, lateral femoral condyle **(LF)**, tibial plateau **(T)**, proximal sesamoid bones **(S)**, and popliteal sesamoid bone **(PS)** (arrow).

2. Supplemental projections:
   a. Craniocaudal projection
   b. Skyline projection (for patella and trochlear groove)
   c. Flexion or extension stress projections

DISEASES/DISORDERS

Cranial Cruciate Ligament Injury

Clinical correlations

1. Can occur from acute or chronic injury. The result is partial to complete instability of the stifle joint.
   a. Associated causes include aging and conformational abnormalities (i.e., patella luxation, genu valgum, genu varum), excessive activity, and immune mediated processes.
2. It is a common cause of lameness in dogs and cats.
3. Is the most common cause of degenerative joint disease in the stifle joint.
4. On palpation, a "cranial drawer" sign is diagnostic, but absence of this sign does not rule out the diagnosis, especially if there is a joint effusion, partial ligament tear, or chronic changes of fibrosis and degenerative joint disease.
5. Avulsion fracture is more common in animals younger than 18 months of age because the cruciate ligament is stronger than the epiphyseal bone.
6. May be concurrent with other stifle disease (i.e., osteochondrosis, osteochondritis dissecans, patella luxation, meniscal tear).

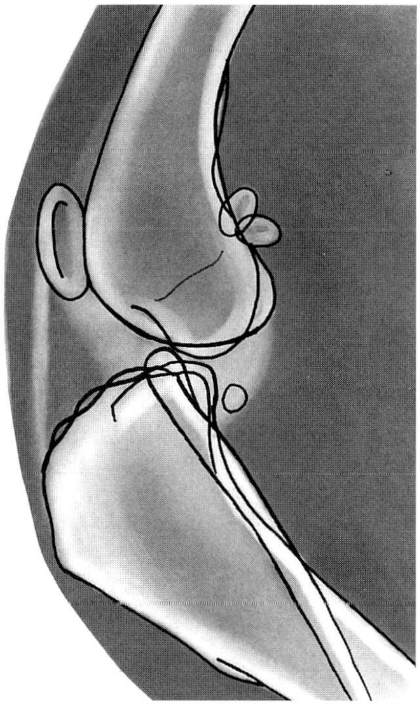

Figure 5.57. Cranial cruciate ligament injury. There is cranial displacement of the proximal tibia relative to the femoral condyles. The popliteal sesamoid is normal in position, but appears relatively more caudal in position because of cranial displacement of tibia.

Radiographic findings (Figures 5.57 and 5.58 A, B)

1. Joint effusion (characterized by partial obliteration of the infrapatellar fat pad), caudal displacement of

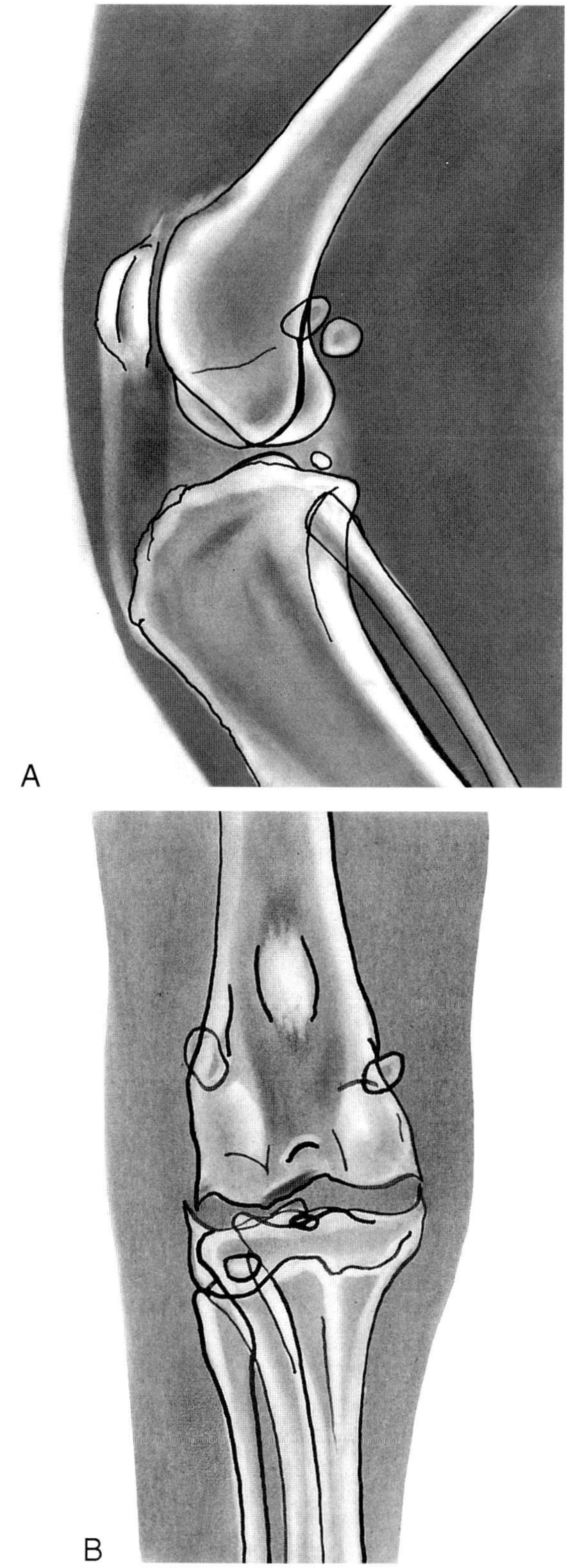

Figure 5.58. Degenerative joint disease secondary to chronic cruciate ligament injury. **A)** Bone spurs are present on trochlea, patella, and tibial plateau. **B)** Bone spurs are present on lateral and medial margins of femoral condyles and tibial plateau.

the joint capsule, and/or cranial displacement of the patella
2. The popliteal sesamoid bone is usually normal in position, but it may be displaced caudally and distally.
3. Secondary degenerative joint disease characterized by osteophytes is commonly seen on the distal border of the patella, the trochlear groove, periarticular medial and lateral margins of the distal femur and the proximal tibia, and on the mid tibial plateau at the site of attachment of the cranial cruciate ligament.
4. Avulsion fractures may occur, usually at the insertion of the cranial cruciate ligament on tibial plateau.

Caudal Cruciate Ligament Injury

Clinical correlations

1. Is a rare injury by itself and is usually associated with concurrent collateral ligament and cranial cruciate ligament injury.
2. May be isolated avulsion fracture of the origin or insertion of the caudal cruciate ligament.

Radiographic findings

1. Radiographs of stifle may appear normal.
2. Joint effusion is often present.
3. Avulsed fragments may be seen in the caudal joint compartment. The origin of the fracture fragment may be difficult to identify.

Osteochondrosis/Osteochondritis Dissecans

Clinical correlations

1. Usually occurs in large breed dogs. Has been reported in many breeds, but is most common in the German Shepherd Dog and Great Dane.
2. Usually affects the medial aspect of the lateral femoral condyle; however, occasionally occurs on the medial condyle or on the lateral trochlear ridge.
3. Is often bilateral.
4. In some dogs, the lameness is minor and the cartilage lesion heals spontaneously. Degenerative joint disease may still occur as a sequel.
5. Affected dogs usually show mild lameness beginning at 5 to 7 months of age, which is often aggravated by exercise.

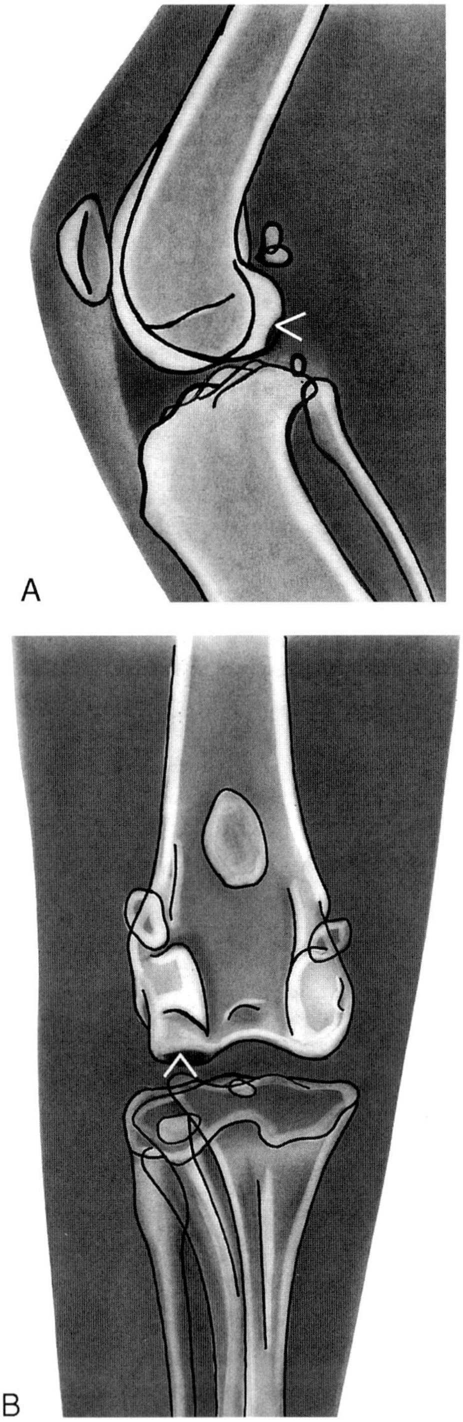

Figure 5.59. Osteochondrosis/osteochondritis dissecans of the lateral femoral condyle (arrow). **A)** Subchondral defect (lateral projection). **B)** Subchondral defect (craniocaudal projection).

Radiographic findings (Figure 5.59 A, B)

1. A flattened or circular radiolucent articular defect with or without a sclerotic margin identified best on lateral oblique and caudocranial projections.
2. Ossified free bodies (joint mice) may be seen in the suprapatellar pouch, cranial, or caudal joint compartments.

3. Increased joint fluid is often present.
4. Secondary degenerative joint disease characterized by subchondral sclerosis and osteophytes may be present.
5. Anatomic structures that can mimic osteochondrosis are:
   a. Normal fossa of the long digital extensor tendon on the craniolateral surface of the lateral femoral condyle
   b. Aberrant origin of the cranial cruciate ligament

Luxation

Clinical correlations

1. Is seen occasionally in cats, and rarely in dogs.
2. Luxation is a combined rupture of the collateral ligaments and both the cranial and caudal cruciate ligaments.

Radiographic findings

1. Malalignment of the femorotibial joint
2. The finding may only be visible on one of two orthogonal projections.
3. Other concurrent injuries may include fractures, patella luxation, and/or soft tissue injuries.

Avulsion of the Tendon of Origin of the Long Digital Extensor

Clinical correlation

1. Occurs most commonly in immature large dogs.
2. Is associated with trauma.

Radiographic finding (Figure 5.60)

1. Avulsed bone fragment is seen adjacent to the fossa of the long digital extensor tendon of the lateral femoral condyle within the cranial joint compartment.

Avulsion of the Origin of the Popliteal Muscle

Clinical correlations

1. Is associated with trauma.
2. May exist concurrently with injury to the cranial cruciate ligament.

Radiographic finding (Figure 5.61)

1. Distal displacement of the popliteal sesamoid bone.

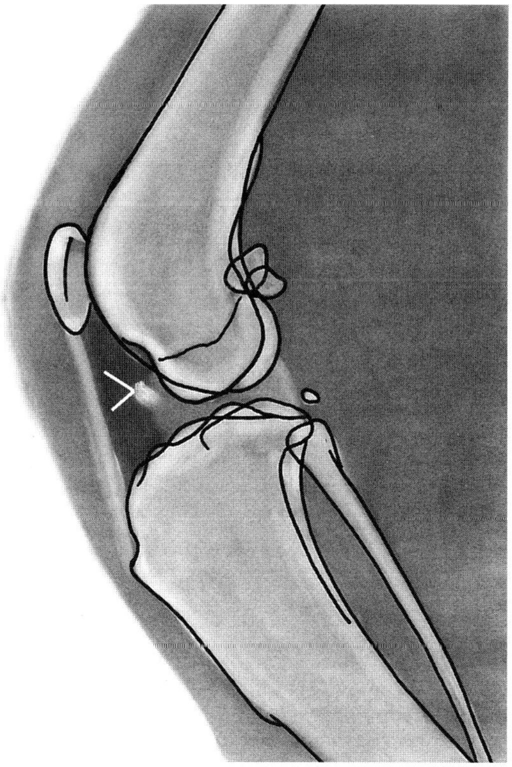

Figure 5.60. Avulsion of the long digital extensor tendon (LDE). The avulsed fragment (arrow) is displaced distally away from LDE attachment site on the lateral aspect of the lateral condyle.

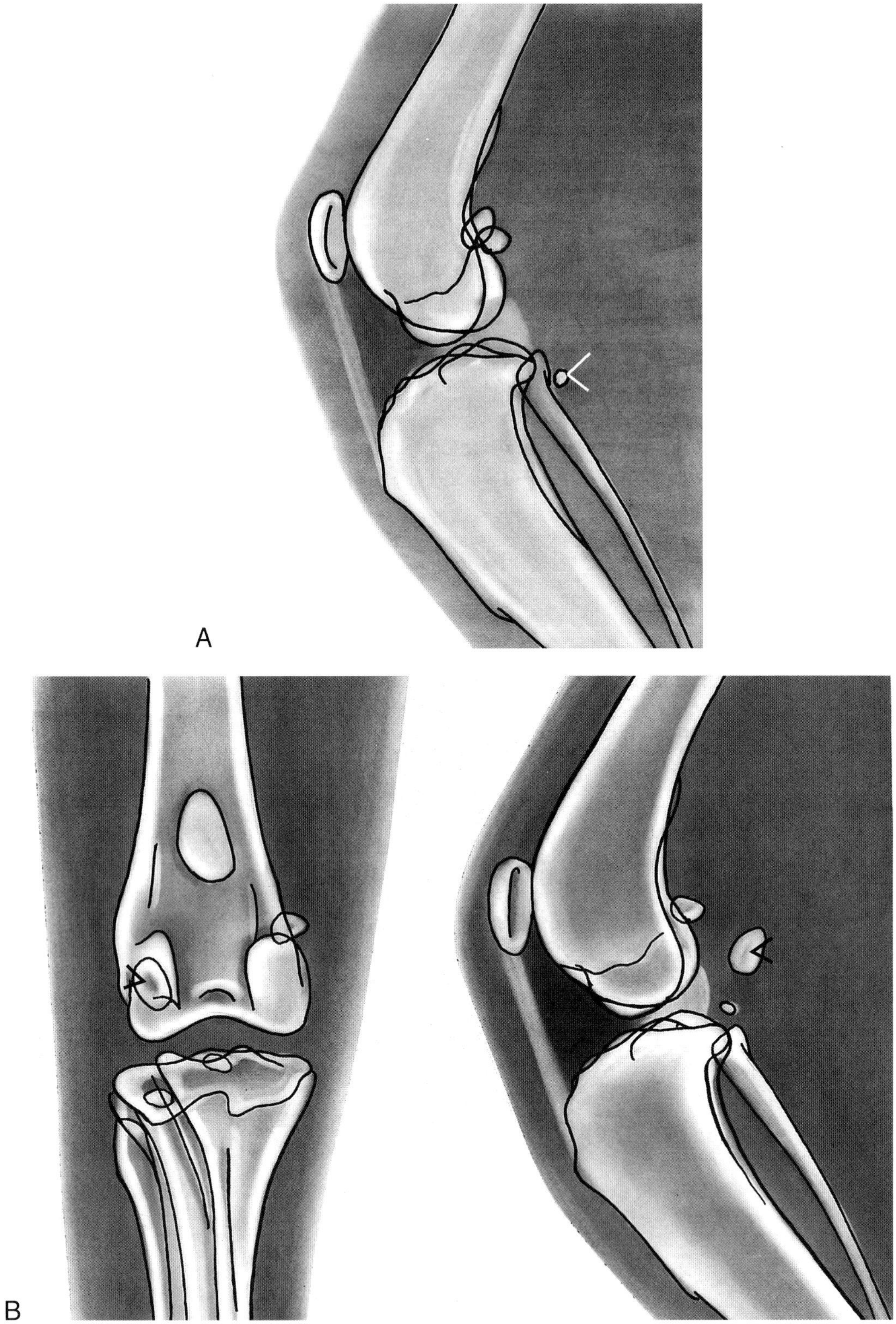

Figure 5.61. **A)** Avulsion of the origin of the popliteal muscle. The popliteal sesamoid bone is displaced distally (arrow). **B)** Ruptured tendon of gastrocnemius muscle with displacement of lateral sesamoid bone (arrow).

Intraarticular ossification

Clinical correlations

1. Ossification may be a sequel of trauma. It represents a mineralization of the meniscus, cruciate ligament, long digital extensor tendon, or infrapatellar fat pad.
2. May represent synovial osteochondromatosis in cats (See Figure 5.5).
3. May represent "joint mice" from osteochondritis dissecans.

Radiographic findings

1. Discrete or irregular mineralizations within the joint compartment.
2. Lateral and caudocranial and/or oblique projections are needed for complete assessment.

Avulsion of the Tibial Tuberosity

Clinical correlations

1. Usually occurs in immature dogs and cats
2. Usually results from a single traumatic episode consisting of blunt trauma and hyperflexion of the stifle.

Radiographic findings (Figure 5.62)

1. Proximal displacement of the tibial tuberosity
2. Proximal displacement of the patella may be seen.
3. A comparison radiograph of the opposite stifle joint enables accurate assessment of the degree of avulsion and patella malposition.

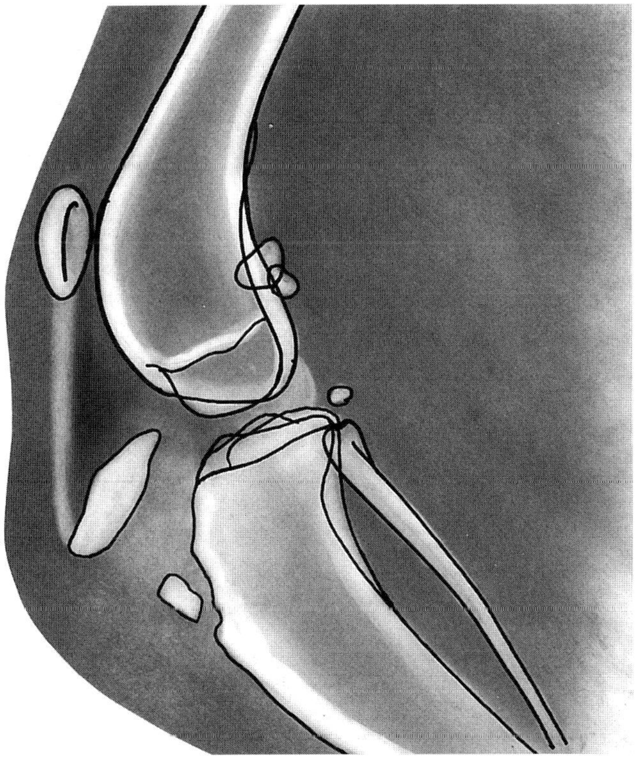

Figure 5.62. Avulsion fracture of the tibial tuberosity. The tibial tuberosity is displaced proximally.

Patellar Luxation/Subluxation

Clinical correlations

1. Medial or lateral displacement of the patella may be a congenital anomaly (most common) or be a secondary consequence of trauma.
2. Is more common in dogs than cats, especially the toy and miniature canine breeds.
3. Congenital or developmental deformities of the rear limb, which predispose to patella luxation, are seen in many affected dogs and cats. These include:
   a. Femoral neck angles (coxo vara, coxo valga, femoral anteversion angle)
   b. Lateral bowing of femur
   c. Hypoplastic medial femoral condyle
   d. Displacement or rotation of the tibial tuberosity and crest
   e. Shallow trochlear groove and rotation of distal femur
   f. External rotation of the tarsus with medial deviation of the paw
4. Medial patella luxation is more common than lateral luxation.
   a. Most affected dogs are bow-legged (genu varum) and the patellas luxate medially.
   b. Small breed dogs, especially toy and miniature breeds, are most commonly affected.
   c. Bilateral luxation is present in approximately 50% of the affected dogs.
5. Lateral patellar luxation usually occurs in large breed dogs that have knock-knees (genu valgum).
6. May have other concurrent and unrelated diseases (i.e., cruciate ligament rupture, chondromalacia of patella, or hip dysplasia).
7. Clinical signs vary with the degree of subluxation/luxation, and gait abnormality can range from minimal to severe. With congenital patella luxation, lameness is rarely acute. Animal exhibits skipping or intermittent carrying of the limb with the stifle flexed.
8. Frequently, patella luxations are actually subluxations in which the diagnosis is best based on palpation.

Radiographic findings (Figures 5.63 and 5.64)

1. Patellar luxation is often intermittent and the patella may appear normal in position on radiographs.
2. A craniocaudal projection provides easier identification of the medial or lateral subluxation/luxation. The hip, femur, and proximal tibia should be included on the radiograph to assess torsion or bowing.
3. On the lateral projection, the luxated patella may be seen superimposed on the femoral condyles.
4. The skyline projection with the stifle flexed will demonstrate the depth of the trochlear groove and the position of the patellar luxation.

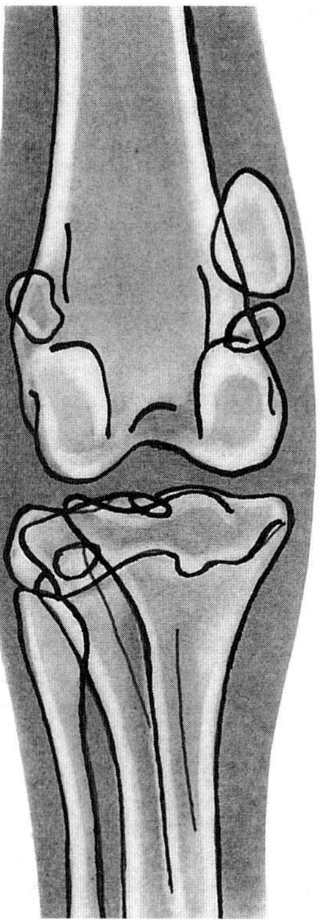

Figure 5.63. Medial patellar luxation.

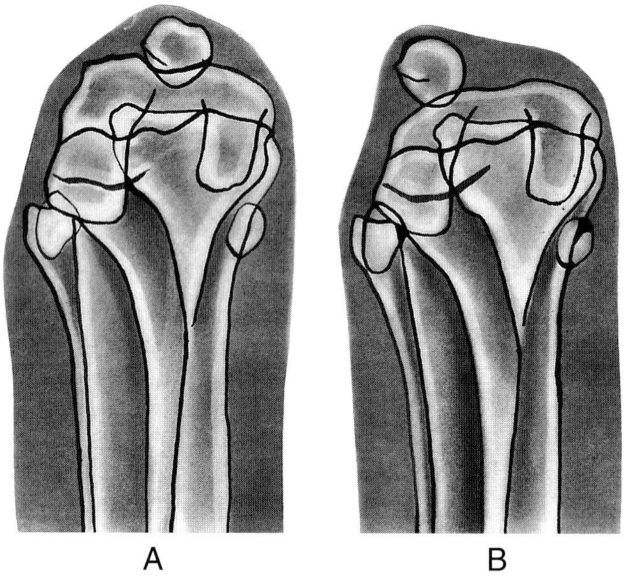

Figure 5.64. Lateral patella luxation. The skyline projection allows evaluation of the patellar groove and position of patella within it; **(A)** is normal and **(B)** is a lateral patella luxation, note the flattened lateral condyle.

5. Degenerative joint disease and/or other conformational abnormalities of the limb may be visible.

Ruptured Patellar Tendon

Clinical correlations

1. This is an acute injury to the stifle with blunt trauma or hyperextension of the stifle.
2. The injured ligament may be associated with a patellar fracture.

Radiographic findings (Figures 5.65 and 5.66)

1. On the lateral projection, the patella is displaced proximally.
2. A flexed lateral projection (as a stress view), will demonstrate the severity of ligament injury. The degree of proximal patellar distraction will be noted, especially when compared to the contralateral normal limb.
3. With some partial tears or contusion of patellar ligament, the patella ligament appears thickened, with caudal displacement of the infrapatellar fat pad.
4. Patellar fracture may also be present.

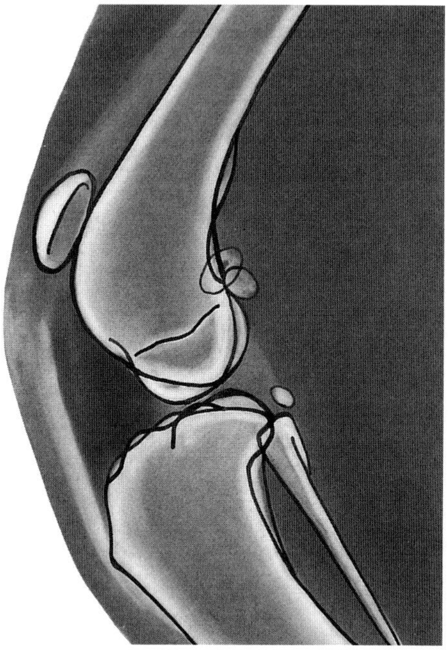

Figure 5.65. Ruptured patellar ligament. The patella is displaced proximally.

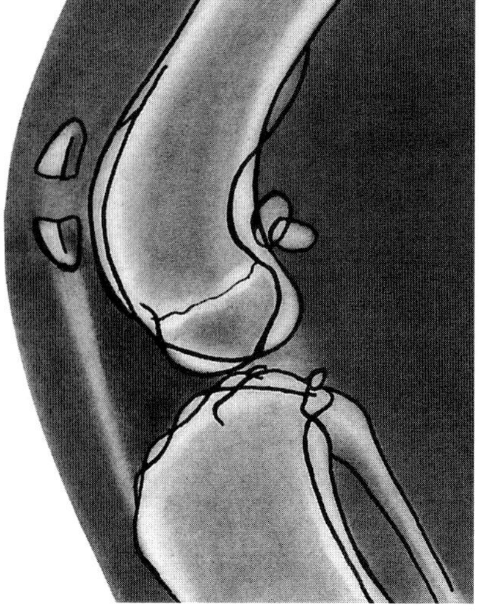

Figure 5.66. Fracture of the patella.

TARSUS (TARSOCRURAL JOINT, TIBIOTARSAL JOINT)

RADIOGRAPHIC TECHNIQUE (Figures 5.67 through 5.70)

1. Standard projections:
   a. Lateral projection
   b. Dorsocaudal projection

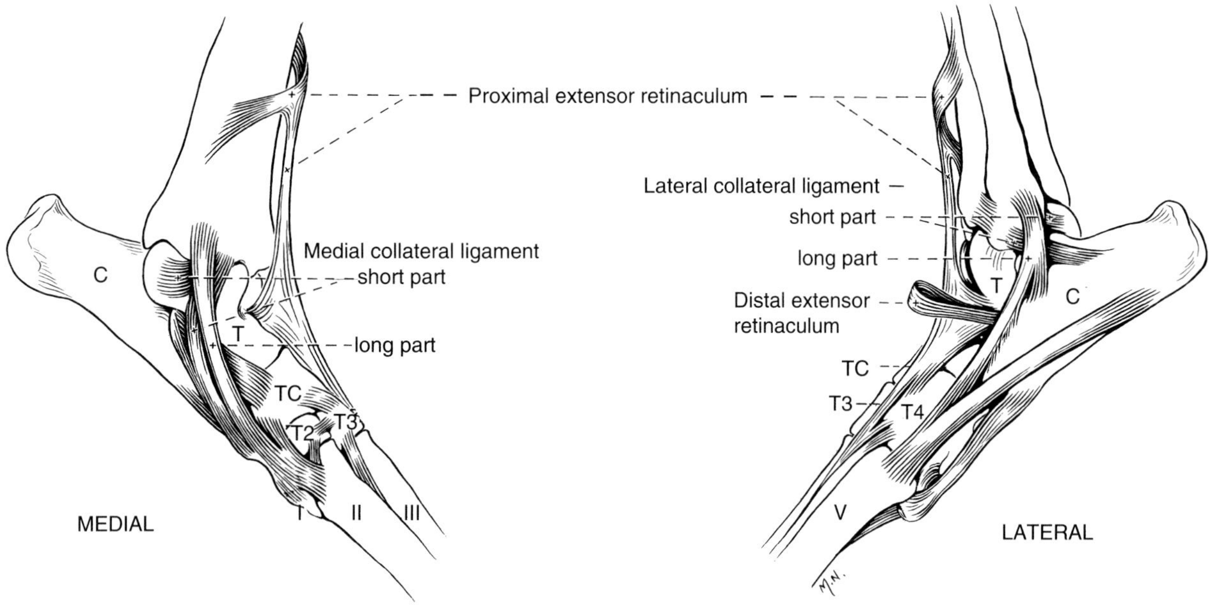

Figure 5.67. Ligaments of left tarsus—lateral and medial views. (From Evans HE. Arthrology. In: Evans HE, ed. Miller's Anatomy of the Dog. 3rd ed. Philadelphia: W.B. Saunders; 1993:254. Courtesy of and with permission of Dr. Howard E. Evans.)

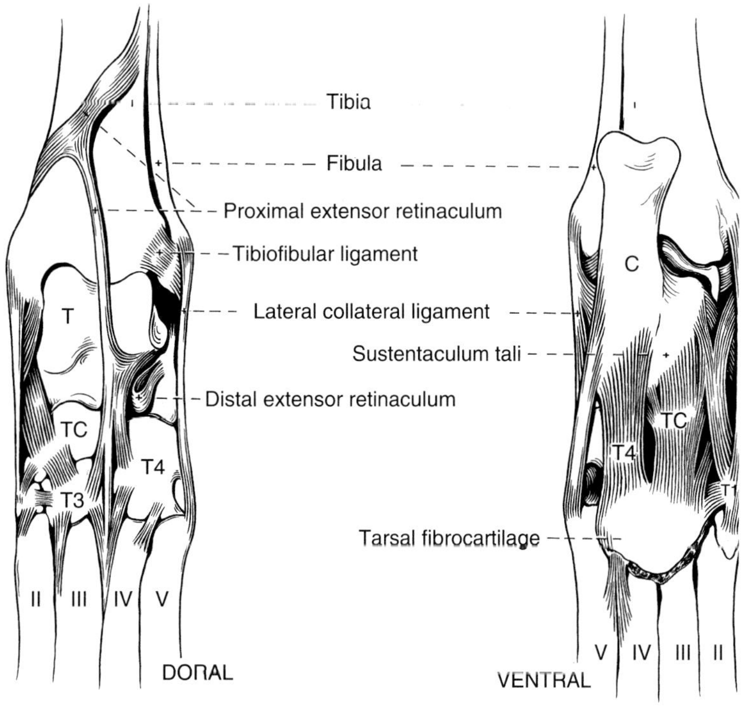

Figure 5.68. Ligaments of left tarsus—dorsal and plantar views. (From Evans HE. Arthrology. In: Evans HE, ed. Miller's Anatomy of the Dog. 3rd ed. Philadelphia: W.B. Saunders; 1993:252. Courtesy of and with permission of Dr. Howard E. Evans.)

2. Supplemental projections:
   a. Flexed lateral projection
   b. Flexed dorsoplantar (skyline) projection
   c. Medial and lateral oblique projections
   d. Standing lateral projection (weight bearing)

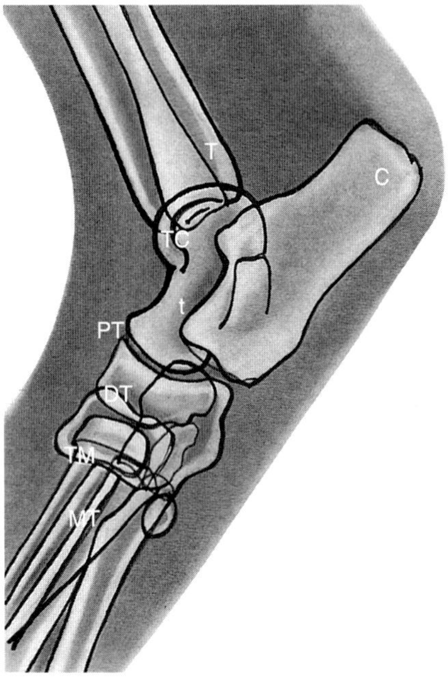

Figure 5.69. Normal canine tarsus (lateral projection). Major landmarks include the tibia **(T)**, calcaneus **(C)**, talus **(t)**, tarsocrural joint **(TC)**, proximal intertarsal joint **(PT)**, tarsometatarsal joint **(TM)**, distal tarsometatarsal joint **(DT)**, and proximal metatarsal bones **(MT)**.

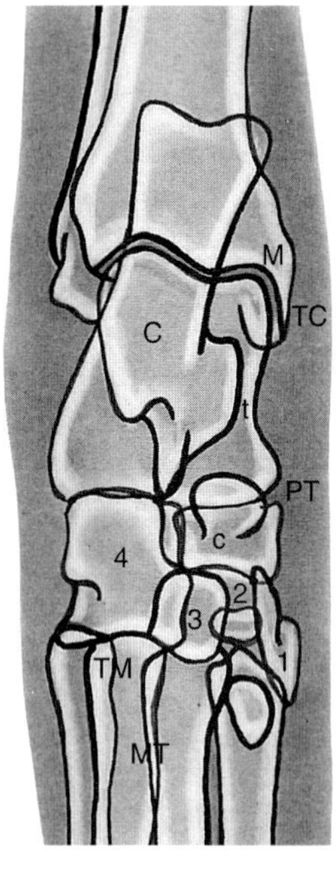

Figure 5.70. Normal canine tarsus (dorsoplantar projection). Major landmarks include the medial malleolus of tibia **(M)**, lateral malleolus of fibula **(L)**, tarsocrural joint **(TC)**, proximal intertarsal joint **(PT)**, tarsometatarsal joint **(TM)**, and proximal metatarsal bones **(MT)**. The tarsal bones are calcaneus **(C)**, talus **(t)**, central tarsal **(c)**, and numbers **1, 2, 3** and 4.

DISEASES/DISORDERS

Luxation/Subluxation

Clinical correlations

1. Tarsocrural luxations often are associated with malleolar fractures.
2. Tarsocrural subluxations occur when one malleolus and its attached collateral ligament are distracted.
3. Intertarsal subluxations can occur secondary to trauma or as a result of degeneration in the plantar ligaments.
4. Obese middle-aged dogs are predisposed (Shetland Sheepdog, Collie, and Samoyed).

Radiographic findings (Figure 5.71 A, B)

1. Usually, standard radiographic projections are adequate for diagnosis.

A
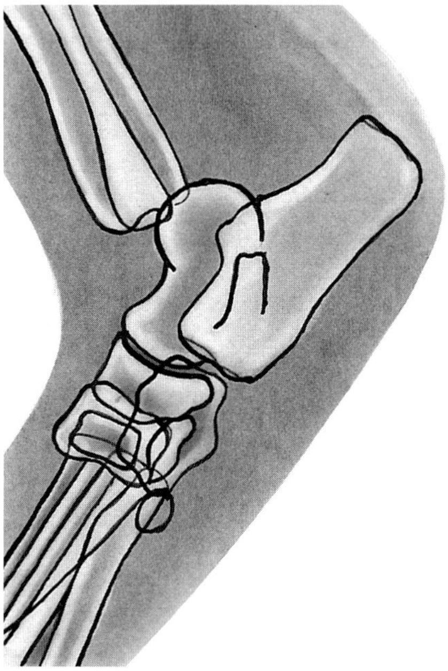

B
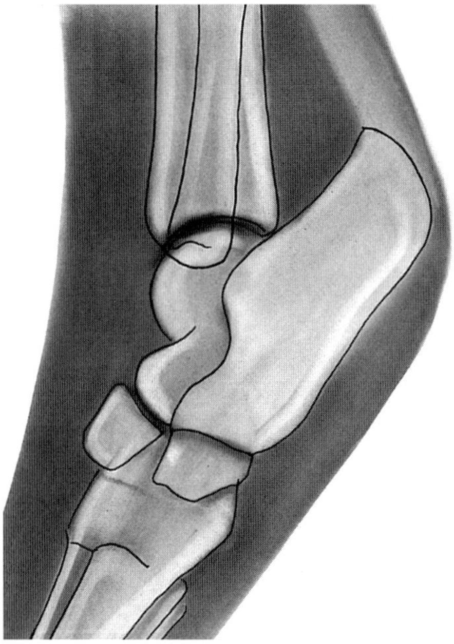

Figure 5.71. **A)** Tarsocrural luxation. **B)** Fractured central tarsal bone.

2. Subluxations may require stress radiographs to demonstrate the instability.
3. Articular fractures commonly are seen in association with the luxation or subluxation.

Calcaneon Tendon Injury:

Clinical correlations

1. The injury can be either acute or chronic.
2. Occurs most often in mature dogs of working breeds. Overweight dogs also are susceptible.
3. Acute injury is associated with hyperflexion of the tarsus, often with concurrent hyperextension of the stifle.
   a. The calcaneon tendon can stretch or tear.
   b. The origin of the lateral or medial head of the gastrocnemius muscle may avulse or tear.
4. Chronic injury causes thickening of the calcaneon attachment, which may involve the tendon of the superficial digital flexor and/or the gastrocnemius tendon.
5. Postural deficits may include a dropped hock (with complete calcaneon injury) or a "claw foot," if contracture of the superficial digital flexor tendon develops.

Radiographic findings (Figure 5.72 A–C)

1. The calcaneon tendon appears thicker than normal.
2. Avulsion of the head of the gastrocnemius muscle causes distal displacement of the associated fabella.
3. An avulsion fracture of the tuber calcis (calcaneal process) may be present.
4. With chronic injuries, mineralization within the calcaneon tendon may be seen, often with irregular periosteal reaction on the tuber calcis.

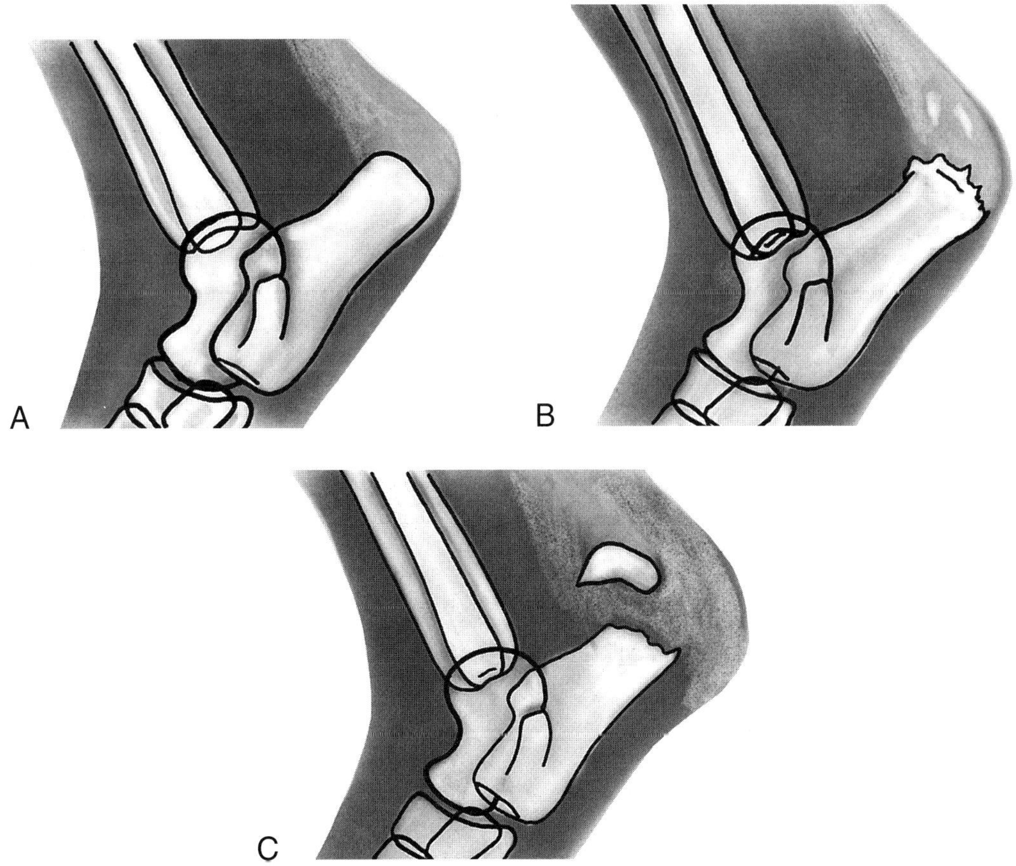

Figure 5.72. Calcaneon tendon injury. **A)** Soft tissue swelling of tendon. **B)** Chronic injury of tendon with dystrophic focal mineralization within tendon and periosteal new bone on calcaneal process. **C)** Avulsion fracture of calcaneal process with proximal distraction of the calcaneon tendon and marked soft tissue swelling.

Osteochondrosis/Osteochondritis Dissecans

Clinical correlations

1. More common in males of large and giant breed dogs, and most commonly is reported in Rottweilers, Labrador Retrievers, and Golden Retrievers.
2. May be unilateral or bilateral.
3. Usually causes mild lameness that is aggravated with exercise, often after 6 months of age.
4. May observe distended joint capsule, especially with periarticular swelling on the medial side.
5. May be associated with a conformational defect involving hyperextension of the tarsocrural joint.

Radiographic findings (Figures 5.73 through 5.75 A, B)

1. Affects the tarsocrural joint, usually the medial ridge of talus, and less commonly, the lateral ridge.
2. On the craniocaudal view, a flattening or radiolucent articular defect may be observed on the medial or lateral ridge of the talus. In some cases, the lesion only is visible on a skyline projection of the tarsocrural joint.
3. Joint capsule distension indicating joint effusion and/or joint capsule thickening is seen best on the lateral projection.
4. In chronic cases, osteophytes, representing degenerative joint disease, may be present with or without joint mice.

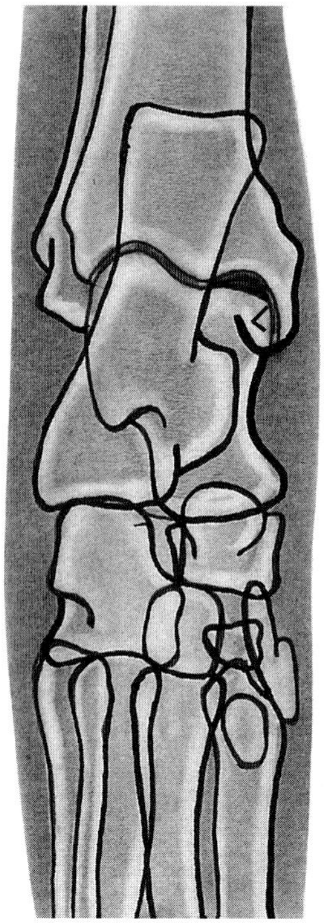

Figure 5.73. Osteochondrosis/osteochondritis dissecans. There is a widening of the medial tarsocrural joint space and subchondral flattening of the medial ridge of talus (arrow).

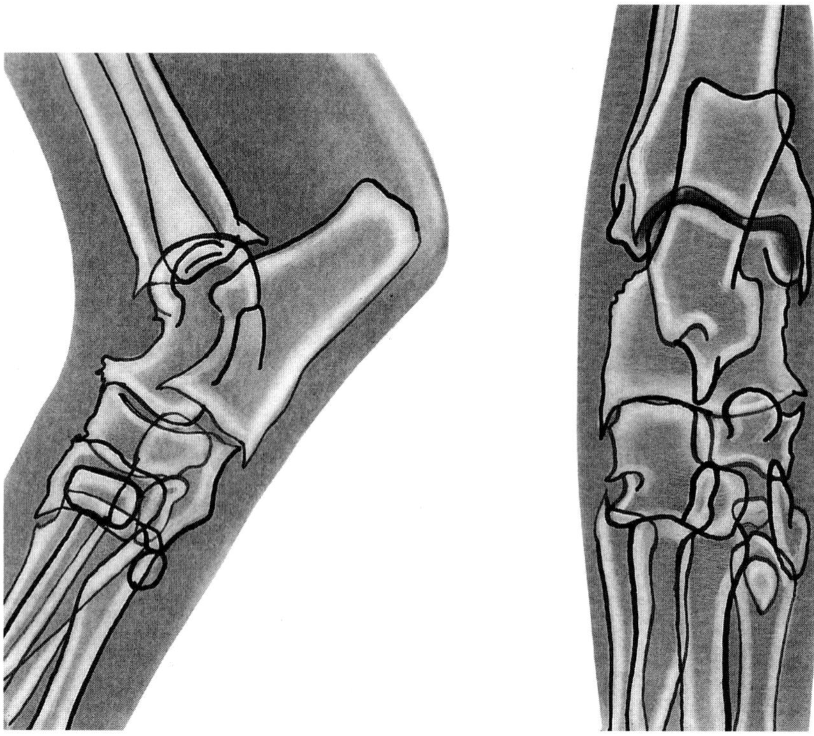

Figure 5.74. Degenerative joint disease of tarsus. Periarticular osteophytes are present.

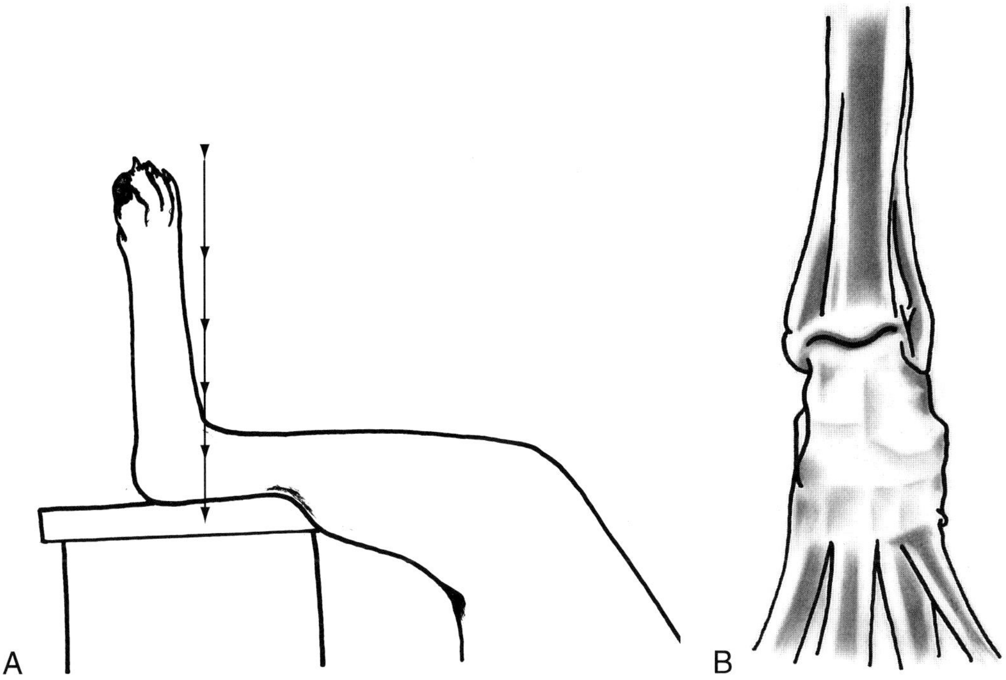

Figure 5.75. Skyline view of tarsocrural joint. **A)** Positioning and direction of x-ray beam. **B)** Normal radiographic appearance.

Chapter 6

6

Skull

RADIOGRAPHIC TECHNIQUE

Radiographic positioning varies greatly between the different skull types owing to anatomic variations of different breeds (Figures 6.1 through 6.15).

1. Standard projections:
   a. Lateral projection.
   b. Dorsoventral (DV) or ventrodorsal projection (VD). A symmetrical view is usually easier to obtain in the DV position, in which the animal is resting on the horizontal rami of the mandible.
2. Supplemental projections:
   a. Additional projections are frequently necessary, depending on the suspected site and/or type of disease problem.
   b. Oblique projections of both the abnormal and the normal sides are frequently helpful.
   c. In Table 6.1, the various areas of the skull are listed

TABLE 6.1

Area of Skull	Radiographic Projections	Figure
Routine skull	Lateral	6.1
	DV	6.2
Mandible	Lateral	6.1
	DV	6.2
	Open-mouth lateral oblique	6.9
Zygomatic bone and orbit	Lateral	6.1
	DV	6.2
	Frontal	6.3
	Lateral oblique	6.4
	Open-mouth VD	6.7
Temporomandibular joints	DV	6.2
	Sagittal oblique	6.5
Tympanic bullae	DV	6.2
	Lateral oblique	—
	Rostroventral-caudodorsal open mouth	6.6A
	10° Ventrodorsal	6.6B
Foramen magnum	Rostrocaudal	6.8
Nasal Cavities and Sinuses	Lateral recumbent	6.1
	DV	6.2
	Occlusal DV	6.11B
	Open-mouth VD	6.7
	Lateral oblique open mouth	6.4
	Frontal	6.3
Teeth:		
Maxillary teeth	Open-mouth lateral oblique	6.10
	Open mouth VD	6.7
Mandibular teeth	Open-mouth lateral oblique	6.9
Incisor teeth	Occlusal DV (Premaxilla)	6.11A
	Occlusal VD (Mandible)	6.12
	Bisecting and Parallel techniques	6.13, 6.14, 6.15

DV, dosal ventral; VD, ventrodorsal.

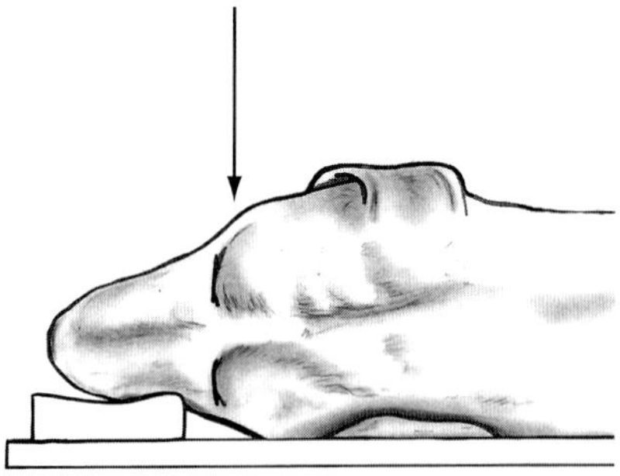

Figure 6.1. Lateral projection.

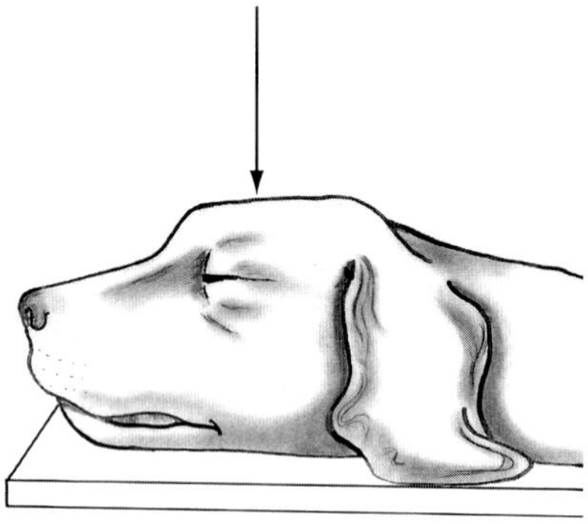

Figure 6.2. Dorsoventral projection.

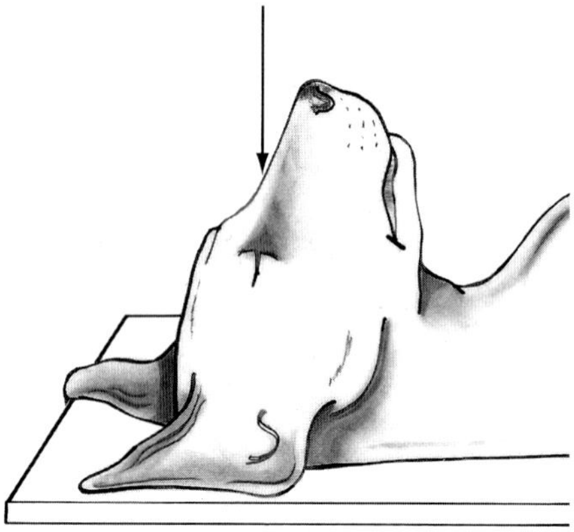

Figure 6.3. Frontal projection.

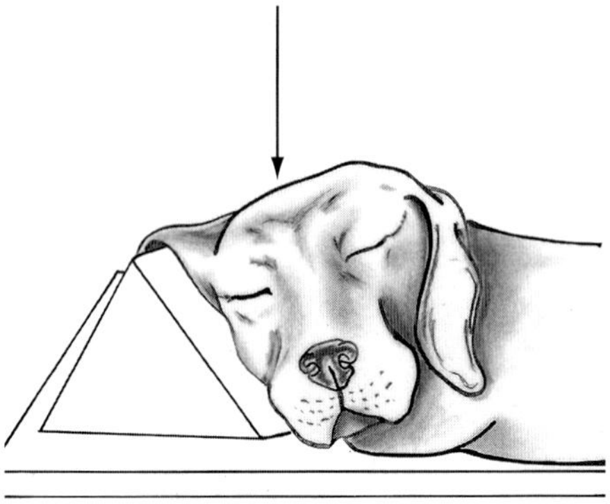

Figure 6.4. Lateral oblique projection for frontal sinuses.

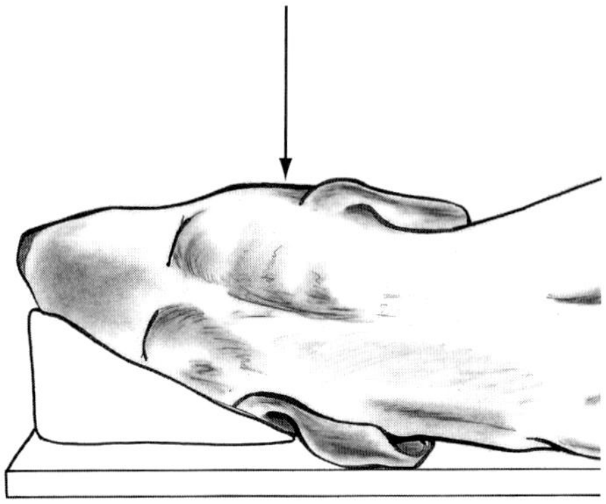

Figure 6.5. Sagittal oblique projection for temporomandibular joint.

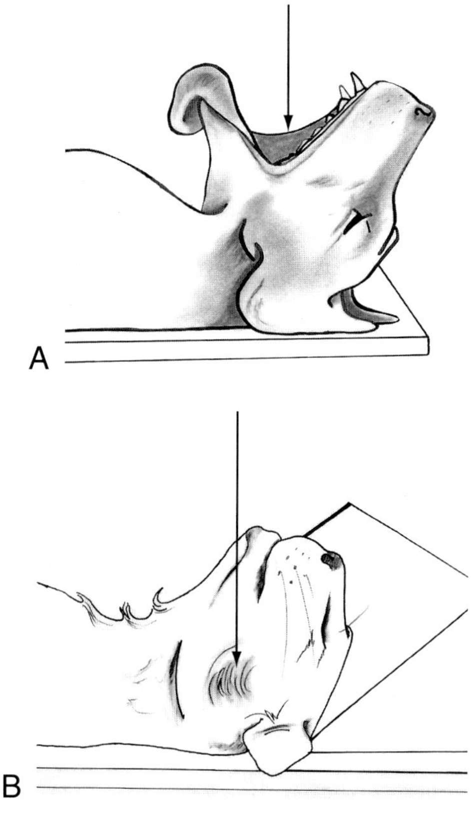

Figure 6.6. **A)** Open mouth rostrocaudal projection for tympanic bullae. **B)** 10° ventrodorsal.

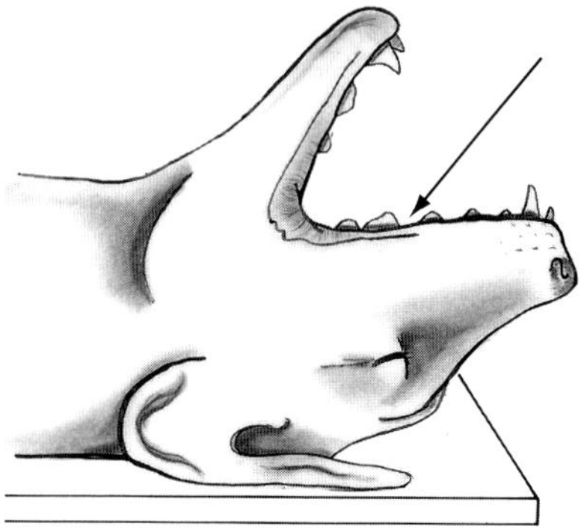

Figure 6.7. Open mouth ventrodorsal projection nasal cavity.

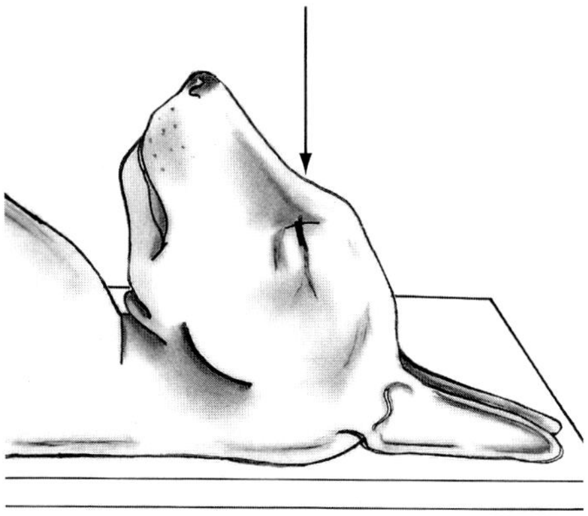

Figure 6.8. Rostrocaudal projection for foramen magnum.

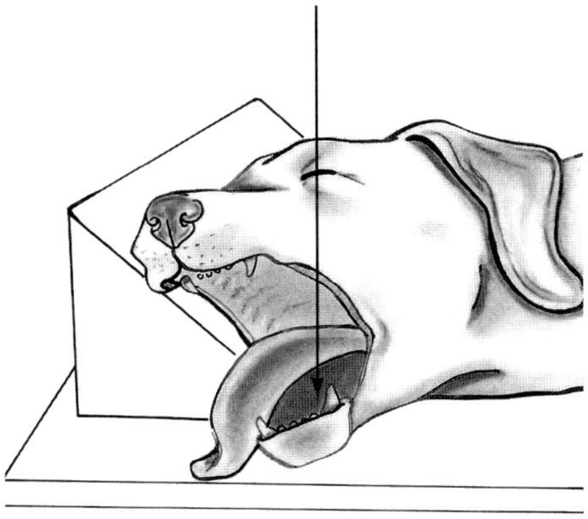

Figure 6.9. Open mouth lateral oblique projection for mandible.

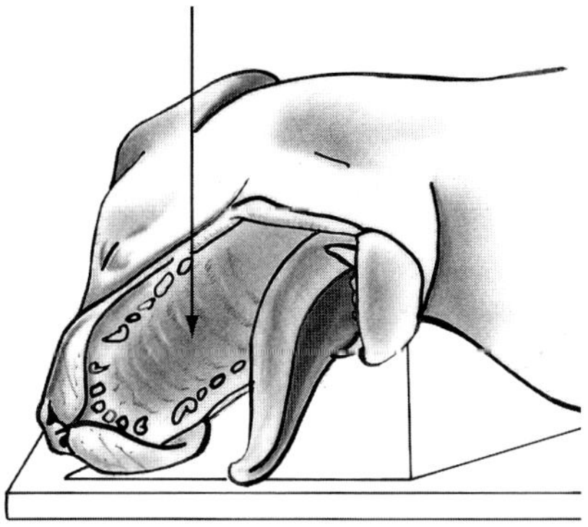

Figure 6.10. Open mouth lateral oblique projection for maxilla.

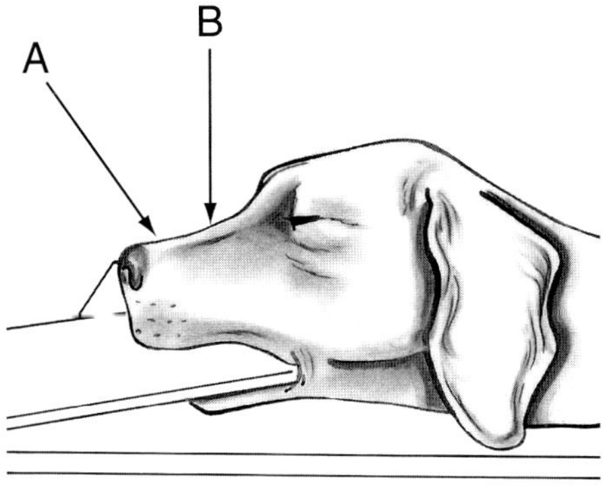

Figure 6.11. Occlusal dorsoventral projection. **(A)** Direction of x-ray beam for premaxilla and **(B)** direction of x-ray beam for nasal cavity.

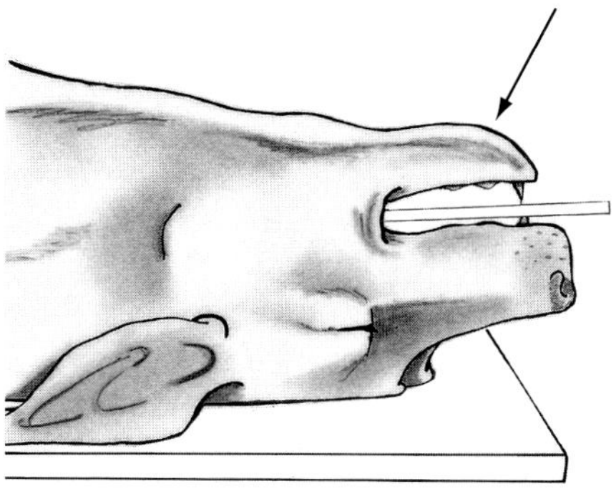

Figure 6.12. Occlusal ventrodorsal projection for rostral mandible.

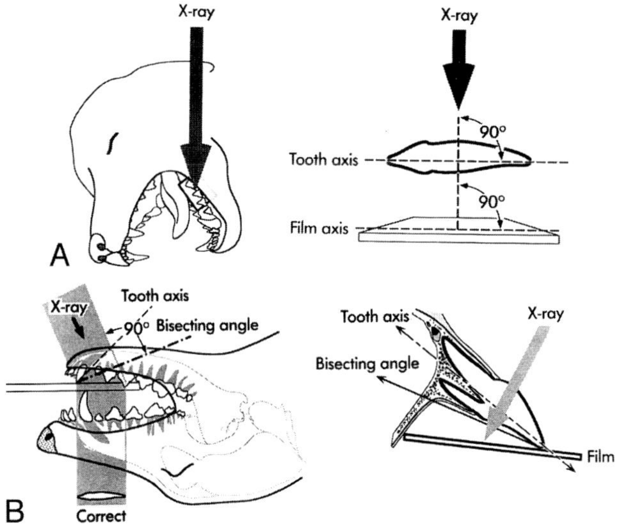

Figure 6.13. Intraoral dental techniques. **(A)** Parallel technique and **(B)** bisecting angle technique. (From Harvey CE and Emily PP. Small Animal Dentistry. 1993:806, 808. Used with permission Mosby-Year Book, Inc., St. Louis.)

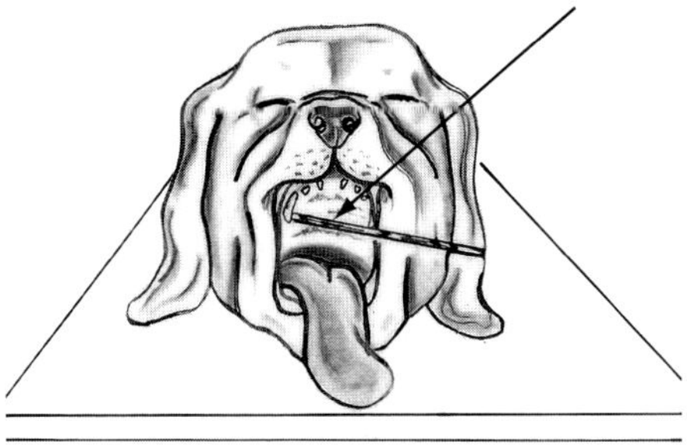

Figure 6.14. Approximate angle for x-ray beam for bisecting angle technique of premolar and molar teeth in maxilla.

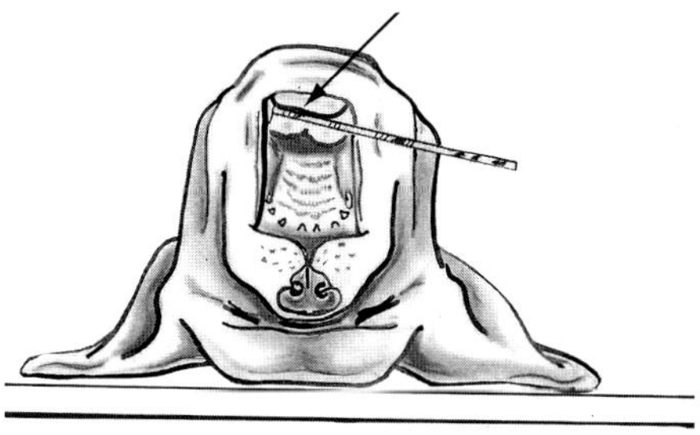

Figure 6.15. Approximate angle for x-ray beam for bisecting angle technique of premolar and molar teeth in mandible.

with the suggested radiographic projections for each area.

3. Optimal positioning usually requires general anesthesia or heavy sedation.

It is not always necessary to obtain all of the different projections for each area examined. One must choose the most appropriate projections that would best demonstrate the radiographic lesion.

OTHER IMAGING

Many of the radiographic studies of the skull, particularly the contrast studies (e.g., orbital venography, cerebral arteriography, pneumoventriculography) have been replaced by computed tomography (CT), magnetic resonance imaging (MRI), and ultrasound. These other imaging modalities provide improved imaging and diagnostic sensitivity for many diseases.

RADIOGRAPHIC ANATOMY

1. The radiographic anatomy of the skull is complex because of the superimposition of many bones and extensive compartmentalization. The external bony anatomy is illustrated in Figures 6.16 through 6.18.
2. There is variability in anatomy (e.g., shape and size) of the normal skull for the many dog and cat breeds. Major radiographic anatomy features of the canine and feline skulls are illustrated in Figures 6.19 through 6.22.

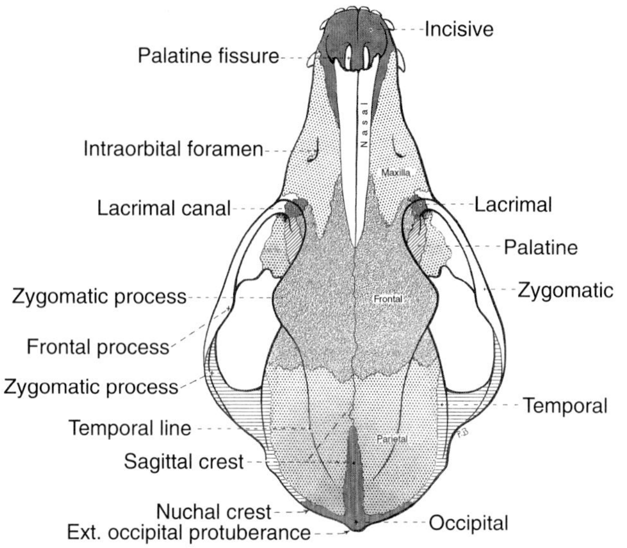

Figure 6.17. Bones of the skull, dorsal aspect. (From Evans HE. The skeleton. In: Evans HE, ed. Miller's Anatomy of the Dog. 3rd ed. Philadelphia: W.B. Saunders; 1993:129. Courtesy of and used with permission of Dr. Howard E. Evans.)

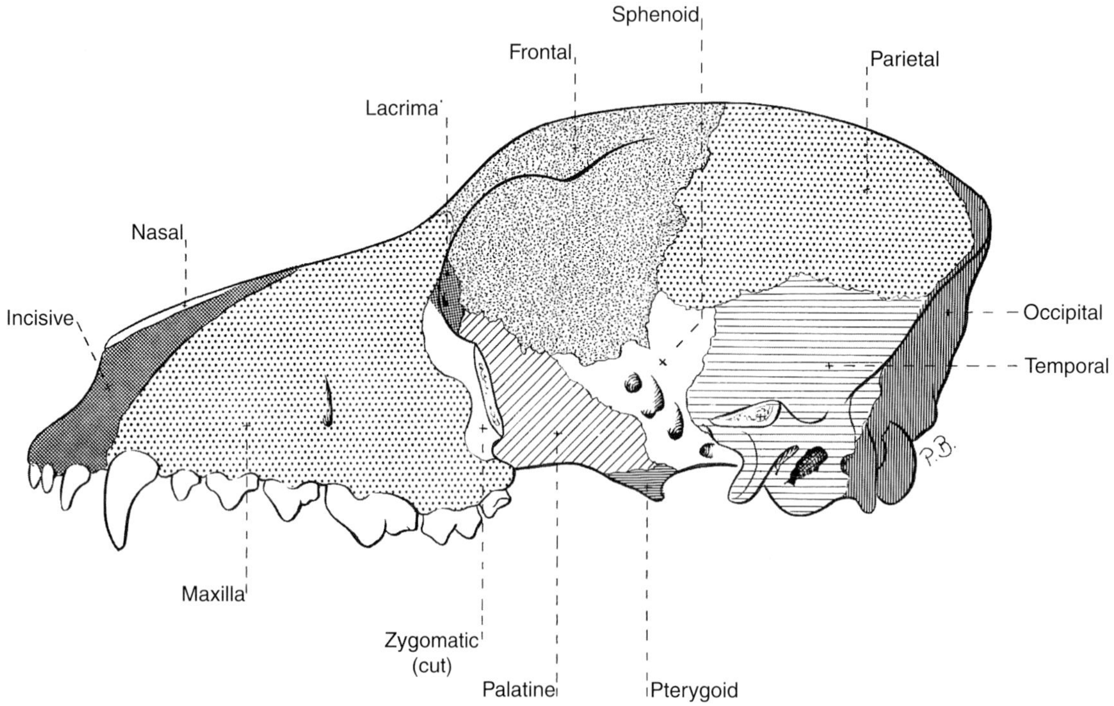

Figure 6.16. Bones of the skull, lateral aspect (Zygomatic arch and mandible removed). (From Evans HE. The skeleton. In: Evans HE, ed. Miller's Anatomy of the Dog. 3rd ed. Philadelphia: W.B. Saunders; 1993:128. Courtesy of and used with permission of Dr. Howard E. Evans.)

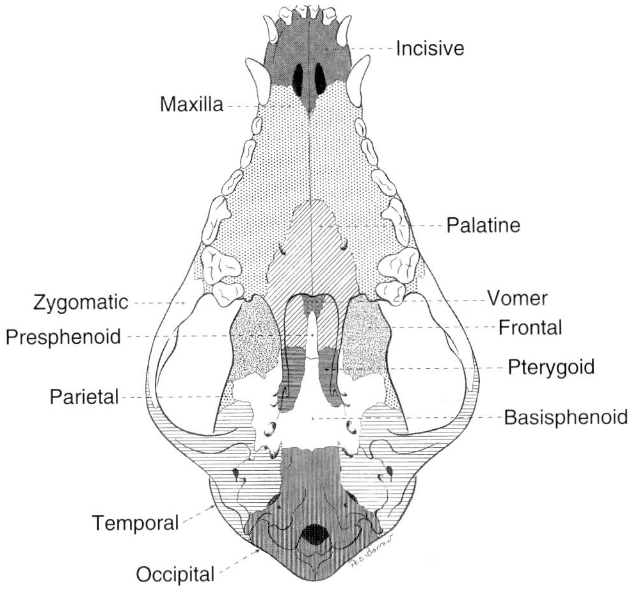

Figure 6.18. Bones of the skull, ventral aspect. (From Evans HE. The skeleton. In: Evans HE, ed. Miller's Anatomy of the Dog. 3rd ed. Philadelphia: W.B. Saunders; 1993:130. Courtesy of and used with permission of Dr. Howard E. Evans.)

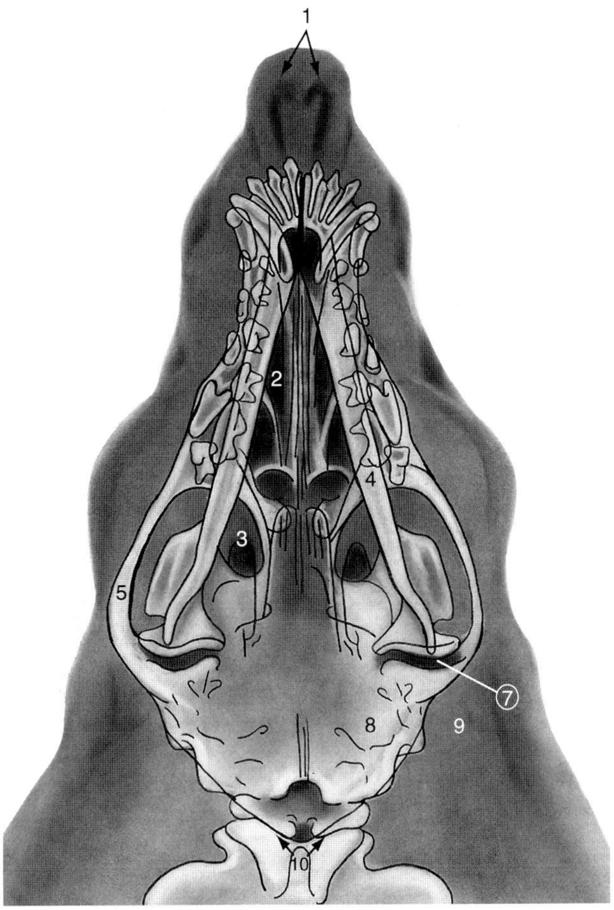

Figure 6.20. Normal canine skull (dorsoventral projection). Major landmarks are **1)** external nares, **2)** nasal cavity, **3)** frontal sinus, **4)** mandible, **5)** zygomatic process, **6)** coronoid process of mandible, **7)** temporomandibular joint, **8)** petrous temporal bone and tympanic bulla, and **9)** occipital condyle.

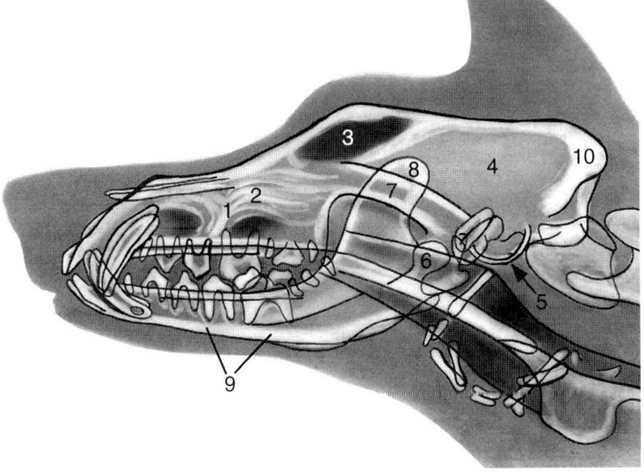

Figure 6.19. Normal canine skull (lateral projection). Major landmarks are **1)** nasal cavity, **2)** ethmoid turbinates, **3)** frontal sinus, **4)** cranial cavity and calvarium (arrow), **5)** tympanic bulla, **6)** temporomandibular joint, **7)** zygomatic arch, **8)** coronoid process of mandible, **9)** mandible, and **10)** nuchal crest.

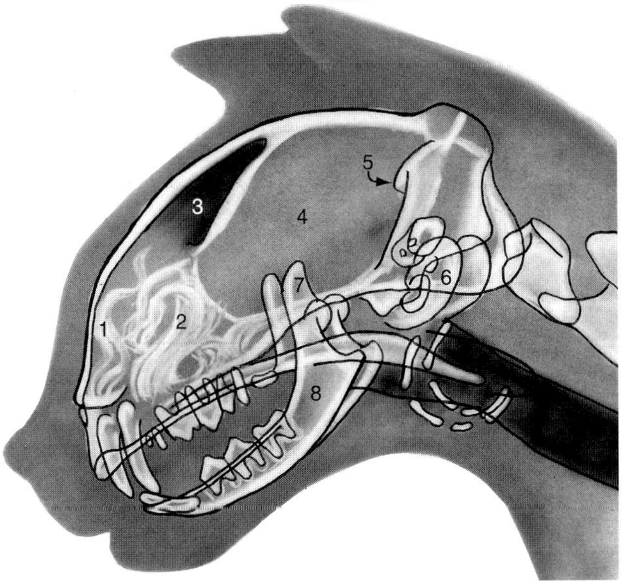

Figure 6.21. Normal feline skull (lateral projection). Major landmarks are **1)** nasal cavity, **2)** ethmoid turbinates, **3)** frontal sinus, **4)** cranial cavity **5)** tentorium cerebelli, **6)** petrous temporal bone and tympanic bulla, **7)** coronoid process of mandible, and **8)** horizontal ramus of mandible.

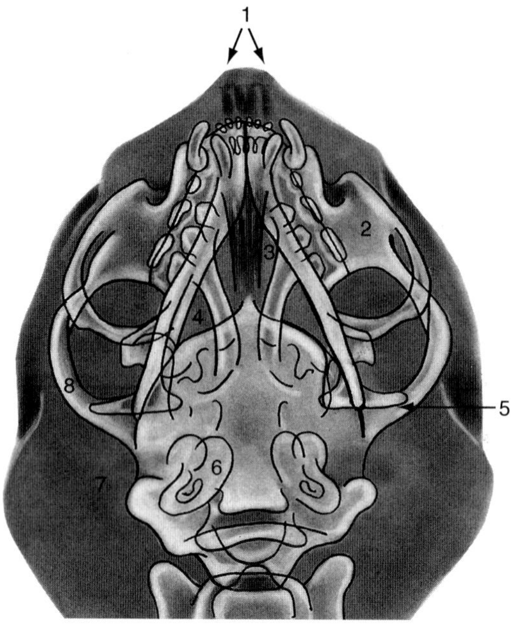

Figure 6.22. Normal feline skull (dorsoventral projection). Major landmarks are **1)** external nares, **2)** maxilla, **3)** nasal cavity, **4)** frontal sinus, **5)** temporomandibular joint, **6)** petrous temporal bone and tympanic bulla, **7)** external ear canal, and **8)** zygomatic process.

RADIOGRAPHIC INTERPRETATION

As with other regions of the body, a systematic examination should be made of each radiograph.

1. The soft tissues should be evaluated for enlargement, deficit, or abnormal opacity.
2. Symmetry of the skull should be carefully evaluated. Variations in size, shape, opacity, or position should be noted. Radiographic techniques must be varied to adequately image portions of skull of different thicknesses.
3. It is beneficial to refer to textbooks of anatomy and radiology. It is also helpful to have bone specimens available to understand the three-dimensional anatomy of the skull and to aid in the radiographic interpretation of abnormal radiographic findings.

The following discussion on the diseases of the skull is divided into four sections

1. The cranial vault and temporomandibular joints
2. The nasal cavity and paranasal sinuses
3. The teeth
4. The salivary glands and nasolacrimal duct

THE CRANIAL VAULT (CALVARIUM)

Radiographic Anatomy

1. The cranial vault contains the brain and the organs of hearing and equilibrium in the petrous part of the temporal bone.
2. The bony calvarium is formed by 14 bones (four paired and six unpaired); these bones are joined together by sutures.

DISEASES/DISORDERS

Hydrocephalus

Clinical correlations

1. Hydrocephalus represents pathologic accumulation of fluid within the ventricular system of the brain.
2. Obstructive (noncommunicating) hydrocephalus, the more common form, is caused by ventricular obstruction, usually by congenital anomalies (e.g., stenosis, septum formation), trauma, viral and bacterial infections, parasitic migration, and neoplasia.
3. Nonobstructive (communicating) hydrocephalus is a result of the failure of the arachnoid villi to absorb cerebral spinal fluid (CSF) at an adequate rate. It is the least common form of hydrocephalus in dog and cat, but has been reported in cats with feline infectious peritonitis and dog with other neural anomalies such as spinal cord dysgenesis and cerebellar ataxia.
4. Small, toy, and brachycephalic breeds of dogs (e.g., Yorkshire Terrier, Chihuahua, Maltese, Toy Poodle, Boston Terrier, English Bulldog, Pekinese, Lhasa Apso) are at increased risk for hydrocephalus. In Siamese cats hereditary hydrocephalus is an autosomal recessive trait.
5. The most common clinical signs of hydrocephalus may include an enlarged dome-shaped cranium, open fontanelles, visual and auditory deficits, vocalization, and an uncoordinated gait.

Radiographic findings

1. Survey radiographs (Figure 6.23):
   a. Enlargement of the cranium with a dome shape and cortical thinning of bony calvarium.
   b. Decreased prominence of normal calvarial convolutional markings.
   c. Open fontanelles and cranial sutures.
   d. Skull may appear normal, particularly if the hydrocephalus is acquired or in its early stages
   e. Most severe radiographic changes occur in congenital hydrocephalus. Minimal to no changes may be visible in cases of acquired hydrocephalus, especially after ossification is complete.
2. Contrast radiographs
   a. Ventriculography
   b. Pneumoventriculography
3. Other imaging
   a. Ultrasound
   b. CT
   c. MRI

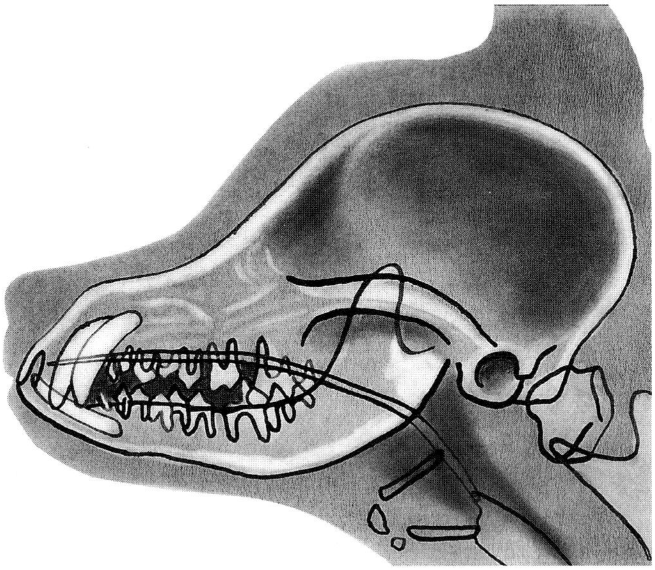

Figure 6.23. Hydrocephalus with enlarged cranial cavity and thinning or calvarium.

Occipital Dysplasia

Clinical correlations

1. Developmental malformation of the occipital bone with enlargement and dorsal extension of the foramen magnum.
2. More common in toy and miniature breed dogs
3. Affected animals may appear normal clinically unless herniation of the brain stem or cerebellum occurs through the enlarged foramen magnum.
4. Often accompanied by other anomalies such as hydrocephalus, shortening of C1, and atlantoaxial malformation.

Radiographic findings (Figure 6.24 A, B)

1. Slight to marked enlargement of the foramen magnum may be present with the major defect in the dorsal occipital border.
2. The foramen magnum is best visualized on a frontal occipital (foramen magnum) projection (see Figure 6.3).

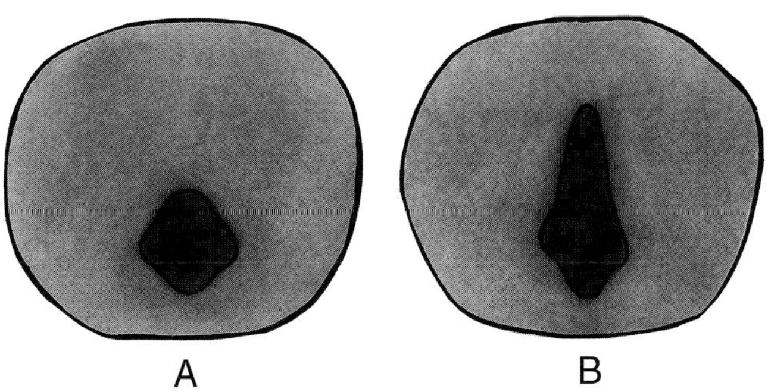

Figure 6.24. Occipital dysplasia (rostrocaudal projection for foramen magnum). **A)** Normal appearance of foramen magnum. **B)** Occipital dysplasia with enlarged foramen magnum.

Fractures

Clinical correlations

1. Usually the result of blunt trauma.
2. Less common than maxillary and mandibular fractures.
3. Central nervous system involvement may occur as the result of the fracture or as a result of brain contusion, extradural hemorrhage, or subdural hemorrhage.

Radiographic findings (Figures 6.25 and 6.26)

1. Adjacent soft tissue swelling is usually present.

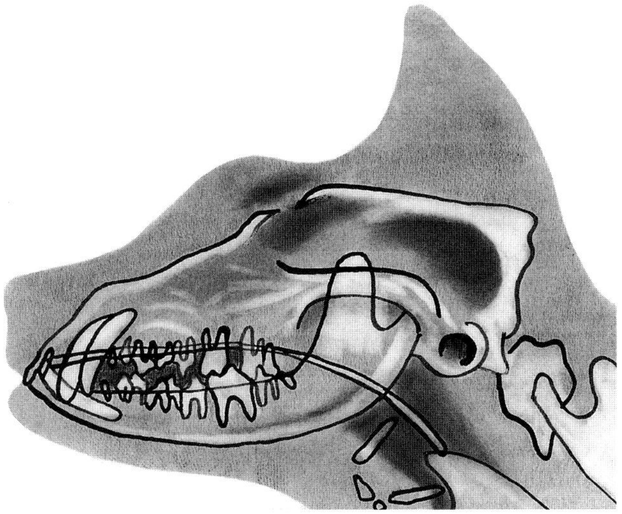

Figure 6.25. Comminuted fracture of frontal bone with adjacent soft tissue swelling and subcutaneous.

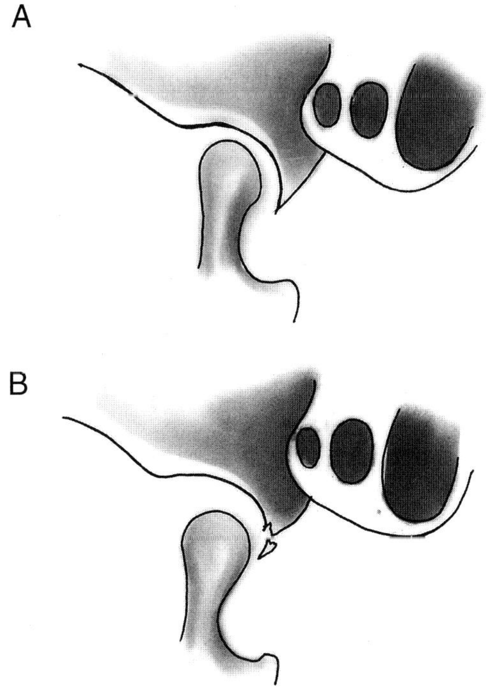

Figure 6.26. Temporomandibular fracture and luxation (lateral oblique projection). **A)** Normal. **B)** Subluxation of joint with fracture of retroarticular process of glenoid.

2. Subcutaneous emphysema may be present, especially if the fracture involves the nasal cavity or frontal sinus.
3. Fractures can be classified as linear, depressed/nondepressed, comminuted, simple, or compound.
4. Many skull fractures are small, linear, and nondisplaced.
5. Multiple radiographic projections, including tangential views, may be necessary to visualize the fracture lines.

Temporomandibular Subluxation or Luxation

Clinical correlations

1. There is unilateral and/or bilateral malocclusion and palpable instability of the temporomandibular joint.
2. Frequently associated with fracture of the mandibular symphysis or ramus.

Radiographic findings (See Figure 6.26):

1. Luxation of the temporomandibular joint may occur cranially, caudally, or laterally. Most commonly the mandibular condyle is displaced cranially.
2. The retroglenoid process of the temporal bone may be fractured with caudolateral luxation of the condyle.

Infection (Osteomyelitis)

Clinical correlations

1. Most infections are the result of sinus infections, external penetrating wounds, or previous surgery.
2. Bacterial or mycotic nasal infections may extend into the cranium through the cribiform plate and cause central nervous system disease.

Radiographic findings

1. If the infection occurs as the result of trauma, soft tissue swelling, a fracture, and/or a sequestrum may be seen.
2. Bone lysis and/or proliferation is usually seen at the site of the osteomyelitis.
3. If the infection extends through the ethmoid, increased radiopacity may be apparent in the nasal cavity, frontal sinuses, or ethmoid region.

Craniomandibular Osteopathy (CMO)

Clinical correlations

1. Is also known as temporomandibular osteodystrophy and mandibular periostitis.
2. A proliferative, nonneoplastic disorder of dogs that almost exclusively affects the bones of the cranium and mandibles. Occasionally produces a periosteal reaction on the periosteal long bones.
3. Predominantly affects terrier breeds, especially West Highland White, Scottish, and Cairn Terriers, but has also been reported in other terrier breeds, Labrador Retrievers, Doberman Pinschers, German Shepherd Dogs, and Boxers.
4. Reported as autosomal recessive trait in West Highland White Terriers and as a probable hereditary predisposition in other breeds.
5. A similar syndrome involving the frontal areas (Cranial Hyperostosis) has also been described in the Bull Mastiff.
6. Affected individuals usually show clinical signs at 3 to 8 months of age, consisting of mandibular swelling, drooling, prehension difficulties, pyrexia, and/or pain when opening the mouth.
7. The disease is self-limiting with regression of clinical signs. Proliferation of the new bone usually slows after the dog is 7 to 8 months old. Subsequently, the bony lesions tend to regress, although radiographic abnormalities or impaired function sometimes remains.

Radiographic findings (Figure 6.27):

1. Radiographic changes are usually bilateral.
2. Irregular and rough new bone proliferative changes

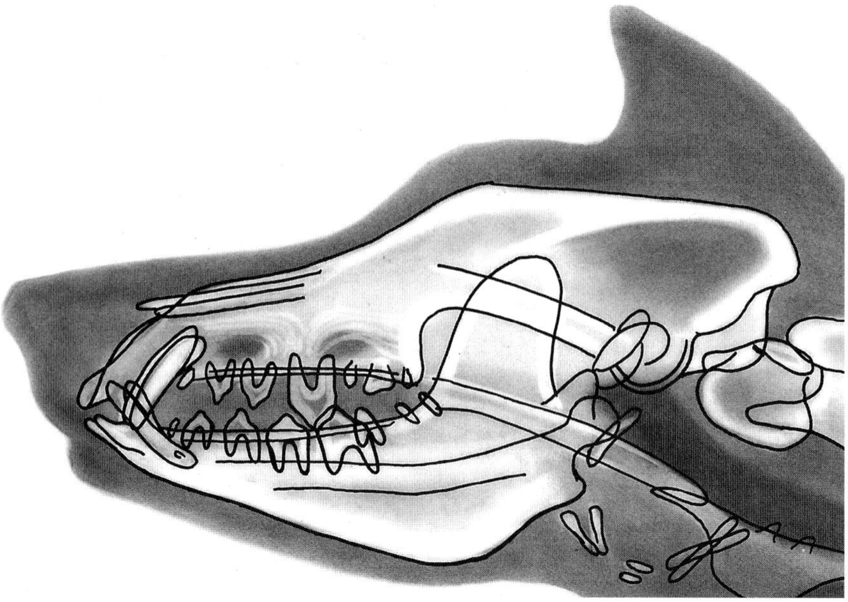

Figure 6.27. Craniomandibular osteopathy with bony proliferative changes on mandibles and calvarium.

involving the mandibles, usually originating near the angular process of the mandibles, the petrous tympanic regions of the skull, and occasionally the parietal, frontal, or maxillary bones. The calvarial thickening has no disruption of the inner or outer tables.
3. Bony proliferation of the tympanic bulla and temporomandibular joint ankylosis.
4. Occasionally there is a periosteal reaction on a long bone.

Lesions of the External, Middle, and Inner Ear

Clinical correlations

1. Inflammation involving the external, middle, and/or inner ear, usually caused by bacterial infection.
2. Middle and internal ear infection is frequently an extension of chronic otitis externa, but may also be a result of oral, nasopharyngeal, and systemic infection.
3. Nasopharyngeal polyps and auricular polyps are associated with inflammatory ear and nasal disease, with clinical signs of nasal discharge, sneezing, or stridor.
4. Polyps, more common in cats, may be cause of or sequel to otitis media.
5. Other causes include trauma and bone or soft tissue neoplasia (e.g., osteosarcoma, squamous cell and ceruminous carcinomas, fibrosarcoma).

Radiographic findings (Figures 6.28 A, B and 6.29)

1. Acute otitis and otitis interna commonly have no radiographic abnormality.
2. Chronic otitis externa may have:
   a. Mineralization and/or narrowing of the external auditory canal.
   b. Partial or complete occlusion of the normally radiolucent ear canal caused by exudates or hyperplastic tissue.

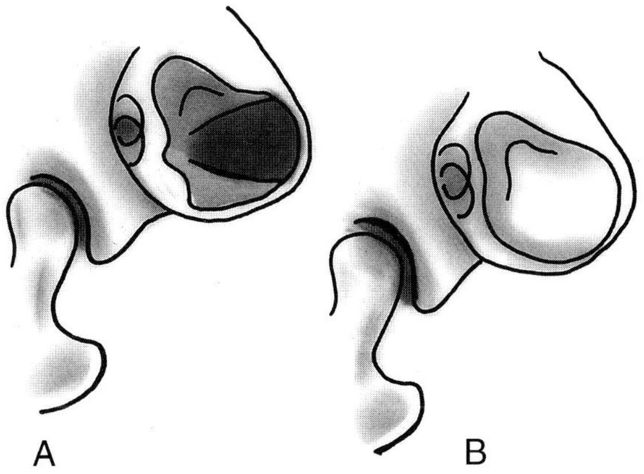

Figure 6.29. Tympanic bulla. **A)** Normal air-filled tympanic bulla. **B)** Infection with fluid-filled bulla and bony thickening.

3. Chronic otitis media and interna may have:
   a. Soft tissue/fluid radiopacity of the normally air-filled tympanic bulla.
   b. Osseous changes in the tympanic bulla, including lysis, sclerosis, thickening, and/or periosteal new bone formation.
   c. Enlargement of the bulla (uncommon).
4. Nasopharyngeal polyps may be single or multiple and occasionally visible as a soft tissue mass in the nasopharynx (Figure 6.30). Most often, there is thickening of one or both bony bullae and radiopacity within the bulla.
5. In aged animals, sclerosis of the petrous temporal bone may be present, but it is not representative of inflammatory ear disease and probably has no clinical significance.
6. Other diseases such as craniomandibular osteopathy may also produce bony proliferation and an increased opacity to the tympanic bullae; this is usually bilateral

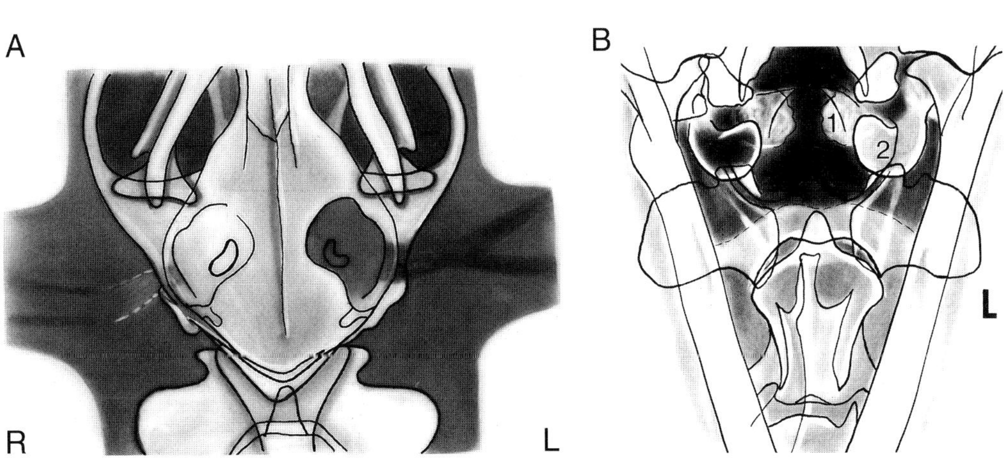

Figure 6.28. **A)** Chronic otitis (dorsoventral projection). There is increased opacity to the right petrous temporal bone and tympanic bulla (otitis media) and obliteration and mineralization of the external auditory canal (otitis externa). **B)** Chronic otitis (open mouth bulla projection). There is increased opacity in left petrous temporal bone **(1)** and left tympanic bulla **(2)**.

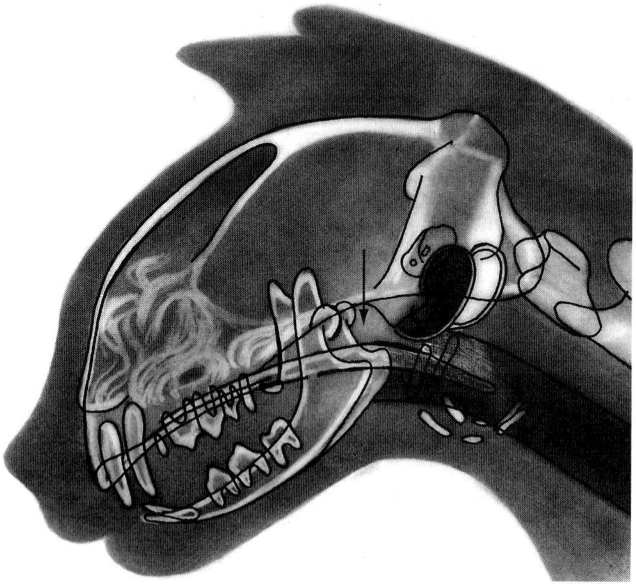

Figure 6.30. Nasopharyngeal polyp is visible in nasopharynx (arrow), and one tympanic bulla has an increased opacity associated with otitis media.

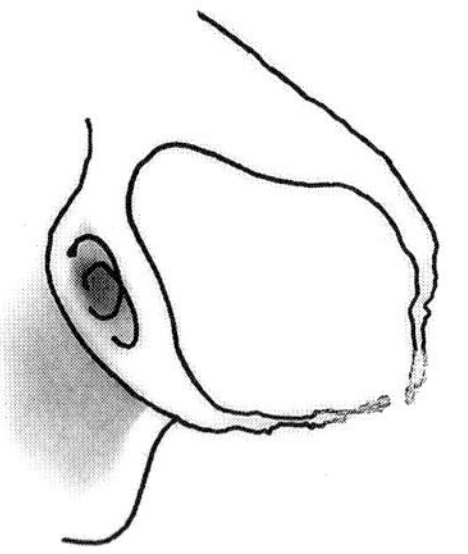

Figure 6.31. Tumor of tympanic bulla with bone lysis.

and concurrent with mandibular periosteal proliferation.

7. Neoplasms produce a variety of soft tissue and bony changes, depending on tumor type and location (Figure 6.31).

Neoplasms

Clinical correlations

1. Most commonly seen in middle aged and older dogs and cats.
2. Clinical signs are commonly related to the location of the tumor (e.g., nasal, oral, brain, cranial vault):
   a. External mass or enlargement.
   b. Seizures, common with intracranial tumors.
   c. Endocrinologic changes, common with pituitary tumors (e.g., polydypsia, polyuria, haircoat changes, obesity), visual deficits and sometimes seizures.
   d. Vestibular signs (e.g., head tilt, tremor, ataxia).
   f. Nasal discharge and upper airway obstruction.

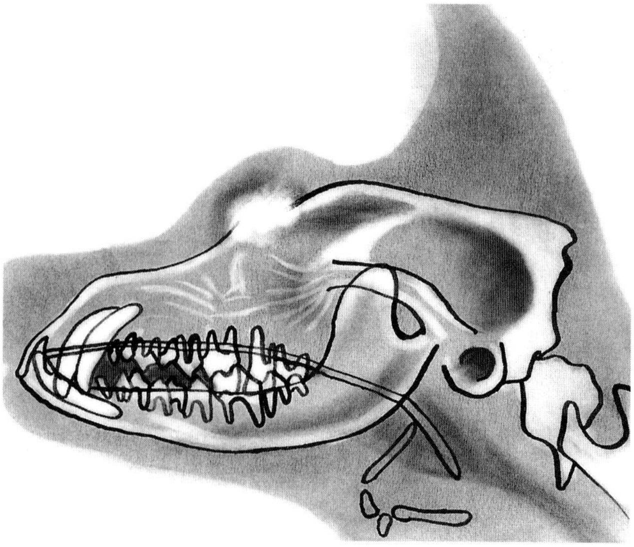

Figure 6.32. Osteosarcoma. There is marked bone lysis with periosteal proliferation of the frontal bone and adjacent soft tissue swelling.

Radiographic findings

1. Primary bone tumors resemble the clinical and radiographic appearance of similar tumors in the appendicular skeleton.
   a. Osteosarcoma is the most common primary malignant tumor. Osteosarcomas are usually osteoblastic with an aggressive periosteal reaction (Figure 6.32).
   b. Osteoma is the most common benign bone tumor. Osteomas are usually smooth, sclerotic, and well-marginated (Figure 6.33).
   c. Other bone tumors include chondrosarcoma, osteochondroma, and multilobular osteoma/chondroma.
   d. Multilobular osteoma and chondroma (chondroma rodans) is usually a locally invasive lytic lesion with a lobulated soft tissue mass containing diffuse amorphous mineralization. The most common locations include the parietal crest, the temporooccipital regions, and the zygomatic bone (Figure 6.34).
2. Soft tissue tumors often invade adjacent bone with varying amounts of bone destruction and proliferation (Figure 6.35).
3. Metastatic malignant tumors rarely occur in the skull and mandible. An exception is multiple myeloma, which is usually seen as multiple "punched out" lytic lesions (Figure 6.36).
4. Brain tumors, primary and metastatic, are usually not visible on survey radiographs:
   a. Some meningiomas may mineralize and be visible on survey radiographs; adjacent hyperostosis of the adjacent calvarium may sometimes be seen (Figure 6.37).
   b. CT and MRI are preferable for the diagnosis of intracranial neoplasms. These imaging procedures are less invasive and more definitive than cerebral

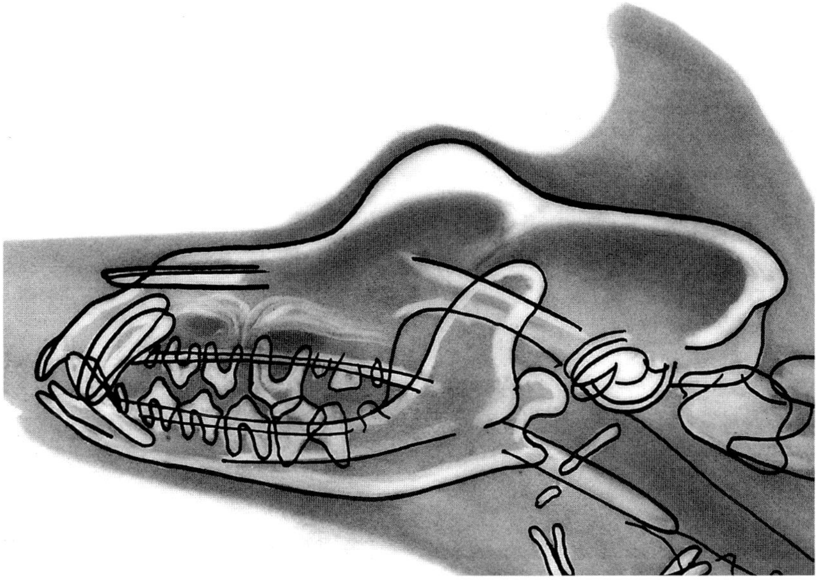

Figure 6.33. Osteoma. There is a smooth and sclerotic thickening of the frontal bone.

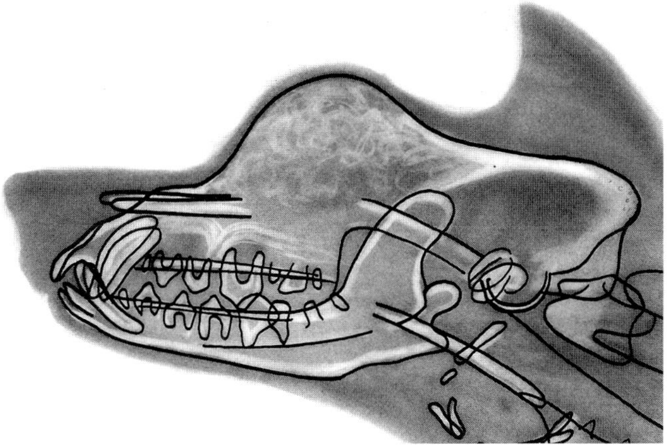

Figure 6.34. Multilobular osteoma/chondroma. There is an invasive lobulated lytic lesion with diffuse amorphous calcification of the frontal and parietal regions.

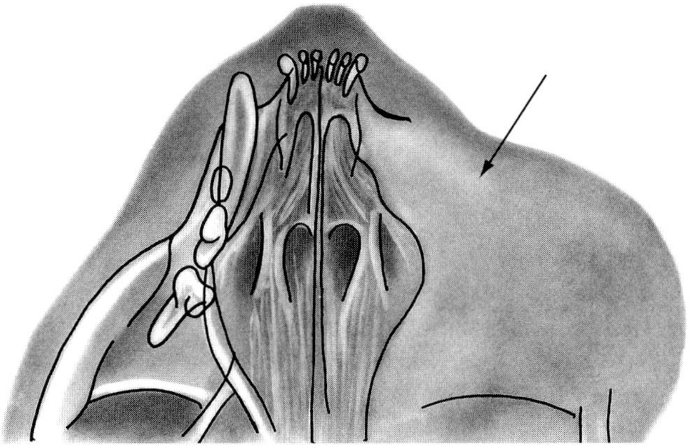

Figure 6.35. Soft tissue tumor infiltrating maxilla with bone destruction (arrow).

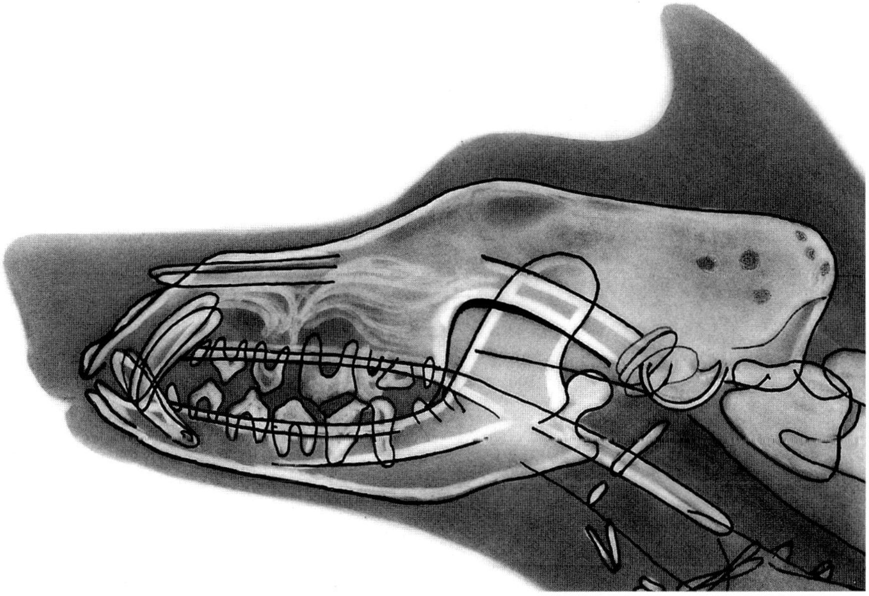

Figure 6.36. Multiple myeloma. Multiple lytic lesions (punched-out) are visible in the bones of the cranium.

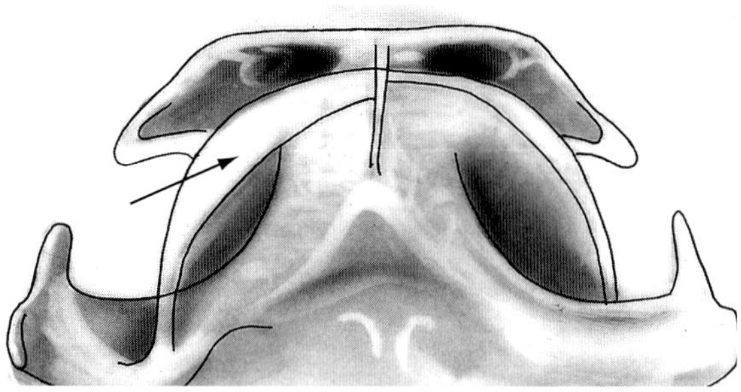

Figure 6.37. Meningioma. Hyperostosis of the calvarium is visible on a rostrocaudal projection (arrow).

angiography, pneumoventriculography, and cranial sinus venography.

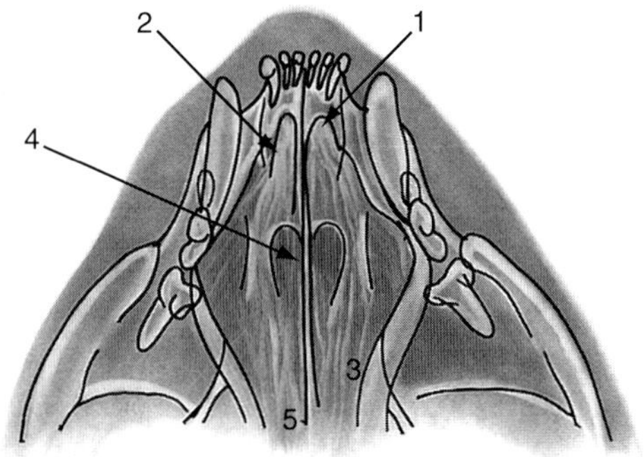

Figure 6.39. Normal feline nasal cavity (open mouth ventrodorsal occlusal projection). Major landmarks are **1)** palatine fissure, **2)** nasal turbinates, **3)** ethmoid turbinates, **4)** vomer bone, and **5)** frontal sinus.

NASAL CAVITY AND PARANASAL SINUSES

RADIOGRAPHIC ANATOMY (Figures 6.38 and 6.39):

1. The nasal cavity is divided into two symmetrical compartments (right and left) by a nasal septum. The vomer bone is located in the middle of the floor of the nasal cavity and forms the ventral portion of the nasal septum.
2. The primary four air passages of the nasal cavity are:
   a. the dorsal nasal meatus lying between the nasal bone and dorsal nasal concha
   b. the middle nasal meatus lying between the dorsal nasal concha and the ventral nasal concha
   c. the ventral nasal meatus lying dorsal to the hard palate
   d. the common nasal meatus lying on each side of the nasal septum.
3. The turbinates include the more cranially located maxillary turbinates and the more caudally located ethmoid turbinates.
4. The paranasal sinuses include the frontal sinus and maxillary recess and communicate with the nasal cavity. In the cat, the maxillary sinus is nonexistent.

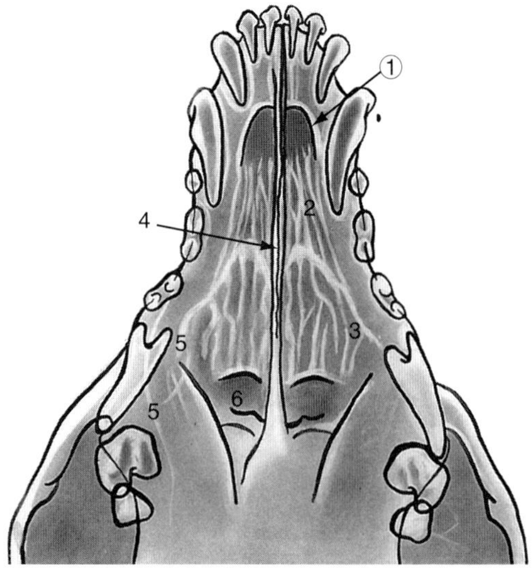

Figure 6.38. Normal canine nasal cavity (open mouth ventrodorsal projection). Major landmarks are **1)** palatine fissure, **2)** maxillary turbinates, **3)** ethmoid turbinates, **4)** vomer bone, **5)** maxillary sinus, and **6)** frontal sinus.

DISEASES/DISORDERS

Fractures of the Face and Frontal Area

Clinical correlations

1. Are frequently open fractures.
2. Fractures tend to involve multiple bones.
3. Asymmetry of the facial area is common.

Radiographic findings (See Figure 6.25)

1. Fractures are usually associated with adjacent soft tissue swelling.
2. Subcutaneous emphysema is frequently associated with fractures extending into the nasal cavity or frontal sinus.
3. There is frequently increased radiopacity at the fracture site because of overlapping of the fracture fragments and associated hemorrhage and soft tissue swelling.
4. Many fractures cannot be readily identified from only the standard lateral and DV projections, necessitating oblique projections to fully identify the fractures.

Infections

Clinical correlations

1. Infections commonly involve the paranasal sinuses and mucous membranes of the nasal cavity.

2. Infectious causes include:
   a. herpes and caliciviruses in cats
   b. adenovirus and influenza viruses in dogs
   c. mycotic infections
      1) Cryptococcus in cats
      2) Aspergillus in dogs
   d. bacteria (e.g., Pasteurella)
   e. parasites (e.g., Cuterebra in cats)
3. Acute infections are frequently secondary to:
   a. Upper respiratory diseases.
   b. Inhalation of a foreign body (e.g., plant awn).
4. Chronic infections are usually caused by:
   a. Chronic bacterial infections.
   b. Mycotic infections.
   c. Inhaled foreign body.
   d. Oronasal fistula.

Radiographic findings

1. Acute (Figure 6.40)
   a. In bacterial and mycotic infections, the radiographs may be normal or have an increased radiopacity involving one or both nasal cavities and/or frontal sinuses.
   b. In fungal disease, there may be focal areas of turbinate bone (concha) lysis.
   c. Radiopaque foreign bodies can usually be seen.
   d. Radiolucent foreign bodies (e.g., plant awns) are usually not visible, however in some cases, a localized increased radiopacity may be seen adjacent to the site of the foreign body associated within a soft tissue mass or localized fluid accumulation.

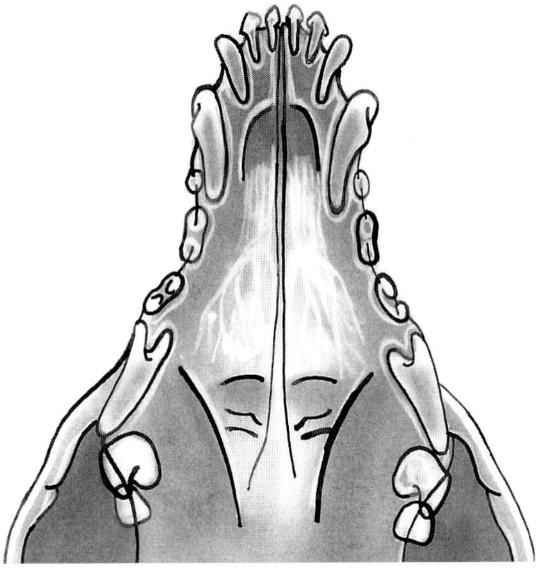

Figure 6.41. Chronic rhinitis (open mouth ventrodorsal projection). There is increased opacity to both nasal turbinates without evidence of bone destruction.

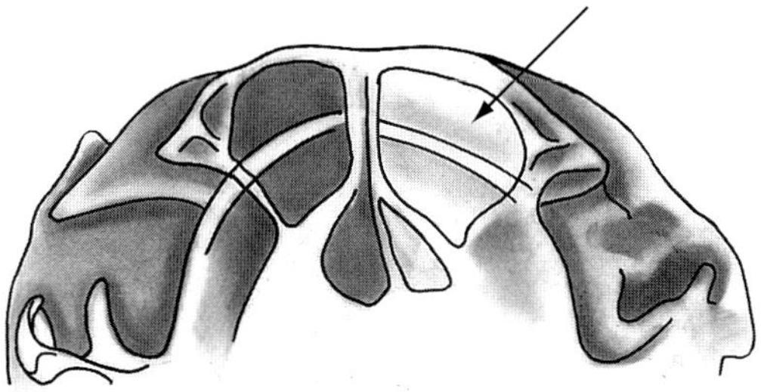

Figure 6.42. Frontal sinusitis (rostrocaudal frontal projection). There is an increased soft tissue opacity to the left frontal sinus with no bone lysis (arrow).

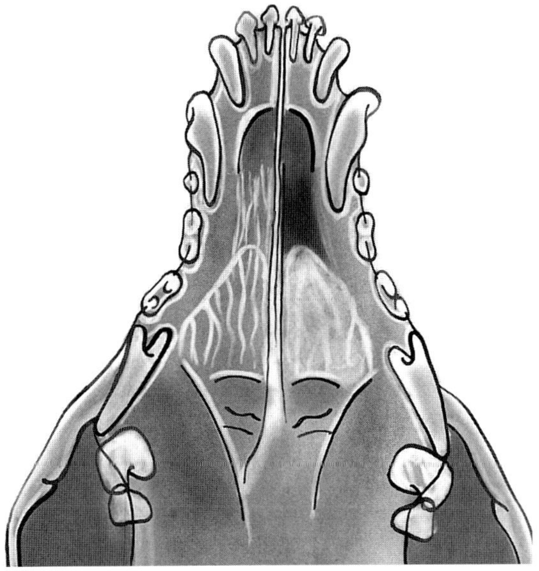

Figure 6.40. Fungal rhinitis (open mouth ventrodorsal occlusal projection). There is osteolysis of the nasal turbinates and increased opacity of the ethmoid turbinates on the left side.

2. Chronic (Figures 6.41 and 6.42):
   a. Complete or partial unilateral or bilateral opacification of the nasal cavity, and/or frontal sinuses.
   b. Blotchy opacification and blurring of the turbinate margins involving one or both sides of the nasal cavity.
   c. Nasal septum is usually intact.
   d. Bone sclerosis, if present, is usually localized with smooth borders.
   e. Soft tissue swelling or facial deformity is rare; if present is usually due to a mycotic infection or neoplasia.

Neoplasms Involving the Nasal Cavity

Clinical correlations

1. More frequent in dogs than cats, with reported higher frequency in dolichocephalic dogs.
2. Most common tumors are adenocarcinomas and squamous cell carcinomas in dogs and lymphosarcoma in cats; other primary tumors include epithelial and mes-

enchymal tumors (e.g., chondrosarcoma, fibrosarcoma, osteosarcoma, and hemangiosarcoma).
3. Most common clinical sign is unilateral or bilateral nasal discharge with or without epistaxis.

Radiographic findings (Figures 6.43 and 6.44)

1. In the early stage of disease, the radiographic findings may mimic infection:
   a. Blotchy increased radiopacity in the nasal cavity and/or frontal sinus.
   b. Diffuse radiopacity of the nasal cavity and/or frontal sinus, usually unilateral.
2. In the later stages of the disease, the common radiographic findings are:
   a. Irregular radiopacity within the nasal cavity and/or frontal sinus.
   b. Bone erosion (lysis) of the nasal turbinates (conchi) and/or cortical bone.
   c. Deviation and/or lysis of the nasal septum and vomer bone. Lysis may extend caudally through the cribiform plate into the cranial vault.
   d. Enlargement of the nasal cavity or frontal sinus with facial deformity, missing teeth, and/or external soft tissue swelling/mass.

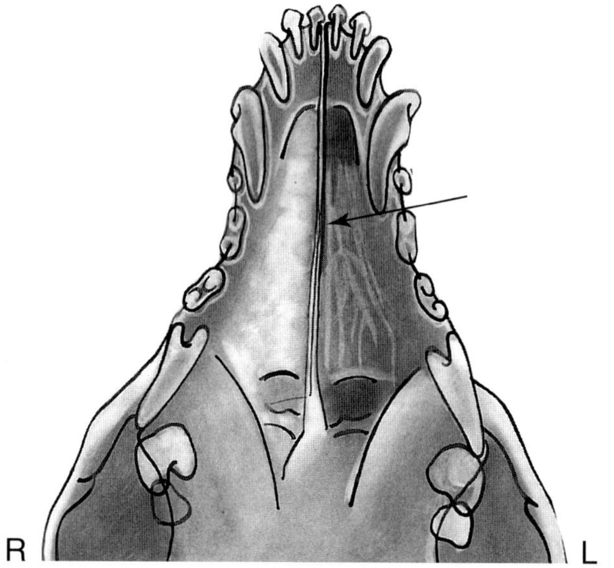

Figure 6.43. Nasal neoplasia (open mouth ventrodorsal projection). There is an increased soft tissue opacity to the entire right nasal cavity with lysis of the midvomer bone (arrow). No turbinate detail is seen.

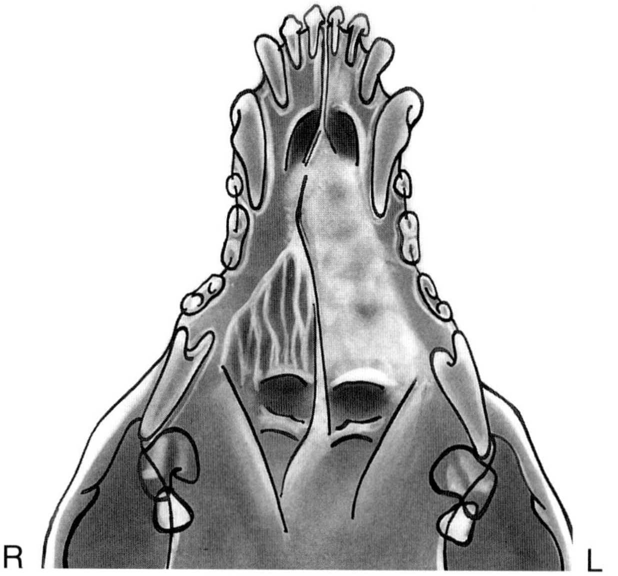

Figure 6.44. Nasal neoplasia (open mouth ventrodorsal projection). There is a mass in the left nasal cavity with lysis and deviation of the vomer bone and septum to the right side.

TEETH

RADIOGRAPHIC ANATOMY (Figure 6.45)

1. All teeth are similar structurally, although they differ in size and shape and may have one or more roots. The crown and root structures of the tooth and adjacent bone differ in radiographic opacity.
2. The dental enamel covering the tooth crown is the most radiopaque. Dentine, which composes most of the tooth substance and roots, is less radiopaque than enamel.
3. Each tooth root is surrounded by a thin radiolucent line representing the periodontal ligament, which at-

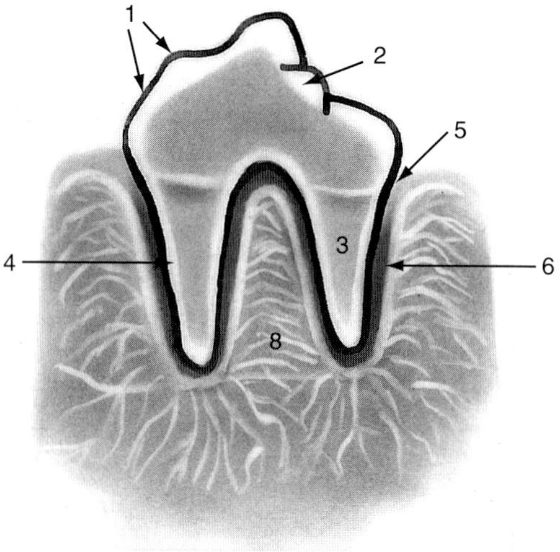

Figure 6.45. Normal tooth: **1)** crown, **2)** enamel, **3)** pulp cavity, **4)** dentin, **5)** amelocemental junction, **6)** periodontal membrane, **7)** lamina dura, and **8)** trabecular bone.

TABLE 6.2

Dental Formula for Dog

$$\text{Deciduous: } 2 \times \frac{\overset{\text{I C P}}{3\ 1\ 3}}{3\ 1\ 3} = 28$$

[Some authors refer to the last upper and lower premolar teeth as the molars]

$$\text{Permanent: } 2 \times \frac{\overset{\text{I C P M}}{3\ 1\ 4\ 2}}{3\ 1\ 4\ 3} = 42$$

Dental Formula for Cat

$$\text{Deciduous: } 2 \times \frac{\overset{\text{I C P}}{3\ 1\ 3}}{3\ 1\ 2} = 26$$

$$\text{Permanent: } 2 \times \frac{\overset{\text{I C P M}}{3\ 1\ 3\ 1}}{3\ 1\ 2\ 1} = 30$$

taches the tooth to the adjacent cortical bone. The cementum and periodontal ligaments, which attach to the tooth, are radiolucent and not visible.

4. The lamina dura is the thin radiopaque cortical layer of the normal bone visible next to the periodontal ligament.
5. The bone of the maxilla and mandible adjacent to the lamina dura usually has a trabecular pattern. Bone between adjacent teeth and between multiple tooth roots is termed the interradicular bone. Bone between roots of multirooted teeth is also called furcatin bone (Table 6.2).

EFFECT OF AGE (Figure 6.46 A, B):

1. Young animals:
   a. The permanent teeth develop as a bud from the deciduous teeth precursors.
   b. The pulp cavity in young permanent teeth is large, with an open apical foramen.
   c. Eruption times for deciduous and permanent teeth vary within a narrow range of weeks and months. Teeth of female dogs often erupt earlier than those of males and teeth of large breed dogs erupt earlier than small breed dogs.

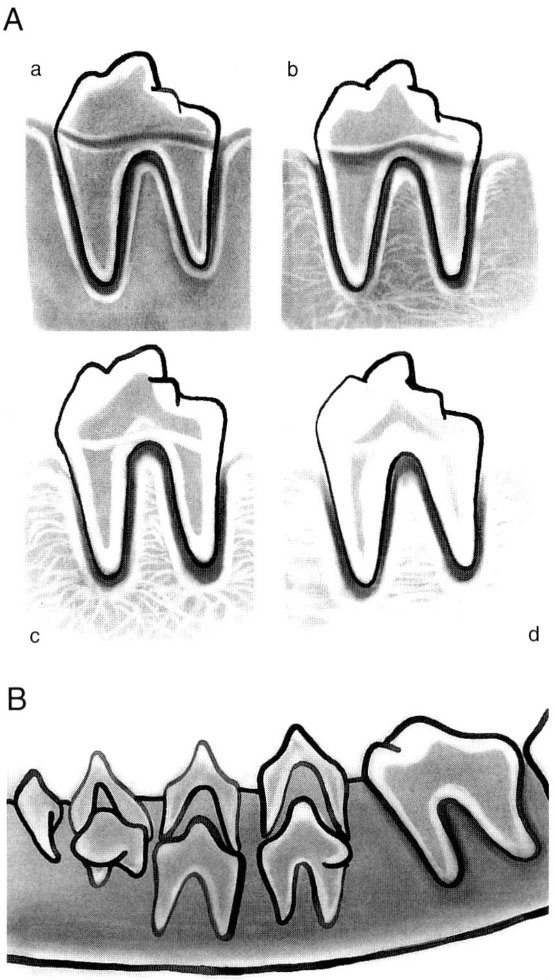

Figure 6.46. **A)** Effect of age in dogs. Note the open apical foramen in **A** and the progressive decreased size of the pulp cavity that occurs with age: **a)** 4 months old, **b)** 1 year old, **c)** 3 years old, and **d)** 10 years old. **B)** Deciduous teeth.

2. Older animals:
   a. All the permanent teeth normally erupt by 7 months of age. The root lengthens until the apex of the root closes.
   b. Predictable radiographic changes affecting the normal teeth and the adjacent structures occur after eruption:
      1) The apical foramen "closes" several months after eruption of the permanent tooth.
      2) The pulp cavity and root canal become narrower during the animal's life; in aged animals, the pulp cavity and root canal may be nearly nonexistent.
      3) The lamina dura, identified as a smooth radiopaque line bordering the periodontal membrane, becomes less distinct as the animal ages.
      4) The bone trabeculae of the supporting alveolar bone changes from a fine and distinct trabecular appearance in young animals to a more sclerotic and dense trabeculation in older animals.

RADIOGRAPHIC EXAMINATION

1. A dental x-ray machine with a small focal spot and universal joint mounting is ideal for obtaining oral radiographs.
2. Nonscreen film for intraoral and extraoral radiographs provides better detail than screen film techniques.
3. For the best detail and least distortion, the plane of the film should be placed parallel to the long axis of the tooth and perpendicular to the plane of the x-ray beam. Because this is difficult to do in many dogs and cats because of anatomic variations, frequently a bisecting angle technique is used in which the central ray beam is directed perpendicular to an imaginary line bisecting the angle formed by the plane of the long apex of the tooth and film surface (see Figure 6.13B).

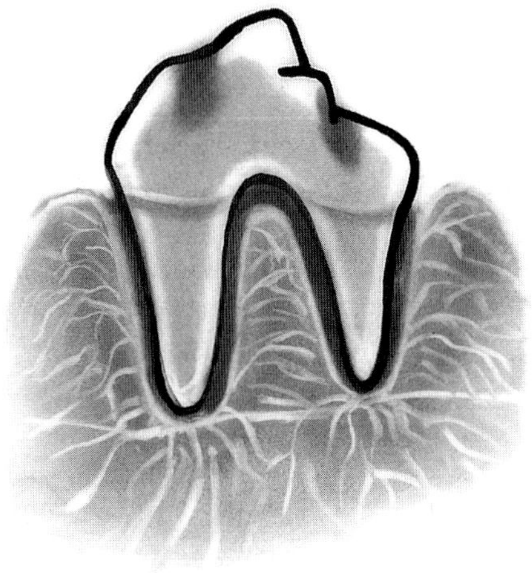

Figure 6.47. Dental caries in enamel of tooth.

DISEASES/DISORDERS

Dental Anomalies

1. Congenital and inherited anomalies in size, shape, and number of teeth are common in the dog and cat. These anomalies may be clinically significant and inheritable.
2. Anomalies include supernumerary teeth, hypodontia (absence of a tooth), conjoined or divided crown (gemini tooth), and retained deciduous teeth.
3. Congenital anomalies and systemic disease can cause variations in eruption times of deciduous and permanent teeth and in enamel and dental formation. Abnormal placement of teeth may cause malocclusion. Large teeth may cause crowding and periodontal disease later in life.
4. Malocclusion of teeth may occur as sequel to anomalies of tooth or bone development, temporomandibular luxation or dysplasia, fracture or callus of the mandible or maxilla, craniomandibular osteopathy, or other masses causing mechanical obstruction.
5. Dental radiographs can be made at a young age to determine the presence of the crowns before eruption.

Dental Calculus

Clinical correlations

1. Sequel to accumulation of dental plaque.
2. Common in dogs and cats, related to type of diet, and often associated with periodontal disease.

Radiographic findings

1. Mineralization of dental plaque, usually visible above the gingival crest or below the crest on the tooth root.
2. Commonly present on the buccal surfaces of the maxillary fourth premolar and mandibular first molar teeth in dogs.
3. May create a roughened and irregular appearance to the tooth surface.

Dental Decay (Caries)

Clinical correlations

1. Uncommon in dogs and rare in cats.
2. When present in dog, the upper fourth premolar, first and second molar and lower first molar are most commonly affected.
3. If present, may be painful and lead to pupal death and root abscess.

Radiographic findings (Figure 6.47)

1. Radiolucent defects in the enamel of the tooth.
2. Variable degrees of enamel erosion.
3. Periapical radiolucency around roots when pulp is penetrated (abscess).

Tooth Resorption

Clinical correlations

1. Common lesions in cats and occasionally seen in dogs.
2. Commonly begins as external resorption at the gingival margin involving the crown and/or root. May progress to erosion of the dentin and the pulp with loss of adjacent bone.
3. Gingiva usually appears irregular, hyperplastic, inflamed, and often covers lesion.
4. Strong correlation between radiographic extent of tooth destruction and peridontal disease.
5. Resorptive process often results in extrusion of the teeth.

Radiographic findings (Figure 6.48 A, B)

1. Varying degrees of crown and root resorption.
2. Secondary loss (lysis) of alveolar crest or furcation bone and occasionally a pathologic fracture.

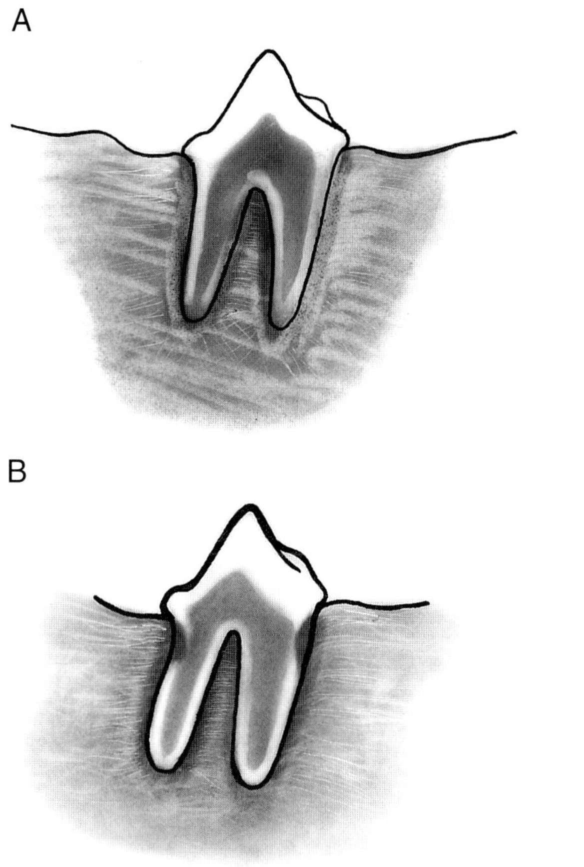

Figure 6.48. Tooth resorption. **A)** Normal feline tooth **B)** Root resorption.

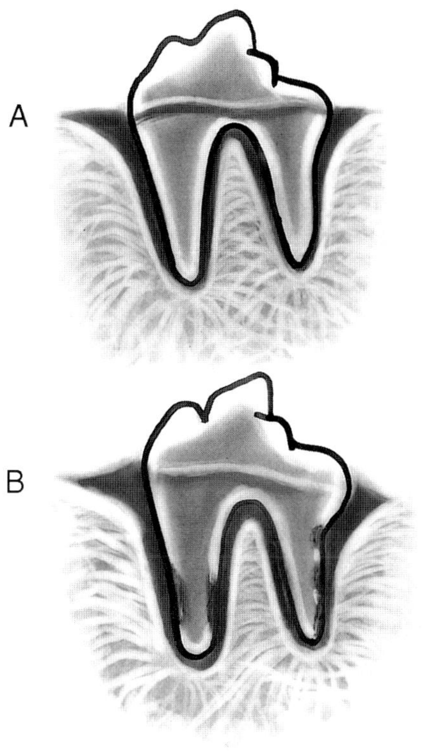

Figure 6.49. Periodontal disease. **A)** Early changes. **B)** Later changes.

Periodontal Disease

Clinical correlations

1. The most common dental disease in the dog and the cat.
2. Composed of gingivitis, vasculitis, loss of perivascular collagen, and infection by periodontal pathogens.
3. Can be associated with other diseases such as chronic nephritis.
4. Periodontitis commonly leads to tooth loss in the dog, often without clinical evidence of pain or other disabling side effects.
5. Results in bone resorption, including regression of the alveolar crest or furcation bone.
6. Osteomyelitis, pathologic fractures, and oronasal fistula may be sequelae.

Radiographic findings (Figure 6.49 A, B)

1. Changes usually visible only in the later stages of the disease.
2. Loss of sharpness and density of the crestal bone.
3. Loss of crestal bone, beginning with early furcation involvement and progressing to the root apex.
4. Widening of the periodontal space.
5. Loss of the radiopaque lamina dura, commencing coronally.
6. Moderate to severe horizontal, oblique, or vertical bone loss.
7. Cavitation, resorption, and/or exfoliation of a tooth.
8. Root resorption.
9. Pathologic fracture of tooth root or adjacent bone.

Apical Infection

Clinical correlations

1. Infection of the apex of the root may occur secondary to:
   a. Periodontal disease.
   b. Fractures of the tooth or alveolar bone.
   c. Dental or oral neoplasms.
   d. Hematogenous infection.
2. Frequently, an apical abscess of the tooth in the dog involves the upper fourth premolar tooth (carnassial tooth). This infection may extend into the maxillary sinus recess or be evident as an externally draining fistulous tract or facial swelling.

Radiographic findings (Figure 6.50 A, B)

1. Widening of the radiolucent space surrounding and centered on the apex of the root.
2. Bone lysis or sclerosis adjacent to the apex.
3. Progressive reabsorption of the tooth root.
4. Osteomyelitis of adjacent bone.

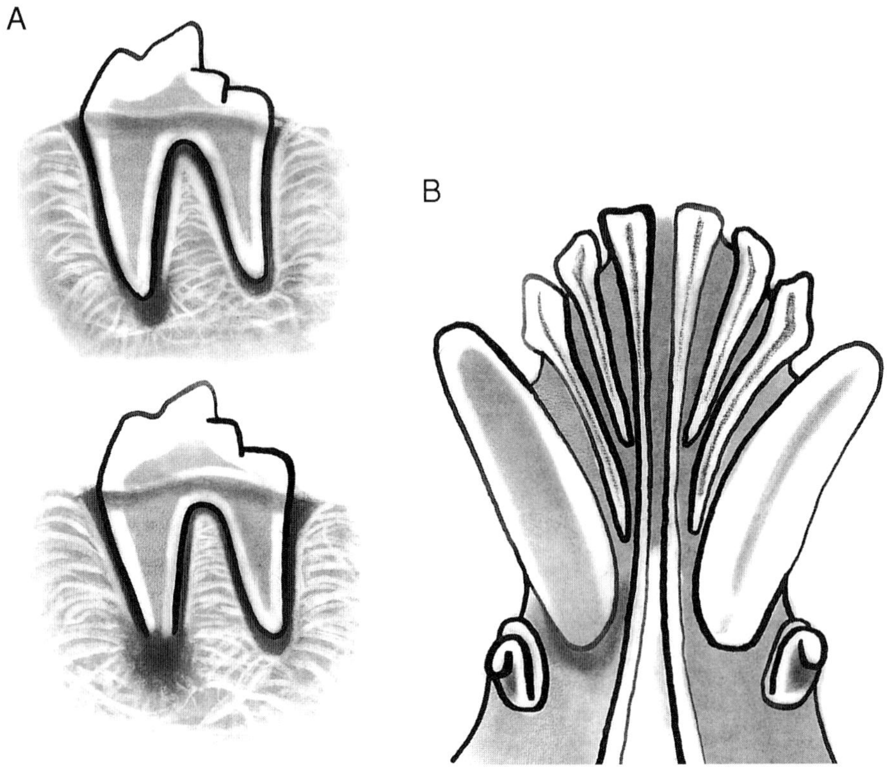

Figure 6.50. Apical tooth abscess. **A)** Early and later tooth changes of pulp/root resorption. **B)** Chronic apical abscess with enlargement of pulp cavity indicative of tooth death.

5. Differential diagnosis is apical cyst, which has a lytic lesion surrounded by a sclerotic margin. This cyst is derived from epithelial cells trapped in the periodontal ligament tissue.

Fractures of Tooth

Clinical correlations

1. Usually the result of chewing on hard objects or the result of external trauma.
2. If the pulp cavity is exposed, infection invariably extends into the root of the tooth, eventually causing an apical abscess.

Radiographic findings (Figure 6.51 A, B)

1. Small, linear cracks or fissures are usually readily identified in the affected teeth.
2. Fractures may involve the tooth below the gingiva.

Metabolic Diseases

Clinical correlations

1. Diseases that affect calcium metabolism (e.g., primary hyperparathyroidism, secondary hyperparathyroidism, or tertiary hyperparathyroidism) may cause loss of bone, especially in the mandibles and maxillae.
2. Calcium resorption occurs, starting with the lamina dura and cortical bone of the tooth alveolus.

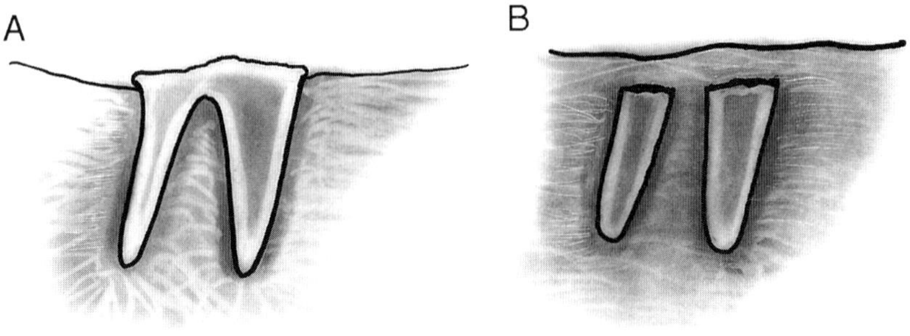

Figure 6.51. Tooth fracture. **(A)** Fractured crown and **(B)** retained roots.

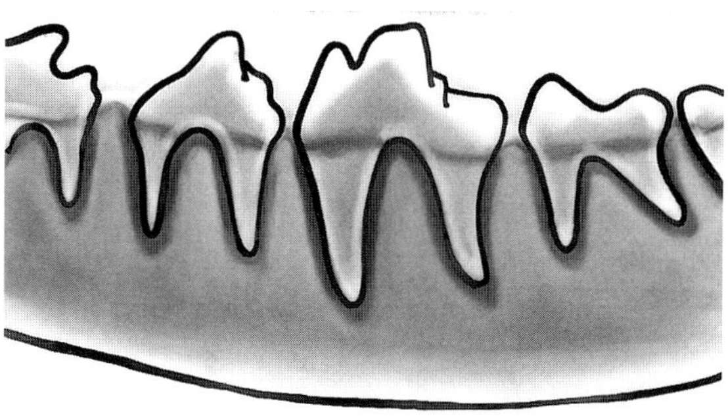

Figure 6.52. Secondary hyperparathyroidism. Loss of lamina dura and osteoporosis of the trabecular bone.

3. In advanced disease there may be generalized demineralization of the entire skull, the spine, and the limb bones.

Radiographic findings (Figure 6.52)

1. Loss of the radiopaque lamina dura and replacement with fibrous tissue.
2. Diffuse osteoporosis or uniform loss of bone, especially in the mandibles and maxillas. Bone is replaced by soft tissue radiopacity and teeth appear to "float."

Neoplasms of the Teeth and the Oral Cavity

Clinical correlations

1. The oral cavity is a common site of malignant and benign neoplasms.
2. The teeth can be affected with tumors originating from dental elements or, secondarily, from an adjacent soft tissue or bony neoplasm.
   a. Some of the more common dental tumors include ameloblastoma, ameloblastic fibroodontoma, and odontoma.
   b. The most common types of malignant gingival soft tissue tumors are: squamous cell carcinoma, fibrosarcoma, and malignant melanoma.
   c. The most common benign oral tumors are dentigerous cyst, fibromatous epulis, ossifying epulis, acanthomatous epulis, and viral induced papilloma. Although not malignant, acanthomatous epulis is aggressive locally and mimics a malignant tumor grossly and radiographically.
3. Must differentiate dental tumors from odontogenic inflammatory and developmental cysts. Cysts (e.g., odontogenic keratocyst and primordial cyst) are benign, but can mimic the clinical and radiographic appearance of tumors.

Radiographic findings (Figures 6.53, 6.54, 6.55, and 6.56)

1. Ameloblastoma and adamantinoma:
   a. May involve one or more teeth
   b. May appear solid or cystic

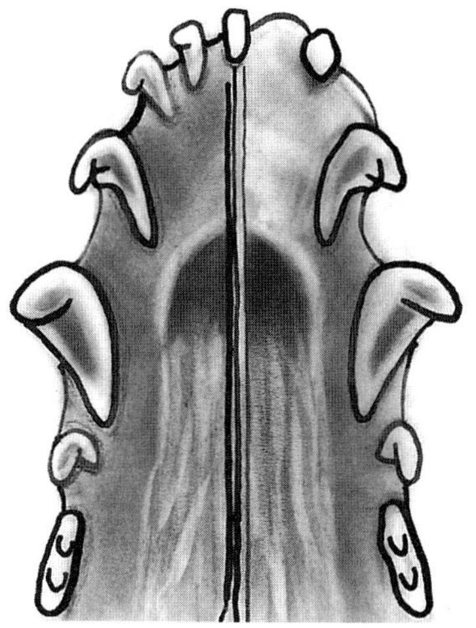

Figure 6.53. Adamantinoma. There is a poorly demarcated lytic lesion of the rostral left premaxilla with displacement and loss of several teeth.

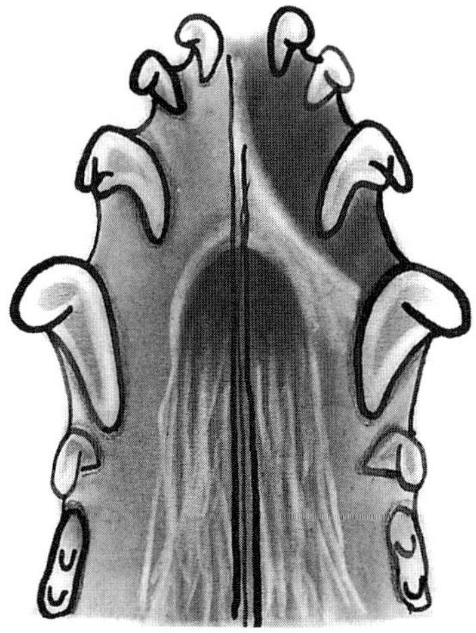

Figure 6.54. Dentigerous cyst. Well-demarcated and expansile lytic lesion of the rostral left premaxilla.

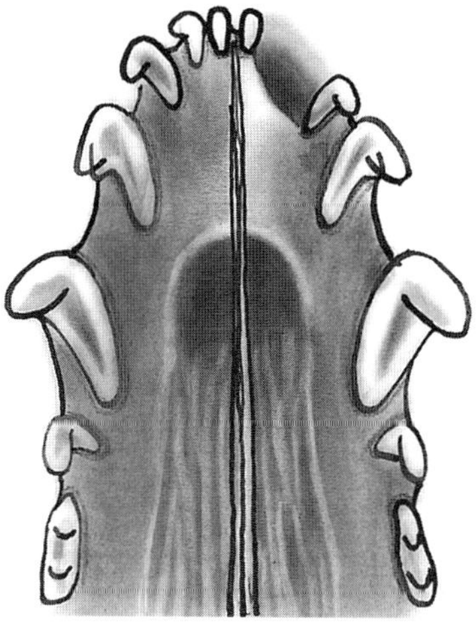

Figure 6.55. Squamous cell carcinoma. Poorly demarcated lytic lesion of the rostral left premaxilla with loss of teeth.

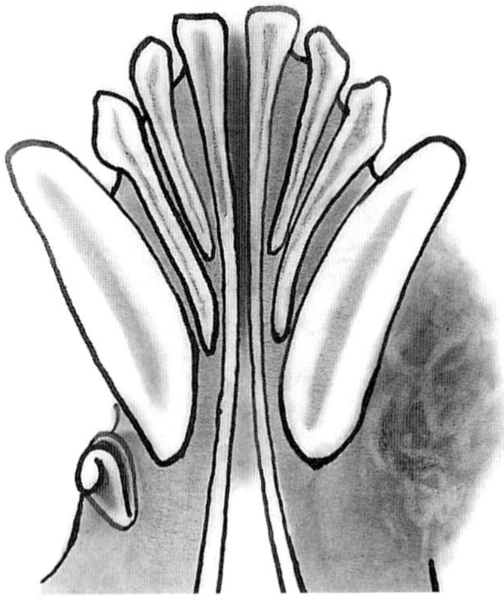

Figure 6.56. Acanthomatous epulis. An expansile bony lesion adjacent to the left canine tooth with irregular mineralization.

   c. Frequently expansile with adjacent bone destruction
   d. Usually associated with an adjacent soft tissue mass
2. Odontoma:
   a. Usually lytic and expansile with smooth borders.
   b. Often contains focal mineralized opacities
3. Dentigerous cyst:
   a. Usually lytic and expansile with a well-defined margin.
   b. May involve the roots of one or more teeth.
   c. May have "teeth" in the lesion.
4. Nonodontogenic malignant tumors:
   a. Most arise from soft tissues (e.g., gingiva, hard palate) or bone of the mandible or maxilla. Common tumors include carcinomas, firbrosarcoma, malignant melanoma, and acanthomatous epulis.
   b. Irregular and poorly demarcated with lysis of bone.
   c. Variable degrees of bony proliferation, from none to a "sunburst" type of periosteal reaction.
   d. May extend into the alveolar bone of one or more teeth.
   e. A pathologic fracture may occur if bone lysis is extensive.

SALIVARY GLANDS

RADIOGRAPHIC ANATOMY

1. In the dog and cat there are four pairs of salivary glands: the parotid, zygomatic, mandibular, and sublingual glands, and multiple areas of smaller gland acini, sometimes referred to as the dorsal and ventral buccal glands. The location of the salivary glands and salivary ducts is shown in Figure 6.57.
2. The salivary glands are not visible on survey radiographs.
3. Sialography, using iodinated contrast media, is necessary to evaluate the salivary ducts and glands.

DISEASES/DISORDERS

Sialolithiasis

Clinical correlations

1. Rare in the dog and cat.
2. Usually associated with chronic inflammation.

Radiographic findings

Small, round, or rod-shaped radiopaque calculi within the salivary ducts.

Sialocoele

Clinical correlations

1. Usually occur spontaneously, probably from self-trauma during chewing or swallowing. A sialocoele has no epithelial lining.
2. May be associated with neck trauma after rupture of the gland or duct.
3. The sublingual salivary gland is most frequently involved; commonly, a fluctuant soft tissue mass or swelling is present in the ventral submandibular region, less often as sublingual swelling (ranula). A pharyngeal mucocoele is least common.

Radiographic findings

1. Survey radiographs:
   a. Radiographs may be normal.
   b. Soft tissue swelling at site of sialocoele.
2. Contrast radiographs
   a. All of the salivary ducts can be cannulated.
   b. Sialography may demonstrate a rupture of the duct or salivary gland.

Salivary Duct Fistula

Clinical correlation

1. Usually associated with parotid duct and secondary to facial trauma.
2. May be secondary to neoplasia

Radiographic findings

1. Survey radiographs
   a. Radiographs may be normal.
   b. Soft tissue swelling may be seen.
2. Contrast radiographs
   a. Sialography will demonstrate patency of duct.
   b. A fistulogram may demonstrate communication with the salivary gland or the salivary gland.

Neoplasms

Clinical correlations

1. Tumor type is usually adenocarcinoma.
2. May metastasize to the regional lymph nodes or lungs.

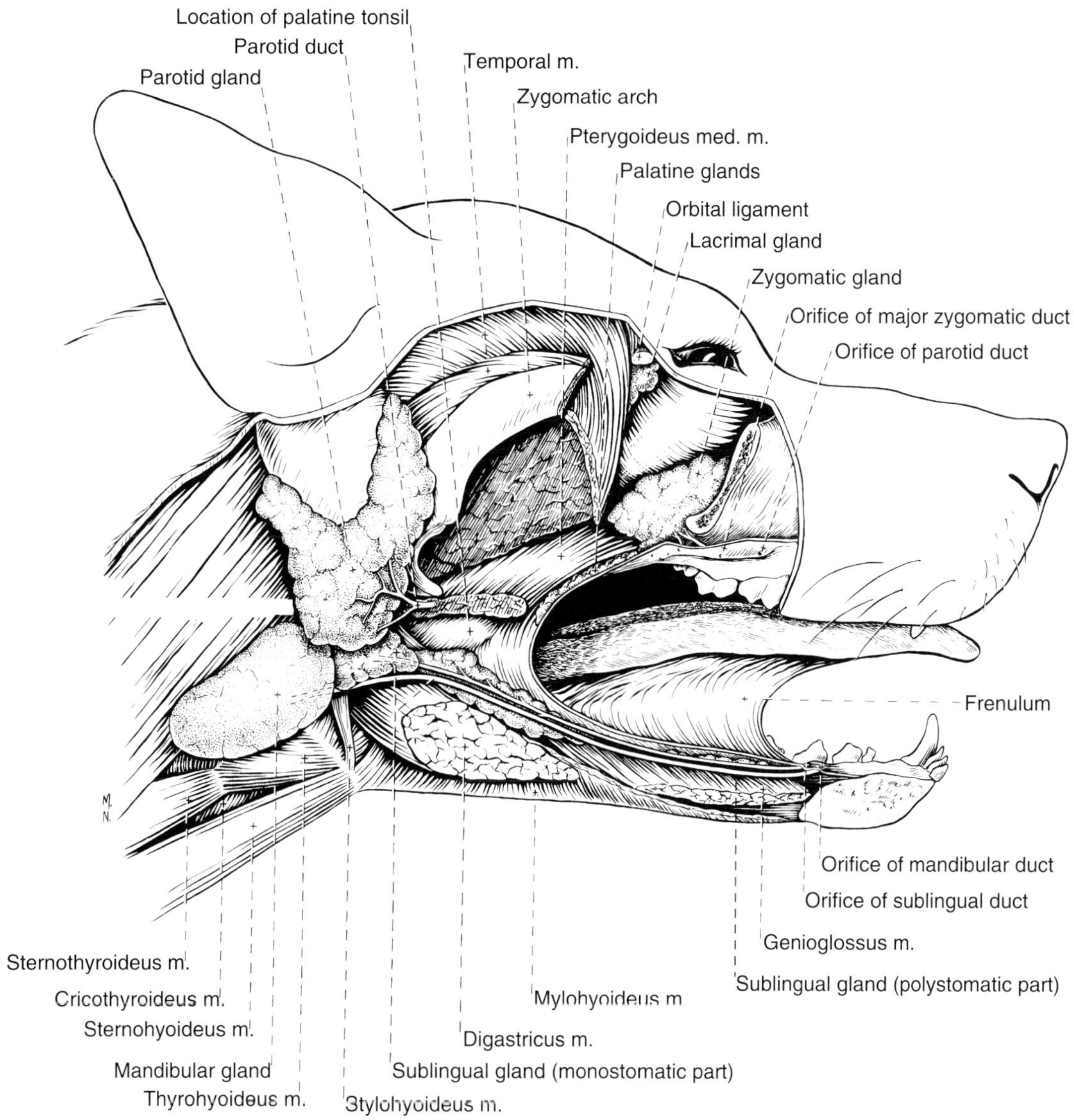

Figure 6.57. Salivary glands and ducts. (From Evans HE. The digestive apparatus and abdomen. In: Evans HE, ed. Miller's Anatomy of the Dog. 3rd ed. Philadelphia: W.B. Saunders; 1993:386. Courtesy of and used with permission of Dr. Howard E. Evans.)

Radiographic findings

1. Soft tissue enlargement at tumor location.
2. Bone lysis may be present adjacent to the tumor.
3. Sialography may be beneficial in demonstrating displacement or infiltration of structures by a tumor.

Nasolacrimal Duct Abnormalities

Clinical correlations

1. Epiphora is usually present.
2. Types of conditions include:
   a. Cysts of the orbital adnexal tissues (e.g., lacrimal duct or gland, gland of the third eyelid).
   b. Maxillary or nasal cavity cyst.
   c. Congenital or acquired stenosis or dilation of the nasolacrimal duct.
   d. Dacryocystitis.
   e. Neoplasia obstructing the nasolacrimal duct from the nasal cavity, facial bones, or orbit.

Radiographic findings

1. Survey radiographs
   a. Usually normal.
   b. Bone destruction or increased soft tissue opacity may be present involving the maxilla, nasal cavity, or orbit.
2. Contrast radiographs (Dacryocystorhinography):
   a. Using iodinated contrast media, location, size, and patency of the nasolacrimal duct can be evaluated.
   b. Sites of obstruction, displacement, dilation, or rupture may be seen.

chapter seven

7

Spine

VERTEBRAL DEVELOPMENT

Each vertebra develops from primary and secondary ossification centers that fuse during the first year of life. Knowledge of these centers of ossification fosters an appreciation of the complex anatomy of the vertebrae and an understanding of how congenital anomalies may develop.

1. Primary ossification centers:
   a. Vertebral body (one or two separate centers)
   b. Paired lateral arches (right and left sides)
2. Secondary ossification centers (Figures 7.1 and 7.2):
   a. Dorsal spinous process
   b. Paired epiphyses of vertebral body (cranial and caudal)
   c. Paired transverse processes
   d. Paired cranial articular processes
   e. Paired caudal articular processes

VERTEBRAL ANATOMY

The vertebral column is divided into five regions: cervical (C), thoracic (T), lumbar (L), sacral (S), and coccygeal (Cy). The vertebral formula for the dog and cat is: C7, T13, L7, S3, Cy 6–20. The number of coccygeal vertebrae varies among breeds and is affected by cosmetic tail amputations. Individual vertebra in each region differs in anatomy and radiographic appearance.

Major radiographic landmarks of the spine are identified in Figures 7.3 and 7.4.

RADIOGRAPHIC TECHNIQUE

1. The radiographic anatomy of the spine is complex. High-quality radiographic technique is critical for a complete and accurate radiographic examination. Film/screen systems with appropriate collimation and the smallest focal spot are preferred, so that structures, such as intervertebral disk spaces, can be more accurately exposed and evaluated.
2. Sedation or preferably general anesthesia is usually necessary for adequate animal restraint to reduce positional artifacts and motion. Positioning devices, such as sand bags and foam cushions, are helpful. Position the area of interest parallel to the table top and perpendicular to the "central" x-ray beam.
3. The radiographic examination should include all regions of the spine that may be a cause for the clinical signs. Separate radiographs of the spinal regions (cervical, thoracic, thoracolumbar, lumbar, and lumbosacral) usually are preferred, especially in larger dogs.
   a. Standard radiographic projections:
      1) Lateral projection (left or right)
      2) Ventrodorsal projection
   b. Supplemental projections:
      1) Oblique lateral or ventrodorsal projections
      2) Flexion and extension lateral projections
         a) These projections are used to assess spinal instability and spinal cord compression (e.g. atlantoaxial subluxation, cervical spondylopathy, cauda equina syndrome).
         b) Often, they are used in conjunction with myelography for evaluation of the caudal cervical region and with epidurography and/or myelography for the lumbosacral region.

Other Imaging

1. Myelography is useful in evaluating the spinal cord and determining the presence of cord compression or swelling.
2. Epidurography is useful in evaluating for cauda equina compression.
3. Discography is useful as a supplemental procedure in evaluating for disk extrusion, usually in the lumbosacral region.

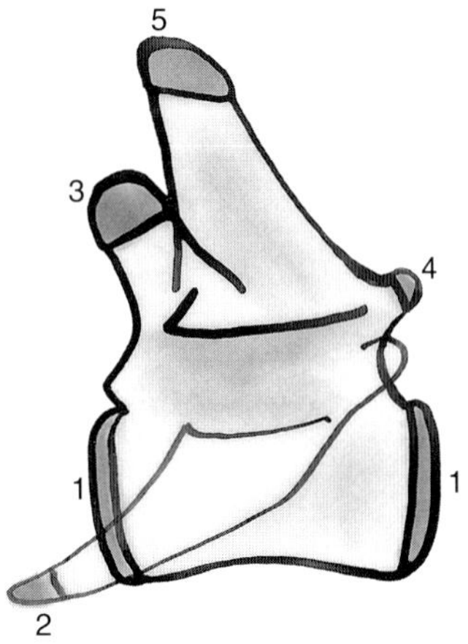

Figure 7.1. Secondary ossification centers lateral projection: **1)** epiphysis, **2)** transverse process, **3)** cranial articular process, **4)** caudal articular process, and **5)** dorsal spinous process.

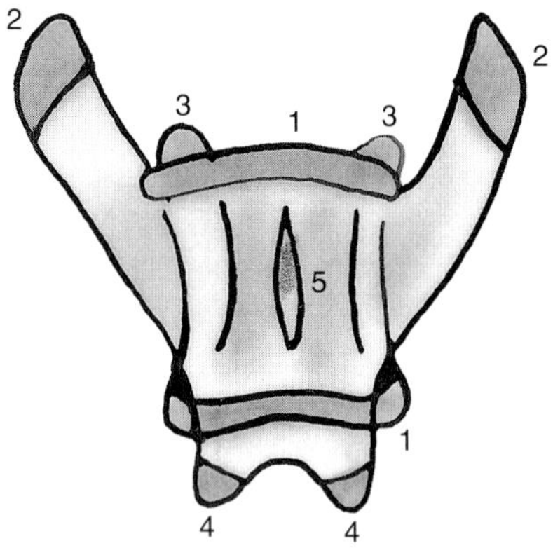

Figure 7.2. Secondary ossification centers ventrodorsal projection: **1)** epiphysis, **2)** transverse process, **3)** cranial articular process, **4)** caudal articular process, and **5)** dorsal spinous process.

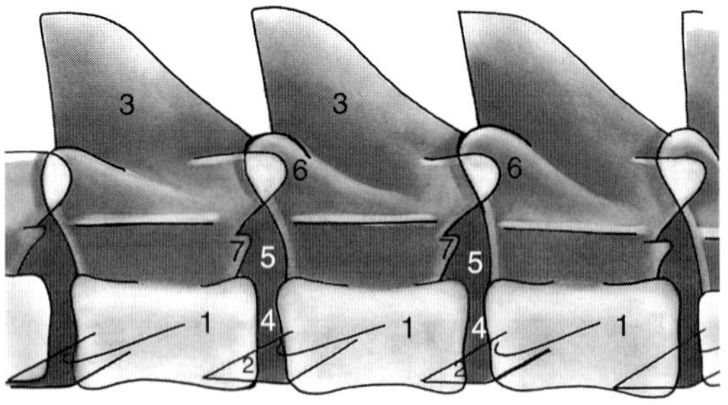

Figure 7.3. Normal vertebral anatomy, lateral projection: **1)** vertebral body, **2)** transverse process, **3)** dorsal spinous process, **4)** intervertebral disk space, **5)** intervertebral foramen, **6)** joint space of interarticular facets, and **7)** accessory process.

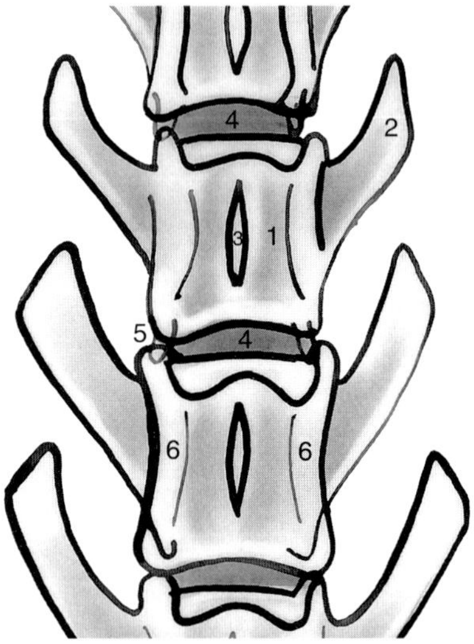

Figure 7.4. Normal vertebral anatomy, ventrodorsal projection: **1)** vertebral body, **2)** transverse process, **3)** dorsal spinous process, **4)** intervertebral disk space, **5)** interarticular facets, and **6)** pedicle.

4. Computed tomography (CT) is useful for evaluating the vertebrae, spinal canal, and spinal cord.
5. Magnetic resonance imaging (MRI) is useful for evaluating the parenchyma of the spinal cord, the intervertebral disks, and the nerve roots.

RADIOGRAPHIC INTERPRETATION

1. Systematically examine radiographs for:
   a. Alteration in alignment of the vertebral column
      1) Spinal curvature (e.g., scoliosis, kyphosis, or lordosis)
      2) Traumatic fracture or luxation
   b. Abnormalities in the shape or contour of the vertebrae:
      1) Congenital anomaly (e.g., hemivertebra)
      2) Fracture
      3) Infection
      4) Neoplasia
   c. Changes in the radiographic opacity of the vertebrae:
      1) Increased radiopacity as can occur in:
         a) Osteopetrosis
         b) Osteomyelitis
         c) Neoplasia
         d) Healing or healed fracture
      2) Increased radiolucency as can occur in:
         a) Osteoporosis
         b) Primary neoplasia (e.g., osteosarcoma)
         c) Metastatic neoplasia
         d) Osteomyelitis
   d. Variation in the width of the intervertebral disk spaces:

1) Decrease in width of the intervertebral disk space as can occur in:
   a) Protruded or extruded intervertebral disk
   b) Chronic diskospondylitis
   c) Fracture or luxation involving the intervertebral disk space
   d) Positional artifact
2) Increase in width of the intervertebral disk space as can occur in:
   a) Acute diskospondylitis
   b) Fracture or luxation involving the intervertebral disk space

e. Changes in the radiographic opacity of the intervertebral disk spaces:
   1) Increased radiopacity to the intervertebral disk space can be caused by:
      a) Mineralized disk
      b) Superimposition of lateral spondylosis deformans
   2) Increased radiolucency to the intervertebral disk space can be caused by:
      a) Acute diskospondylitis
      b) Gas bubble as a result of vacuum phenomenon (usually related to making stress view radiographs)

2. Make a tentative or definitive diagnosis by correlating the identified radiographic abnormalities with the clinical data.

Myelography

1. Myelography is indicated when a diagnosis of spinal disease cannot be made from the survey radiographs. It is used when the diagnosis of spinal cord compression is clinically suspected and surgical intervention is contemplated or when a prognosis is desired.
2. Myelography is an invasive procedure, consisting of a spinal tap and the infusion of radiopaque contrast media into the subarachnoid space. (See Chapter 3: Radiographic Contrast Procedures). The nonionic contrast media (e.g., Iohexol and Iopamidol) used in myelography have a low morbidity and provide excellent radiographic contrast.
3. The contrast medium is injected into the subarachnoid space at the cisterna magna or within the caudal lumbar region at the L4–5, L5–6, or L6–7 interarcurate spaces. The dose of contrast injected is determined, in part, by clinical localization of the lesion and the site of the injection.
   a. The cisterna injection is preferred for most cervical spinal cord evaluations. To visualize the cervical region, a dose of 0.30 mL/kg body weight is recommended. For visualization of the entire cervical, thoracic, and lumbar regions a recommended dose is 0.45 mL/kg body weight.
   b. When a lumbar injection is used for visualizing the lumbar region, a recommended dose is 0.30 mL/kg body weight. When visualizing all of the spinal cord, a dose of 0.45 mL/kg body weight is recommended.
   c. The initial radiographs should be made immediately after the infusion of contrast media. Some lesions may be missed should there be a time delay.
   d. After infusion of the contrast media, it usually is beneficial to reposition the animal by elevating or lowering the head/neck or lumbar region to aid the gravitational movement of contrast (e.g., lower the pelvis for greater contrast filling of the lumbosacral region).

Interpretation

1. The normal subarachnoid space is visualized as thin radiopaque columns of contrast surrounding the spinal cord (Figures 7.5 and 7.6). The columns are nearly

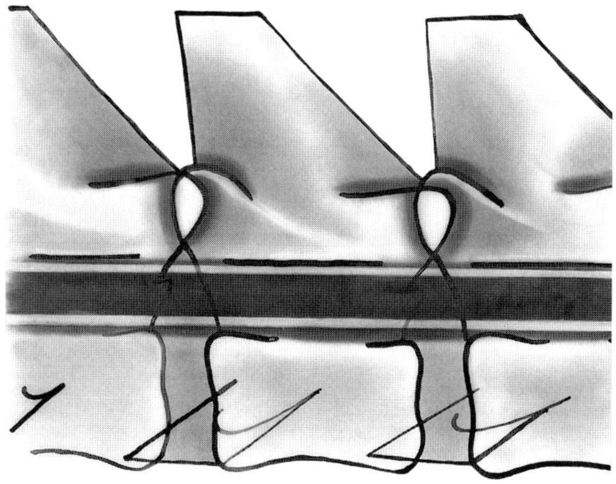

Figure 7.5. Normal myelogram (lateral projection). Contrast media in subarachnoid space outlines the spinal cord.

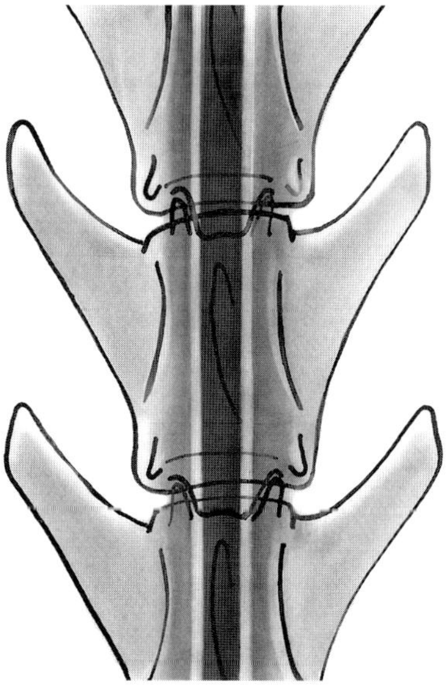

Figure 7.6. Normal myelogram (ventrodorsal projection). Contrast media in subarachnoid space outlines the spinal cord.

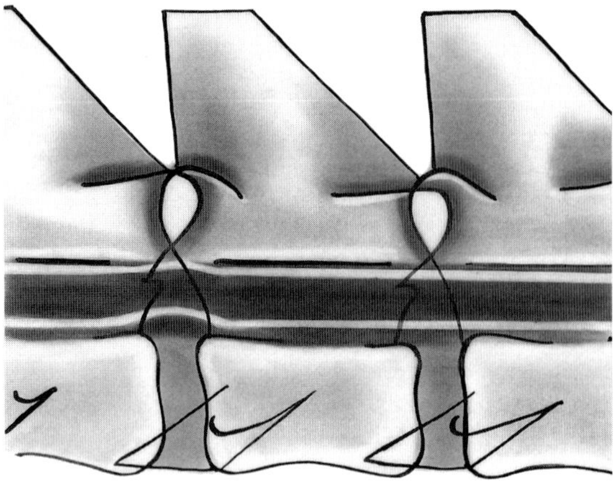

Figure 7.7. Extradural lesion, lateral projection of myelogram. A ventral extradural lesion caused by disk extrusion causing cord compression. There is dorsal deviation of the ventral subarachnoid space with thinning of the dorsal and ventral subarachnoid spaces at the extradural lesion site.

parallel except at the cauda equina where the subarachnoid space tapers to form the dural sac. Normally, the spinal cord is slightly wider in the caudal cervical and caudal lumbar regions associated with the brachial and lumbosacral intumescences. In many animals, the ventral subarachnoid space may be thinner than the dorsal subarachnoid space (e.g., common on lateral projection over C2–C3 intervertebral disk space).

2. Common myelographic lesions include obstruction of contrast flow or changes in size, shape, or position of the spinal cord and the subarachnoid space.
3. Localization and extent of the lesions are based on myelographic findings:
   a. Extradural lesions are outside the dura mater. At the site of spinal cord compression, the contrast column in the subarachnoid space is usually thinned with displacement of the spinal cord away from the site of compression. The spinal cord is usually narrowed in at least one projection (Figures 7.7 and 7.8).
      - Differential diagnosis:
      1) Disk protrusion or extrusion (most common extradural lesion)
      2) Enlarged or hypertrophied vertebral ligaments
      3) Vertebral neoplasia (primary or metastatic)
      4) Hemorrhage or hematoma
      5) Vertebral fracture or luxation
      6) Extradural tumor (e.g. lymphosarcoma)
      7) Subarachnoid cyst
   b. Intradural-extramedullary lesions are within the dura mater. The subarachnoid space is usually widened at the lesion site with a filling defect within the subarachnoid space. Because of its appearance, this defect is often referred to as "golf tee" sign. Usually, the subarachnoid space opposite the lesion is narrowed because of cord compression. In the

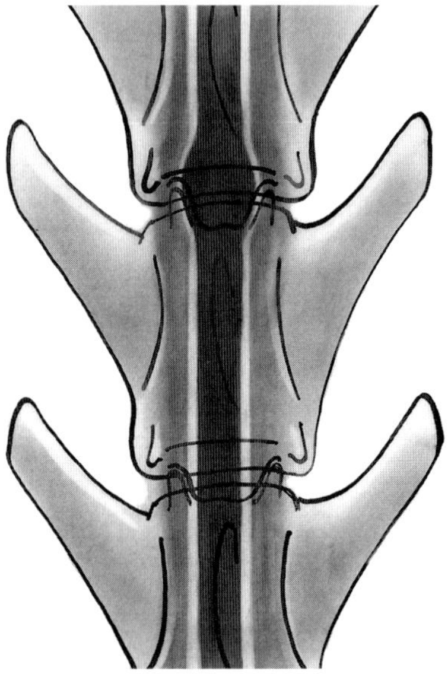

Figure 7.8. Extradural lesion, ventrodorsal projection on myelogram. The spinal cord is widened as a result of the effect of the ventral compression by the disk extrusion with thinning of both lateral subarachnoid contrast spaces.

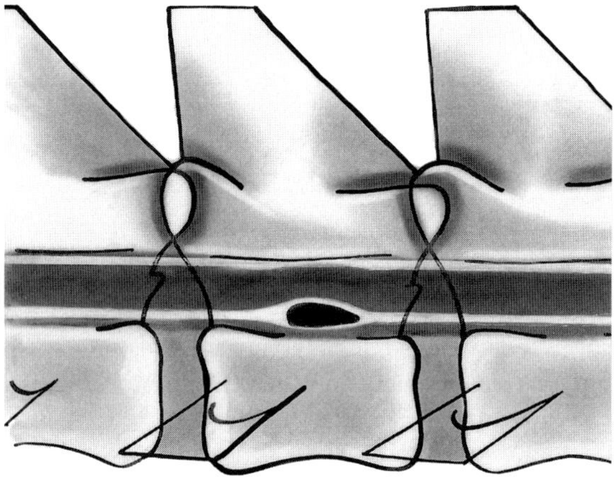

Figure 7.9. Intradural extramedullary lesion, lateral projection on myelogram. The intradural mass causes widening of the subarachnoid space adjacent to the lesion with dorsal displacement and compression of the spinal cord. The dorsal subarachnoid space is thinned.

orthogonal projection, the spinal cord may be widened with thinning of the subarachnoid contrast column (Figures 7.9 and 7.10).
      - Differential diagnosis
      1) Primary tumor (e.g. neurofibroma, neurofibrosarcoma or meningioma)
      2) Metastatic tumor (e.g. lymphoma)
      3) Hemorrhage or hematoma
      4) Subarachnoid cyst
   c. Intramedullary lesions are within the spinal cord. A lesion within the spinal cord produces a uniform and symmetrical widening of the spinal cord on all projections. If compression is severe, there may be an area of total absence of contrast media within

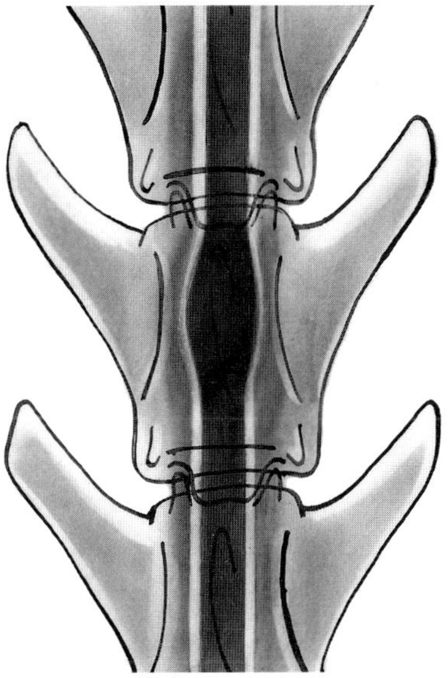

Figure 7.10. Intradural extramedullary lesion, ventrodorsal projection on myelogram. The spinal cord is widened at the site of cord compression with thinning of both lateral subarachnoid spaces.

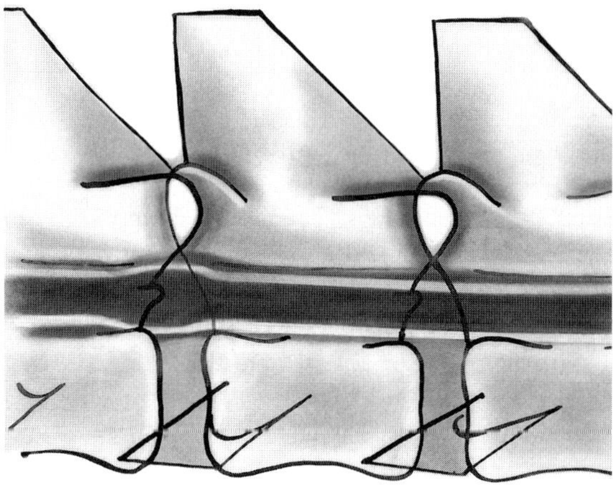

Figure 7.11. Intramedullary lesion, lateral projection on myelogram. The spinal cord is widened with thinning of the ventral and dorsal subarachnoid spaces.

the subarachnoid space at the site of the lesion (Figures 7.11 and 7.12).

- Differential diagnosis:

1) Spinal cord edema, usually associated with trauma or disk herniation
2) Spinal cord tumor (e.g., astrocytoma, glioma)
3) Granulomatous meningoencephalitis (GME)
4) Hemorrhage
5) Ischemic myelopathy and fibrocartilaginous embolization

4. Artifactual myelographic findings may occur if the contrast medium is not injected into the subarachnoid space.
   a. Extradural injection of contrast medium:

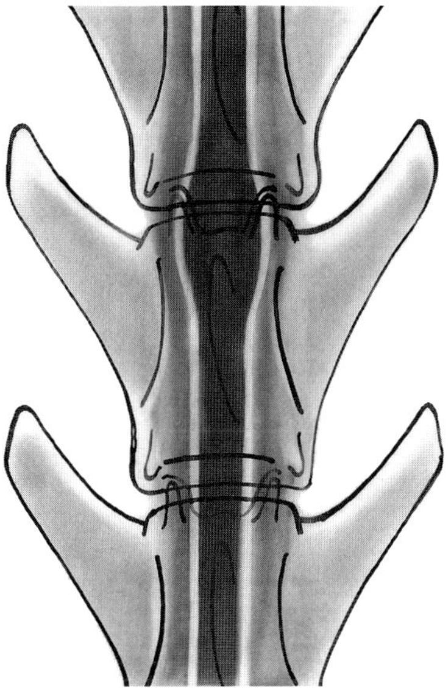

Figure 7.12. Intramedullary lesion, ventrodorsal projection on myelogram. The spinal cord is widened with thinning of both lateral subarachnoid spaces.

1) The contrast column may appear wider than normal.
2) The contrast column may "drape" over the intervertebral disk spaces adjacent to the venous sinuses.
3) The nerve roots may be outlined with contrast.
4) The contrast column may appear irregular and incomplete.
5) Commonly, the presence of contrast media in the extradural space prevents accurate assessment of the subarachnoid space and spinal cord.

   b. Intramedullary injection of contrast medium:

1) Contrast blush appears within the spinal cord. In cord malacia there can be a patchy or irregular appearance of the contrast media within the cord.
2) Contrast within the central canal of the spinal cord. This can be caused by:
   a) Incorrect injection site
   b) Leakage of contrast media through the needle tract during spinal puncture
   c) Spinal cord malacia
   d) Some congenital anomalies (e.g., hydromyelia)

5. Absence of an abnormality on a myelogram does not exclude a spinal cord lesion. Some cord lesions may have no abnormality on a myelogram (e.g., ischemic myelopathy, degenerative myelopathy, fibrocartilaginous embolization).

DISEASES/DISORDERS

Spinal Bifida

Clinical correlations

1. Spinal bifida is caused by developmental failure of the lateral arches to fuse dorsally, causing incomplete development of the dorsal spinous process.

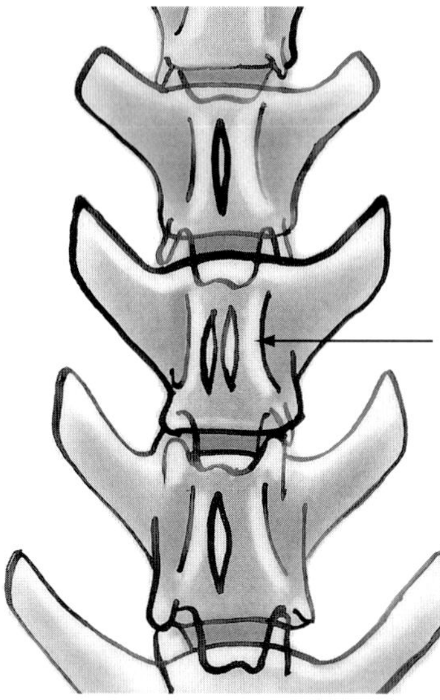

Figure 7.13. Spina bifida. The dorsal spinous process is not fused and is seen as a midline cleft (arrow).

2. Affected animal may have no clinical signs.
3. If clinical signs occur, they are noticed most frequently when the animal begins to walk and may include rear limb ataxia and paresis, fecal and urinary incontinence, perineal analgesia, and flaccid anal sphincter.
4. May cause neural abnormalities (if the meninges protrude through the dorsal spinal defect).
   a. Meningocoele (sac contains meninges)
   b. Myelocele (sac contains spinal cord)
   c. Meningomyelocoele (sac contains meninges and spinal cord or nerve roots)
5. Most commonly occurs in the thoracic and lumbar regions, but may occur anywhere in the spine, including coccygeal vertebrae of "screw tail" breeds (e.g., Bulldog, Boston Terrier, Pug).
6. Probably is inheritable.
7. In the Manx cat, it commonly involves the sacral and coccygeal vertebral segments.
8. May be associated with other anomalies (e.g., hemivertebra, tethered spinal cord).

Radiographic findings (Figure 7.13)

1. On the ventrodorsal projection, a radiolucent line is seen on the midline between the two unfused sides of the dorsal spinous process, or a cleft spinous process may be present. This may involve incomplete separation of the vertebral body, arch, or the entire vertebra.
2. With myelography, CT, or MRI, a protrusion of spinal cord, meninges, or both may be observed.

Block Vertebra

Clinical correlations

1. Block vertebra is caused by developmental failure of somite segmentation and may involve the arch or all of the vertebral body.
2. Rarely produces clinical signs.
3. If block vertebra is associated with other anomalies causing spinal angulation or instability, pain or neurologic deficits may occur.
4. As a result of the vertebral fusion, there is potentially increased risk of intervertebral disk extrusion cranial and caudal to the fused segments.

Radiographic findings (Figure 7.14)

1. There is partial to complete fusion of two or more adjacent vertebral bodies.
2. Intervertebral disk space usually is absent or only partially developed.
3. The block vertebra is usually longer in length than adjacent normal vertebrae.
4. Abnormal angulation of the spine or stenosis of the spinal canal may be present.

Hemivertebra

Clinical correlations

1. Hemivertebra is caused by developmental hemimetameric displacement of vertebral somites or by altered vascularization and ossification resulting in only a partial development of the vertebral body.
2. Rarely produces clinical signs.
3. If clinical signs are present, they often are associated with other congenital malformations (e.g., sacrococcygeal dysgenesis in the Manx cat).
4. May be associated with spinal canal stenosis, angulation, or instability of the spine, which may be exacerbated by trauma or degenerative disk disease.
5. Is most common in the Manx cat and "screw tail" dog breeds, such as the English bulldog, Boston terrier, French bulldog, and Pug.

Radiographic findings (Figures 7.15 and 7.16)

1. Wedged shape. The affected vertebra is usually wedged shaped, with the base oriented dorsally, medially, or ventrally (depending on the portion of the vertebra that does not form). The disk spaces are usually normal

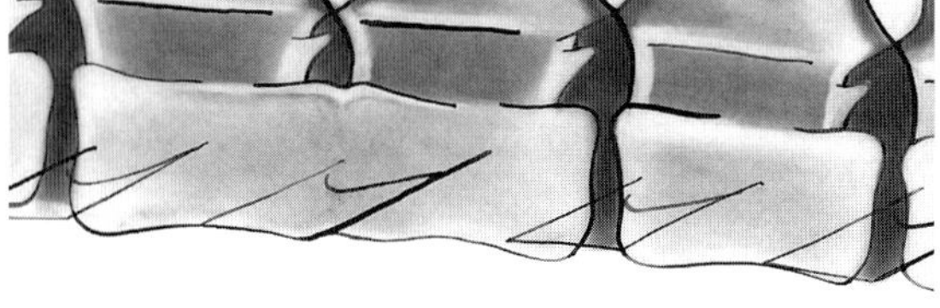

Figure 7.14. Block vertebra. There is fusion of two vertebral bodies with no intervertebral disk space.

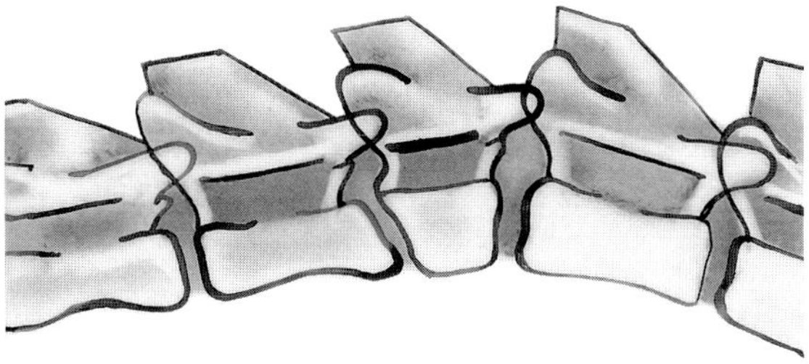

Figure 7.15. Hemivertebra. The wedge shaped hemivertebra causes a kyphosis to the affected spinal region.

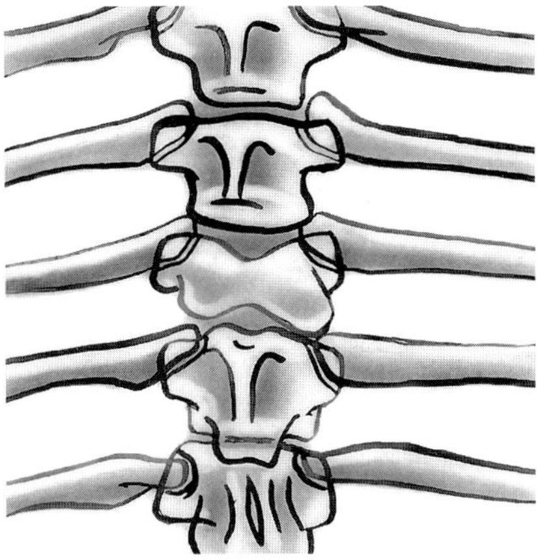

Figure 7.16. Hemivertebra. The misshapen "butterfly" vertebra has incomplete development of the vertebral body causing a cleft to form.

but conform to the abnormal shape of the vertebra. The vertebral end-plates are smooth and of normal thickness.

2. Butterfly. A "butterfly" segment may be seen if the central portion of the vertebra does not form, causing right and left segments to be recognized.
3. An angular deformity of the spine may be present, secondarily to the hemivertebral malformation, causing a lordosis, scoliosis, or kyphosis.
4. On myelography, if spinal cord compression is present, the deformity will have extradural compression of the spinal cord over one or more anomalous vertebra.

Transitional Vertebrae

Clinical correlations

1. Transitional vertebrae is a developmental anomaly in which the vertebra has some anatomic characteristics of an adjacent region.
2. Usually occurs at junctions of spinal regions.
3. Usually causes no clinical signs, but may:
   a. Be a cause of scoliosis.
   b. Prevent symmetrical positioning for the ventrodorsal view of the pelvis and hips.
   c. Predispose the ipsilateral coxofemoral joint to degenerative joint disease.

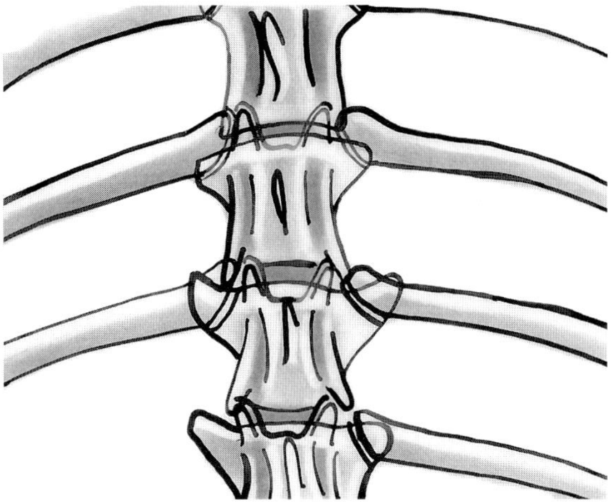

Figure 7.17. Thoracolumbar transitional vertebra. There is lumbarization of T13 with a rib only on the left side.

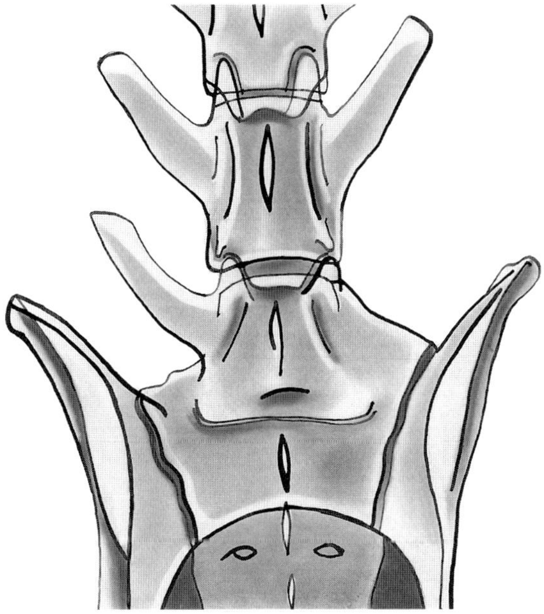

Figure 7.18. Lumbosacral transitional vertebra. There is sacralization of the 7th lumbar vertebra with an absence of the left transverse process and the union of L7 with the pelvis forming a portion of the sacroiliac joint.

   d. Have an association in the lumbosacral region with degenerative disk disease and caudal equina syndrome.
   e. Transitional vertebrae may cause error of anatomic localization (e.g., on palpation the absence of rib on T13 could be diagnosed erroneously as L1).

Radiographic findings (Figures 7.17 and 7.18)

1. Cervicothoracic transitional vertebrae:
   a. Thoracoization of C7 has a unilateral or bilateral rib development on C7.
   b. Cervicoization of T1 has a unilateral or bilateral rib absence on T1.

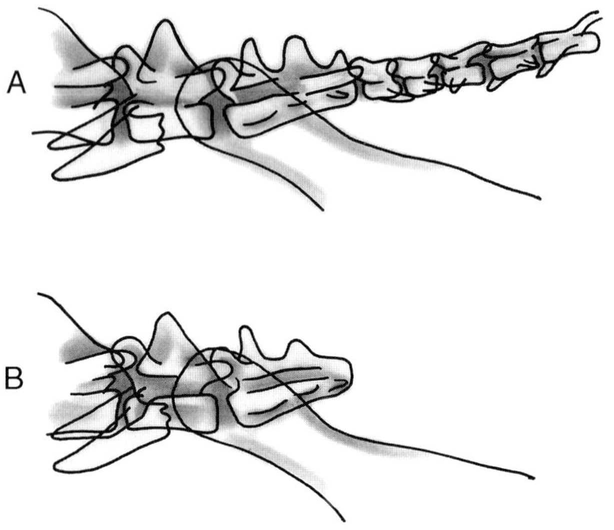

Figure 7.19. **A)** Normal feline lumbosacral spine. **B)** Sacrococcygeal dysgenesis.

2. Thoracolumbar transitional vertebrae:
   a. Lumbarization of T13 has a unilateral or bilateral rib absence on T13.
   b. Thoracoization of L1 has a unilateral or bilateral rib development on L1.
3. Lumbosacral transitional vertebrae:
   a. Lumbarization of S1 has a unilateral or bilateral transverse process on the sacrum.
   b. Partial to complete transition causes shortening of the sacrum.
   c. Sacralization of L7 has a unilateral or bilateral absence of the transverse processes of the lumbar vertebra. The lumbar vertebra commonly articulates with the sacrum and the ilium (unilaterally or bilaterally).

Sacrococcygeal Dysgenesis

Clinical correlations

1. Sacrococcygeal dysgenesis, also referred to as anury, is a developmental anomaly consisting of an absence of one or more vertebra.
2. It is usually recognized as animal without a tail.
3. It is transmitted as an autosomal dominant trait in the Manx cat.
4. Clinical signs vary depending on the extent of anurous vertebra and presence of other associated bony and neurologic abnormalities. Signs may include gait abnormalities, limb paresis or paraplegia, fecal and urinary incontinence, and perianal sensory loss.
5. Affected animals may have meningocoele, myelocoele, myelomeningocele, syringomyelia, shortening of spinal cord, absence of cauda equina, and anomalies of the dorsal horn.

Radiographic findings (Figure 7.19 A, B)

1. There is an absence of one or more vertebra.
2. Other anomalies also may be present (e.g., hemivertebra, transitional vertebra).

Spinal Curvature Deformities

Clinical correlations

1. Curvature deformities of the vertebral column usually are the result of a congenital malformation of one or more vertebrae but may be acquired after traumatic spinal injury.
2. Types of curvature deformities:
   a. Scoliosis (lateral deviation)
      1) Common causes:
         a) Hemivertebrae
         b) Transitional vertebrae
         c) Muscle spasm
         d) Vertebral luxations and fractures
         e) Malunion vertebral fractures
      2) Less common causes:
         a) Spinal cord aplasia
         b) Hypoplasia or myelodysplasia with syringomyelia
         c) Hydromelia or central cord canal abnormalities
   b. Kyphosis (dorsal deviation)
      1) Common causes:
         a) Hemivertebrae
         b) Malunion vertebral fractures
         c) Vertebral luxations and fractures
         d) Muscle spasm
         e) Abdominal pain (causing arching of the back)
         f) Back pain caused by disk protrusion
      2) Less common causes:
         a) Spinal cord aplasia or hypoplasia
         b) Myelodysplasia (with syringomyelia, hydromelia, or central cord canal abnormalities)
   c. Lordosis (ventral deviation)
      - Common causes:
         a) Hemivertebrae
         b) Malunion vertebral fractures
         c) Vertebral luxations and fractures

Radiographic findings (Figure 7.20)

1. Deviation of the spinal region is apparent.
   a. Scoliosis, lateral deviation
   b. Kyphosis, dorsal deviation
   c. Lordosis, ventral deviation

Osteoporosis

Clinical correlations

1. Osteoporosis, also referred to as osteopenia, is a condition of diminished bone quantity, but the bone is otherwise normal.
2. Usually, the entire skeleton is involved; however, the radiographic changes are often most pronounced in the spine, mandible, and maxilla.
3. Osteoporosis may be caused by many conditions, but is frequently seen in systemic disorders of calcium and phosphorus metabolism.
4. Differential diagnosis (Table 7.1)

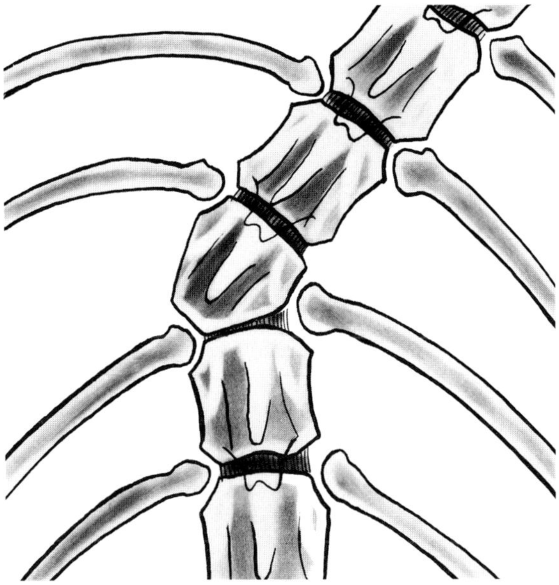

Figure 7.20. Scoliotic deviation of spine secondary to congenital hemivertebra.

TABLE 7.1

Differential Diagnosis of Osteoporosis

1. Hyperparathyroidism
   a. Primary hyperparathyroidism (functional parathy roid adenoma or carcinoma)
   b. Secondary nutritional hyperparathyroidism
   c. Secondary renal hyperparathyroidism
   d. Pseudohyperparathyroidism
2. Hyperadrenocorticism
3. Diabetes mellitus
4. Hypothyroidism
5. Diffuse malignancies
   a. Multiple myeloma
   b. Lymphosarcoma
6. Senile osteoporosis
7. Steroid therapy
8. Disuse atrophy
9. Malnutrition (including calcium and protein deficiency)

Radiographic findings

1. Thinning of the cortices
2. Decrease in bone radiopacity.
3. Prominent coarse bone trabeculae (e.g., double cortical sign)
4. Vertebral endplates may appear more radiopaque in contrast to the vertebral bodies.
5. Radiographic technique may cause artifact of "apparent" osteoporosis.
   a. Excessive scatter radiation in obese animals (e.g., nongrid versus grid)
   b. Radiographic exposure factors (e.g., overexposure and low scale contrast)

Hypervitaminosis A in the Cat

Clinical correlations

1. Also referred to as deforming cervical spondylosis and nutritional osteodystrophy.
2. It is a crippling, degenerative, and proliferative bone disorder in cats, affecting primarily the cervical and thoracic vertebra and the long appendicular bones and joints.
3. Caused by excessive intake of vitamin A and usually is seen in cats fed primarily a liver diet.
4. Frequently, affected cats have concurrent secondary nutritional hyperparathyroidism.
5. Clinical signs that are often present in older adult cats include lameness, depression, scoliosis, and rigidity of cervical spine, muscle atrophy, and cervical hyperesthesia.

Radiographic findings

1. Generalized osteoporosis
2. Extensive new bone proliferation, often including lateral and ventral spondylosis of the spine
3. Intraarticular mineralization and/or ankylosis of the appendicular joints (e.g., shoulder, elbow, and hip) and the articular facets of the cervical and thoracic vertebra
4. Laminar periosteal reaction on the long bones of legs.
5. Differential diagnosis:
   a. Mucopolysaccharidosis (MPS)
   b. Polyarthritis
   c. Hypertrophic osteopathy

Mucopolysaccharidosis

Clinical correlations

1. Mucopolysaccharidosis is a group of recessively inherited lysomal diseases in dogs and cats that result from metabolic deficits of different glycosaminoglycans.
2. The different glycosaminoglycan enzyme deficiencies cause a variety of abnormalities
3. Clinical signs depend on the form and severity of the mucopolysaccharidosis. Common clinical signs include neurologic disorders, stunted growth, joint stiffness and luxation, incontinence, abnormal facies, sternal concavity, and corneal clouding.
4. Affected cats are usually smaller than their littermates. The physical deformities are often seen by 8 weeks of age.
5. Neurologic signs attributed to spinal cord compression (e.g, paresis, paraplegia) are often noticed at 4 to 7 months of age.

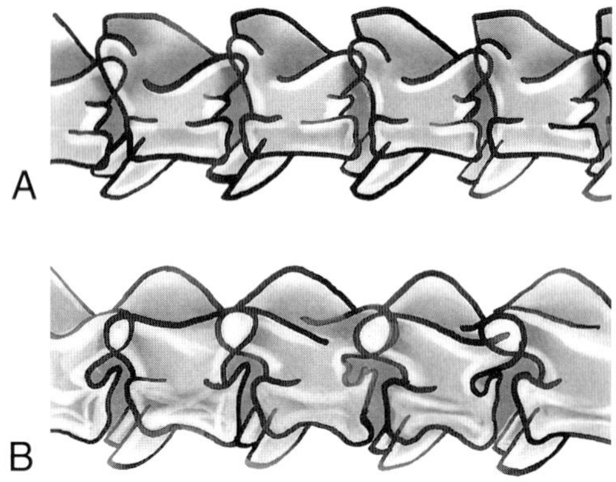

Figure 7.21. Feline mucopolysaccharidosis. **A)** Normal feline lumbar spine. **B)** Shortening and irregularity of the vertebral bodies with deformity of the endplates caused by mucopolysaccharidosis.

Radiographic findings (Figure 7.21) (See also appendicular and skull chapters)

1. Osteoarthrosis of the vertebral articular facets
2. Spondylosis deformans
3. Hypoplasia and/or fragmentation of dens
4. Fused, shortened, and/or misshapen vertebra (especially in the cervical and lumbar regions)

Atlantoaxial Subluxation

Clinical correlations

1. Atlantoaxial subluxation is a developmental anomaly with separation, malformation, hypoplasia, or absence of the odontoid process.
2. It may occur as an acquired lesion caused by trauma, associated with fracture of the odontoid process or the transverse ligament.
3. The congenital form usually is recognized in dogs younger than 1 year of age and most commonly is seen in miniature and toy breeds (e.g., Yorkshire Terrier, Chihuahua, Toy Poodle, or Pekinese), and some large breeds (e.g., Rottweiler and Doberman Pinscher).
4. Some dogs also have concurrent occipitoatlanto malformation.
5. In affected dogs, clinical signs usually occur before 1 year of age and are a result of cord compression by abnormal rotation of axis into the vertebral canal.
6. Clinical signs vary according to the degree of luxation, ranging from mild cervical pain to cervical rigidity, spastic paraparesis, and tetraplegia. Signs may be acute, chronic, or episodic.

Radiographic findings (Figures 7.22 through 7.24)

1. The degree of atlantoaxial instability is assessed from the lateral projection, bearing in mind that flexion of the cranial cervical spine may accentuate spinal cord compression and cause further injury. When suspected, minimal and cautious manipulation should be done when making the appropriate radiographs.

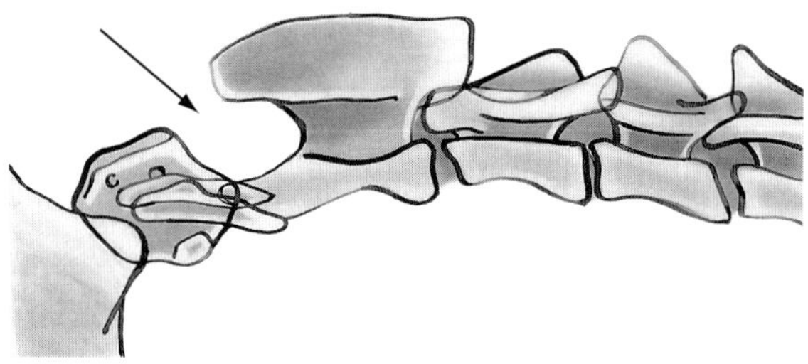

Figure 7.22. Atlantoaxial subluxation. The joint space between the atlas and the axis is wider than normal indicating tearing or stretching of the atlantoaxial ligament (arrow).

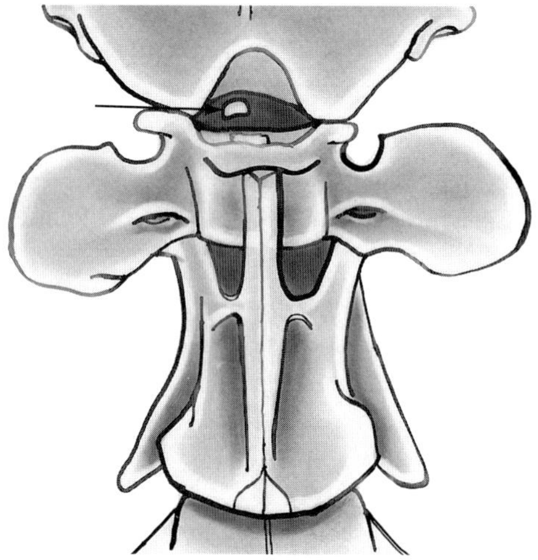

Figure 7.23. Odontoid process fracture. On the ventrodorsal projection, the tip of the odontoid process is fractured and displaced to the right (arrow).

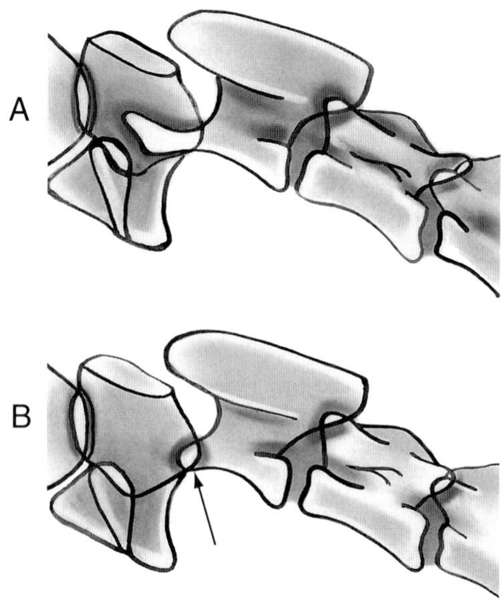

Figure 7.24. Oblique projection of atlantoaxial vertebra. **A)** Normal odontoid process. **B)** Hypoplasia of the odontoid process (arrow).

2. Between the arch of atlas and spinous process of the axis, the space is widened on the lateral view and/or there is an abnormal angulation of the axis relative to the atlas.
3. The hypoplastic, fractured, or absent dens may be seen best on a ventrodorsal, oblique lateral projection or an open mouth rostrocaudal projection.

Cervical Spondylopathy

Clinical correlations

1. Also referred to as wobbler syndrome, cervical vertebral instability, cervical vertebral malformation/malarticulation syndrome, or vertebral subluxation.
2. Has been reported in many dog breeds but is most common in Great Danes (usually less than 2 years of age) and Doberman Pinschers (usually older than 2 years of age).
3. Common clinical signs include ataxia, weakness, and paralysis.
4. Characterized by deformity of the vertebral bodies, narrowing of the vertebral canal, vertebral instability, and malarticulation with resultant varying degrees of spinal cord compression.
   a. Vertebral canal stenosis results from malformation of the vertebral laminae, ligamentous hypertrophy of the ligamentum flavum, enlargement of the articular facets and/or hypertrophy of the dorsal longitudinal ligament and interarcuate ligament.
   b. The vertebral bodies and endplates become malaligned. Often this is associated with intervertebral disk space collapse and disk extrusion, and spinal cord compression.
   c. The degree of spinal canal stenosis and cord compression varies, and is attributed to a combination of abnormal vertebral development and the degenerative changes secondary to instability.

Radiographic findings (Figures 7.25 and 7.26)

1. Survey radiographs (May have none, one, or any combination of the following):
   a. Malformation of one or more vertebral bodies, frequently C5, C6, or C7
   b. Degenerative disk disease (e.g., disk space narrowing, disk mineralization, and/or disk protrusion or extrusion)
   c. Spinal canal stenosis at the affected site (affecting the dorsoventral dimension or the lateral dimension of the spinal canal)
   d. Malalignment of one or more vertebral bodies.
   e. The articular facets are often thickened and irregular with proliferative degenerative changes. The articular processes may encroach into the vertebral canal.
   f. Spondylosis deformans and end-plate sclerosis is often present.

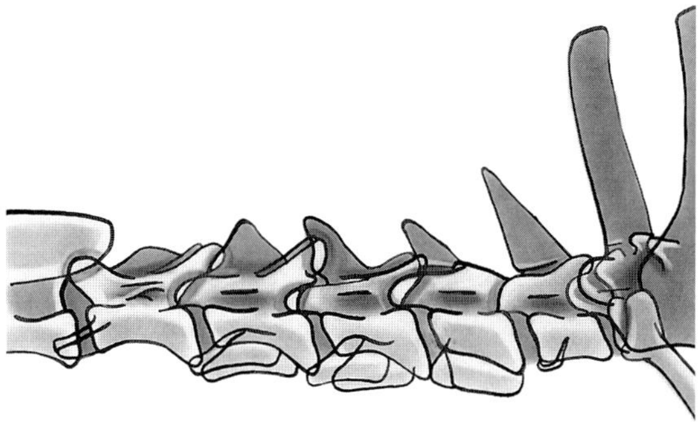

Figure 7.25. Normal cervical spine (lateral projection). Vertebra are numbered 2.7 and transverse processes are identified with arrows.

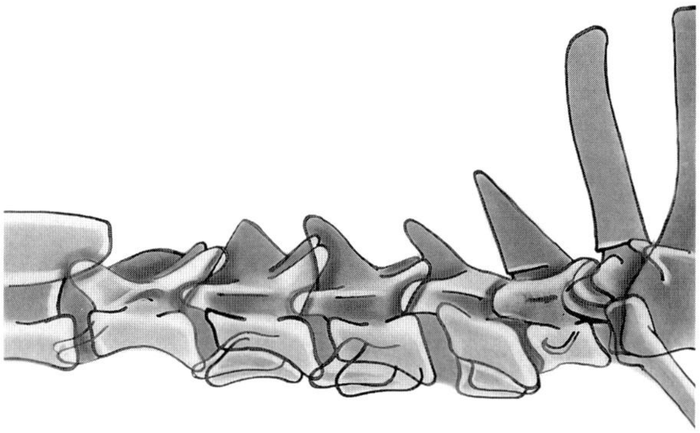

Figure 7.26. Cervical spondylopathy. Notice the malformation of the C6 vertebral body and the malalignment of C5 and C6.

Contrast radiography

1. Myelography
   a. Ventroflexion, hyperextension, and traction positioning of the spine may be necessary to demonstrate the lesion sites and the degree of spinal cord compression.
2. Other imaging:
   a. CT
   b. MRI

Lumbosacral Instability

Clinical correlations

1. Also referred to as cauda equina syndrome, lumbosacral stenosis, or lumbosacral malarticulation.
2. Characterized by narrowing of the vertebral canal and/or intervertebral foramina causing compression of the nerve roots that form the cauda equina.
3. May be congenital or an acquired degenerative disorder. Usually seen in large breed dogs, and most commonly is reported in German Shepherd Dogs. Also occurs in the cat.

4. May develop in association with disk degeneration or protrusion, lumbosacral subluxation, lumbosacral fracture, osteochondrosis, hypertrophy, and hyperplasia of the interarcuate ligament, thickening of the vertebral arch and pedicles, spondylosis deformans, diskospondylitis, and vertebral malformation.
5. Common clinical signs related to cauda equina compression include pain on palpation of the lumbosacral region, hyperesthesia, difficulty rising, and pelvic limb lameness or weakness. Unilateral signs are common. In chronic disease, urinary and/or fecal incontinence may be present.

Radiographic findings (Figures 7.27 and 7.28)

1. On survey radiographs, there may be none, one, or any combination of the following:
   a. Spondylosis deformans at the L7-S1 articulation
   b. Sclerosis of the L7-S1 vertebral endplates
   c. Narrowing of the L7-S1 disk space, including wedging
   d. Degenerative joint disease of the articular facets
   e. Ventral displacement of the sacrum relative to the body of L7. A flexed lateral projection may demonstrate functional subluxation.

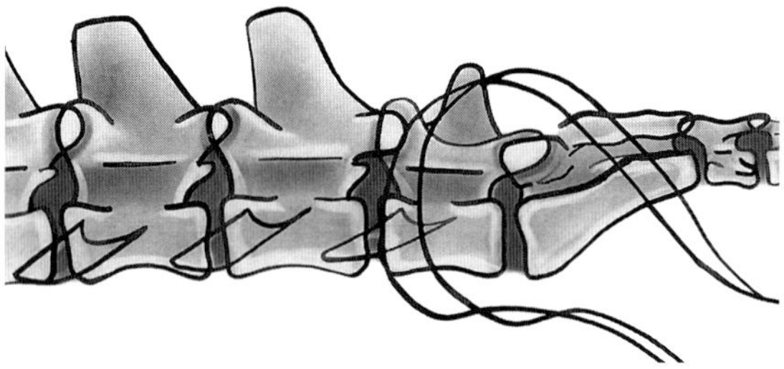

Figure 7.27. Normal lumbosacral spine (lateral projection).

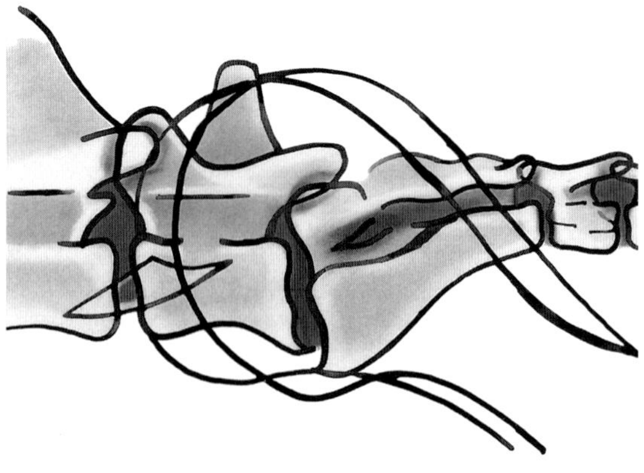

Figure 7.28. Lumbosacral instability demonstrated by L7-S1 subluxation on a flexed lateral projection. There is also a diminished dorsoventral dimension to the spinal canal and ventral spondylosis.

   f. Diminished dorsoventral dimension of the caudal lumbar or cranial sacral spinal canal.
   g. Evidence of diskospondylitis, fracture, or congenital vertebral anomaly.
2. Contrast radiography frequently is used to establish an accurate diagnosis.
   a. Myelography allows filling of the cauda equina for assessment of the cauda equina over the lumbosacral articulation. In some dogs, however, the subarachnoid space does not extend far enough caudally to accurately assess the cauda equina at the LS region.
      1) Supplemental stress radiographs, including hyperextension and hyperflexion lateral projections, may demonstrate the lesion site and degree of compression.
      2) It is preferable to inject the contrast medium through the cisterna tap to avoid extradural leakage of contrast that commonly occurs with a lumbar puncture.
   b. Epidurography of the caudal lumbar canal may demonstrate compression or displacement of the cauda equina. Extended and flexed lateral projections may aid in demonstrating dynamic compression of the cauda equina associated with ligamentous hypertrophy.
   c. Diskography of the L7-S1 disk may demonstrate ruptures of the anulus fibrosis and disk protrusion into the spinal canal.
2. Other imaging:
   a. CT
   b. MR

Osteochondrosis

Clinical correlations

1. An uncommon condition, but most often is reported in large breed dogs, especially the German Shepherd.
2. Recognized most often at L7-S1 with clinical signs referable to cauda equina compression.

Radiographic findings (Figure 7.29)

1. Irregular lysis affecting one vertebral endplate. At L7-S1, more commonly affecting the craniodorsal portion of S1.
2. Sclerosis is usually present at the base of the osteochondral defect.
3. May have an associated fragment of bone, which may extend into the spinal canal and cause cauda equina compression.

Calcinosis Circumscripta

Clinical correlations

1. Also referred to as tumoral calcinosis or apocrine cystic calcinosis.

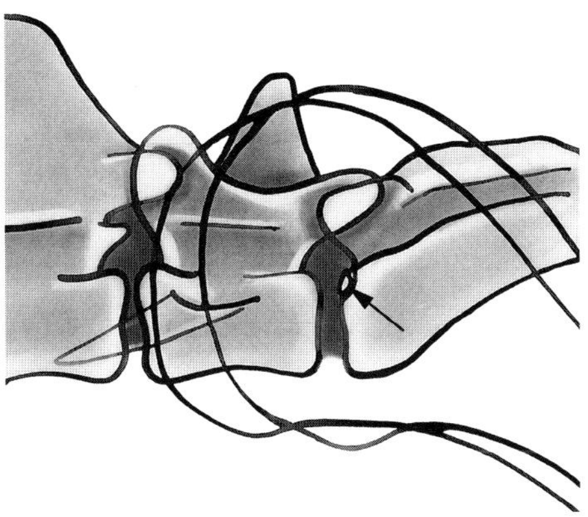

Figure 7.29. Osteochondrosis of the spine. There is irregular radiolucent defect affecting the dorsal portion of the cranial endplate of the sacrum with a bone fragment (arrow) displaced away from the osteochondral defect.

2. An idiopathic condition with single or multiple circumscribed calcium deposits in the cutaneous and connective tissue (refer to Chapter 4).
3. Most prevalent in large breed dogs (e.g., German Shepherd, Great Dane, Viszla, Rottweiler, St. Bernard).
4. Affected dogs and cats are usually less than 1 year of age.
5. Clinical signs of spinal cord compression are rare.

Radiographic findings (See Figure 4.45)

1. Well-circumscribed area of mineralization within the soft tissues, usually adjacent to the transverse process of a vertebral body.
2. Differential diagnosis:
   a. Myositis ossificans
   b. Ossified hematoma
   c. Foreign body

Spinal Trauma

Clinical correlations

1. Trauma can be internal or external.
   a. Internal causes include intervertebral disk extrusion, pathologic fractures, congenital anomalies, and spinal instability.
   b. External causes include vehicular accidents, projectiles (e.g., gunshot wounds), or other external blunt trauma.
2. Injuries can lead to compression or concussion.
   a. Intervertebral disk extrusion can cause concussion of the cord initially or compression if the lesion persists.
   b. Spinal fractures and luxations cause a variable degree of compression and concussion depending on the time and the degree of instability of the spine at the trauma site.
3. Most spinal luxations and fractures occur at the junction of mobile and immobile segments of the spine (i.e., atlantooccipital, atlantoaxial, cervicothoracic, thoracolumbar, and lumbosacral junctions).
   a. Fractures result from forces that cause hyperflexion, hyperextension, or torsion of the affected portion of the spine.
   b. Variable degrees of subluxation or luxation occur depending on the degree of instability.
   c. The severity of spinal trauma is determined by correlative assessment of the clinical status, the neurologic examination, and radiographic findings.

Radiographic examination

1. If severe spinal trauma is suspected and the patient is recumbent, minimal patient manipulation is advised for obtaining radiographic projections (e.g., if patient is in lateral recumbency, use cross table horizontal projections to obtain the ventrodorsal view).
2. Usually, a minimum of two radiographic projections are necessary to assess the spine for trauma.
3. Depending on the initial radiographic findings, a more complete spinal series under general anesthesia may be needed.
4. The use of additional imaging modalities, such as myelography, CT, or MRI, may be indicated to provide additional diagnostic and prognostic information.

Radiographic findings

1. Fractures of the vertebral body (Figures 7.30 and 7.31):
   a. Commonly also involve the intervertebral disk space and may cause narrowing or widening of the disk space.
   b. Abnormal abrupt angulation of the spine may be seen on one or more radiographic projections.
   c. Loss of continuity of the lateral, ventral, or dorsal margins of the vertebral body
   d. Chip fractures are seen most often at the ventral or dorsal margins of the vertebral bodies.
   e. Separation or avulsion of the articular facets

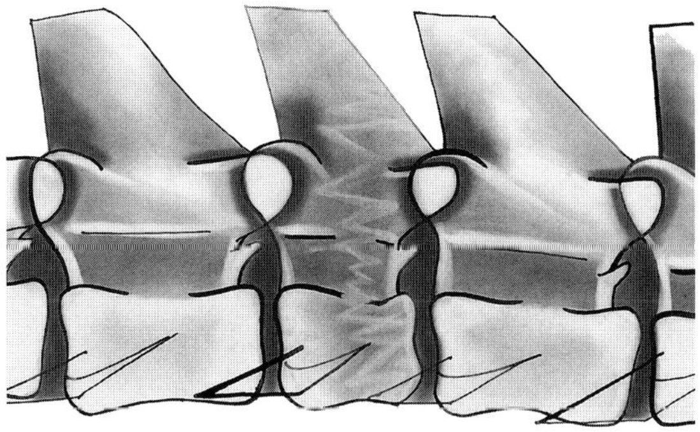

Figure 7.30. Compression type fracture of a lumbar vertebra.

f. Change in size or shape of the vertebral body or neural arch as compared with adjacent vertebrae.
2. Epiphyseal fracture (Figures 7.32 and 7.33):
   a. This fracture occurs in an immature animal in which the vertebral physis is open.
   b. Is identified best by comparing the widths and appearances of the epiphyses of the adjacent vertebral bodies. The physis is usually widened and irregular at the fracture site.
   c. The fractured epiphysis may be displaced dorsally or ventrally depending on whether the injury was caused by a flexion or extension force.
3. Dorsal spinous process fracture (Figure 7.34):
   a. This fracture is most common in the thoracic and lumbar vertebrae.
   b. Fractures are usually horizontal, multiple, and sequential.
4. Transverse process fracture (Figure 7.35):
   a. These fractures are usually longitudinal, multiple, and sequential.
   b. Is often unilateral.
   c. Concurrent intraabdominal or intrathoracic trauma is common.

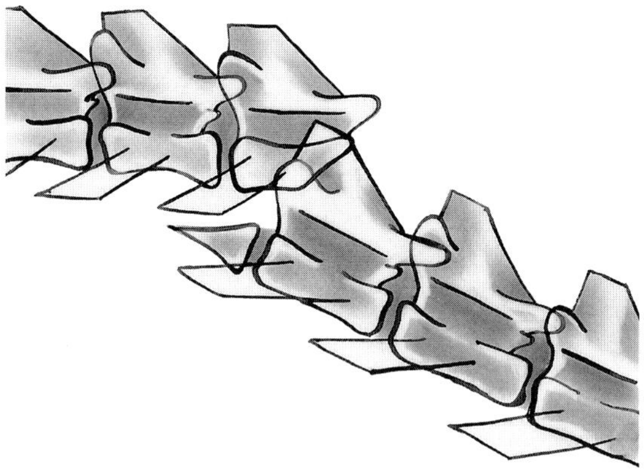

Figure 7.31. Fracture with luxation involving the lumbar vertebral body with marked ventral and cranial displacement of the caudal fracture fragment and adjacent vertebra.

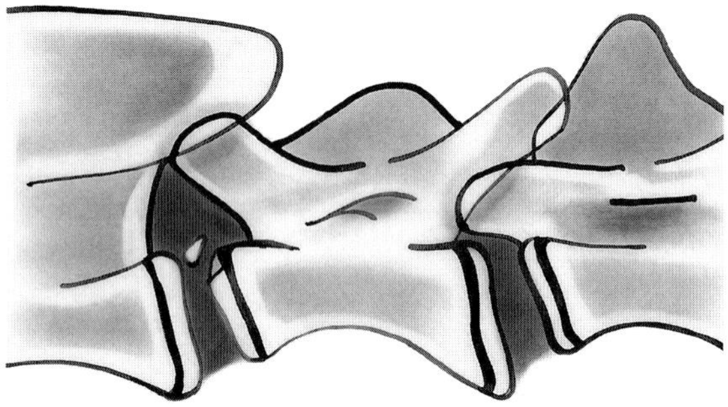

Figure 7.32. Epiphyseal fracture involving the dorsal portion of the epiphysis of C3. The chip-like fracture fragment is displaced dorsally and cranially.

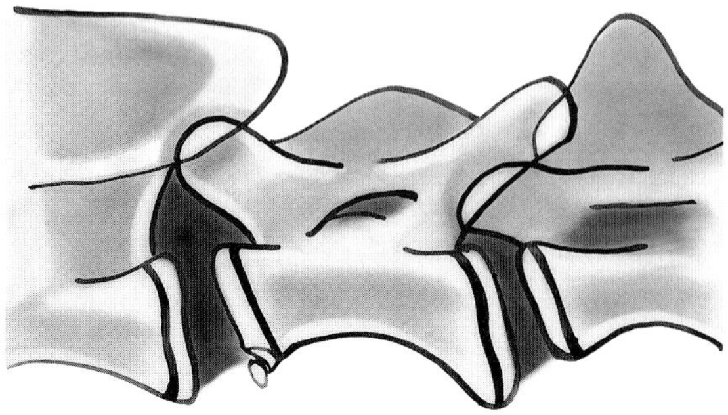

Figure 7.33. Epiphyseal fracture involving the ventral portion of the epiphysis of C3 with minimal displacement of the fracture fragment.

Intervertebral Disk Disease

Clinical correlations

1. Intervertebral disk disease also is referred to as ruptured disk, prolapsed disk, or disk herniation.

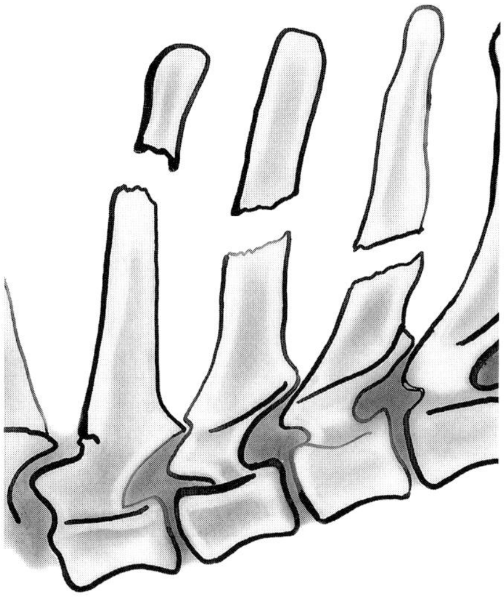

Figure 7.34. Fractures of three vertebral dorsal spinous processes.

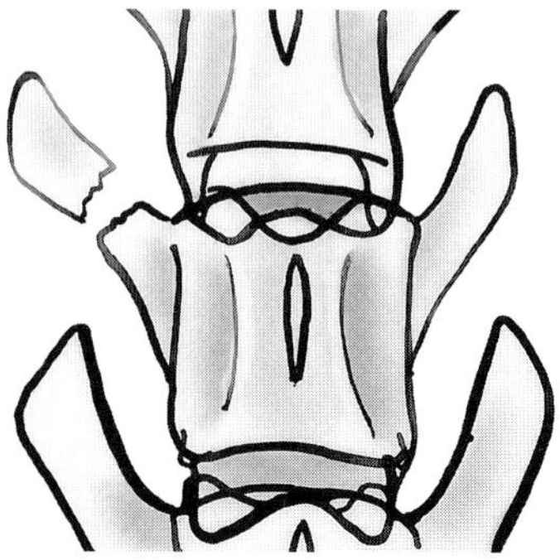

Figure 7.35. Transverse process fracture.

2. Involves degenerative changes in the morphology and biochemical parameters of an intervertebral disk, which result in extrusion or protrusion of disk material into the spinal canal and resultant compression of the spinal cord and/or nerve roots.
   a. Protrusion is bulging of the disk into the vertebral canal as a result of the nucleus shifting while its outer fibrous envelope remains intact.
   b. Extrusion indicates that the outer fibrous layers have ruptured and the nucleus has been extruded into the vertebral canal.
3. Disk degeneration may occur in any of the intervertebral disks. However, disk protrusion or extrusion is most common in the cervical, caudal thoracic, and lumbar spinal regions.
4. The thoracic disks, between T2 and T10 in dogs and between T2 and T9 in cats, are less likely to protrude or extrude because additional ligamentous support is provided by the intercapital ligaments between the rib heads and the conjugal ligaments on the floor of the spinal canal.
5. The clinical signs of disk disease, which causes cord compression, are usually neurologic. Affected animals often have pain with or without paresis or paralysis.
6. The disease is more common in dogs that are chondrodystrophoid, such as the Dachshund, Beagle, Cocker Spaniel, and Pekinese. In these breeds chondroid metaplasia of the nucleus occurs at a young age and progresses with aging. In nonchondrodystrophoid dogs, disk degeneration is usually caused by fibroid metaplasia of the nucleus.
7. Pathogenesis of intervertebral disk disease:
   a. There is progressive dehydration of the nucleus pulposus.
   b. Subsequent fibroid or chondroid metaplasia of the nucleus occurs. In chondroid metaplasia, the nucleus becomes more cartilaginous and granular and may mineralize.
   c. Rupture or tearing of the annulus allows the nucleus to extrude or prolapse into the epidural space of the spinal canal. The extruded disk material may be gelatinous, fibrous, or mineralized.
8. There are two types of disk herniation as described by Hansen.
   a. Type I disk herniation
      1) Disk herniation is associated with degeneration and rupture of the dorsal annulus. The nucleus pulposus extrudes through the ruptured anulus into the spinal canal.
      2) Is most commonly associated with chondroid disk degeneration.
      3) Is frequently a more acute condition and has more severe clinical signs than Type II.
   b. Type II disk herniation
      1) Disk protrusion is characterized by bulging of the intervertebral disk without complete rupture of the annulus.
      2) Is often a gradual progressive process.

Radiographic findings (Figures 7.36 and 7.37)

1. Mineralization of the nucleus pulposus: in situ is a degenerative process, but is not a finding of disk protrusion or extrusion.
2. Intervertebral disk space is narrowed (as compared with adjacent spaces).
   a. The space may be uniformly narrowed.
   b. The space may be wedge shaped. Often the most narrowed portion is dorsal, indicating that the dorsal portion of the disk has ruptured and the more ventral portion of the disk is still intact.
   c. The T10–11 disk space, or anticlinal disk space, is normally more narrow than the other disk spaces.
3. Decreased size and/or altered shape of the intervertebral foramen

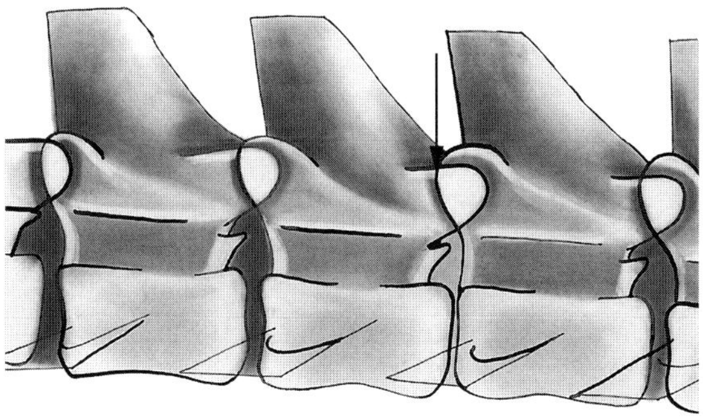

Figure 7.36. Extruded intervertebral disk. The intervertebral disk space is collapsed, the intervertebral foramen is reduced in size, and there is increased radiopacity within the intervertebral foramen. The joint space between the articular facets is often also narrowed (arrow).

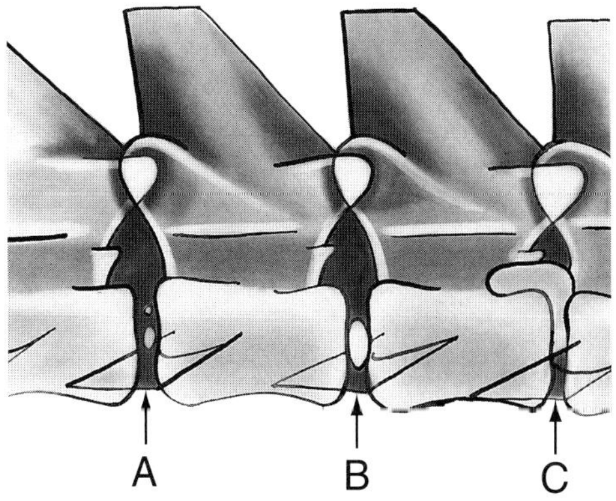

Figure 7.37. Intervertebral disk disease. **A)** Partial mineralization of the disk with no extrusion. **B)** Complete mineralization of the nucleus with no extrusion. **C)** Extrusion of mineralized disk into the spinal canal with narrowing of the intervertebral disk space.

4. Narrowing of the joint space between the articular processes
5. Increased radiopacity (soft tissue or calcified disk material) within the spinal canal, usually seen superimposed over the intervertebral foramina. The radiopacity is caused by the presence of disk material in the spinal canal.
6. Sclerosis of the vertebral endplates with collapse of the intervertebral disk space is indicative of chronic disk collapse. There also may be associated spondylosis deformans.
7. In some cases, especially acute extrusions, there may be no abnormal findings on the survey radiographs.

Contrast radiography

1. Myelography
   a. Most protruded or extruded disks cause an extradural lesion, which results in cord compression.
   b. Intramedullary swelling caused by edema or hemorrhage may be identified with or without an extradural lesion.

Other imaging

1. CT
2. MRI

Schmorl's Nodes

Clinical correlations

1. Characterized by a small smooth defect in midportion of vertebral endplates.
2. Is thought to represent herniation of nucleus pulposus through a weakened or incompletely ossified endplate of the vertebral body.
3. Is a rare condition in dogs and cats with no known clinical significance.

Radiographic findings (Figure 7.38)

1. A break in the vertebral endplate, referred to as "fish-shaped" disk space.
2. Differential considerations:
   a. Acute diskitis
   b. Diskospondylitis

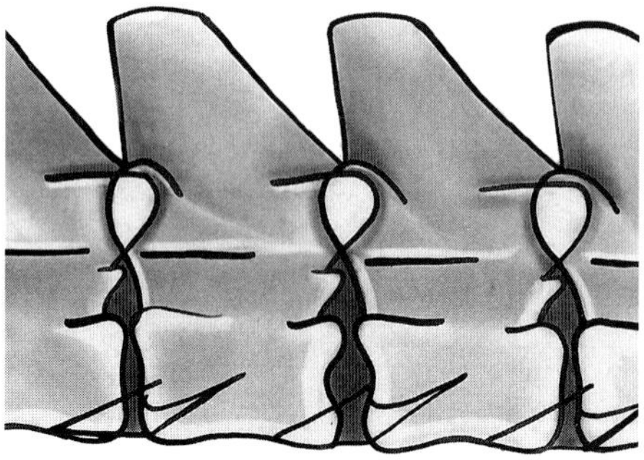

Figure 7.38. Schmorl's node. There is a smooth defect of the opposing vertebral endplates.

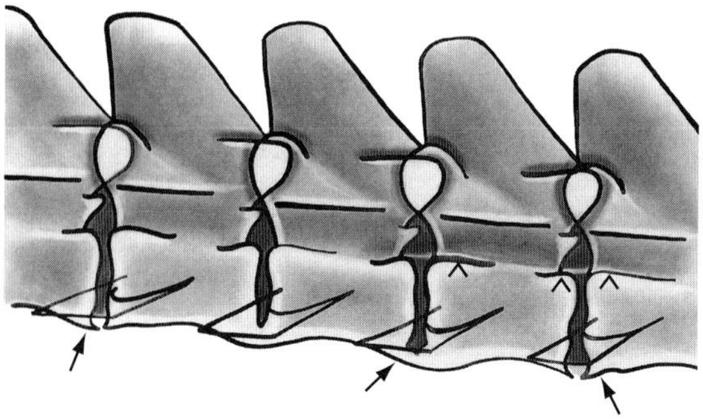

Figure 7.39. Spondylosis deformans (straight arrows) and calcified dura mater (half arrows).

Dural Ossification

Clinical correlations

1. Is also known as osseous metaplasia of dura mater and ossifying pachymeningitis.
2. Is a degenerative process in dogs that is usually an incidental finding and of no clinical significance. The etiology is unknown.
3. Is characterized by bony plaques on the inner surface of dura mater.
4. Reported to occur in more than 60% of large breed dogs, and occasionally is seen in small breed dogs.
5. Most commonly recognized in the cervical and lumbar regions.

Radiographic findings (Figure 7.39)

1. Thin radiopaque line in the neural canal most easily seen ventrally and at levels of the intervertebral foramina.
2. Must be differentiated from mineralization of the intervertebral disk and lateral spondylosis deformans.

Spondylosis Deformans

Clinical correlations

1. Spondylosis deformans is a degenerative change associated with the intervertebral joints and characterized by osteophytes originating at the margins of the vertebral endplates.
2. Is common in both dogs and cats.
3. Is thought to be related to intervertebral joint instability and degeneration.
4. The incidence and size of the osteophytes increase with age.
5. Osteophytes occur singly or multiply and locate most frequently in the midthoracic, lumbar, and lumbosacral regions.
6. Is rarely of clinical significance.

Radiographic findings (See Figures 7.39 and 7.40)

1. Bony changes vary from small curved beak-like osteophytes (spurs) to large solid bone bridging or interdig-

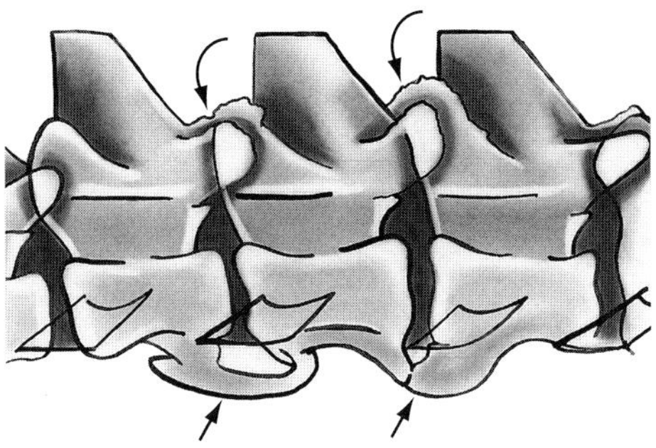

Figure 7.40. Spondylosis deformans (straight arrows) and osteoarthritis of the interarticular facets (curved arrows).

itation, singly or multiple, which originate from the ventral and lateral margins of the vertebral bodies (endplates). The osteophytes are smooth and sharply marginated.
2. Interdigitation of large adjacent bony osteophytes can appear to be solid bony bridges of two or more vertebrae.
3. Osteophytes are more commonly visible on the lateral view, but also may be seen on the ventrodorsal view.
4. Osteophytes on the dorsolateral aspect of the vertebral endplates may be seen superimposed over the intervertebral disc space on a lateral radiograph and may be misinterpreted as intervertebral disc mineralization.
5. Must differentiate radiographic findings of spondylosis deformans from osteoarthritis, spondylitis, diskospondylitis, and neoplasia.

Disseminated Idiopathic Skeletal Hyperostosis (DISH)

Clinical correlations

1. Is an ossifying condition characterized by bony hyperostosis at tendon and ligament attachments in axial and extraxial sites.
2. The etiology is unknown.
3. Reported in young large and giant breed dogs, especially Great Dane, Boxer, and Bulldog.
4. Rarely of clinical significance.
5. May be associated with other diseases (e.g., hyperthyrocalcitoninism, hyperthyroidism, or hyperparathyroidism).
6. Diagnosis is usually based on the presence of at least four radiographic findings.

Radiographic findings

1. "Flowing" mineralization and ossification along the ventral and lateral aspects of three or more contiguous vertebral bodies
2. Intervertebral disk spaces appear normal and there is an absence of degenerative disk disease.
3. Periarticular osteophytes of the synovial vertebral joints (articular facets)
4. Formation of pseudoarthrosis between the bases of spinous processes
5. Mineralization in the soft tissue attachments near joints
6. Sclerosis and ankylosis of the sacroiliac joints and the pubis

Osteoarthritis

Clinical correlations

1. Also referred to as degenerative joint disease or osteoarthrosis.
2. Includes primary and secondary degenerative joint disease involving the synovial articular joints.
3. Most commonly seen in the cervical and lumbar spinal region.

Radiographic findings (Figure 7.40)

1. Degenerative changes of this joint appear similar to other synovial joints affected with osteoarthritis or osteoarthrosis.
2. Periarticular bone spurs and subchondral bone sclerosis are seen in more chronic cases.
3. Spondylosis deformans frequently exists concurrently.

Spondylitis

Clinical correlations

1. Spondylitis is an infection of the vertebral bodies.
   a. Bacterial infection (most common cause)
   b. Fungal infections
   c. Protozoal infection (e.g., Hepatozoon)
2. Common causes:
   a. Direct extension from adjacent infected soft tissues
   b. Secondary to regional infection (e.g., kidney)
   c. Migrating foreign body (e.g., plant awn)
   d. External wound or surgical complication
3. Common clinical signs include fever, pain, and discomfort.

Radiographic findings (Figure 7.41)

1. Proliferative periosteal reaction is observed involving one or more vertebral bodies.

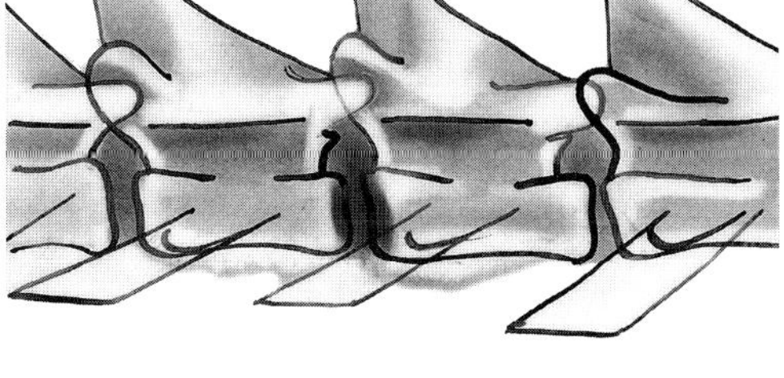

Figure 7.41. Spondylitis. Irregular new bone is seen on the ventral portions of the vertebral bodies.

2. Most commonly involves the ventral and/or lateral aspects of one or more vertebral bodies.
3. May extend into the intervertebral disk space causing diskospondylitis.
4. Differential considerations:
   a. Metastatic carcinoma
   b. Atypical hypertrophic osteopathy

Diskospondylitis

Clinical correlations

1. An infection of the intervertebral disk space and secondarily the contiguous vertebral body.
2. May involve one or more disk spaces, commonly not adjacent to each other.
3. Common causes:
   a. Hematogenous infection associated with endocarditis, dental disease, and urogenital infections
   b. Migrating foreign body (e.g., plant awn). Proposed mechanisms include:
      1) Inhalation into the lung and migration through the lungs along the crura of the diaphragm into the muscular insertion of the crura to the ventral vertebra of L2–L4.
      2) Penetration of skin with migration into the paravertebral musculature.
      3) Ingestion and penetration through the bowel wall, migrating along the mesenteric root, and extending into the paravertebral musculature and spine.
   c. Postoperative complication after spinal cord and vertebral surgery.
4. The most common organism cultured is *Staphylococcus spp*. Other infections, such as *Brucella canis,* mycoses, and mycobacterium.
5. Immunosuppression may predispose some breeds (e.g., German Shepherd Dog, Basset Hound, Airedale Terrier).
6. The clinical signs vary depending on the location, severity, and other systems involved with the infection.
   a. Common signs include fever, anorexia, pain, stiffness, and spinal hyperesthesia.
   b. Lameness, paresis or paralysis may occur if the spinal cord is affected secondarily by infection, cord compression, or vertebral instability.

Radiographic findings (Figures 7.42 and 7.43)

1. Radiographic changes commonly lag behind the onset of the clinical signs.
2. More than one disk may be affected. It is advisable to obtain radiographs of the entire spine.
3. Depending on the virulence of the infection, variable degrees of osteolysis of the vertebral bodies and osteoblastic bone reaction may be seen.
4. Early findings:

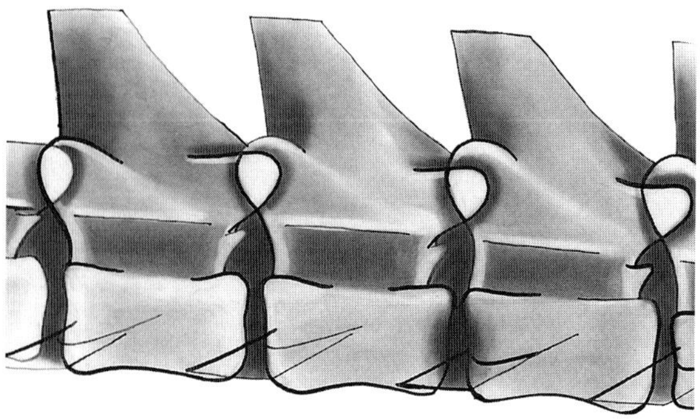

Figure 7.42. Acute diskospondylitis. There is irregular lysis of the endplates with widening of the intervertebral disk space.

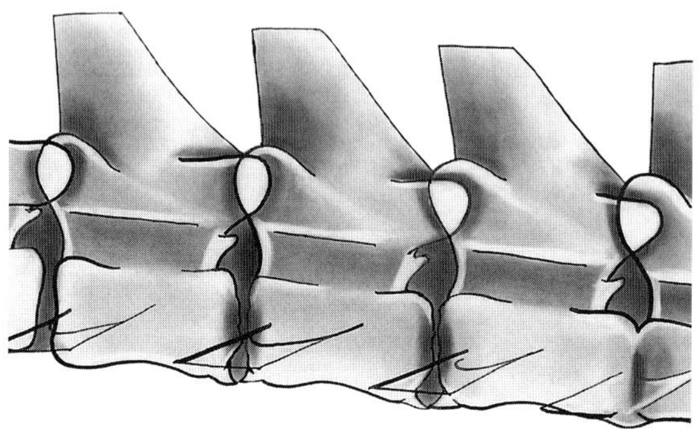

Figure 7.43. Chronic healing diskospondylitis. During healing, there is progressive narrowing of two intervertebral disk spaces resulting from endplate destruction and sclerotic remodeling of the bone. Secondary spondylosis deformans is also present.

   a. Irregular lysis at one or both endplates of the affected disk
   b. Widening or collapse of the intervertebral disk space
5. Later findings:
   a. Collapse of the intervertebral disk space
   b. Sclerosis of the vertebral endplates
   c. Osteophyte formation at the margins of the vertebral bodies
   d. Fusion of adjacent vertebral bodies may occur with healing.
6. Complete vertebral fusion may occur with a healed infection; however, many infections can become inactive without complete vertebral fusion.
   a. Serial radiographs (over time) aid in differentiating active from inactive infections.

Osteochondromatosis

Clinical correlations

1. Also referred to as multiple cartilaginous exostoses.
2. Results from abnormal differentiation of cartilage cells that give rise to exostoses in the axial and appendicular skeleton.
3. Exostosis may be monostotic (solitary osteochondroma) or polyostotic (osteochondromatosis). Most

commonly affects the vertebra, ribs, long bones, and flat bones such as scapula and pelvis.
4. Usually, is seen before 1 year of age in cats and dogs (more commonly reported in Yorkshire and other terriers, German Shepherd Dog, and Alaskan Malamute).
5. Although uncommon, neurologic signs may result from spinal cord compression secondary to the exostosis.

Radiographic findings (Figure 7.44)

1. Cartilage capped bony exostosis can be observed arising from the surface of a bone formed by endochondral ossification.
2. Lesions usually appear nonaggressive (e.g., smooth, spherical, and with sclerotic margins).
3. Lesions may be solitary or multiple.

Neoplasia

Clinical correlations

1. Neoplasms can occur in the vertebra, the extravertebral soft tissues, or in the spinal cord and meninges. These tumors may be primary or metastatic lesions.
2. Clinical signs commonly include pain, paresis, lameness, or paralysis, depending on the degree and location of compression and the involvement of spinal cord and nerve roots.
3. Tumors of the vertebrae
   a. Benign tumors:

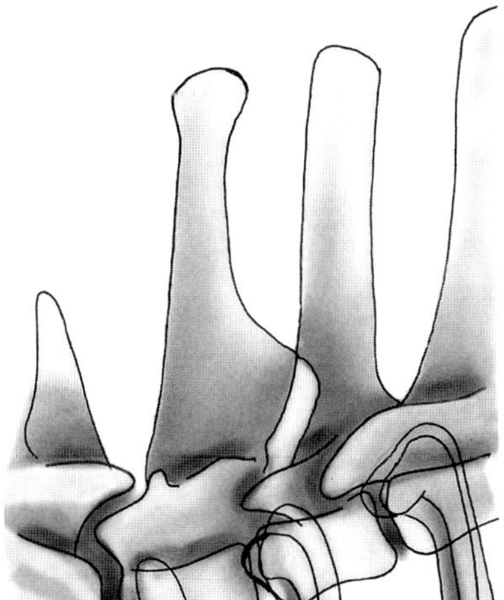

Figure 7.44. Osteochondromatosis. There is a smooth expansile lesion of the dorsal spinous process of the first thoracic vertebra.

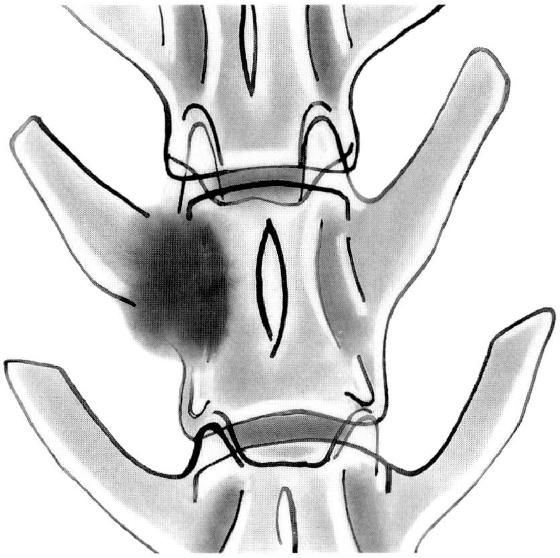

Figure 7.45. Malignant primary sarcoma of a lumbar vertebra. There is an irregular osteolytic and osteoblastic lesion of the right side of the vertebral body extending from the pedicle into the transverse process.

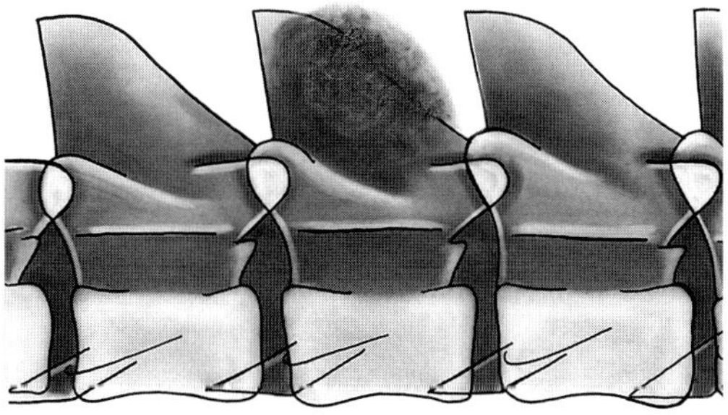

Figure 7.46. Malignant primary sarcoma of a lumbar vertebra. There is irregular osteolysis of the dorsal spinous process.

      1) Osteoma
      2) Osteochondroma (solitary or multiple)
   b. Malignant tumors (more common types):
      1) Osteosarcoma
      2) Chondrosarcoma
      3) Fibrosarcoma
      4) Hemangiosarcoma
      5) Plasma cell myeloma
   c. Metastatic tumors:
      1) Carcinoma (e.g., prostate, mammary, lung)
      2) Lymphosarcoma
      3) Hemangiosarcoma
4. Tumors of spinal cord:
   a. Most intramedullary cord tumors are glial cell types.
   b. Most intradural-extramedullary tumors are meningiomas or nerve sheath tumors (e.g., neurofibroma, neurofibrosarcoma).
   c. Metastatic tumors to the cord are rare.

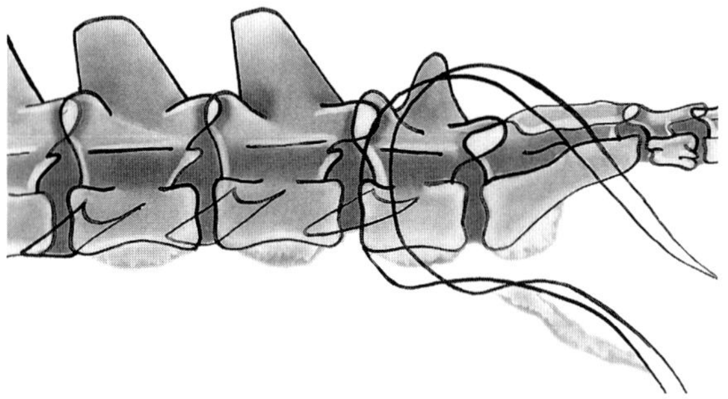

Figure 7.47. Metastatic carcinoma involving multiple vertebra. There is irregular periosteal proliferation on the ventral border of the several lumbar vertebrae and the sacrum. The intervertebral disk spaces are unaffected.

Radiographic findings

1. Tumors of the spinal cord, spinal nerves, and meninges
   a. Usually, no abnormality is seen on survey radiographs.
   b. Some cord tumors may cause enlargement of the bony spinal canal, erosion of the lamina, or erosion of a pedicle.
   c. Some tumors of the nerve roots may cause enlargement of the intervertebral foramen. Right and left oblique projections are made to compare the size and shape of the intervertebral foramen.
2. Benign tumors of vertebra
   a. Osteoma is usually a well-circumscribed bony mass.
   b. Osteochondroma is an expansile smooth bony mass with a sclerotic border and rarely a periosteal reaction.
3. Malignant tumors of vertebra (primary and metastatic) (Figures 7.45 through 7.47):
   a. Primary tumors usually involve only one vertebra and usually appear aggressive with osteolytic, osteoblastic, or mixed changes.
   b. Metastatic tumors commonly involve more than one vertebrae and/or other bones.
      1) Metastatic tumors usually are osteolytic.
      2) Metastatic carcinoma (through paravertebral venous plexus from the bladder, urethra, prostate, or rectum) often cause a productive bony lesion often involving the caudal lumbar and sacral vertebrae, the pelvis, adjacent vertebra, and the femurs.
   c. Uncommonly extends into the intervertebral disk space.
   d. May have a paraspinal soft tissue mass.
   e. A pathologic fracture of the vertebral body often causes collapse and shortening of the vertebra.

Contrast radiography

1. Myelography
   a. Allows evaluation of the spinal cord
   b. Can determine the degree and type of cord compression.
      1) Intramedullary compression: tumors of the spinal cord
      2) Intradural and extramedullary compression: tumors of the nerve roots
      3) Extradural compression: tumors of the vertebral body, some meningiomas and metastatic tumors

Other imaging

1. CT allows imaging of the vertebral bodies and intervertebral disk spaces and may identify some tumors of the spinal cord, nerve roots, and vertebrae.
2. MRI allows imaging of the spinal cord, nerve roots and intervertebral disk spaces.

chapter eight

8

Thorax (Noncardiac)

RADIOGRAPHIC TECHNIQUE

Standard Projections

1. Lateral recumbent projection exposed at peak inspiration.
   a. A right or left lateral projection should be used routinely.
   b. With consistent projection, the normal relationships between the heart, the caudal vena cava, and the diaphragm will be less variable. The normal heart has a more consistent position on the right lateral projection.
   c. Use of both lateral views is commonly recommended, especially for lung diseases (e.g., pneumonia, primary, and metastatic tumors). Because the nondependent lung usually is more inflated, lung lesions are usually more visible in the nondependent lung lobes. Dependent lung lesions are often obscured by positional atelectasis.
   d. Appearance of normal thorax varies because of variations in size and shape of thorax and because of partial collapse of the dependent lung, especially in anesthetized, heavily sedated, or obese animals.
2. The dorsoventral (sternal recumbent) or ventrodorsal (dorsal recumbent) projection exposed at peak inspiration.
   a. The ventrodorsal projection is frequently preferable for symmetrical positioning of the animal and usually enables a better inspiratory effort for examination of the lungs.
   b. The dorsoventral projection provides for greater consistency of the heart's position and better visualization of the caudal lobar vessels.
   c. The dorsoventral projection may be less compromising to an animal in hypovolemic shock or severe respiratory distress.
   d. If a pleural effusion is present, the lung and heart are better visualized on a ventrodorsal view. On a dorsoventral view, pleural effusion commonly obscures the heart.

Supplemental Projections

1. Right and left ventrodorsal oblique projections are useful in the evaluation of mediastinal, pleural, and extrapleural masses
2. Horizontal beam projections (standing lateral, erect, ventrodorsal, and recumbent lateral) are useful in the evaluation of fluid or air within the pleural cavity.
3. Expiratory phase radiographs
   a. May aid in the detection of small amounts of pleural fluid or pneumothorax.
   b. May aid in the diagnosis of tracheal and/or bronchial collapse.
4. Lateral and ventrodorsal projections are useful in evaluation of larynx, cervical tracheal, and cervical soft tissues.

RADIOGRAPHIC ANATOMY (Figures 8.1 and 8.2):

1. The trachea is an air-filled structure within the neck and cranial mediastinum extending to the bifurcation of the trachea (carina).
   a. The tracheal rings are cartilaginous and radiolucent in the young animal. In chondrodystrophoid breeds or with age the rings frequently mineralize.
   b. The trachea bifurcates into the right and left main stem bronchi at the hilus dorsal to the heart base.
2. Usually the normal bronchi are only seen in the hilar area as air-filled structures contrasted against the fluid opacity of the adjacent pulmonary vessels. The bronchial walls become more visible when they are thickened, mineralized, or have increased endobronchial secretions. The location of the normal bronchial tree in the dog and cat is illustrated in Figures 8.3 and 8.4.
   a. The left primary bronchus has two major divisions:
      1) Proximal common bronchus to the cranial and caudal segments to the left cranial lung lobe
      2) Distal bronchus to the left caudal lung lobe.

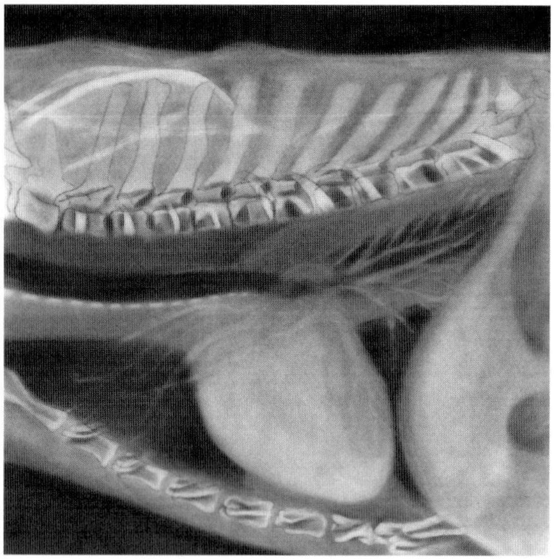

Figure 8.1. Normal canine thorax.

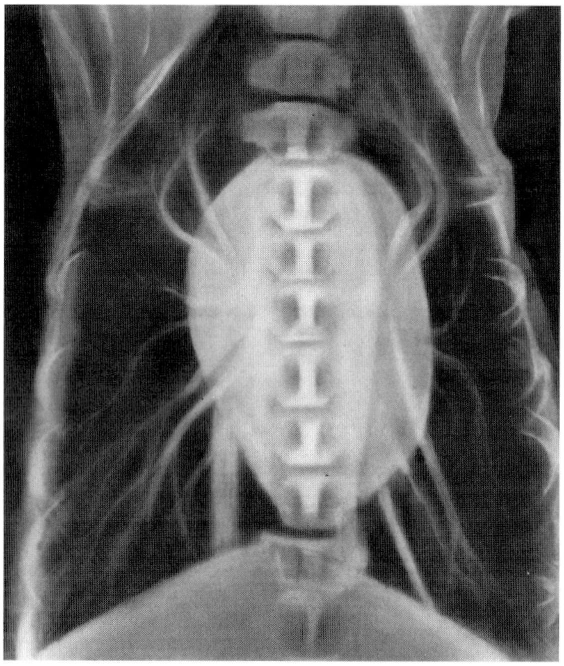

Figure 8.2. Normal canine thorax.

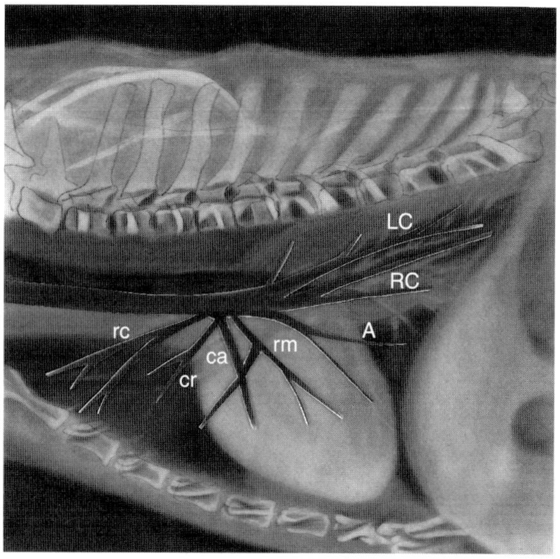

Figure 8.3. Normal bronchial anatomy. The normal lobar bronchi are labeled: right cranial lobe (**rc**), right middle lobe (**rm**), right caudal lobe (**RC**), accessory lung lobe (**A**), left cranial lobe, cranial segment (**cr**), left cranial lobe caudal segment (**ca**), and left caudal lobe (**LC**).

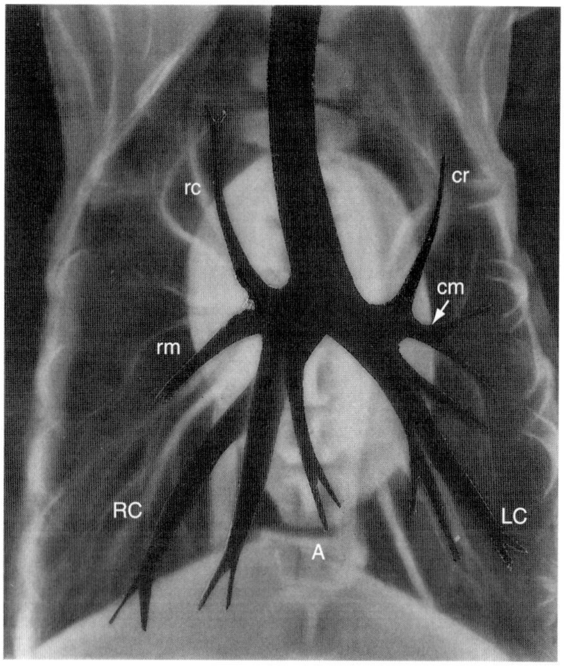

Figure 8.4. Normal bronchial tree. The normal lobar bronchi are labeled: right cranial lobe (**rc**), right middle lobe (**rm**), right caudal lobe (**RC**), accessory lung lobe (**A**), left cranial lobe, cranial segment (**cr**), left cranial lobe caudal segment (**ca**), and left caudal lobe (**LC**).

b. The right primary bronchus has four major divisions:
   1) Right cranial lung lobe bronchus
   2) Right middle lung lobe bronchus
   3) Accessory lung lobe bronchus
   4) Right caudal lung lobe bronchus

3. The normal pulmonary vessels are usually visible in the hilar area and middle third of the lung fields as branching soft tissue radiopacities, contrasted against the radiolucency of the air-filled lung (Figure 8.5).

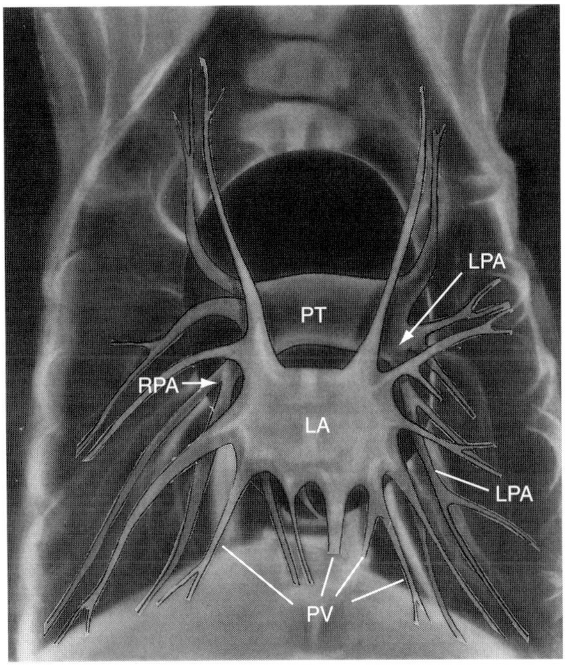

Figure 8.5. Normal pulmonary vasculature: pulmonary trunk (**PT**), left pulmonary artery (**LPA**), right pulmonary artery (**RPA**), left atrium (**LA**), and pulmonary veins (**PV**).

a. The position, size, and shape of the pulmonary arteries and veins are important for disease recognition. The normal artery and vein should be equivalent in size and branch with smooth and gradual tapering.
b. On the lateral projection:
   1) Origins of the pulmonary arteries are usually visible at the level of the tracheal bifurcation.
   2) The left pulmonary artery lies dorsal to the tracheal bifurcation.
   3) The right pulmonary artery lies ventral to the tracheal bifurcation.
   4) When an artery, bronchus, and vein are seen, the artery is dorsal to the bronchus and vein.
   5) The right cranial lung lobe artery, bronchus, and vein are routinely visible, especially on the left lateral recumbent projection. They are commonly used as reference vessels for evaluation of the pulmonary circulation.
c. On a dorsoventral or ventrodorsal projection:
   1) The left and right pulmonary arteries can usually be seen superimposed over the heart and extending caudolaterally from the midcardiac region.
   2) The left pulmonary artery extends beyond left heart border at approximately the 4 o'clock position.
   3) The right pulmonary artery extends beyond right heart border at approximately the 8 o'clock position.
   4) The lobar pulmonary arteries are usually seen lateral to the vein with bronchus located between the two vessels.
d. The pulmonary veins can usually be seen as they enter the atrium over the heart base medial to the corresponding pulmonary arteries.
   1) The lobar pulmonary veins are usually ventral and medial to the corresponding bronchi and pulmonary arteries, as seen on both the lateral and ventrodorsal projections.

4. The lungs are the largest organ in the thorax.
   a. The cranial aspect of each lung is called the apex and the caudal aspect adjacent to the diaphragm is called the base.
   b. As seen from the lateral projection, each lung has four borders: the cranial, dorsal, caudal (basal), and ventral.
   c. There are six lung lobes in the dog and cat.
      1) The left lung has two lobes: the cranial lobe (with cranial and caudal segments) and the caudal lobe.
      2) The right lung has four lobes: the cranial, middle, caudal, and accessory lobes.
5. The lung parenchyma consists of air-filled spaces (alveoli) contained within the supporting interstitial structures.
   a. Within this interstitium are bronchi, blood vessels, alveolar walls, lymphatics, and nerves.
   b. The blood vessels and bronchi are seen as tubular structures radiating from the hilum. The soft-tissue radiopaque vessels are seen more peripherally than the air-filled bronchi.
   c. Each lung can be divided into three regions: hilar, central, and peripheral. The normal bronchi usually are seen only in the hilus, and pulmonary vessels are usually only seen in the hilar and central regions.
   d. In some projections, a normal bronchus may be observed end-on, and have mineralized walls. This is seen especially in chondrodystrophoid and older normal dogs and cats.
6. The mediastinum is formed by the reflection of the parietal pleura and the space and structures between them that divides the right and left hemithorax.
   a. The mediastinum contains the trachea, esophagus, and heart, the aorta and its major branches, the cranial and caudal vena cavae, the azygous vein, the thoracic duct, lymph nodes (cranial mediastinal, sternal, and tracheobronchial), and nerves.
7. The pleural space is located between the visceral pleura covering the lungs, parietal pleural lining the chest wall, mediastinum and diaphragm, and the interlobar fissures between lung lobes.
   a. Normally is not visible on radiographs because the inflated lungs are in contact with the parietal pleura of the chest wall.
   b. If negative pressure in the pleural space is lost because of the presence of fluid or air, the lungs will

collapse and be separated from the chest wall, creating a true pleural space.

8. The thoracic wall is formed by the rib cage. It is composed of skin, fat, subcutaneous muscles and fat, ribs, intercostal muscles, parietal pleural, and numerous vessels and nerves. The ribs have intercostal muscles between them and are lined internally by parietal pleura. The sternum and vertebrae are also components of the thoracic wall.
9. The diaphragm, a musculocutanous partition between thoracic and abdominal cavities, attaches to the sternum (called the cupola). It extends dorsocaudally as the crura (right and left crus) to attach to the ribs and to the ventral aspect of the lumbar spine.
   a. The diaphragm is seen radiographically as a convex soft tissue opacity. Visualization depends on differing radiopacity of adjacent structures. Normally, only the thoracic surface of the diaphragm is visible because of contrasting air in the adjacent lung.
   b. Only a small part of the diaphragm is visible (on one view), and its appearance is variable based on body shape, phase of respiration, radiographic projection, and presence of abdominal or thoracic disease.
   c. On the lateral recumbent projection, the diaphragm is usually dome shaped with the dependent crus located more cranially. In left lateral recumbency the crura may appear to cross. In right recumbency they are more likely to appear parallel.
   d. On the ventrodorsal or dorsoventral projection, the diaphragm usually appears as a dome-shaped structure, or as two or three separate domed structures, usually related to the centering of the x-ray beam and phase of respiration.

RADIOGRAPHIC INTERPRETATION: SYSTEMATIC EVALUATION

1. Recognition of thoracic disease requires proper viewing of the radiographs on the illuminator.
   a. Orient the lateral radiographic projections (left and right) on the illuminator with the animal's head toward the left.
   b. Orient the dorsoventral and ventrodorsal radiographic projections on the illuminator with the animal's left side to the observer's right.
2. Evaluate the radiographs for their technical quality (symmetrical positioning and proper exposure factors).
3. Observe the position of the diaphragm relative to the heart to determine whether the radiograph was made during inspiration or expiration.
4. Evaluate the extrathoracic structures including the soft tissues, spine, sternum, diaphragm, ribs, thoracic wall, and liver.
5. Evaluate the position and diameter of the trachea and the tracheal bifurcation.
6. Evaluate the cranial and caudal mediastinum, including all its pleural reflections for widening, abnormal opacity, or the presence of a mass.
7. Evaluate the entire aorta, aortic arch, and the caudal vena cava.
8. Evaluate the position of the cardiac silhouette for size, shape, opacity, and position relative to the thoracic shape.
9. Evaluate the esophagus or region where it is normally located.
10. Evaluate the main pulmonary arteries and the size and shape of the lobar pulmonary arteries and veins.
11. Evaluate the lung for areas of overall or localized alterations in radiopacity.

THE LARYNX AND HYOID BONES

RADIOGRAPHIC INTERPRETATION

1. The larynx is best evaluated with a symmetrical lateral projection, centered over the larynx. The neck should be extended, preferably with an approximately 135° angulation between the vertebral canal and horizontal rami of the mandibles. Anesthesia or sedation is usually necessary for proper positioning.
2. A ventrodorsal view is rarely helpful because the larynx is superimposed over the skull and cervical spine. If the animal is anesthetized, the endotracheal tube can also obscure structures.
3. Major anatomic landmarks of the larynx are depicted in Figure 8.6. The normal larynx is usually at the C1 and C2 level, but can vary depending on the phase of respiration and the position of the neck. If the head is extended, the larynx is pulled cranially and closer to the spine. If the head is flexed, the larynx may be as far caudal as C4.
4. In the dog, the laryngeal structures that can usually be identified include the epiglottis, the lateral ventricles, the corniculate process of the arytenoid cartilage, the thyroid cartilage, and the cricoid cartilage. The vocal folds cannot be visualized. Depending on the phase of respiration and the effect of swallowing, the tip of the normal epiglottis may be located dorsal, ventral, end-on to the soft palate, or on the floor of the pharynx.
5. In the cat, usually only the epiglottis is seen.
6. Mineralization of the laryngeal cartilages, most notably the cricoid cartilage, commonly occurs as part of the normal aging process. The mineralization is more com-

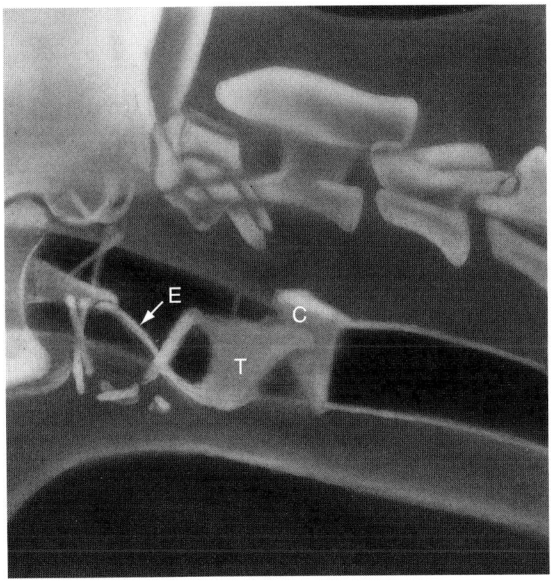

Figure 8.6. Normal laryngeal anatomy. Normal radiographic landmarks include epiglottis (**E**), thyroid cartilage (**T**), and the cricoid cartilage (**C**).

mon in large breed and chondrodystrophoid dogs and is rare in the cat.
7. The hyoid bones are well-defined and usually identified on radiographs of the laryngeal region. Variations in the positioning of the head and neck cause variations in the angles of the hyoid bones.
8. Displacement from a normal position is usually caused by abnormal soft tissue masses associated with the pharynx, esophagus, retropharyngeal, retrolaryngeal, or paratracheal structures.

DISEASES/DISORDERS

Clinical correlations

1. Most diseases of the larynx cause respiratory distress, possibly because of functional disruption (e.g., laryngeal paralysis) or airway obstruction that result from intraluminal, mural, or extraluminal masses or from scarring or stenosis secondary to trauma related to intubation.
2. Respiratory distress varies depending on the cause and severity of the laryngeal obstruction. However, inspiratory stridor is most common in animals with fixed upper airway obstruction (e.g., laryngeal tumors); inspiratory and expiratory stridor may occur.
3. Definitive diagnosis is made through combination of the radiographic examination, laryngoscopy, and if needed, laryngeal biopsy.

Laryngeal Hypoplasia

Clinical correlations

1. Common in brachycephalic dog breeds (e.g., Bulldog, Boston Terrier).
2. Laryngeal cartilages are soft and often underdeveloped.
3. Respiratory distress is caused by narrowing of the laryngeal lumen and dysfunction of the abductors.
4. The degree of hypoplasia is best assessed by laryngoscopy.

Radiographic findings

1. The dorsoventral diameter is narrowed on the lateral projection.
2. The pharynx is often smaller than normal and the soft palate is thick and elongated.

Laryngeal Paralysis

Clinical correlations

1. Laryngeal paralysis is characterized by the failure of the vocal folds and/or the arytenoid cartilage to abduct on inspiration, because of loss of innervation of intrinsic musculature of the larynx.
2. Occurs most commonly in dogs, rarely in cats, and is most often seen in large breed dogs (e.g., Labrador Retriever, Golden Retriever, and Saint Bernard).
3. Is often idiopathic.
4. Has been reported as an inheritable disease in Bouvier des Flandres, Siberian Husky, English Bulldog, and Dalmatian.
5. Other causes include trauma, inflammation, neoplasia, and systemic neuromuscular disease (e.g., polyneuropathy, myasthenia gravis, hypothyroidism).

Radiographic findings

1. The radiographs of the larynx and cervical trachea are usually normal.
2. Occasionally, with dilation of the pharynx, the air containing lateral ventricles may become obliterated or more rounded than normal.
3. In some dogs with severe paralysis, the resistance to air flow may cause narrowing of the cervical trachea, dilation of the intrathoracic trachea, and/or pulmonary hyperinflation.
4. Aspiration pneumonia is occasionally seen as a sequel.
5. Pulmonary edema may be present if respiratory distress is severe, probably because of noncardiogenic pulmonary edema.

Laryngeal Neoplasia

Clinical correlations

1. In the dog, the most common tumor is squamous cell carcinoma. Less common tumors in the dog include: leiomyoma, lymphosarcoma, and rhabdomyosarcoma.
2. In the cat, most laryngeal tumors are squamous cell carcinoma and lymphosarcoma.
3. Thyroid and tonsillar carcinomas may invade the larynx.
4. The degree and extent of disease is best assessed by laryngoscopy. One must differentiate it from other

mass-like lesions (i.e., lymphadenopathy, abscess, foreign body, polyp, and granulation tissue).

Radiographic findings

1. Large tumor masses may cause partial occlusion of the larynx or laryngeal opening.
2. If the cartilage of the larynx is involved, a soft tissue or mineralized mass may be seen adjacent to the larynx, with or without laryngeal displacement.
3. If a mass lesion is large, it may cause displacement of normal adjacent structures.

The Hyoid Bones

Clinical correlations

1. Fracture and luxation caused by trauma are the most common abnormalities.
2. Tumors (e.g., osteosarcoma) are rare.
3. May have concurrent injury to the larynx.

Radiographic findings

1. Fracture or displacement of one or more of the hyoid bones.
2. Irregular new bone production, bone lysis, and/or periosteal reaction may be present.

TRACHEA AND MAJOR AIRWAYS

RADIOGRAPHIC INTERPRETATION

1. The lumen of the trachea contains air and is easily recognized.
2. Normal size of the tracheal lumen (Rules of thumb)
   a. The ratio of tracheal diameter to the thoracic inlet diameter ranges from approximately 0.20 in non-brachycephalic breed to 0.16 in non-bull dog brachycephalic dogs. Bulldogs have the smallest ratio of 0.07 to 0.21. The ratio in dogs younger than 1 year of age is slightly smaller.
   b. Tracheal diameter should be slightly smaller than the diameter of larynx.
   c. Tracheal diameter should be wider than the width of proximal one third of third rib.
3. The intraluminal diameter of the normal trachea varies slightly with the phase of respiration in different breeds.
   a. Effect of phase of respiration.
      1) On inspiration, the intrathoracic portion of the normal trachea widens slightly and the cervical portion of the trachea narrows.
      2) On expiration, the intrathoracic portion of the normal trachea narrows slightly and the cervical portion of the trachea widens.
4. Upper respiratory obstructions, which cause abnormal widening of the trachea, include: laryngeal edema, laryngeal paralysis, tracheal foreign body, or tumor.
5. Causes for abnormal narrowing of the trachea include:
   a. Hypoplasia of the trachea (See Figure 8.7)
   b. Stenosis of the trachea (See Figure 8.8)
   c. Tracheal collapse (See Figure 8.9)
6. Position of the trachea should be evaluated for any displacement away from a normal position. The trachea is a midline structure, but as a variant of normal in some dogs (i.e., English Bulldog, Boston Terrier), especially obese animals, it can be slightly to the right of the midline in the cranial mediastinum.
   a. Causes for ventral or lateral deviation of the cervical trachea
      1) Enlarged retropharyngeal lymph nodes
      2) Foreign body abscesses or granulomas
      3) Megaesophagus, esophageal foreign bodies
      4) Tumors in the neck (e.g., thyroid carcinoma)
   b. Causes for dorsal deviation of the thoracic trachea
      1) Cranial mediastinal mass
      2) Excessive fat in the cranial mediastinum
      3) Right heart enlargement
      4) Anomalous position secondary to pectus excavatum
      5) Positional artifact
         a) Oblique projection
         b) As a result of flexed position of the head and neck
         c) Expiratory radiograph (expiratory hump sign)
   c. Ventral deviation of the thoracic trachea
      1) Megaesophagus or esophageal mass
      2) Dorsal cranial mediastinal mass
   d. Lateral deviation of the thoracic trachea
      1) Cranial mediastinal mass (e.g., lymphadenopathy, heart base tumor)
      2) Excessive mediastinal fat
      3) Pulmonary mass
      4) Mediastinal shift caused by atelectasis
      5) Positional artifact
         a) Oblique projection
         b) As a result of flexed position of the head and neck
         c) Expiratory radiograph
7. The walls of the tracheal wall and major bronchi should be evaluated for irregularity, mineralization, or thickening.
   a. Tracheal rings and bronchial walls (bronchial markings) are often mineralized and/or are more prominent in:
      1) Normal young chondrodystrophic and large breed dogs
      2) Normal older animals (normal aging)
      3) Chronic bronchitis and/or bronchiectasis
      4) Dystrophic mineralization secondary to steroid therapy or hyperadrenocorticism

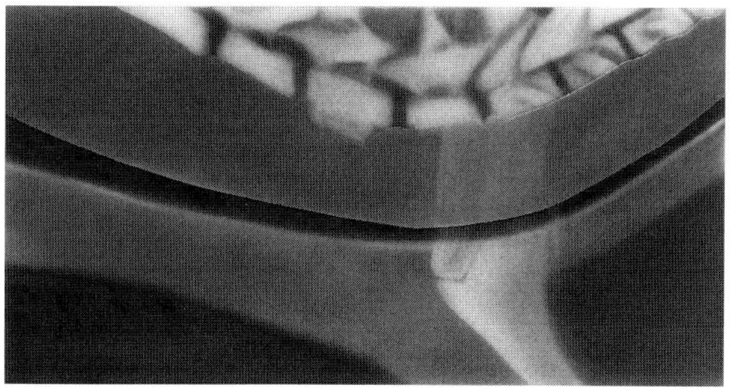

Figure 8.7. Hypoplastic trachea.

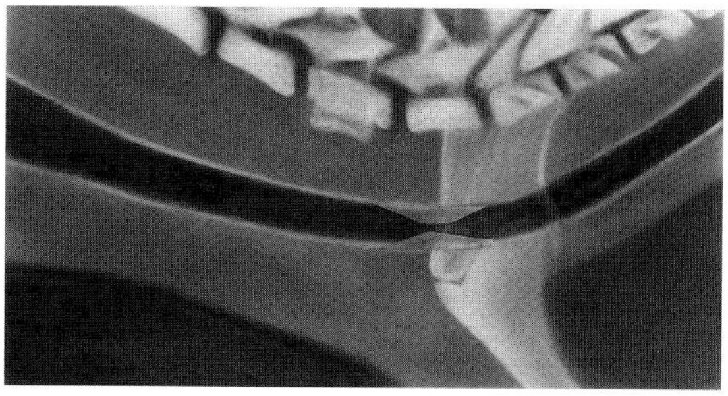

Figure 8.8. Tracheal stenosis.

DISEASES/DISORDERS

Hypoplastic Trachea

Clinical correlations

1. Is a congenital defect, resulting in incomplete or anomalous development of the tracheal rings.
2. Most common in brachycephalic breeds (e.g., English Bulldog).
3. Affected animals may have recurrent airway infections and/or decreased exercise tolerance.

Radiographic findings (Figure 8.7)

1. Diminished tracheal diameter in the lateral and the ventrodorsal projections. Usually the entire length from larynx to the tracheal bifurcation is uniformly smaller than normal.
2. The shape is normal ovoid compared to elliptical shape that usually occurs with tracheal collapse.

Tracheal Stenosis

Clinical correlations

1. Usually segmental
2. May be congenital in small breeds.
3. May be acquired from previous tracheal trauma (e.g., bite wounds, overinflated endotracheal tube cuff).
4. Narrowing can also be caused by inflammation and fibrosis.
5. Must be differentiated from intramural and intraluminal mass lesions.

Radiographic findings (Figure 8.8)

1. Segmental narrowing of the tracheal lumen, usually involving only one to several rings
2. Tracheal rings may be deformed.

Trachea Collapse

Clinical correlations

1. Is a congenital or acquired weakness of the trachea with a range of dynamic variations in the size of the trachea.
2. Most frequently seen in toy and miniature dog breeds (e.g., Yorkshire Terriers, Poodles, Chihuahuas, Pomeranians). It is rarely reported in cats.
3. Commonly a chronic "honking" cough will be present.

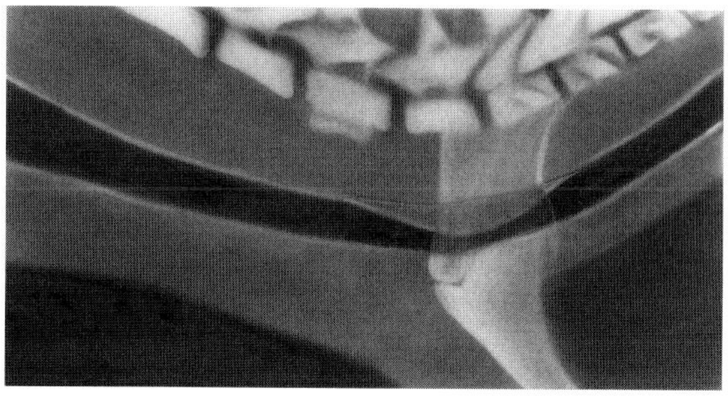

Figure 8.9. Tracheal collapse.

4. May have concurrent collapse of the main stem bronchi, commonly near the carina.

Radiographic findings (Figure 8.9)

1. There are variable degrees of collapse on expiratory and inspiratory radiographs. More than 50% narrowing of the lumen during respiration or coughing is usually considered abnormal.
2. Commonly involves the caudal cervical trachea or thoracic trachea at the carina
3. The narrowed diameter is usually more apparent on a lateral expiratory radiograph, preferably with the head and neck in neutral position. A tangential cross-sectional projection at the thoracic inlet may be helpful.
4. Occasionally, the abnormal trachea may "balloon" rather than collapse.
5. Must differentiate narrowing of trachea from superimposition of the esophagus and soft tissues of the shoulder and from folding of trachealis muscle into lumen of the trachea.
6. Because the disease is dynamic, fluoroscopy or endoscopy is usually necessary for confirmation.
7. Many dogs frequently have right-sided cardiac enlargement as compensatory effect (cor pulmonale), and chronic bronchial lung disease.

Endotracheal Masses

Clinical correlations

1. Endotracheal masses may be granulomas, polyps, thickened mucosal folds, or tumors.

2. Granulomas may occur secondary to surgical trauma (e.g., posttracheostomy, overinflation of an endotracheal tube cuff) or secondary to a foreign body.
3. Filaroides spp. granulomas most often occur in young dogs.
4. Neoplasms are uncommon.
   a. Benign tumors include chondroma, osteoma, or osteochondroma
   b. Malignant tumors include squamous cells carcinoma, lymphosarcoma, osteosarcoma, and adenocarcinoma.
5. Clinical signs vary depending on the size, location, and associated inflammatory changes.
   a. Cough, when present, is usually nonproductive.
   b. If the lesion causes significant obstruction of the tracheal lumen, inspiratory and expiratory distress may be present.
6. Is best assessed by endoscopy.

Radiographic finding

1. There is an irregular filling defect or mass on the intraluminal surface of the trachea.
2. Large masses may cause narrowing of the tracheal lumen.

Tracheal Rupture

Clinical correlations

1. Is usually caused by external trauma, puncture wounds, foreign bodies, or secondary to over inflation of endotracheal tube cuff.
2. Most ruptures occur in the cervical trachea.
3. May develop or have concurrent subcutaneous emphysema, pneumomediastinum, pneumoretroperitoneum, or pneumothorax.
4. Can often be assessed by tracheoscopy

Radiographic findings

1. There is interruption in the tracheal wall from slight to complete avulsion. The avulsed ends may be widely separated or seen with a thin line connecting the ends.
2. There is subcutaneous emphysema in the neck and usually a pneumomediastinum.
3. May also have pneumothorax and/or pneumoretroperitoneum.

Tracheal Foreign Body

Clinical correlations

1. Usually sudden onset of respiratory distress caused by aspiration of a foreign body.
2. Small foreign bodies commonly lodge and obstruct a bronchus, most commonly the right caudal lobe bronchus. Larger foreign bodies may lodge at the tracheal bifurcation.

Radiographic findings

1. Most radiopaque foreign bodies are easily recognized.
2. May need two or more radiographic projections to localize the foreign body.

Tracheitis

Clinical correlations

1. Tracheitis most often is caused by the inflammatory effect of viral, bacterial, or parasitic infections, allergies, or secondary to the inhalation of dust, irritating gases, smoke, food, or gastric contents.
2. Is often seen concurrent with bronchitis or bronchopneumonia.
3. Inflammation often is associated with edema, increased secretions of mucus, or exudate. With more chronic inflammatory disease, proliferation of the mucosa and submucosa may occur.
4. Major clinical signs include coughing that varies from a dry paroxysmal cough in mild cases to a more productive cough in more severe cases.

Radiographic findings

1. In mild tracheitis, the radiographs are usually normal.
2. With more severe or chronic disease, the intraluminal diameter may be decreased and the tracheal wall may appear indistinct or irregular as a result of increased secretions.

Bronchial Collapse

Clinical correlations

1. Animals usually have chronic cough, often "honking" similar to collapsing trachea.
2. May occur concurrently with collapsed trachea.
3. The severity and location of the collapse is best assessed by endoscopy.

Radiographic findings (Figure 8.10)

1. Narrowed bronchial luminal diameter near carina.
2. May be best demonstrated on a lateral radiograph during expiration or cough.
3. Can be assessed with fluoroscopy.

Bronchitis

Clinical correlations

1. May be acute or chronic.
2. The severity of the clinical signs do not always correlate with the radiographic findings.
3. May be caused by
   a. infection
   b. allergy
   c. irritation (e.g., inhaled dust, smoke, gases, or other environmental irritants)
4. Disease of the bronchi can be caused by:
   a. Endobronchial exudate
   b. Bronchial wall thickening
   c. Peribronchial infiltration

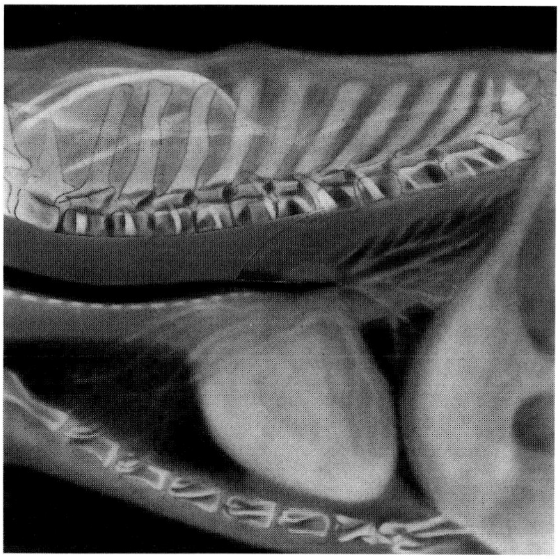

Figure 8.10. Bronchial collapse at carina.

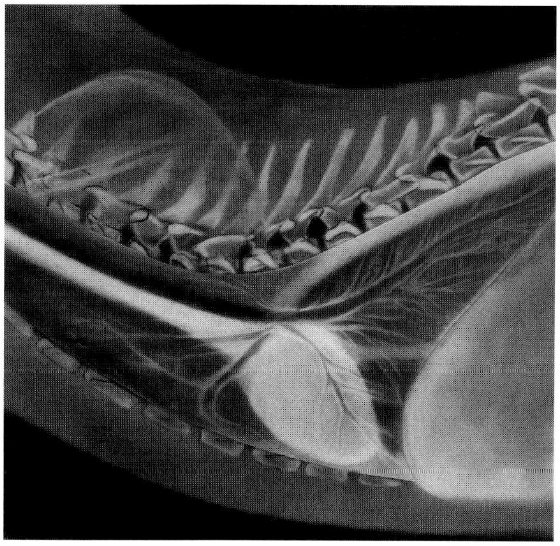

Figure 8.11. Bronchitis. The bronchi are thickened and prominent. Many end-on bronchi are seen.

Radiographic findings (Figure 8.11)

1. Radiographs are usually normal in acute bronchitis.
2. With chronic disease, the bronchial walls may be more prominent than normal and seen as either:
   a. Bronchi on end "donut sign"
   b. Bronchi on end with adjacent pulmonary vessel "signet ring sign"
   c. Parallel bronchial markings extending into central lung region, sometimes referred to as "tram lines" or "railroad tracks"
   d. Smudging or increased soft tissue opacity of the bronchial markings
3. With chronicity, airways may be dilated and irregular because of bronchiectasis.

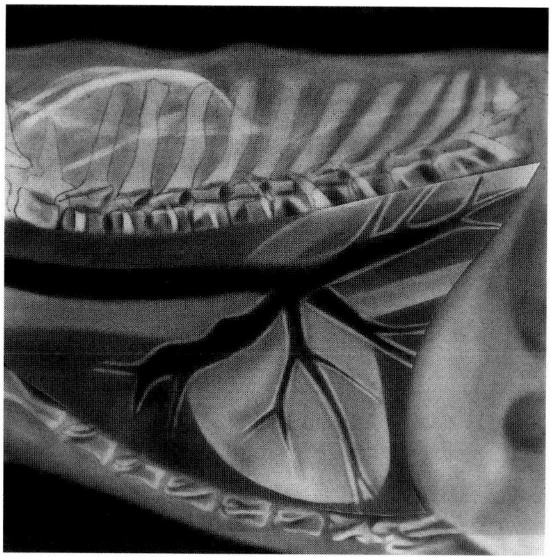

Figure 8.12. Bronchiectasis. There is severe dilation and irregularity of the major bronchi.

Bronchiectasis

Clinical correlations

1. Is usually an irreversible bronchial dilatation with loss of the normal tapering of bronchial airways.
2. Is usually secondary to destructive inflammatory bronchial disease.
3. Predisposes the animal to recurrent airway and pulmonary infections.
4. Direct examination by bronchoscopy is frequently necessary for diagnosis.

Radiographic findings (Figure 8.12)

1. The radiographs may be normal.
2. Cylindrical or tubular form has dilated central bronchi, which appear to have blunted ends and do not taper normally into the periphery of the lung.
3. Saccular form has focal dilations along the bronchi with round or ovoid-shaped radiolucent areas of trapped air.
4. May be localized or generalized.
5. May have associated increased bronchial markings, hyperlucent lung caused by air trapping or emphysema, and focal areas of consolidation caused by bronchopneumonia.
6. Bronchography can confirm the abnormal size and shape of the airways.

Bronchial Obstruction

Clinical correlations

1. Is usually caused by mucus plugs or inhaled foreign bodies (e.g., plant awn, marble, pebble).
2. Less commonly associated with neoplasm occluding the bronchus or lung torsion.
3. May be acute or chronic.

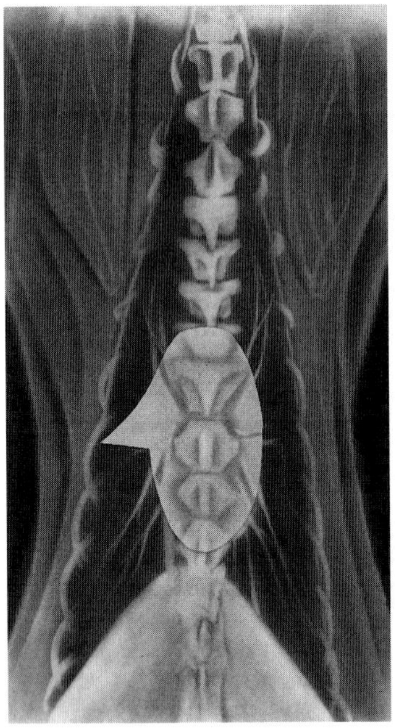

Figure 8.13. Bronchial obstruction. There is consolidation and atelectasis of the right middle lung lobe secondary to bronchial obstruction.

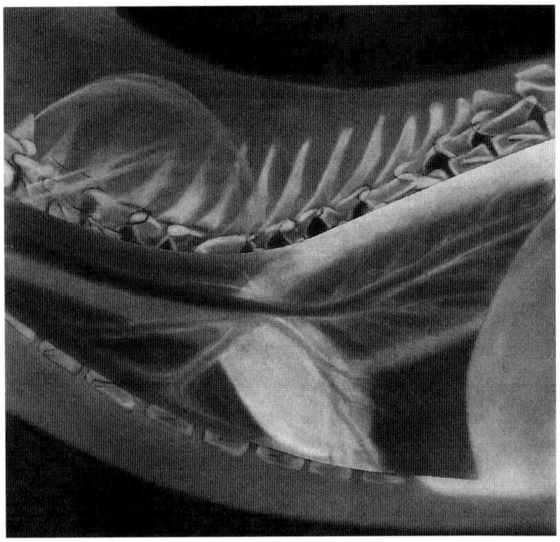

Figure 8.14. Lower airway disease (feline asthma). There is hyperinflation of the lungs with slight flattening of the diaphragm. The bronchial markings are accentuated. The hyperlucency of the caudal lobes is caused by air trapping.

Radiographic findings (Figure 8.13)

1. Opaque foreign bodies are usually seen.
2. Secondary pulmonary changes may be focal or lobar, depending on the degree of obstruction and location of the obstruction within the lung lobe.
3. Atelectasis occurs with total bronchial obstruction often with mediastinal shift.
4. With partial bronchial obstruction, hyperinflation of the affected lung lobe may be seen. This is the result of a valve effect that allows air to enter the lobe on inspiration, but blocks its effective release on expiration.
5. Pleural effusion may be present secondarily, especially if pneumonia is present or if the bronchial obstruction is caused by lobar torsion.

Lower Airway Disease

Clinical correlations

1. Common in the cat, less common in the dog.
2. Commonly known as feline allergic bronchitis or feline asthma.
3. May have peripheral eosinophilia.
4. Cats usually exhibit episodic acute dyspnea with forceful prolonged expiration, and often a cough. Severely affected cats may be cyanotic.

Radiographic findings (Figure 8.14)

1. In mild cases, radiographs may be normal.
2. The earliest changes seen radiographically are usually related to a mild bronchial and interstitial lung pattern.
3. In more advanced cases, there is an increased radiolucency of the lung because of hyperinflation (trapping of air), often with a flattened diaphragm.
4. Thoracic size is increased (barrel-chested appearance), which may make the heart appear disproportionately smaller than normal.
5. The bronchi may be ill-defined because of increased endobronchial secretions.
6. May have concurrent chronic lobar disease, especially in cats with partial or complete collapse of the right middle lung lobe.

LUNG

RADIOGRAPHIC INTERPRETATION

1. Common ways to assess the lung for diagnosis or differential diagnoses include:
   a. Assessing changes in the radiographic opacity of the lung parenchyma as being more radiolucent or more radiopaque than normal.
   b. Evaluating the distribution and appearance of pulmonary patterns.
2. Diseases may also appear localized or generalized and solitary, multiple, or diffuse.

TABLE 8.1

Diseases Causing Increased Focal Radiopacity of the Lung

Solitary Pulmonary Lesions

1. Well-defined, circumscribed, distinct borders "mass" lesion:
   a. Primary neoplasm of lung
   b. Metastatic neoplasm of lung (rare)
   c. Hematoma
   d. Fluid-filled cyst
   e. Granuloma
   f. Abscess
2. Ill-defined or indistinct:
   a. Focal pneumonia (abscess, foreign body)
   b. Infarct (Dirofilariasis, neoplasm, thromboembolism)
   c. Granuloma (fungal, bacterial, foreign body)
   d. Focal hemorrhage or contusion
   e. Focal atelectasis
   f. Primary neoplasm of lung

TABLE 8.2

Diseases Causing Multiple Focal Radiopacity of the Lung

1. Neoplasms usually greater than 3 mm in diameter
   a. Primary multicentric
   b. Metastatic (adenocarcinoma, lymphosarcoma, hemangiosarcoma)
2. Granulomatous diseases
   a. Fungal (Coccidioidomycosis, Histoplasmosis, Blastomycosis)
   b. Parasitic (Aeleurostrongylus)
   c. Eosinophilic granulomas
   d. Lymphoid granulomas
3. Vascular disease: Dirofilariasis
4. Heterotopic bone formation (pulmonary osteomas)
5. Differentiate from:
   a. Nipples
   b. Subcutaneous nodules
   c. End-on view of normal pulmonary vessels

TABLE 8.3

Diseases Causing Multiple Ill-Defined Radiopacity of the Lung

1. Hematogenous pneumonia
   a. Embolic spread of bacterial or fungal infections
   b. Opportunistic pneumonia caused by reduced host resistance
   c. Parasitic (e.g., toxoplasmosis)
2. Granulomatous pneumonia
   a. Fungal infection active disease
   b. Parasitic (e.g., toxoplasmosis, Aeleurostrongylus)
3. Neoplasia
   a. Metastatic neoplasia with edema or hemorrhage in adjacent alveoli (e.g., hemangiosarcoma)
   b. Primary multicentric
4. Infarcts (with edema, hemorrhage, or necrosis in adjacent alveoli)
   a. Dirofilariasis
   b. Pulmonary thromboembolism

TABLE 8.4

Diseases that may Cause Generalized or Diffuse Lung Radiopacity

1. Pulmonary edema (cardiogenic or noncardiogenic)
2. Pneumonia (aspiration or hematogenous)
3. Pulmonary hemorrhage
   a. Trauma (e.g., contusion)
   b. Coagulopathy (e.g., disseminated intravascular coagulation, rodenticide)
4. Acute respiratory distress syndrome (ARDS)
5. Atelectasis
6. Neoplasia (uncommon)
   a. Lymphosarcoma
   b. Bronchioalveolar carcinoma
7. Interstitial edema
8. Interstitial pneumonia
9. Eosinophilic pneumonia
10. Interstitial hemorrhage
11. Pulmonary fibrosis
12. Neoplasia
    a. Lymphosarcoma
    b. Lymphangitic metastasis (e.g., mammary adenocarcinoma)

TABLE 8.5

Diseases that may Cause Increased Radiopacity of the Lung

Generalized

1. Overinflation by air trapping secondary to airway obstruction (e.g., chronic bronchitis, bronchial foreign bodies, allergic airway disease)
2. Compensatory hyperinflation secondary to volume loss of other lung lobes (e.g., atelectasis, lobectomy)
3. Emphysema related to increased air content usually with decreased perfusion
4. Undercirculation (Oligemia)
   a. Right to left shunts
   b. Pulmonary thromboembolism without infarction
   c. Hypovolemic shock or severe dehydration
   d. Hypocorticism
5. Radiographic techniqual artifact (overexposure)

Localized

1. Bleb, bulla, pneumatocoele
2. Parasitic cyst (e.g., paragonimus)
3. Cavitation (tumor, abscess, or infarct)
4. Dilated bronchus

TABLE 8.6

Diseases that may Cause Mineralization or Calcification of the Lung (Focal or Diffuse)

1. Heterotopic bone formation (pulmonary osteomas)
2. Granulomas from fungal disease or foreign material
3. Inhaled foreign material (e.g., aspiration of barium sulfate)
4. Hypervitaminosis D in cats
5. Dystrophic mineralization within abscess or tumor
6. Dystrophic mineralization from systemic disease (e.g., hyperadrenocorticism)
7. Microlithiasis

Examples include:
   a. Diffuse hyperlucency: asthma, emphysema,
   b. Localized hyperlucency: bulla, lobar emphysema, parasitic cyst
   c. Localized increased radiopacity: pneumonia, neoplasm, infarct, foreign body.
   d. Generalized increased radiopacity: pulmonary edema, atelectasis, pneumonia, hemorrhage, or neoplasia (Tables 8.1 through 8.6)
3. The pulmonary pattern approach can be used to describe the abnormal radiographic changes as being in the alveoli, interstitium, bronchi, or vascular structures of the lung.
4. When there is a mixture of different lung patterns, the one most involved or severe is usually chosen. Based on recognizing different lung patterns, one can then prioritize one or more diseases as being most likely.
5. However, pattern recognition is nonspecific and not always accurate because there is commonly an overlap of patterns, a limited number of ways that the lung can respond to numerous etiologies, and the patterns can change from time to time.

PATTERNS OF LUNG DISEASE

Alveolar Pattern

Clinical correlations

1. In the alveolar pattern of pulmonary disease, the alveoli are filled with fluid and/or cellular debris or are collapsed because of atelectasis.
2. Alveolar infiltrates often have "rapid timing" in which the infiltrates progress and regress rapidly.
3. The most common causes of alveolar disease in the dog and cat are bronchopneumonia, atelectasis caused by pneumothorax, pulmonary contusion, and pulmonary edema.

Radiographic findings

1. There is fluffy, ill-defined increased radiopacity with obliteration of pulmonary vessels and other structures having the same opacity (e.g., Silhouette Sign).
2. Coalescence of infiltrates
3. Frequently involves one or more lung lobes (lobar distribution).
4. Presence of an air-bronchogram
   a. The air-filled bronchus is seen because the adjacent fluid-filled or collapsed alveoli have a greater opacity "air bronchogram sign."
   b. If the bronchus is also filled with fluid or collapsed, an air-bronchogram may be absent in alveolar disease.
5. Occasionally, smaller end airways are visible similar to air bronchograms and are referred to as air alveolograms.

Interstitial Pattern

Clinical correlations

1. The interstitium of the lung surrounds and supports the alveoli, pulmonary vessels, and bronchi, and includes the alveolar and interlobar septae.
2. The interstitial pattern results in the filling of the interstitial space with fluid, exudate, fibrosis, or mass lesions such as primary or metastatic tumors.
3. This may represent chronic or acute changes associated with interstitial edema, interstitial pneumonia, eosinophilic pneumonia, interstitial hemorrhage, pulmonary fibrosis, or neoplasia.
4. The interstitial pattern can be classified radiographically as having a nodular pattern or an unstructured pattern.

Radiographic findings

1. Interstitial Nodular Pattern
   a. The ability to recognize interstitial nodules depends on the size, number, distribution within the lung, margination, and degree of radiopacity.
   b. Nodules smaller than 3 to 5 mm in diameter are difficult to identify unless they are numerous, mineralized, or superimposed over the heart or the diaphragm.
   c. Interstitial nodules having a smooth and well-defined border are usually caused by primary or metastatic tumors, but benign masses such as an abscess, fluid-containing bulla, granulomas, and some peribronchial pneumonias can mimic a tumor.
   d. If the nodules are indistinct, a more active process is suggested as the adjacent alveoli are involved or edema, infection, and/or hemorrhage is also present. This often occurs in granulomatous pneumonias, some metastatic and primary lung neoplasms, and in acute embolic pneumonia.
   e. Must differentiate the normal end-on view of pulmonary vessels from pulmonary interstitial nodules. Usually vessels seen end-on are more numerous in the hilar area, can be associated in terms of size and location with a vessel from which they branch, and become smaller and less numerous in the lung periphery as they branch.
   f. Superimposed subcutaneous nodules, nipples, and heterotopic bone must also be differentiated from pulmonary nodules. Heterotopic bone or pulmonary osteoma is commonly associated with aging and is more common in some breeds (e.g., Collie).
2. Unstructured Pulmonary Pattern
   a. The unstructured interstitial pulmonary pattern has a hazy appearance with the lung appearing more radiopaque than normal with smudging or blurring of the vascular shadows and a decreased contrast to the lung field.
   b. A fine, indistinct linear or reticulonodular opacity may also be seen. As the disease becomes chronic or resolves, the linear opacities may become thinner and better defined with improved visualization of the vascular structures.
   c. The apparent appearance of interstitial pulmonary disease can be artifactual caused by patient motion, underexposure or underdevelopment of the film, and poor lung inflation (i.e., expiration, positional atelectasis).

Bronchial Pattern

Clinical correlations

1. The bronchial wall is thickened and/or irregular because of the presence of fluid, chronic cellular allergic or inflammatory infiltrates.
2. The bronchial pattern of pulmonary disease is usually associated with bronchitis or bronchiectasis.
3. Normal bronchial mineralization must be differentiated from bronchial disease. Many normal chondrodystrophoid breeds and older animals commonly have prominent bronchi with mineralized walls.

Radiographic findings

1. In the bronchial pulmonary pattern, normal bronchi, which are not normally seen, are visible.
2. Bronchial walls are more prominent or thicker than normal. When seen end-on there is a ring-like appearance because the air within the lumen contrasts with the surrounding increased bronchial wall thickening or mineralization (e.g., donut sign, signet ring sign).
3. Bronchi may not taper normally into the periphery of the lung (described as railroad tracks or tram lines).
4. In bronchiectasis, the bronchi may be abnormally dilated or saccular in appearance.

Vascular Pattern

Clinical correlations

1. Normal pulmonary arteries and veins are seen as being of soft tissue radiopacity with smooth walls and even branching as they extend into the periphery of the lung.
2. Normal end-on views of vessels have a spherical shape with a diameter similar to other vessels visible in the opposite plane in the same region of the lung.
3. The normal vessels are larger and usually easier to see in the hilar and central portions of the lung.
4. Changes in size, shape, or number of vessels is helpful for differentiating some diseases.
5. Enlargement of the arteries and veins may be caused by over circulation (e.g., left to right shunts such as patent ductus arteriosis, ventricular and atrial septal defects, peripheral arteriovenous shunts), feline cardiomyopathy, and hypervolemia.
6. Enlargement of the arteries may be caused by parasitic diseases (e.g., Dirofilariasis), thromboembolic disease,

and chronic lung diseases with pulmonary hypertension.

7. Enlargement of the veins may be caused by left heart failure (e.g., mitral insufficiency, cardiomyopathy), iatrogenic fluid overload, or left atrial obstruction (e.g., neoplasia, thrombus).

Radiographic findings

1. The vascular pattern of normal arteries and veins are paired and usually similar in size.
2. On the lateral projection, the right cranial lobar artery and vein should be approximately the same size. The diameter of each should not exceed the smallest diameter of the right fourth rib.
3. On the dorsoventral projection, the caudal lobar arteries and veins should be similar in size and their diameters caudal to the ninth rib should not exceed the diameter of the ninth rib.

DISEASES/DISORDERS

Pulmonary Edema

Clinical correlations

1. Pulmonary edema is the accumulation of abnormal quantities of fluid in the lung. The edema can be within interstitial connective tissues (interstitial edema) or within the alveoli and terminal airspaces of the lung (alveolar edema).
2. Pulmonary edema is common and occurs secondary to many disorders, including cardiogenic and noncardiogenic causes.
3. Physiologic factors include the following:
   a. Increased capillary hydrostatic pressure
      1) Cardiogenic edema
      2) Pulmonary venous-occlusive disease
      3) Overinfusion of crystalloid fluids or blood
   b. Decreased capillary osmotic pressure (hypoproteinemia)
      1) Chronic liver disease
      2) Protein losing nephropathy
      3) Protein-losing enteropathies
      4) Severe malnutrition
   c. Obstruction of pulmonary lymphatic flow
      1) Lymphangitic metastasis
      2) Interstitial metastasis
      3) Hilar lymph node enlargement
   d. Increased pulmonary alveolar-capillary membrane permeability
      1) Pulmonary infections (edema protein content high)
      2) Toxic damage to membrane
         a) Inhaled toxins (e.g., smoke, aspirated gastric acid)
         b) Exogenous toxins (e.g., snake venom, spider venom, alpha-naphthyl thylthiourea (ANTU), or paraquat)
         c) Endogenous toxins (uremia, pancreatitis, vasoactive substances released from thrombosis or shock)
      3) Drowning or near drowning
      4) Disseminated intravascular coagulation (DIC) caused by damage to the capillary endothelial membrane
      5) Shock and pulmonary hemorrhage (shock lung)
      6) Immunologic reactions and anaphylaxis (drug, contrast media, transfusion reactions)
   e. Mixed or undetermined causes
      1) Neurogenic (seizure disorder, head trauma, encephalitis, brain tumor, electric shock)
      2) Postoperative of diaphragmatic hernia repair (rapid reexpansion of atelectatic lung favors pulmonary capillary ultrafiltration and alters surface tension)
4. Noncardiogenic (e.g., idiosyncratic reaction)
   a. Laryngeal edema (e.g., airway obstruction)
   b. Foreign body
   c. Laryngeal paralysis
5. Causes of cardiogenic edema with radiographically visible cardiomegaly (left heart failure) include:
   a. Chronic mitral valve insufficiency
   b. Cardiomyopathy
   c. Ruptured chordae tendinae
   d. Heart block
   e. High output failure in left to right shunts
6. Causes of cardiogenic edema without radiographically visible cardiomegaly include:
   a. Electric shock
   b. Cardiomyopathy (some cases)
   c. Trauma
   d. Tachyarrythmias or heart block
   e. Myocardial depressants (exogenous or endogenous in origin)

Radiographic findings

1. Cardiogenic edema (Figures 8.15 and 8.16)
   a. Usually, enlargement of the left ventricle and the left atrium is seen.
   b. Enlarged ill-defined pulmonary veins, in the hilar region, as they enter the left atrium, and occasionally in the central lung region (e.g., right cranial lobar vein on the lateral projection).
   c. The infiltrate is predominantly in the perihilar area, with a more normal appearance to the more peripheral portions of the lungs.
   d. The infiltrate is usually symmetrical, but may be unilateral because of hypostasis (e.g., animal lying on one side for a prolonged period of time).
   e. The pulmonary infiltrate is frequently a mixed interstitial and alveolar pattern.

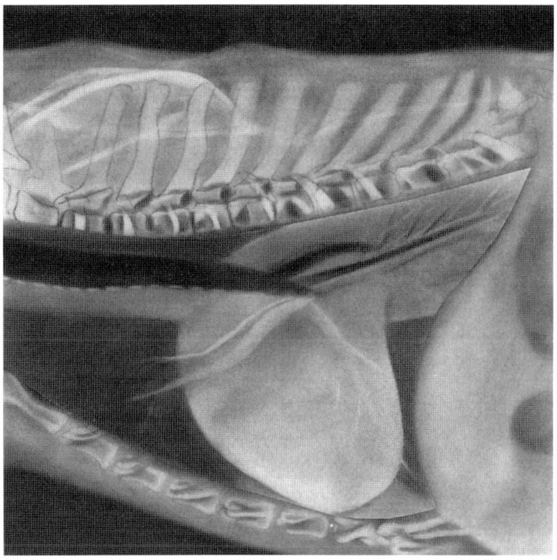

Figure 8.15. Cardiogenic edema caused by left heart failure from mitral insufficiency. There is moderate left heart enlargement with hilar edema present causing blurring of the left atrial border and pulmonary veins.

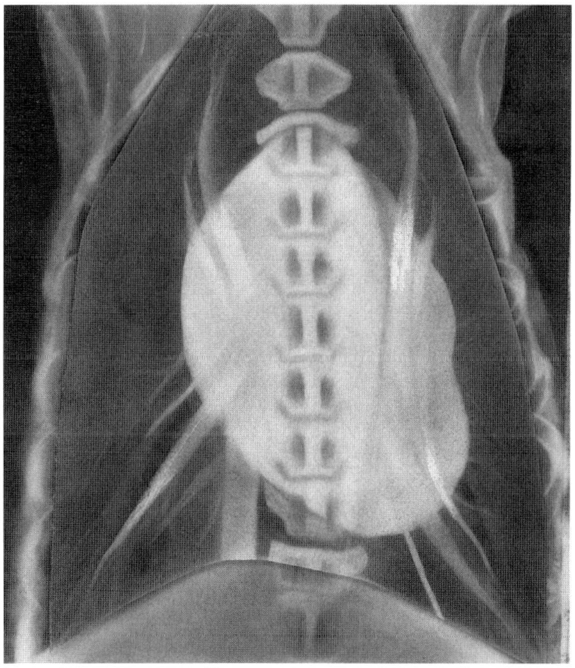

Figure 8.16. Cardiogenic edema caused by left heart failure from mitral insufficiency. There is moderate left heart enlargement with engorgement of the pulmonary veins in the hilus.

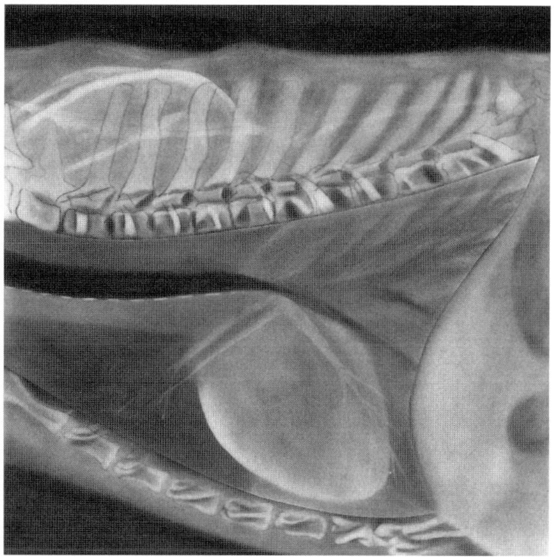

Figure 8.17. Noncardiogenic edema. The heart size is normal. There is marked alveolar infiltrate in the caudal lung lobes with prominent air bronchograms.

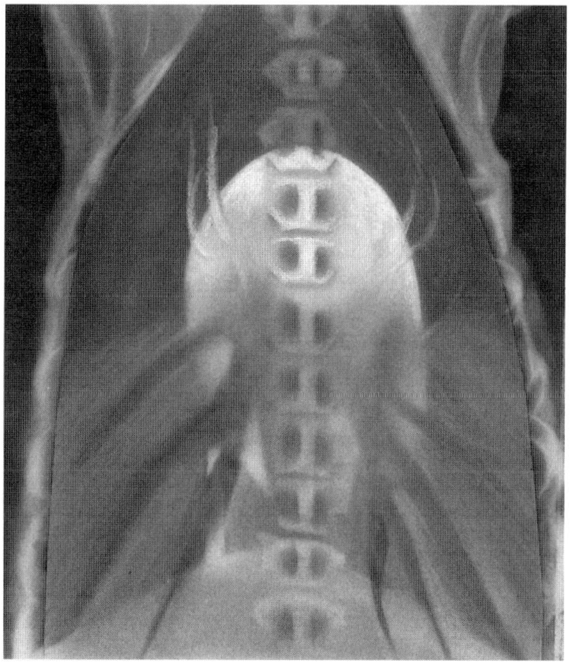

Figure 8.18. Noncardiogenic edema. The heart size is normal. There is marked alveolar infiltrate in the caudal lung lobes with prominent air bronchograms.

f. In some animals with acute left heart failure (e.g., heart block or tachyarrhythmia), cardiomegaly may not be apparent.

2. Noncardiogenic pulmonary edema (Figures 8.17 and 8.18)
   a. Cardiac silhouette is normal in size.
   b. The edema may be characterized by variable degrees of interstitial and/or alveolar infiltrates.
   c. Alveolar pulmonary infiltrates often are more severe in the caudal lung lobes
   d. There is usually a fairly rapid change in the type, extent, and location of the pulmonary pattern of disease, as seen on sequential radiographs over time.

Pulmonary Hemorrhage

Clinical correlations

1. Usually traumatic in origin (pulmonary contusion):
   a. Usually occurs within 6 hours after trauma.
   b. Usually improves within 24 to 48 hours and is usually completely resolved within 3 to 10 days.
   c. Persistence of infiltrates suggests complication such as atelectasis or secondary pneumonia.
   d. The severity of clinical signs depends on the extent of lung injury (one lobe or several lobes) and concurrent lesions (e.g., pneumothorax, fractured ribs).
2. Pulmonary hemorrhage may also occur secondary to:
   a. Coagulopathies (e.g., DIC, rodenticides)
   b. Neoplasia (e.g., hemangiosarcoma)

Radiographic findings

1. Irregular patchy areas of a mixed alveolar and interstitial lung pattern
2. May appear diffuse with extensive lung consolidation.
3. Not usually lobar and often affects the entire lung

Pulmonary Hematomas and Pneumatoceles

Clinical correlations

1. Usually a sequel to trauma.
2. Hematomas are caused by focal laceration of the lung.
3. Often associated with pulmonary contusions, pneumothorax, hemothorax, and subcutaneous emphysema.
4. Usually resolves in 3 to 6 weeks and rarely persists.

Radiographic findings (Figure 8.19)

1. Initially, a hematoma and cyst may be difficult to detect, but is easier to see later as a more well-defined lesion.

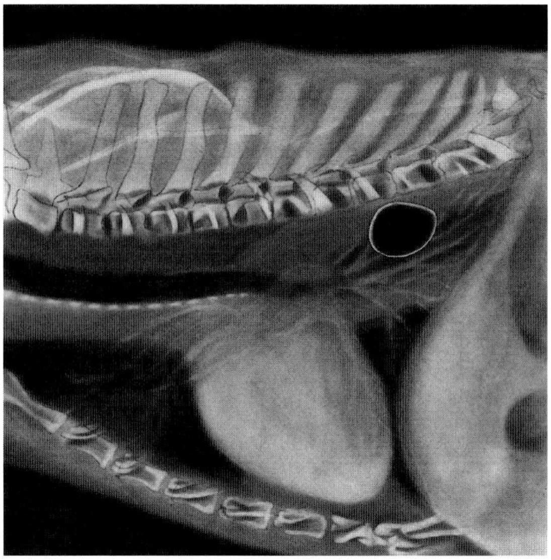

Figure 8.19. Emphysematous bulla.

2. A traumatic cyst is usually seen as an ill-defined spherical structure containing air. A horizontal beam radiograph may demonstrate an air-fluid level better.

Pneumonia

Clinical correlations

1. Pneumonia is an acute or chronic inflammation of the lung that may be acute or chronic. Most pneumonias are caused by viral infections, parasitic infections, or secondary to aspiration of foreign material.
2. Common clinical signs include cough (usually productive), mucopurulent nasal discharge, exercise intolerance, and respiratory distress. Other common signs include anorexia, weight loss, fever, and lethargy. A neutrophilic leukocytosis is commonly present.
3. Bacterial pneumonia most commonly affects the more dependent portions of the affected lung lobes. Underlying disease often predisposes an animal to bacterial infection.
   a. Decreased clearance of normally inhaled debris as seen in
      1) Chronic bronchitis
      2) Bronchiectasis
      3) Ciliary dyskinesia
   b. Immunosuppression
      1) Secondary to drugs (e.g., during chemotherapy)
      2) Malnutrition
      3) Stress
      4) Other infections such as:
         a) Feline immunodeficiency virus (FIV)
         b) Canine distemper
   c. Aspiration pneumonia (e.g., megaesophagus, dysphagia)
   d. Neoplasia
   e. Fungal infections
   f. Parasitic infections
   g. Inhaled foreign bodies
4. Mycotic infections that cause pneumonia include Blastomycosis, Histoplasmosis, Coccidioidomycosis, and Cryptococcosis. The fungal organisms enter the respiratory tract, and often the infection is successfully eliminated with minimal or no clinical signs. However, the infection may progress to cause a more severe pulmonary involvement or spread systemically to other organs. (The individual fungal infections are discussed later in this chapter.)
5. May result as a complication of:
   a. Viral pneumonia (e.g., canine distemper, feline calicivirus, rarely rhinotracheitis). Viruses that can affect the lower respiratory tract include canine adenovirus 2, parainfluenza virus, and distemper virus in the dog; and the calicivirus, mycoplasma, and feline infectious peritonitis in the cat.
   b. *Bordatella bronchiseptica* (kennel cough)
   c. Aspiration pneumonia or inhalation of a foreign body (e.g., plant awn).

6. The specific diagnosis is usually based on the results of cytology and culture from a tracheal or bronchial lavage or wash.

Radiographic findings (Figure 8.20 and 8.21)

1. Mixed pulmonary infiltrates, but primarily an alveolar pattern of disease with air bronchograms

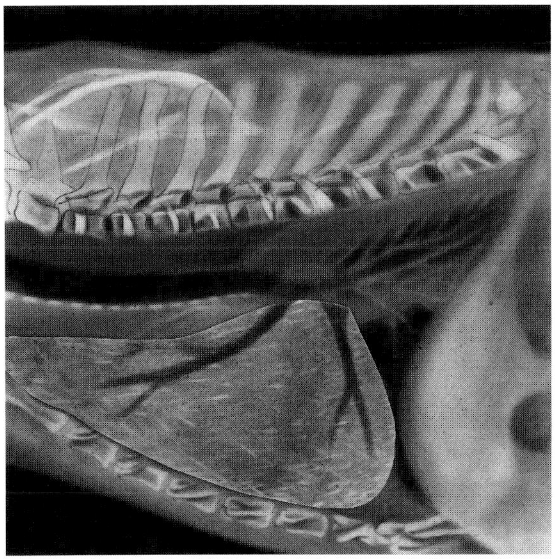

Figure 8.20. Lobar consolidation. There is alveolar consolidation with prominent air bronchograms involving the right cranial and middle lung lobes.

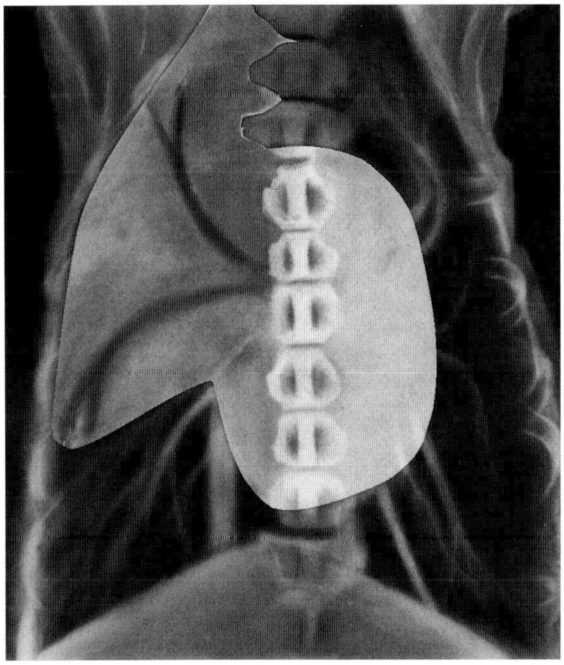

Figure 8.21. Lobar consolidation. There is alveolar consolidation of the right cranial and middle lobes with prominent air bronchograms.

2. Usually involves one or more lung lobes.
3. Often the disease is most severe in the dependent portions of the lung lobes.

Interstitial Pneumonia

Clinical correlations

1. Is usually a manifestation of generalized systemic disease.
   a. Septicemia
   b. Embolic pneumonia
   c. Migrating parasitic larvae
   d. Viral pneumonia
2. Is frequently complicated by bacterial bronchopneumonia.

Radiographic findings (Figure 8.22):

1. Diffuse interstitial pulmonary pattern consisting of a hazy appearance to the lung with blurring/smudging of the bronchial and vascular structures.
2. Absence of alveolar pulmonary infiltrate and other abnormalities, unless complicated by infection, infarction, or edema.

Aspiration Pneumonia

Clinical correlations

1. Refers to the pulmonary inflammation resulting from the inhalation of liquid or particulate matter, such as food and gastric contents, fresh or salt water (near drowning), mineral oil (lipid pneumonia), or hydrocarbons (petroleum distillates, kerosene).
2. Frequently occurs as a sequel to megaesophagus.
3. May occur in recumbent or comatose patients or as a complication of anesthetic recovery.
4. Pulmonary pathology depends on the type and quan-

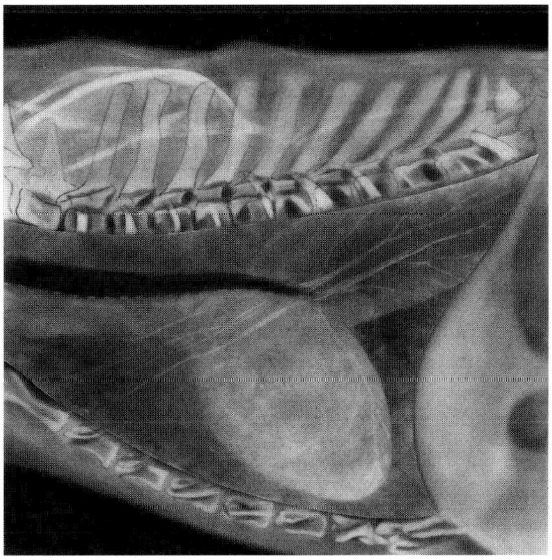

Figure 8.22. Diffuse interstitial infiltrate.

tity of material aspirated and its distribution within the lung.
5. Gastric acid contents causes collapse of the alveoli, bronchoconstriction, pulmonary edema, and systemic hypotension if aspiration is severe.
6. Particulate matter may cause airway obstruction. The degree of obstruction depends on the size and amount of inhaled particulate material.
7. Infection can occur immediately after aspiration of contaminated material, or may occur at a later time as the result of injury to the normal pulmonary defense mechanisms.

Radiographic findings

1. Similar to bronchopneumonia with an alveolar or mixed pulmonary pattern. The alveolar pattern is usually more prominent with visible air bronchograms.
2. May involve entire lobe or lung.
3. Usually located in the dependent lung lobes (depending on the position of the animal during the time of aspiration).

Eosinophilic Pneumonia

Clinical correlations

1. Is also referred to as pulmonary infiltrates with eosinophilia (PIE).
2. Is usually seen as a hypersensitivity reaction caused by pulmonary parasites, Dirofilariasis, drugs, or inhaled allergens.
3. A peripheral eosinophilia is usually present.
4. Bacteria, fungal infections, and some neoplasms may cause an eosinophilic infiltration.
5. Eosinophilic granulomatosis is a specific entity and is usually caused by Dirofilariasis.
6. Coughing is common; other clinical signs include weight loss, lethargy, and anorexia.
7. The diagnosis is confirmed from either a bronchial lavage, fine needle aspirate, or biopsy of the lung.

Radiographic findings (Figure 8.23)

1. The radiographic pulmonary pattern is predominantly interstitial; however, patchy alveolar infiltrates and occasionally well-defined interstitial nodules may also be seen.
   a. In eosinophilic granulomatosis nodules can be large (10 to 20 cm in diameter). Hilar lymphadenopathy is also common.
2. In Dirofilariasis, the main pulmonary arteries and the pulmonary artery segment are usually enlarged and the peripheral arteries are tortuous and attenuated. Right heart enlargement is usually present.
3. May appear similar to bronchopneumonia with a mixed bronchial, interstitial, and alveolar pattern of pulmonary disease.
4. Differential diagnosis considerations include mycotic pneumonia, lymphosarcoma, and metastatic neoplasia.

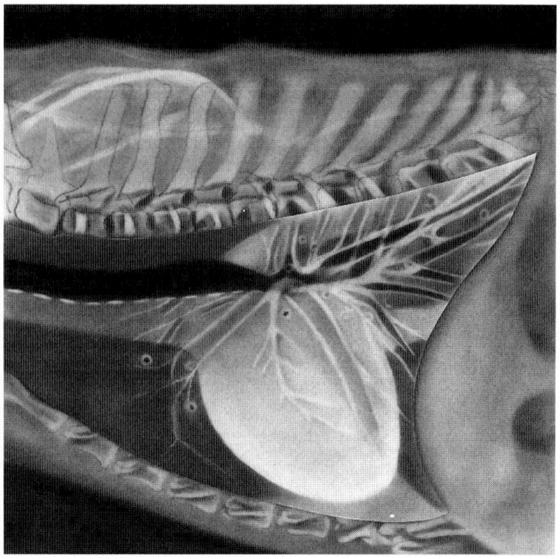

Figure 8.23. Eosinophilic bronchitis. There is marked bronchial thickening with a diffuse increased interstitial lung opacity from pulmonary infiltrates with eosinophilia (PIE).

Pulmonary Abscess

Clinical correlations

1. Pulmonary abscesses are usually either complications of or secondary to:
   a. Bronchiectasis or bacterial bronchopneumonia
   b. Embolus (dirofilaria, bacterial, fungal)
   c. Trauma
   d. Bronchial obstruction caused by foreign body
   e. Neoplasm
   f. Parasitic infection

Radiographic findings (Figure 8.24)

1. May be solitary or multiple.
2. May involve the entire lung lobe.
3. Lesion may cavitate and be air filled.

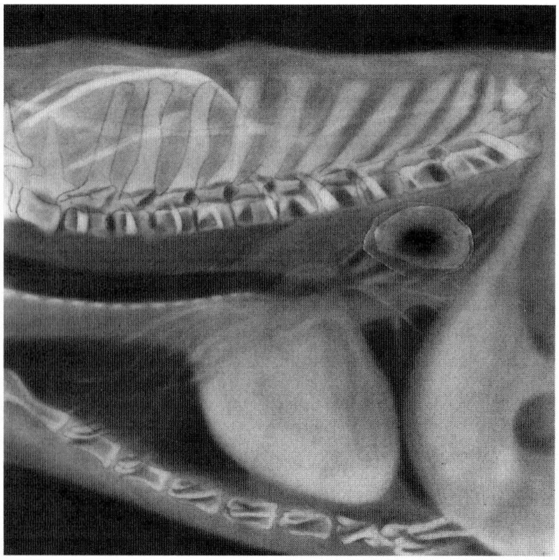

Figure 8.24. Cavitated pulmonary mass.

Atelectasis

Clinical correlations

1. May be congenital (e.g., incomplete expansion of one or more lung lobes at birth) or acquired (e.g., partial or complete collapse of the lung).
2. Frequently is secondary to external compression resulting from pleural effusion or pneumothorax.
3. May occur secondary to airway obstruction by exudate, foreign body, tumor, or torsion of the lung lobe. With bronchial obstruction, air within the lobe is absorbed, causing atelectasis of the lung lobe.
4. May occur as a result of positioning, especially if the animal is sedated or anesthetized. This form of atelectasis is reversible and referred to as positional atelectasis.
5. In cats, there is a predisposition for atelectasis of the right middle lung lobe, possibly associated with chronic upper respiratory diseases and bronchial obstruction.

Radiographic findings (See Figure 8.31)

1. Homogenous, soft tissue radiopaque appearance to the lung. Occasionally, there is an alveolar pulmonary pattern, often with a lobar distribution.
2. Air bronchograms may be present early with partial atelectasis, but are not present with complete atelectasis.
3. Mediastinal shift toward the side of atelectasis with compensatory hyperinflation of the other lung lobes.
4. Pneumonia may develop as a sequel to atelectasis.

Emphysema

Clinical correlations

1. Is a focal or diffuse pulmonary condition characterized by an abnormal increase of the airspaces distal to the terminal bronchioli, usually associated with destruction of the alveolar walls.
2. May occur as a congenital anomaly or, more commonly, secondary to bronchial obstruction or chronic obstructive lung disease.
3. The major clinical sign is an accentuated expiratory effort.

Radiographic findings

1. Increased radiolucency of the lung field as the result of hyperinflation.
2. The cardiac silhouette may appear small relative to the size of the thorax.
3. Flattened diaphragm
4. Increased distance between the heart and the diaphragm
5. A "barrel-chested" appearance
6. Bullae, if present, are seen as well-defined air-filled cavities in the lung. These bullae may rupture with the sequel of pneumothorax.

Pulmonary Cysts, Bullae and Blebs, and Other Cavitating Lung Lesions

Clinical correlations

1. Bronchogenic cysts are greatly dilated bronchioles. Thought to be congenital, resulting from failure of maturation of the terminal air passages.
2. A pulmonary cyst is not associated with the bronchus, and if infected, may become an abscess (associated with a mycotic, bacterial, or parasitic infection).
3. Bullae result from the destruction of the alveolar walls, which results in confluence of airspaces. It may be associated with trauma or chronic obstructive pulmonary disease.
4. Blebs are subpleural in location and form. They are secondary to ruptured alveoli, which dissect through the interstitial tissue into the fibrous layer of the visceral pleura.
5. A pneumatocoele is a large bulla located in the lung parenchyma, usually from trauma, but can occur secondary to bronchial obstruction from infection or mucus plugs (in which focal hyperinflation develops from collateral ventilation).
6. Cavitary pulmonary lesions containing gas occur within nodules or masses usually associated with abscesses or necrotic neoplasms.
7. No clinical signs are present if the lesion remains intact and is uninfected. Abnormal respiration or clinical illness may be present if the cystic lesion becomes enlarged and compromises pulmonary inflation, becomes infected, or ruptures causing pneumothorax.

Radiographic findings (See Figure 8.19)

1. Cavitary lesions can be classified according to:
   a. Their location relative to the pleura
   b. Location of gas within the lesion
   c. The number and size of the lesions
   d. The type of fluid within the cystic mass
2. Large radiolucent lesions are usually cysts or abcesses; a cyst is thin walled, an abscess usually is thick walled and contains some fluid.
3. Multiple irregular cavitated lesions most likely represent focal abscessation caused by necrosis within a primary or metastatic tumor, or parasitic granuloma.
4. Blebs are usually small and subpleural in location.
5. Bullae are usually small, thin walled, and are located within the lung parenchyma; some may contain fluid.
6. A horizontal beam radiograph will demonstrate whether a fluid level exists in the cystic lesion.

Chronic Obstructive Pulmonary Disease

Clinical correlations

1. Results from chronic disease of the peripheral airways and pulmonary parenchyma, and is often associated with chronic bronchitis, emphysema and bronchiectasis.

2. Small airway obstruction can be associated with edema or cellular infiltration of the bronchial walls, increased endobronchial mucus, spasticity of the bronchial smooth muscle, or secondary to interstitial fibrosis.
3. Mismatch of ventilation and perfusion that causes chronic hypoxemia.
4. Clinical signs vary according to the degree and duration of the bronchial obstruction. Coughing, wheezing, decreased exercise tolerance, cyanosis, and an accentuation of expiratory effort are commonly seen.

Radiographic findings

1. Radiographic findings vary depending on the severity of peripheral airway obstruction and abnormal ventilation.
2. Bronchial dilation, bronchial wall thickening, and/or mineralization are commonly seen.
3. Hyperinflation with areas of focal or diffuse hyperlucency may be seen, depending on the location and severity of the airway obstruction. Hyperlucent areas can be caused by air trapping or emphysema.
4. Lobar atelectasis may be present if the bronchus is completely occluded, especially common in the right middle lobe in cats.
5. A diffuse, unstructured interstitial pattern may be seen if pulmonary fibrosis is present.
6. Intercostal muscles may appear concave because of fatigue and sternabra may become deviate.
7. Right heart enlargement is common as a sequel (cor pulmonale).

Lung Torsion

Clinical correlations

1. Is more common in the dog, and reported most frequently in large, deep-chested dogs.
2. Lobar torsion most often affects the right middle lung lobe in the dog and cat. The right cranial lobe and the left cranial lobe occur less often. Caudal lobe torsion is rare.
3. After torsion, the venous return is compromised and the twisted lobe becomes congested. Fluid and alveolar blood diffuses into the pleural space as an obstructive type of pleural effusion.
4. In small dogs and cats, is often associated with pleural effusion, trauma (e.g., diaphragmatic hernia), or a sequel to thoracotomy.
5. Bronchoscopy may aid in the diagnosis.

Radiographic findings

1. The radiographic findings vary depending on duration of the torsion.
2. There is lobar consolidation of affected lobe. An air bronchogram may be seen early in the disease course, but not identified later.
3. Pleural effusion is common. Drainage of the pleural effusion and follow-up radiographs will allow better evaluation of the lobar consolidation.
4. The affected lobe or its vessels may be oriented in an abnormal position and the bronchus at the carina may appear twisted.
5. Differential considerations:
   a. Pneumonia
   b. Pulmonary neoplasia
   c. Pleural neoplasia or encapsulated fluid
6. In many cases, a thoracotomy may be necessary for diagnosis.

Pulmonary Thrombosis and Thromboembolism

Clinical correlations

1. Results from obstruction of pulmonary arteries and arterioles, either as a primary disease (thrombosis) or because of emboli from an extrapulmonary site.
2. Emboli are usually fragments of clots, but can also consist of bacteria, foreign bodies (e.g., intravenous catheter), air, fat, or parasites.
3. Thromboembolism results in an abnormal ventilation perfusion relationship within the lung. Ventilated regions with poor perfusion result in areas of alveolar dead space. Hyperperfused regions cause pulmonary hypertension and increased work on the right heart.
4. Infarction occurs if the thromboembolic disease results in necrosis and cell death because of ischemia.
5. The most common cause of pulmonary thromboembolism in the dog and cat is Dirofilariasis, both before and after therapy.
6. Other diseases that have an increased incidence of associated pulmonary thromboembolism include:
   a. Nephrotic syndrome
   b. Immune mediated hemolytic anemia
   c. Hyperadrenocorticism
   d. Neoplasia
   e. Sepsis
   f. Pancreatitis
   g. Disseminated intravascular coagulation (DIC)
   h. Hyperlipidemia
   i. Heart disease
      1) Dilated cardiomyopathy
      2) Chronic valvular regurgitation
      3) Endocarditis
7. The most common clinical sign is peracute respiratory distress and tachypnea, which responds poorly to routine supportive therapy.

Radiographic findings

1. The thoracic radiographs are often normal.
2. Variable degrees of pulmonary changes may be present.
3. Focal areas of hyperlucency may be present because of oligemia.
4. The pulmonary artery segment may be increased in size and a right heart enlargement may be present.

5. Enlarged and attenuated (pruned) pulmonary arteries may be present.
6. Other common findings include focal alveolar infiltrate and a small pleural effusion.
7. Definitive diagnosis can be obtained by pulmonary angiography (selective or nonselective) or by scintigraphy (ventilation perfusion scan).

Adult Respiratory Distress Syndrome (ARDS)

Clinical correlations

1. Is a syndrome also referred to as ARDS characterized by respiratory failure occurring as sequel to another disease condition. Potential causes include:
   a. Shock
   b. Infection
   c. Trauma
   d. Aspiration pneumonia
   e. Inhaled gas (smoke, chemicals)
   f. Disseminated intravascular coagulopathy (DIC)
   g. Pancreatitis
   h. Post cardiac arrest and resuscitation
   i. Complications associated with mechanical ventilation
2. The diffuse pulmonary injury consists of edema, vasoconstriction, and microembolization with resultant reduction in functional lung capacity, pulmonary compliance and severe hypoxemia with a severe ventilation and perfusion imbalance.
3. The most common clinical signs include dyspnea and hyperinflation (often unresponsive to oxygen therapy), tachycardia, and anxiety. In most instances the disease is progressive and fatal.

Radiographic findings

1. The radiographs may appear normal in the early phase of disease.
2. With progression, a diffuse interstitial opacity of the lung field will be seen, often associated with hyperinflation.
3. Bronchial cuffing and ill-defined alveolar consolidations tend to occur, often spreading over wide areas. The lung volume often becomes decreased.
4. Differential diagnosis:
   a. Other causes of noncardiogenic pulmonary edema
   b. Pneumonia
   c. Pulmonary hemorrhage
   d. Pulmonary thromboembolism

PARASITIC PNEUMONIA

Toxoplasmosis

Clinical correlations

1. Is caused by *Toxoplasma gondii;* more often seen in cats than dogs.

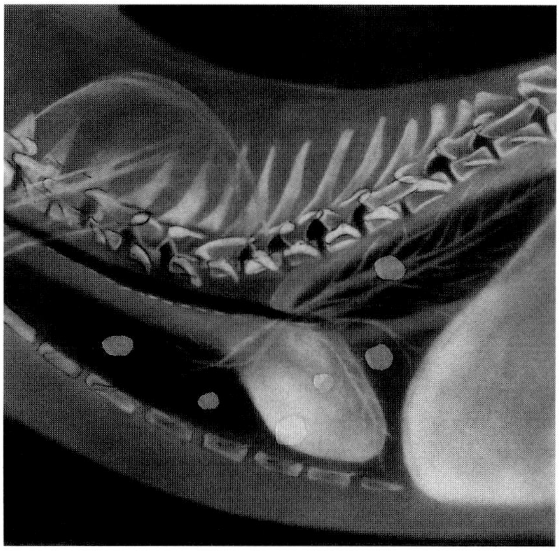

Figure 8.25. Multiple irregular interstitial nodules. Differential considerations include granulomatous pneumonia (e.g., Toxoplasmosis, Cryptococcosis), lungworm, or atypical metastasis.

2. May occur in an acute infection or as a relapsing disease.
3. Common clinical signs include fever, malaise, weight loss, anorexia, and variable degrees of dyspnea.

Radiographic findings (Figure 8.25)

1. An embolic type of pneumonia.
2. Multiple ill-defined, blotchy, coalescing alveolar opacities.
3. The infiltrates are usually bilateral and not symmetrical.

Paragonimus

Clinical correlations

1. Is caused by lung flukes, *Paragonimus kellicotti.*
2. Occurs in both dogs and cats.
3. Common clinical signs include chronic cough and weight loss.
4. Acute dyspnea may occur secondary to rupture of cavitary lesions with pneumothorax or atelectasis.
5. Adult flukes may invade the lung parenchyma or lower airways causing variable degrees of obstruction, inflammation, and interstitial emphysema.
6. The diagnosis is made by finding parasitic ova in the feces or tracheal aspirate.

Radiographic findings (Figure 8.26)

1. Solitary or multiple ill-defined nodular lung opacities
2. Focal lesions may be cavitated or cystic.
3. A prominent peribronchial or interstitial lung infiltrate may also be seen.

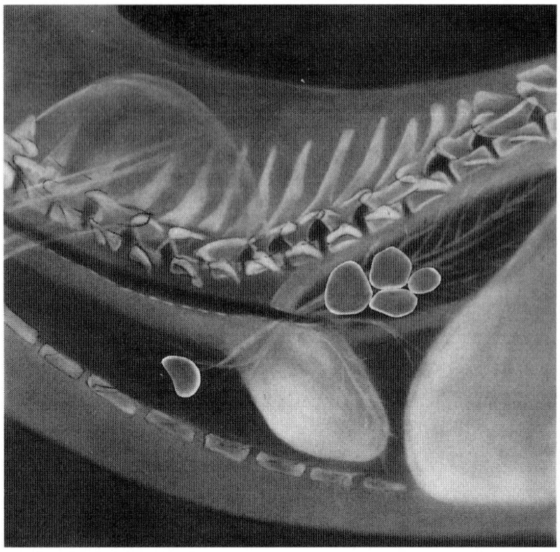

Figure 8.26. Paragonimus. There are multiple air-filled cystic lesions in the lung.

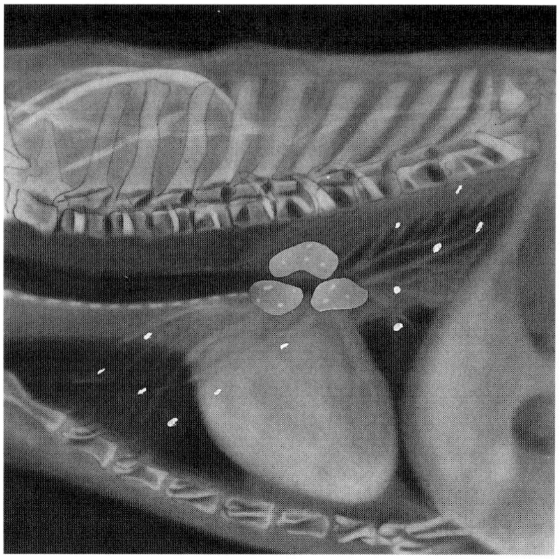

Figure 8.27. Chronic histoplasmosis. There is enlargement of the tracheobronchial lymph nodes containing focal areas of mineralization and multiple mineralized pulmonary nodules.

Aeleurostrongylus

Clinical correlations

1. Is caused by *Aeleurostrongylus abstrusus*, a lung worm.
2. Is seen in cats, most often 1 to 3 years of age.
3. Affected cats often have no clinical signs.
4. When present, clinical signs include choking and coughing, dyspnea, and anorexia.
5. The diagnosis is made by identifying first stage larvae in the feces or tracheal aspirate.

Radiographic findings

1. Interstitial pulmonary pattern, with or without indistinct nodules
2. Prominent bronchial markings are often seen.
3. Pulmonary hyperemia may be seen with enlarged pulmonary arteries.

MYCOTIC PNEUMONIA

Mycotic pulmonary infection, also referred to as pneumonomycosis, usually develops as a primary infection. Occasionally, may develop into systemic disease affecting other organs including the appendicular skeleton.

Histoplasmosis

Clinical correlations

1. Caused by *Histoplasma capsulatum* and affects dogs and cats.
2. Is most common mycotic pneumonia in the cat.
3. Is endemic in the Ohio, Mississippi, and Missouri river valleys.
4. The infective mycelium gains entry to the lung through the upper respiratory tract, converts to the yeast phase, and infects the lung.
5. An acute disseminated form of the disease involves multiple organ systems, affecting the skeleton, eye, skin, and reticuloendothelial system.
6. Many infected animals have no clinical signs of disease and the disease may be self-limiting.
7. Common clinical signs when present include cough, dyspnea, weight loss, lethargy, and fluctuating fever.

Radiographic findings (Figure 8.27)

1. Active stage
   a. Interstitial pneumonia with diffuse interstitial infiltrates and/or focal areas of consolidation
   b. Hilar lymphadenopathy may be present.
2. Chronic or healed stage
   a. Multiple well-defined interstitial nodules that may become mineralized.
   b. Mineralization of the hilar lymph nodes

Blastomycosis

Clinical correlations

1. Caused by *Blastomyces dermatitidis* and is more common in dogs than cats. Siamese cats may be predisposed to disease.
2. Is most common in the southeastern and eastern parts of the United States.
3. Characterized by pyogranulomatous inflammation and may be a disseminated disease involving the lung, liver, spleen, lymph nodes, bone, brain, eyes, and skin.
4. The clinical signs vary depending on which organs are involved; dyspnea and cough are common with respiratory infections.
5. Nonpulmonary clinical signs include depression, weight loss, and fever.

6. Major differentials include toxoplasmosis, cryptococcosis, feline infectious peritonitis, and coccidioidomycosis.

Radiographic findings

1. Active stage:
   a. Interstitial pneumonia with small ill-defined pulmonary radiopacities.
   b. Focal lung consolidations may be seen.
   c. Pleural effusion is often present.
   d. Hilar lymphadenopathy is common.
2. Chronic or healed stage:
   a. Multiple nonmineralized interstitial nodules
   b. Hilar lymphadenopathy may be present.

Coccidioidomycosis

Clinical correlations

1. Is caused by *Coccidioides immitis* and is more common in the dog.
2. Highest incidence is in the southwestern and western regions of the United States.
3. May be a mild, self-limiting pulmonary disease or be a disseminated disease, affecting the skeleton, heart, and central nervous system.

Radiographic findings (See following Figure 8.37)

1. Active state:
   a. Interstitial pneumonia
   b. Hilar lymphadenopathy
2. Chronic stage
   a. Disseminated, ill-defined, noncalcified round or oval lung nodules.
   b. Hilar lymphadenopathy is uncommon.

Nocardiosis

Clinical correlations

1. May appear as a cutaneous or systemic disease.
2. The lung is usually the portal of entry.
3. Occurs in dogs and cats.

Radiographic findings

1. Solitary or multiple granulomas that may coalesce or contain abscesses.
2. Frequently have hilar and mediastinal lymphadenopathy is present.
3. Commonly have pleuritis and pleural effusion.

Cryptococcosis

Clinical correlations

1. Is caused by *Cryptococcus neoformans* and is more common in the cat.
2. Usually causes a chronic rhinitis, and may cause a mass-induced nasopharyngeal obstruction.
3. May extend into the brain and cause neurologic signs.
4. May affect the lung primarily or secondarily.

Radiographic findings (See Figure 8.25)

1. Multiple, small, interstitial pulmonary masses.
2. May cause lung consolidation, often with pleural effusion.

Pneumocystis

Clinical correlations

1. Is caused by *Pneumocystis carinii* and is uncommon in dogs and cats.
2. Reported cases have occurred in animals with inherited immune deficiency, but may be as sequel to immune suppression therapy.

Radiographic findings

1. Multiple ill-defined alveolar focal infiltrates
2. No lymphadenopathy
3. Can mimic bacterial and neoplastic diseases of the lung.

PULMONARY NEOPLASIA

Primary Pulmonary Neoplasia

Clinical correlations

1. Usually seen in dogs and cats older than 6 years of age.
2. Tumors commonly metastasize to other areas of the lung and pleural cavity and extrathoracic body sites.
3. Bronchogenic carcinoma and adenocarcinoma are the most commonly reported primary lung tumors in the dog and cat, respectively. Other tumor types include bronchiolar-alveolar cell carcinoma, squamous cell carcinoma, and small cell carcinoma.
4. A primary lung tumor is reported most commonly arising in the right caudal lobe, but may occur in any lobe.
5. Clinical signs commonly include coughing and weight loss; however, many animals are asymptomatic.

Radiographic findings (Figure 8.28)

1. May appear solitary or multicentric.
   a. Solitary mass may have either well-demarcated or ill-defined margins. Often the mass has a smooth cranial margin and an indistinct peripheral margin.
   b. Multicentric tumors may appear nodular or diffusely disseminated.
   c. Cannot distinguish a multicentric primary lung tumor from a solitary lung tumor with intrapulmonary metastasis, or metastatic lung tumors from another primary tumor site.
2. May cavitate (See Figure 8.24) but rarely mineralizes. Tracheobronchial lymphadenopathy is uncommon and more often associated with multicentric lymphosarcoma or granulomatous disease.
3. May cause hypertrophic osteopathy and metastasize to the skeleton and/or other organs.

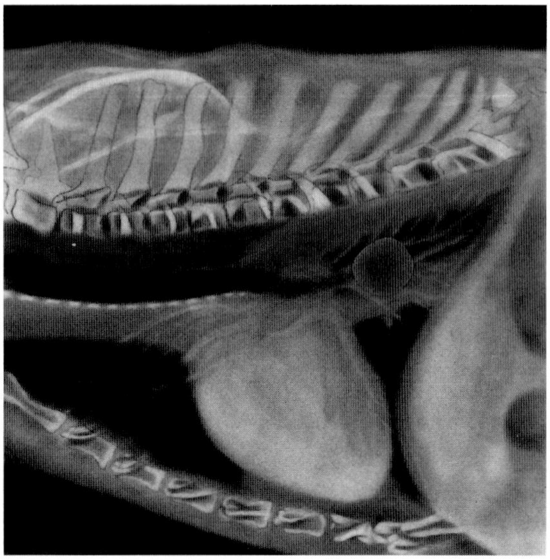

Figure 8.28. Solitary well-defined pulmonary mass.

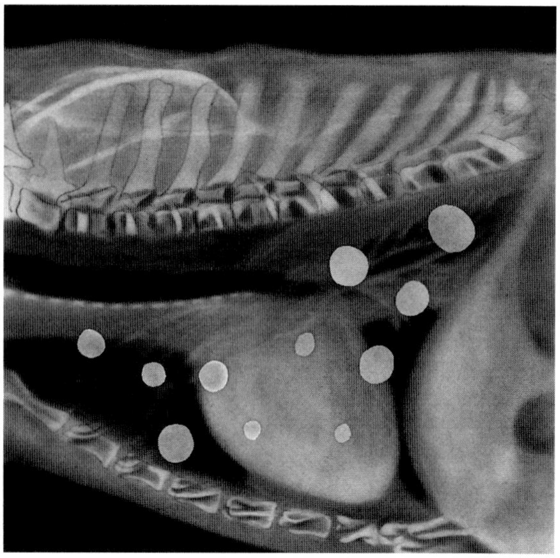

Figure 8.29. Metastatic pulmonary neoplasia. There are multiple, variably sized, well-defined pulmonary nodules throughout the lung.

Metastatic Pulmonary Neoplasia

Clinical correlations

1. Usually seen in older animals.
2. Usually no respiratory signs, but may have other clinical signs of disease, depending on site and type of the primary tumor and other sites of metastatic disease.
3. Respiratory clinical signs, weight loss, and other signs of illness are variable, depending on the location and size of the primary tumor and the extent of the metastasis.
4. Is much more frequent than primary lung tumors.

Radiographic findings (Figures 8.29 and 8.30)

1. Most commonly seen as multiple, noncavitated, discrete, soft tissue pulmonary nodules and masses of varying sizes throughout all lung lobes.
   a. Hemangiosarcoma typically metastasizes as a diffuse nodular interstitial pattern of the lung lobes. The observed nodules commonly vary in size from 3 to 10 mm in diameter.
   b. Other metastatic tumor types usually have fewer and larger nodules. Variations in the radiographic appearances are probably related in part to the characteristics of the primary tumor.
2. The radiographic detection of the metastatic lesions usually depends on the size and location of the lesions.
3. Less common patterns of metastatic lung disease include:
   a. Solitary cavitary or noncavitary mass
   b. Multiple cavitary masses or nodules
   c. Linear interstitial pattern (pulmonary lymphangitic metastasis or septal alveolar wall metastasis), such as may occur in undifferentiated schirrous mammary adenocarcinoma.
   d. Diffuse alveolar infiltrate usually is a result of complicating factors of pneumonia, necrosis, and hemorrhage.

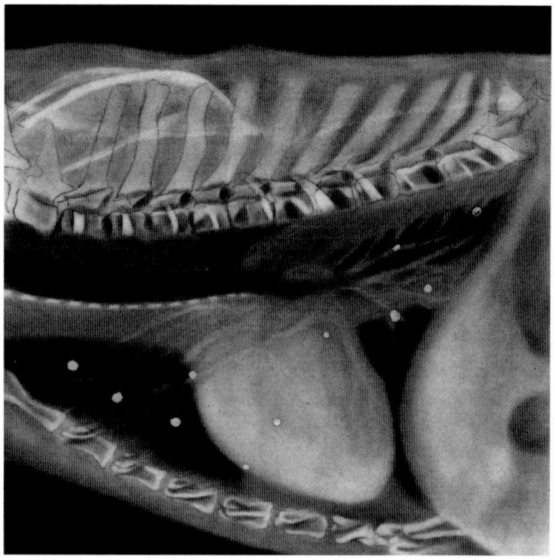

Figure 8.30. Metastatic pulmonary neoplasia. There are multiple small well-defined pulmonary nodules throughout the lung.

MEDIASTINUM

RADIOGRAPHIC ANATOMY

1. The mediastinum is formed by the reflection of the parietal pleura and the space and structures between them, which divides the right and left hemithorax. It extends from the thoracic inlet to the diaphragm. For radiographic purposes, it is usually divided into three sections: a cranial portion between the thoracic inlet and heart, a middle section that includes the heart, and a caudal portion between the heart and the diaphragm.
2. Normally, only the heart, trachea, caudal vena cava, aorta, and occasionally, the esophagus are visible on survey radiographs. The normal thymus may also be seen before involution in young dogs and cats (usually younger than 4 to 6 months of age). The normal thymus has a ''sail sign'' shape on the ventrodorsal projection (See Figure 8.36) and may silhouette and obscure the right side of the heart on the lateral projection.
3. The normal width of the cranial mediastinum varies among dog and cat breeds. The mediastinum is also commonly widened in obese animals that have increased fat in the mediastinum and in young animals with a thymus.
4. On the ventrodorsal or dorsoventral projections, the mediastinum is mainly midline and not visible. The width is usually less than two times the width of a vertebra, but the thickness is affected by the amount of fat it contains. In obese animals, the widened mediastinum caused by fat has smooth borders and no displacement or compression of the trachea.
5. The cranioventral mediastinal reflection is caused by extension of the right cranial lung lobe across the midline, pushing the mediastinum to the left. It is usually visible on the ventrodorsal or dorsoventral projection as a curvilinear soft tissue opacity extending from T1 to the cranial left border of the heart (approximately the level of the pulmonary artery segment). The thymus lies in this reflection. On the lateral projection, the reflection between the left and right cranial lung lobes is visible cranial to the heart and ventral to the cranial vena cava.
6. The caudoventral mediastinal reflection is caused by extension of the right lung's accessory lobe across the midline and is only seen on some ventrodorsal projections. It is seen as a relatively straight, soft tissue opaque line extending from the left apex of the heart caudally to approximately the middle of the left diaphragm.
7. The caudal vena cava mediastinal reflection is not visible.
8. Radiographic abnormalities of the mediastinum are related to:
   a. Mediastinal shift related to a lung volume abnormality or an intrathoracic mass
   b. Mediastinal masses, including dilation of the esophagus
   c. Mediastinal effusion
   d. Pneumomediastinum

DISEASES/DISORDERS

Mediastinal Shift

Clinical correlations

1. Is a condition in which the mediastinum is displaced by pressure differences between the right and left pleural cavities.
2. Common conditions that may cause mediastinal shift:
   a. Unilateral or occasionally bilateral pneumothorax
   b. Unilateral pleural effusion
   c. Diaphragmatic hernia
   d. Bronchial obstruction
   e. Emphysema
   f. Positional atelectasis
   g. Pleural adhesions of the heart or lung to the thoracic wall

Radiographic findings (Figure 8.31)

1. Left or right displacement of one or more mediastinal structures (trachea, heart, aortic arch, cranial and caudal vena cava) as seen on the dorsoventral or ventrodorsal projections of the chest.
2. Increased radiopacity of the lung on the side toward the shift associated with atelectasis.

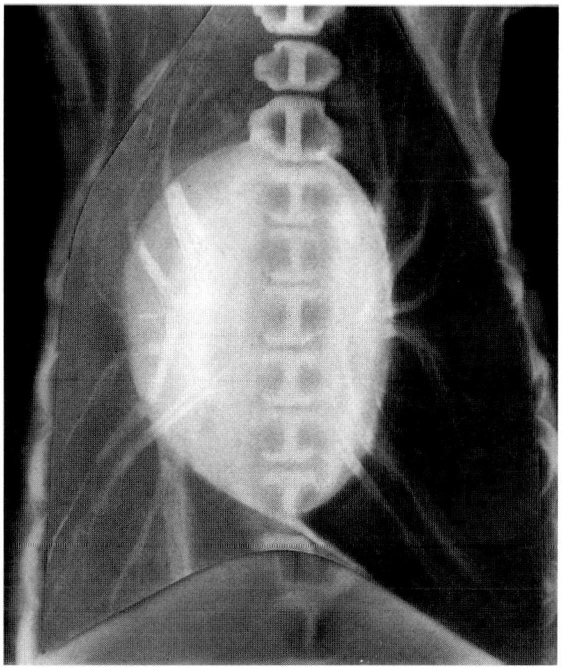

Figure 8.31. Atelectasis with mediastinal shift. There is collapse of the right lung with mediastinal shift. The left lung is hyperinflated.

3. Differential considerations:
   a. Technical artifact (e.g., an oblique projection) may mimic a mediastinal shift.
   b. Congenital abnormalities of the spine
      1) Scoliosis
      2) Lordosis
      3) Pectus excavatum
   c. Increased fat in the mediastinum, usually in obese animals
   d. Dextrocardia

Pneumomediastinum

Clinical correlations

1. There is collection of abnormal free air within the mediastinum.
2. May be caused by a variety of conditions.
   a. Is secondary to interstitial pulmonary emphysema from ruptured alveoli with dissection of air toward hilus of lung and entry into the mediastinal space. This commonly occurs with trauma or after iatrogenic pulmonary hyperinflation, usually with endotracheal intubation for anesthesia or resuscitation.
   b. Secondary to air entering into the mediastinum from fascial planes of the neck or oral cavity as a result of wounds, rupture of the trachea, rupture of the esophagus, as a complication of vena puncture caused by inadvertent penetration of trachea, or after transtracheal aspiration.
   c. Secondary to cranial extension of air from the retroperitoneal space (rare).
   d. Is secondary to mediastinal infections caused by gas-forming organisms.
3. If the increased mediastinal pressure causes rupture of the mediastinal pleura, pneumothorax may occur as a sequel.
4. Dyspnea and coughing may be present, depending on the degree of subcutaneous emphysema and whether pneumothorax is also present.

Radiographic findings (Figure 8.32)

1. There is abnormal radiolucency of the mediastinum because gas is present adjacent to one or more mediastinal structures (e.g., esophagus, azygous vein, the external wall of the trachea, the cranial vena cava, aorta, and/or the brachycephalic artery).
2. There is a range of radiolucency from subtle, patchy gas opacities within the mediastinum to the marked outlining of esophagus, aorta, and other structures with gas.
3. Secondary complications of pneumomediastinum:
   a. Usually when there is a pneumomediastinum and air in the soft tissues of the neck and thoracic wall, a lesion is present in the neck (e.g., tracheal rupture). Dissection of gas from the pneumomediastinum into the fascial planes of the neck and the thoracic wall rarely occurs.

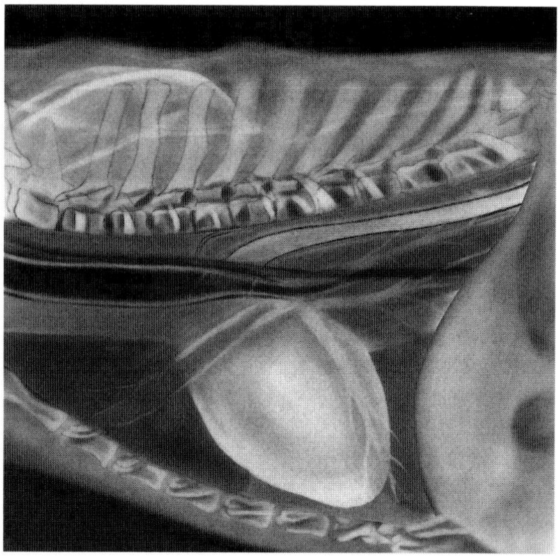

Figure 8.32. Pneumomediastinum. There is gas in the mediastinum outlining the tracheal wall, cranial vena cava, and aorta.

   b. Pneumoretroperitoneum results from the dissection of air around the aorta through the diaphragm into the retroperitoneal space.
   c. Pneumothorax results from traumatic rupture of the mediastinal or pulmonary pleura.
   d. Pneumopericardium is usually associated with trauma.
4. Differential considerations:
   a. Pneumothorax: overall increased radiolucency in the pleural space with pulmonary atelectasis, but mediastinal gas is absent.
   b. Subcutaneous emphysema of the chest wall may be superimposed over the mediastinal area on the lateral projection and mimic pneumomediastinum. The location of the emphysema may be confirmed by making lateral and dorsoventral, or ventrodorsal projections of the chest.

Mediastinal Mass

Clinical correlations

1. The differentiation of mediastinal masses is based on their specific location in one of five regions:
   a. Cranioventral
   b. Craniodorsal
   c. Hilar and perihilar
   d. Caudodorsal
   e. Caudoventral
2. Masses can originate from the thymus or lymph nodes as an extension of a disease process from the lung, heart, spine, esophagus, sternum or chest wall, as a local manifestation of a generalized disease (e.g., lymphosarcoma) or as a congenital anomaly (e.g., branchial cyst).

3. Lymphadenopathy is a common mediastinal mass, usually involving the cranial mediastinal, tracheobronchial and/or sternal lymph nodes.

Radiographic findings (Figures 8.33 through 8.35)

1. Cranial mediastinal lymph node enlargement usually displaces the trachea dorsally and to the right of the midline.
2. Tracheobronchial lymph node enlargement usually displaces the main stem bronchi ventrally at the carina, and there is often narrowing of the trachea and/or main stem bronchus.

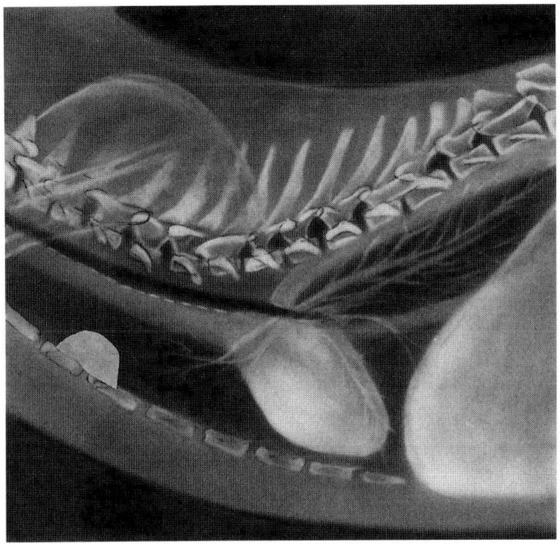

Figure 8.33. Small cranioventral mediastinal mass. There is a well-defined extrapleural mass in the cranioventral thorax, most typical of sternal lymphadenopathy.

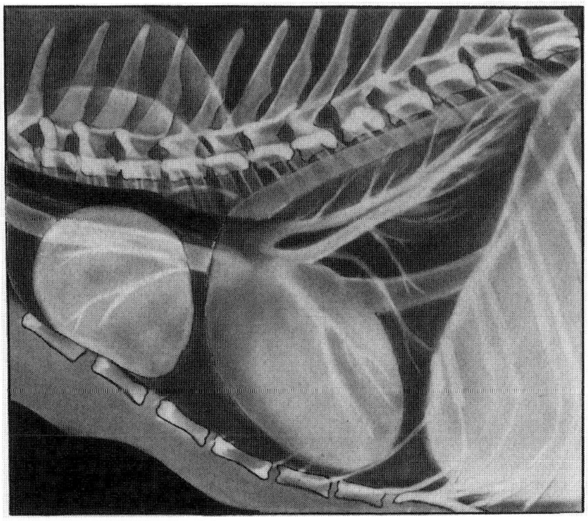

Figure 8.34. Large cranioventral mediastinal mass. There is elevation of the thoracic trachea by the well-defined mediastinal mass.

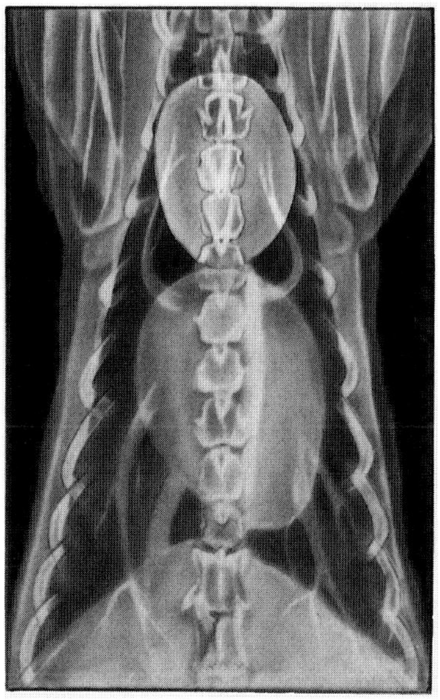

Figure 8.35. Cranioventral mediastinal mass. The large soft tissue mass is seen on the midline within the mediastinum.

3. Retrosternal lymph node enlargement on a lateral projection is usually seen as a convex soft tissue density in the retrosternal region of the cranial ventral mediastinum at the level of the second to fourth sternbra.
4. Cranial mediastinal lymph node enlargement is seen as widening of the cranial mediastinum on the ventrodorsal or dorsoventral projection.

Diffuse Mediastinal Enlargement

Clinical correlations

1. Common conditions include:
   a. Mediastinitis (acute or chronic)
   b. Mediastinal abscess
   c. Mediastinal edema
   d. Mediastinal hemorrhage
2. Anatomic variations:
   a. Brachycephalic dogs normally have a more prominent and wider cranial mediastinum.
   b. Older miniature dogs and some obese dogs frequently accumulate excessive fat within the cranial mediastinum.

Radiographic findings

1. The cranial mediastinum is wider (commonly more than twice the width of the vertebrae on the ventrodorsal projection) with an increased soft tissue radiopacity.
2. Indistinct delineation of the mediastinal and/or cardiac border
3. Widened caudoventral mediastinum
4. Narrowing or displacement of the trachea
5. Depending on the type and location of mediastinal mass, there may be concurrent abnormalities such as pleural effusion, megaesophagus, or bronchopneumonia.

Focal Mediastinal Enlargement

Clinical correlations

1. Common conditions include:
   a. Abscess
   b. Tumor
   c. Lymphadenopathy
   d. Granulomas
   e. Cyst
   f. Esophageal enlargement (e.g., esophageal foreign body or tumor)
2. Clinical signs are variable from no signs to signs of regurgitation, dysphagia, or sepsis depending on cause and extent of disease.

Radiographic findings

1. A mass is often visualized on both the lateral and ventrodorsal projections.
2. A mass is usually well-defined and of soft tissue opacity.
3. Differential diagnosis depends on the mediastinal location of the mass.
   a. Cranioventral mediastinum
      1) Abscess
      2) Cyst
      3) Granuloma
      4) Thymus
         a) Normal in young dogs and cats. When visible on ventrodorsal or dorsoventral projection, is often referred to as "sail sign" (Figure 8.36).
         b) Thymoma
         c) Thymic lymphosarcoma

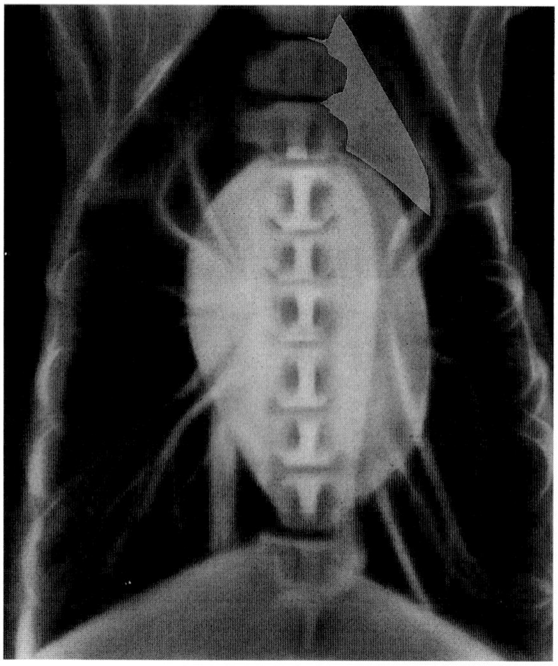

Figure 8.36. Normal thymus with "sail sign."

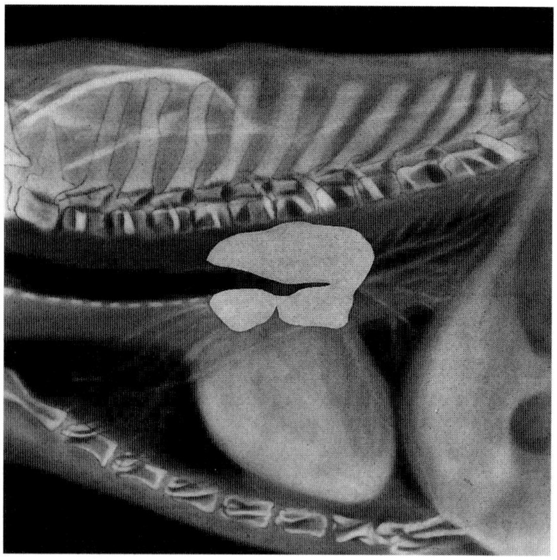

Figure 8.37. Hilar lymphadenopathy.

      5) Lymphadenopathy (Figure 8.37)
         a) Metastatic tumors (e.g., lymphosarcoma)
         b) Systemic mycotic infections
      6) Thyroid and parathyroid tumors
      7) Esophageal enlargement
         a) Megaesophagus
         b) Vascular ring anomaly (e.g., persistent right aortic arch)

PLEURA AND PLEURAL SPACE

NORMAL ANATOMY

1. The pleural space lined by both parietal and pulmonary pleura, form two sacs in the thorax, which are potential spaces in the right and left hemithorax between the chest wall, lung, and mediastinum.
2. Diseases affecting the pleura and pleural space can be subdivided into conditions that cause increased pleural and thoracic radiopacity (e.g., pleural effusion, pleural masses, and pleural thickening) or a decreased pleural and thoracic radiopacity (e.g., pneumothorax).
3. The pleural space normally contains a small volume of fluid that serves as a lubricant, but this normal amount of fluid is not visible radiographically.

RADIOGRAPHIC ANATOMY

The normal pleural is not visualized except for the pleural reflections as part of the caudoventral mediastinum and the cranioventral mediastinum.

DISEASES/DISORDERS

Pleural Effusion

Clinical correlations

1. Fluid present in the pleural space as a result of an exudate, transudate, or modified transudate. This may be unilateral or bilateral.
2. Types of effusions:
   a. Hydrothorax: serous or inflammatory transudate with low fibrin and cell count
      1) Hypoproteinemia
         a) Nephrotic syndrome
         b) Protein-losing nephropathy
         c) Hepatic insufficiency
      2) Fluid overload
      3) Congestive heart failure
         a) Right ventricular failure with systemic venous hypertension
         b) Pulmonary venous hypertension subsequent to chronic mitral valve regurgitation and secondary right ventricular failure
         c) Pericardial effusion and tamponade
      4) Lymphatic obstruction secondary to fibrosis, adhesions, or neoplastic infiltration
   b. Hemothorax: sanguinous effusion
      1) Chest trauma (e.g., lacerated intercostal artery from rib fracture or direct pulmonary laceration)
      2) Eroding neoplasm of chest wall, pleura, lung, or mediastinum
      3) Coagulopathy (e.g., rodenticide)
   c. Pyothorax or empyema: exudative inflammatory effusion with high neutrophil cell count and high fibrin content
      1) Pneumonia or pulmonary abscess
      2) Systemic infection
      3) Penetrating wounds
   d. Chylothorax: chyle or chylous effusion
      1) Erosion of the thoracic duct (neoplasia, abscesses)
      2) Occlusion of the thoracic duct (neoplasia, thrombosis)
      3) Congenital malformations
      4) Lymphangectasia
      5) Pseudochylous effusions: in the cat is most often associated with cardiomyopathy or lymphosarcoma
   e. Exudative pleuritis: effusion with high fibrin and low cell count
      1) Feline infectious peritonitis
      2) Neoplastic effusion
3. Pleural fluid distribution within the thorax conforms to the shape of the lung, mediastinum, chest wall, and diaphragm. Pleural effusion is affected by the forces of gravity and by the positioning of the animal during radiography.
4. Classifications of pleural fluid (based on evaluating distribution of effusion on different radiographic projections):
   a. Free pleural fluid: fluid can be moved freely within the pleural cavity.
   b. Trapped pleural fluid: atypical distribution of the pleural fluid, but the fluid is still capable of being moved under the influence of gravity.
   c. Encapsulated pleural fluid: fluid is loculated by fibrinous deposits or adhesions and unable to be moved by gravity (e.g., as often occurs with pyothorax and chronic pleuritis).

Radiographic findings (Figures 8.38 through 8.41):

1. Amount of pleural fluid recognized on conventional survey radiographic projections:
   a. Is difficult to quantitatively assess the amount of fluid present.
   b. A minimum of approximately 50 mL is necessary in the pleural cavity of a small dog or cat before it is visible on conventional survey radiographs.
   c. A minimum of approximately 100 mL is necessary in the pleural cavity of a medium sized dog before it is visible on conventional survey radiographs.
2. The radiographic signs of unilateral or bilateral pleural effusion are relative to the projection, the location, and the volume of fluid.
3. Lateral recumbent projection:
   a. With small amounts of fluid, the lung border can be seen retracted from the sternum, partially obscuring the ventral border of the heart and ventral diaphragm. Interlobar fissure lines can be seen.
   b. With a moderate amount of fluid, the lung margins will appear rounded and the cardiac borders and diaphragm will be obscured.

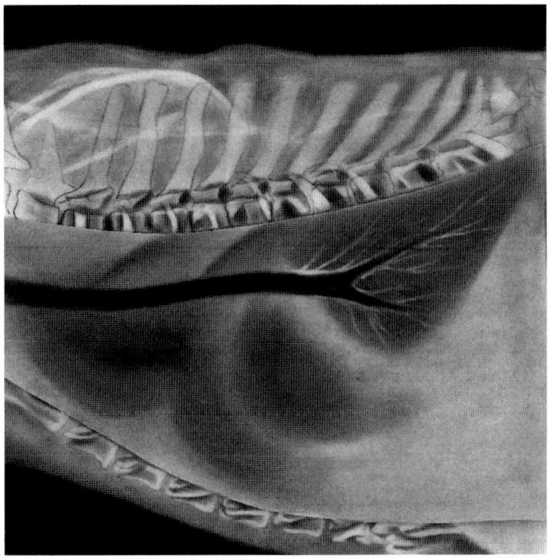

Figure 8.38. Pleural effusion. Marked pleural fluid obscures the heart "silhouette sign."

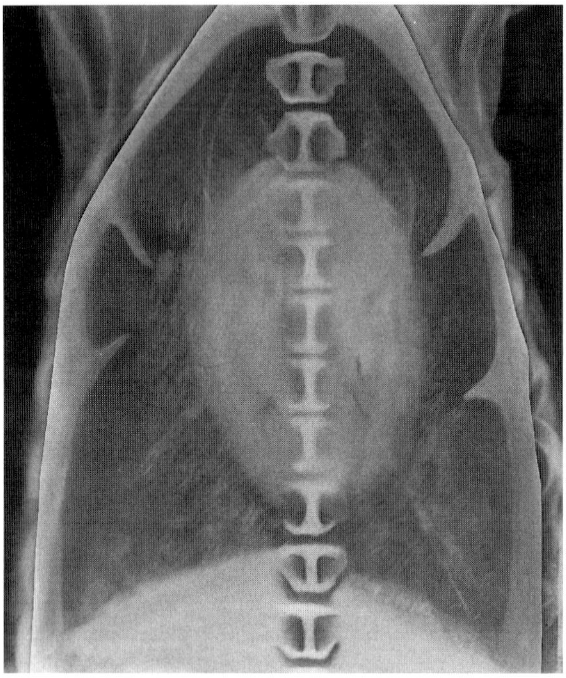

Figure 8.39. Pleural effusion. The bilateral pleural effusion is visible in the interlobar fissures and between lung border and chest wall.

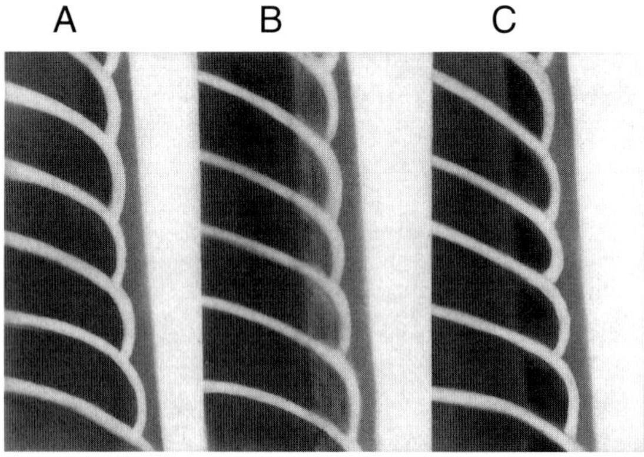

Figure 8.40. The pleural cavity: normal (**A**), pleural effusion (**B**), and pneumothorax (**C**).

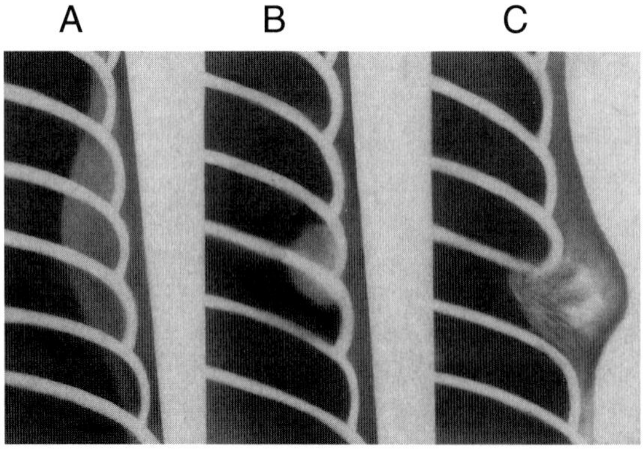

Figure 8.41. Pleural, pulmonary and extrapleural masses-pleural mass or loculated pleural fluid (**A**). Pulmonary mass adjacent to the chest wall (**B**) and an extrapleural mass (**C**) showing rib destruction and an extrathoracic soft tissue and mineralized mass.

   c. Pleural fissure lines are prominent.
   d. With a large amount of pleural effusion, the interlobar fissures are wider and more obvious, and are termed "leafing" of the lung. The diaphragm and cardiac borders may be completely obscured and the trachea and heart displaced dorsally. The diaphragm and liver may also be caudally displaced.
4. Ventrodorsal projection
   a. With a small amount of fluid, pleural fissure lines will be seen. There is mild retraction of the lung (visceral pleura) from the chest wall (parietal pleura) and slight rounding of the costophrenic angle.
   b. With a moderate amount of fluid, the interlobar fissures will be widened, there is moderate retraction of the lung from the chest wall, and the left border of the descending aorta is usually obscured.
   c. With a large amount of fluid, the mediastinum will fasely appear widened, the heart and diaphragm will be partially obscured and the liver may appear caudally displaced.
   d. The cardiac silhouette and lung are usually more visible on a ventrodorsal than on a dorsoventral projection.
5. Dorsoventral projection
   a. With a small amount of fluid, the border of the heart and diaphragm will be partially obscured. The fissures adjacent to the accessory lung lobe will be widened.
   b. With a moderate amount of fluid, the borders of the heart and diaphragm will be completely obscured, the mediastinum will appear fasely widened, and there will be retraction of the lung from the chest wall.
   c. With a large amount of fluid, the lung lobes will appear rounded and retracted from the chest wall. The chest may appear "barrel-shaped" and the heart and other thoracic structures obscured. The diaphragm and liver may be caudally displaced.
6. Horizontal beam radiography (e.g., lateral recumbent or erect positions)
   a. Can enhance the detection of small effusions or changes in the amount of fluid when compared to other projections.
   b. The effusion will be most visible in the more dependent portion of the thorax.

Other imaging

1. Ultrasound
2. Computed tomography (CT)
3. Magnetic resonance imaging (MRI)

Pleural Thickening

Clinical correlations

1. Is a common finding in aged animals, usually without clinical significance.

2. May represent pleural pathology (e.g., pleuritis).
3. Is caused by fibrin and/or calcific deposits on the parietal and/or visceral pleural layers.

Radiographic findings (Figures 8.42 and 8.43)

1. The normal pleura is thin and not visible. Tangential radiographic projections may demonstrate normal interlobar fissures, usually between the middle and cranial lung lobe as seen on the right or left lateral projection.
2. Pleural thickening is usually represented by thin, radiopaque lines between the lung lobes. These lines may or may not extend to the thoracic wall.
3. On the lateral projection, the most common site of pleural thickening is observed between the caudal and middle lobes, superimposed partially over the heart.
4. On the ventrodorsal or dorsoventral projection, the most common site of pleural thickening is often observed between the cranial and caudal lobes on both the right and left sides.
5. If the pleural lines are thin, it is difficult to differentiate between mild pleural thickening and the tangential effect of seeing the normal pleural or a possible small amount of pleural effusion.

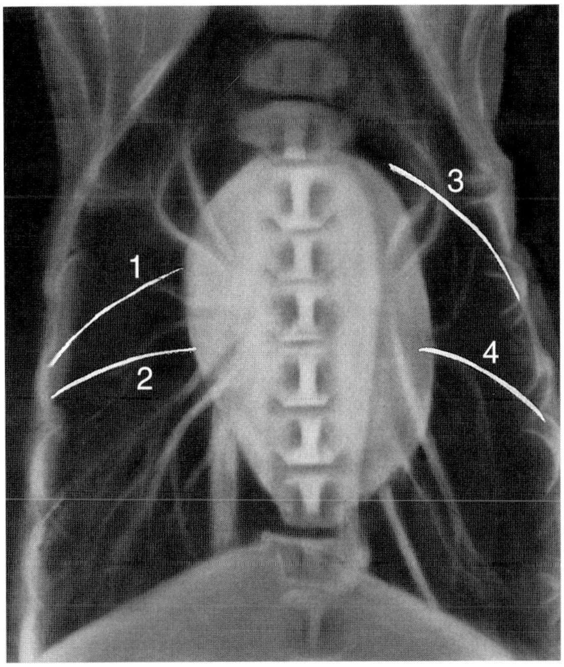

Figure 8.42. Pleural fissure lines. Fissure lines between the right cranial and middle lung lobes (**1**), the right caudal and middle lobes (**2**), between the cranial and caudal segments of the left cranial lobe (**3**), and the left cranial and caudal lobes (**4**).

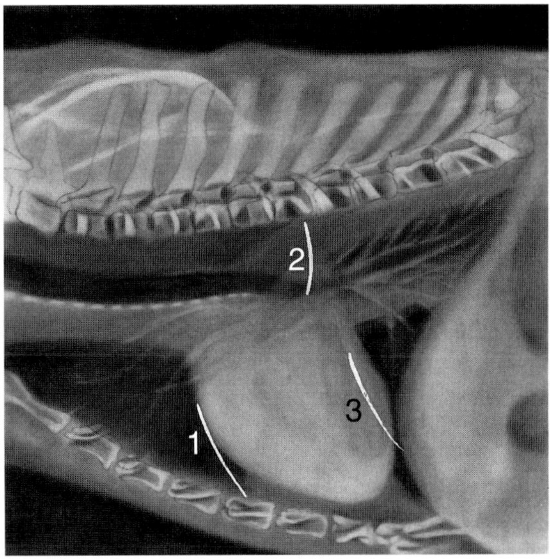

Figure 8.43. Pleural fissure lines. Fissure lines are often seen between the cranial and middle lung lobes (**1**), the cranial and caudal lobes (**2**), and the middle and caudal lobes (**3**).

Pleural Neoplasms

Clinical correlations

1. Often is difficult to diagnose because the presence of concurrent pleural fluid tends to obscure the mass.
2. Benign pleural tumors are often associated with pleural adhesions, hematoma, abscess, pleural peel, or encapsulated fluid (e.g., pyothorax).
3. Pleural neoplasms can be primary or metastatic.
   a. Primary tumor is mesothelioma.
   b. Metastatic neoplasia is usually associated with pulmonary neoplasia (usually carcinoma).
4. A chest wall tumor (e.g., rib tumor) is usually extrapleural but may mimic a pleural mass and can extend through the pleura to involve the lung.

Radiographic findings (See Figure 8.41)

1. May appear similar to or mimic encapsulated fluid.
2. Pleural masses commonly have a convex margin adjacent to the opposed lung and a concave margin at edge adjacent to the chest wall (referred to as the extrapleural sign).
3. Neoplastic masses may produce lysis or proliferative lesions of the rib, dystrophic mineralization, distortion of the intercostal spaces.
4. Pleural masses are best visualized after the pleural fluid has been drained.

Contrast radiography

1. Positive contrast pleurography
2. Diagnostic pneumothorax

Other imaging

1. Ultrasound
2. CT
3. MRI

Other Pleural Masses

Clinical correlations

1. Are often seen associated with rib fractures and secondary soft tissue swelling (e.g., hematoma) or adjacent subcutaneous emphysema.
2. Benign and malignant rib lesions (e.g., osteochondroma, osteosarcoma, chondrosarcoma) and intercostal soft tissue masses (e.g., malignant histiocytoma, fibrosarcoma)
3. Mediastinal and diaphragmatic lesions may mimic extrapleural lesions
   a. Lymphosarcoma of the cranial mediastinal lymph nodes
   b. Esophageal masses (foreign body, granuloma, neoplasm)
   c. Diaphragmatic lesions
      1) Diaphragmatic hernia or eventration
      2) Diaphragmatic tumor or granuloma

Radiographic findings (See Figure 8.41)

1. If pleural fluid is present, an extrapleural mass is best visualized after the pleural fluid has been removed.
2. The size and extent of the mass is best seen with a tangential x-ray beam through the base of the mass.
3. May have rib lesions, dystrophic mineralization, and distortion of intercostal spaces.

Contrast radiography

1. Pleurography
2. Diagnostic pneumothorax

Other imaging

1. Ultrasound
2. CT
3. MRI

Pneumothorax

Clinical correlations

1. There is the abnormal presence of air within the pleural cavity.
2. Types of pneumothorax
   a. Simple pneumothorax: a pneumothorax in which the mean pressure of the gas within the pleural space does not become higher than atmospheric pressure, usually because of chest wall trauma.
      1) Closed pneumothorax: the air within the pleural cavity is contained by an intact chest wall, usually because of ruptured visceral pleura (ruptured lung), ruptured major airway, pneumomediastinum, or esophagus perforation.
      2) Open pneumothorax: air passes freely through an opening in the chest wall; rib fractures are common.
   b. Tension pneumothorax: the pressure within the pleural cavity is greater than the atmospheric pressure, which is a result of a one way valve effect that permits air to enter the pleural space on inspiration but does not allow the air to leave on expiration. The chest wall is intact and the source of air is from severe visceral pleural injury. If unilateral, it will produce a mediastinal shift.
3. Causes of pneumothorax
   a. Common
      1) Trauma
         a) Blunt thoracic trauma
         b) Lung laceration secondary to rib fracture
      2) Iatrogenic
         a) Transthoracic pulmonary aspirate
         b) Sequel to thoracentesis
      3) Secondary to pneumomediastinum
         a) Bite wounds (cervical injury to trachea)
         b) Faulty tracheal intubation
         c) Postoperative to cervical surgery
         d) Esophageal perforation
   b. Uncommon
      1) Spontaneous pneumothorax
         a) Rupture of bleb, bulla, or bronchial cyst
         b) Pulmonary abscess
         c) Necrotic neoplasm
         d) Parasitic diseases
            (1) Paragonimus
            (2) Dirofilariasis
            (3) Filaroides osleri
         e) Esophageal perforation
4. Secondary conditions associated with pneumothorax
   a. Atelectasis
   b. Pulmonary consolidation
   c. Mediastinal shift
5. Mild pneumothorax is usually self-limiting and the pleural air is fairly rapidly absorbed. In more severe pneumothorax, removal of the free pleural air may be necessary. If pneumothorax is persistent, a thoracotomy is usually indicated.

Radiographic findings (Figures 8.44 and 8.45)

1. Lateral projection:
   a. Displacement of the heart dorsally away from the sternum (decreased or no cardiosternal contact).
   b. Retraction of the lung lobes away from the thoracic wall facilitates visibility of the visceral pleura and lung border.
   c. Lack of vascular and bronchial markings beyond the border of collapsed lung lobes
   d. Increased opacity to the lung lobes secondary to atelectasis

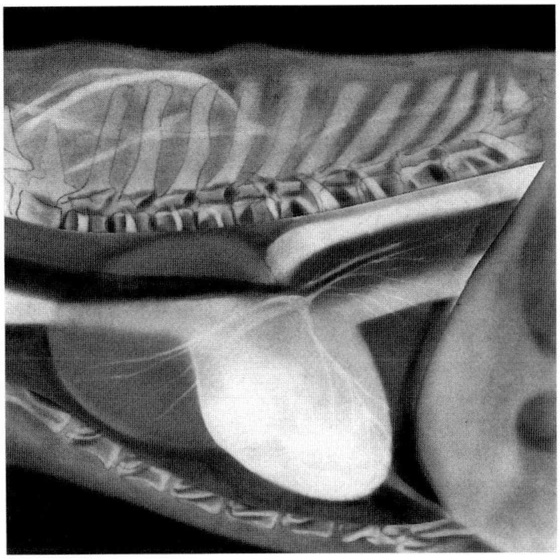

Figure 8.44. Pneumothorax. The lungs are partially collapsed and are more radiopaque because of atelectasis. The heart is displaced away from the sternum and the caudoventral mediastinum is well-visualized.

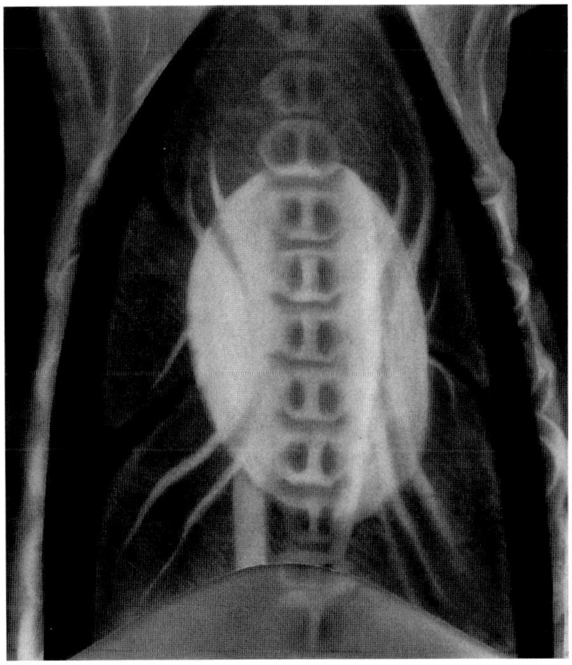

Figure 8.45. Pneumothorax. There is bilateral pneumothorax with retraction of the lung borders away from the chest wall. There is increased radiopacity of thc lungs because of atelectasis.

e. Flattening and/or caudal displacement of the diaphragm
2. Dorsoventral or ventrodorsal projection:
   a. Retraction of the visceral pleura away from the thoracic wall.
   b. Inability to visualize the vascular or bronchial markings extending to the borders of the thorax.
   c. Flattening of the diaphragm in severe pneumothorax; may visualize the scalloped insertions of the diaphragm at the rib attachments.
3. Differential diagnosis:
   a. Superimposed skin folds; skin folds can usually be seen extending beyond the limits of the lung margin and chest wall
   b. In hypovolemic shock, the heart is frequently smaller than normal and may appear to be elevated away from the sternum. However, pulmonary markings appear to extend ventrally to the sternum.
   c. With artifactual overexposure or hyperinflation, the lung markings appear to extend to the margins of the thoracic wall.
   d. On the left lateral recumbent projection (compared to the right lateral recumbent projection), the normal heart can "fall away" from the midline and mimic a pneumothorax.

THORACIC WALL

DISEASES/DISORDERS

Soft Tissue Abnormalities

Clinical correlations

1. Extracostal abnormalities can result from infectious, neoplastic, traumatic, metabolic, degenerative, or other causes.
2. May or may not have clinical significance. Must correlate closely with the history and physical examination to assess the significance.

Radiographic findings

1. Various focal skin or subcutaneous radiopacities may cause variation in visibility (e.g., nipples, abscesses, neoplasms, debris on skin and hair, and foreign bodies).
2. Because many foreign bodies and other extracostal lesions are commonly poorly demarcated and have a homogenous soft tissue/fluid radiopacity, they are not easily identified. Metallic foreign bodies such as bullet fragments are easily identified.
3. Some types of extracostal opacities can be mistaken for other lesions (e.g., a nipple shadow that can mimic a lung mass). Marking the extracostal opacity with a marker (e.g., barium, lead marker) and repeating the radiograph can be helpful for differentiating lesions.
4. Focal subcutaneous radiolucencies are usually caused by gas, commonly from laceration, puncture wounds, gas-forming organisms, or from subcutaneous injections.

5. Tumors vary in radiopacity and definition, ranging from soft tissue dense masses, soft tissue masses containing dystrophic mineralization, or fat-like radiopacities, (e.g., a lipoma in the subcutaneous or interfascial spaces).

Congenital Anomalies of the Chest Wall

Clinical correlations

1. Usually have no clinical significance, but occasionally may be associated with intrathoracic disease (e.g., absent caudal sternabra in some cases of peritoneal pericardial diaphragmatic hernia).
2. May cause alteration in the appearance of intrathoracic structures (e.g., heart position).
3. Anomalies involve variations in size, shape, number, and position of the thoracic vertebra, sternebra, and/or ribs.

Radiographic findings

1. Cervical supernumerary ribs can be unilateral or bilateral and are seen as ribs attached to C7.
2. Transitional vertebrae at T13-L1 may be symmetric or asymmetric. The number of ribs can be increased or decreased with resulting altered number of thoracic and lumbar vertebrae.
3. Rib fusion is more common in chondrodystrophoid dogs and usually is associated with other congenital spinal deformities, such as hemivertebrae or block vertebrae.
4. Variations in costocartilages and costochondral junctions
   a. Young animals have incompletely mineralized costal cartilages.
   b. Mature normal animals, especially dogs, have variable degrees of mineralization of the costal cartilages and costochondral junctions. Commonly is seen as a stippled mineralization.
   c. Chondrodystrophic dogs normally have more prominent and enlarged costochondral junctions.
5. Variations in sternabra
   a. Abnormalities in size, shape, number, position, and radiopacity are usually congenital variants (e.g., sternal dysraphism).
   b. Similar changes can result from neoplasia, chronic inflammation, and trauma.

Pectus Excavatum

Clinical correlations

1. Causes a reduction in the dorsoventral dimension of the thorax because of dorsal intrusion of the sternum.
2. May cause respiratory impairment with exercise intolerance, tachypnea, and weakness because of compromised lung volume.

Radiographic findings (Figure 8.46)

1. On the lateral projection, part or all of the sternum is displaced dorsally (e.g., thoracic sternabra distance is decreased). The sternabrae are commonly superimposed over a portion of the heart on the lateral projection.
2. The ventral ends of the ribs and the costal cartilages form an abnormal curve to join the sternum.
3. On the dorsoventral or ventrodorsal projection, the changes are less obvious. Often there is a mediastinal shift of the heart and trachea to the right or left of the midline (a result of the decreased midline distance between the spine and xyphoid).
4. Differentiate from sternabra deformities that are secondary to hyperinflation of the chest, especially in cats.

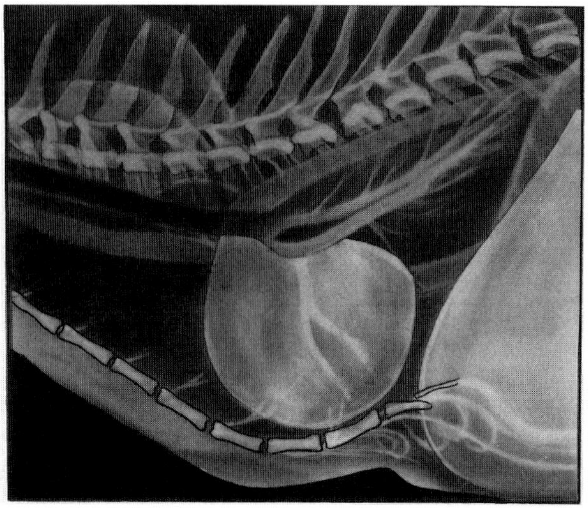

Figure 8.46. Pectus excavatum.

Pectus Carinatum

Clinical correlations

1. Caused by ventral protuberance of the sternum.
2. May be seen in some dogs and cats with cardiomegaly (often associated with congenital heart disease).
3. No reported clinical signs.

Radiographic finding

1. Increased dorsoventral dimension resulting from ventral protrusion of the sternum.

Sternal Dysraphism

Clinical correlations

1. Is caused by faulty development in the right and left cartilaginous sternal precursors, which causes a cleft between the two bony halves.
2. Usually causes no clinical signs.
3. May be associated with abnormal ventral attachment of the diaphragm to the sternum, which results in herniation of abdominal viscera into the thorax (e.g., peritoneomediastinal or peritoneopericardial diaphragmatic hernia).

Radiographic findings

1. On the lateral projection, the xyphoid or sternebrae may appear in two halves or "duplicated." A slightly oblique projection may more readily demonstrate the lesion.
2. Because of superimposition of the spine on the dorsoventral or ventrodorsal projection, the sternal deformity may be difficult to identify.

Fractures of the Sternum and Ribs

Clinical correlations

1. Rib fractures are usually transverse or oblique and are often multiple and sequential.
2. If the fracture is segmental, a flail chest may be present, in which the flailed segment moves inward on inspiration and outward on expiration. This frequently can be life-threatening, especially if the fractures are multiple.
3. Sternal fractures are often associated with luxation and displaced dorsally or ventrally.
4. Depending on the severity of the fractures and intercostal injury, associated complications may include an open or closed pneumothorax, pulmonary contusions, pleural effusion, chest wall hernias, and subcutaneous emphysema.

Radiographic findings (Figures 8.47 and 8.48)

1. Lateral and ventrodorsal projections are necessary to evaluate most rib fractures.
2. Nondisplaced fractures are often difficult to identify; oblique projections may be necessary.
3. Associated radiographic changes of thoracic trauma include subcutaneous emphysema, pneumothorax, pleural hemorrhage, and pulmonary contusions.
4. Healed fractures are usually characterized by smooth bridging callus, but malunion or nonunion of old fractures is commonly seen.
5. Exuberant callus often results secondary to respiratory motion during healing.

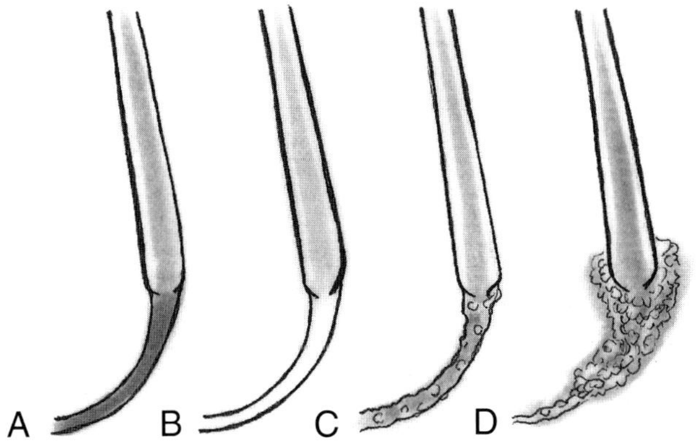

Figure 8.47. Normal costochondral junctions. The costal cartilage is radiolucent in the immature animal (**A**). With aging, the cartilage may ossify (**B**) or show variable degrees of mineralization and ossification (**C, D**).

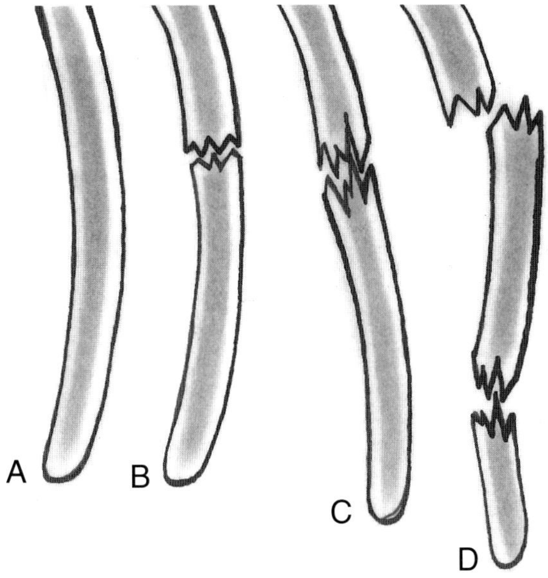

Figure 8.48. Rib fractures. Normal (**A**), transverse nondisplaced (**B**), transverse with slight displacement (**C**), and segmental (**D**).

Masses of the Thoracic Wall

Clinical correlations

1. Extrapleural masses, both benign and malignant, can arise from any element of the thoracic wall including the ribs and intercostal soft tissues.
2. Inflammatory conditions include:
   a. Abscess
   b. Granuloma
   c. Foreign bodies
3. Neoplastic conditions include:
   a. Primary malignant rib tumors
      1) Osteosarcoma (most common)
      2) Chondrosarcoma
      3) Fibrosarcoma
   b. Metastatic tumors (any sarcoma or carcinoma)
   c. Cartilagenous exostosis (osteochondroma)
   d. Soft tissue tumors
      1) Lipoma
      2) Hemangiosarcoma
      3) Neurofibrosarcoma
4. Other conditions:
   a. Hematoma
   b. Healed rib or sternal fractures
   c. Prominent costochondral junctions (a normal variant, especially in chondrodystrophoid dogs)
5. Extrathoracic masses may be palpable; however, most masses tend to enlarge more into the thoracic cavity rather than toward the outside.

Radiographic findings (See Figure 8.41)

1. The soft tissue component usually has a well-defined convex contour facing the lung (called the extrapleural sign).

2. The cranial and caudal margins of the mass are usually tapered or concave and merge with the pleural surface.
3. The widest part of the mass is usually at the site of attachment to the chest wall.
4. The intercostal space may be widened.
5. Periosteal reaction on the affected ribs may be seen.
6. If originating from the rib, irregular lysis, and bone proliferation is often associated with the mass; the rib lesion may also be expansile and/or lytic.
7. Soft tissue masses external to the rib usually may be seen.
8. Pleural effusion may be present if the tumor extends intercostally through the parietal pleura.
9. Differential diagnosis of extrapleural masses:
   a. Pleural abscess
   b. Pleural neoplasm (e.g., mesothelioma, metastatic carcinoma)
   c. Trauma or encapsulated pleural fluid
   d. Pulmonary masses adjacent to the chest wall
10. Additional imaging procedures include tangential views, commonly an oblique projection to visualize the base of the mass.

Contrast radiography
1. Pleurography
2. Diagnostic pneumothorax

Other imaging
1. Ultrasound
2. CT
3. MRI

DIAPHRAGM

RADIOGRAPHIC ANATOMY

1. The diaphragm, a muscular and tendinous structure, separates the abdominal and thoracic cavities.
2. The muscular component is composed of skeletal muscle and attaches to the body wall peripherally, including the ribs (the costal portion), the sternum ventrally (the sternal portion), and the ventral bodies of the third and fourth lumbar vertebrae (the dorsal portion). The dorsal portion forms the crura of the diaphragm.
3. The tendinous component forms the dome of the diaphragm or cupula.
4. Three openings are present in the diaphragm including the aortic hiatus, the esophageal hiatus, and the foramen of the caudal vena cava.

RADIOGRAPHIC INTERPRETATION

1. The appearance of the diaphragm varies with species, breed, and positioning of the animal, the x-ray beam direction, the phase of respiration, and intraabdominal pressure.
2. On any single projection, only a small portion of the diaphragm is visualized. Normally, most of the thoracic surface is visible because of the adjacent gas in the lung, but most of the abdominal surface is not visible because the diaphragm is touching the liver "silhouette sign."
3. In evaluating the diaphragm, one needs to determine whether the diaphragm is in an abnormal position (too far caudal or cranial), whether its shape is symmetric or asymmetric, whether its appearance is continuous or interrupted, and whether there are any irregularities in contour.
4. The positioning is determined by evaluating the distance of the cupula from the heart, the direction and position of the caudal vena cava, the location of the insertions on the ribs, lumbar spine, and sternum, and the shape and location of the costophrenic angles.

Bilateral Displacement of the Diaphragm
1. Causes for cranial displacement:
   a. Obesity
   b. Abdominal distension from peritoneal effusion, pregnancy, abdominal masses, gastric distention, organomegaly (e.g., hepatomegaly)
   c. Pleural adhesions
   d. Severe pain (pleuritis, trauma, peritonitis)
   e. Phrenic nerve paralysis
   f. Bilateral diaphragmatic hernia
   g. Expiration
2. Causes for caudal displacement
   a. Pulmonary hyperinflation (e.g., emphysema, shock, chronic obstructive pulmonary disease, asthma)
   b. Severe pleural effusion or intrathoracic masses
   c. Pneumothorax (especially tension pneumothorax)

Unilateral Displacement of the Diaphragm
1. Causes for cranial displacement of the diaphragm:
   a. Unilateral phrenic paralysis
   b. Diaphragmatic eventration
   c. Diaphragmatic hernia
   d. Unilateral pleural or pulmonary disease with adhesions and/or atelectasis
   e. The effect of spinal or sternal deformities (pectus excavatum, pectus carinatum, scoliosis)
   f. The effect of gastric distension from food or aerophagia
   g. Subdiaphragmatic mass (abdominal abscess, hematoma, or tumor)

2. Causes for caudal displacement of the diaphragm
   a. Unilateral tension pneumothorax
   b. Unilateral pleural effusion
   c. Intrathoracic masses (e.g., pulmonary, pleural, mediastinal)
   d. Bullous emphysema or large pulmonary cysts

DISEASES/DISORDERS

Diaphragmatic Hernia

Clinical correlations

1. Protrusion of the abdominal viscera through the diaphragm into the thoracic cavity
2. Congenital hernias:
   a. Peritoneal-pericardial diaphragmatic hernia
   b. Peritoneal-mediastinal diaphragmatic hernia
   c. Eventration of the diaphragm
   d. Absence of part of the diaphragm
   e. Hiatal hernias
      1) Paraesophageal hernia
      2) Paravenous diaphragmatic hernia (caudal vena cava)
      3) Para-aortic diaphragmatic hernia
3. Acquired hernias:
   a. Usually traumatic and may be associated with other injuries
   b. The diaphragm is often torn along the costal attachment of the diaphragm to the rib cage, but may involve the central portion of the diaphragm.
   c. Variable degree of herniation of abdominal viscera into the pleural cavity
4. Clinical signs:
   a. The degree of respiratory or abdominal visceral embarrassment depends on the degree of internal displacement and the overall affect on the patient's status.
   b. May have no clinical signs.

Radiographic findings (Figure 8.49)

1. Interruption or nonvisualization of the diaphragmatic silhouette in one or more radiographic projections
2. In congenital hernias, there may be:
   a. Enlargement of the cardiac silhouette with or without the presence of gas-filled loops within the pericardial space (peritoneal-pericardial diaphragmatic hernia)
   b. Caudal mediastinal mass (peritoneal-mediastinal diaphragmatic hernia, esophageal, aortic, or paravenous hernia)
   c. Extrapleural mass originating from the diaphragmatic surface extending into the thorax (eventration or true hernia).
   d. Differential diagnosis:
      1) Intrapulmonary mass at the pleural border
      2) Diaphragmatic tumor
      3) Esophageal mass

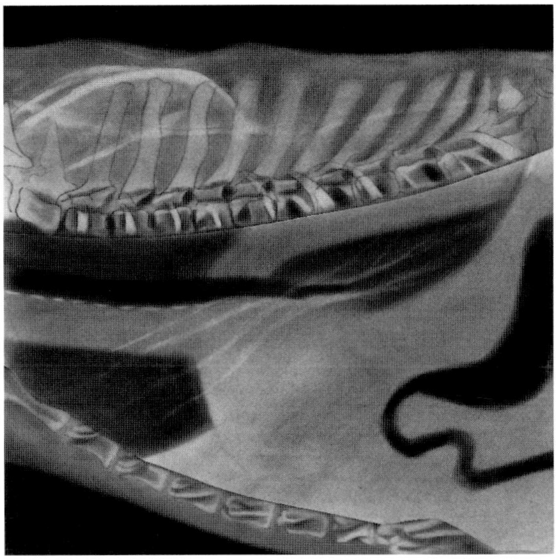

Figure 8.49. Diaphragmatic hernia. The cardiac silhouette is partially obscured because the liver and stomach are herniated into the thorax.

      4) Gastroesophageal intussusception
      5) Hiatal hernia
      6) Paraesophageal hernia
3. Traumatic hernias frequently have associated:
   a. Pleural effusion (unilateral or bilateral)
   b. Cranial displacement or malposition of the abdominal viscera (liver, bowel, etc.)
   c. Other evidence of trauma (e.g., pneumothorax, lung contusion, subcutaneous emphysema, rib fractures)
4. Adjunctive radiographic examinations that may aid in establishing a definitive diagnosis.
   a. If pleural fluid is present, remove the fluid through thoracentesis and then reradiograph the thorax.
   b. Ultrasound is often helpful in evaluating the integrity of the diaphragm and confirming presence and type of herniated viscera.
   c. Upper gastrointestinal examination is useful if the stomach or small bowel is herniated into the chest.
   d. Positive contrast peritoneography (celiography) using iodinated contrast media. If contrast medium is present in the peritoneal and pleural cavities, a hernia is confirmed. A false-negative may result if the hernia is completely obstructed by the herniated viscera.
   e. Pneumoperitoneography is generally not recommended if a hernia is present because a pneumothorax will result.
   f. In chronic hernias in which the hernial opening is totally obstructed with abdominal viscera or scar tissue, a definitive diagnosis may not be possible.

Diaphragmatic Tumors

Clinical correlations

1. Primary and metastatic tumors are uncommon.
2. Most tumors extend into the abdominal cavity.

Radiographic findings
1. Tumors on the peritoneal surface may not be apparent on survey abdominal radiographs.
2. Tumors extending into the thorax will appear as an extrapleural mass. Differentiation from diaphragmatic hernia or eventration should be made.

Contrast radiography
1. Celiography
2. Pneumoperitoneography

Other imaging
1. Ultrasound
2. CT
3. MRI

Diaphragmatic Abscess
Clinical correlations
1. Usually secondary to a walled-off abdominal abscess caused by peritonitis or a migrating plant awn (e.g., foxtail).
2. Usually affects the peritoneal surface of the diaphragm, but can affect the pleural side of the diaphragm and involve the lung or mediastinum.

Radiographic findings
1. May appear as a mass on the diaphragm, but often not visible on the survey radiographs.

Contrast radiography
1. Celiography
2. Pneumoperitoneography

Other imaging
1. Ultrasound
2. CT
3. MRI

chapter nine

9

Heart

Thoracic radiography is an integral part of the cardiovascular examination. The clinician must understand the normal radiographic anatomy, including the variables of age, breed, and conformation, as well as phases of the respiratory and cardiac cycles, and the abnormal radiographic anatomy of the heart in disease. In the abnormal state, it is essential to correlate the compensatory and pathophysiologic mechanisms of heart disease and heart failure.

RADIOGRAPHIC TECHNIQUE

Exposure Technique and Film Quality

1. Use short exposure time (preferably 1/60 or 1/120 second) to minimize motion artifact.
2. A grid is used to improve image quality when the chest is thicker than 10 cm.
3. 400 speed high latitude film-screen systems are recommended for most thoracic radiographs.
4. Radiographic exposures should be made at the peak of inspiration.

Standard Projections

1. Lateral projection (right or left recumbent position):
   a. The right lateral is reported to result in less distortion of the cardiac silhouette.
   b. The left lateral commonly results in less contact of the cardiac silhouette with the sternum.
2. Dorsoventral projection:
   a. The position and shape of the heart in the dog is less variable on a dorsoventral projection than on a ventrodorsal projection (e.g., normal cardiac apex tends to be oriented more toward the midline or right side on a ventrodorsal projection).
   b. If pleural effusion is present, the cardiac silhouette is commonly obscured on a dorsoventral but not on a ventrodorsal projection.
   c. The ventrodorsal projection is commonly recommended for assessment of the lung.

Supplemental Projections

1. Opposite lateral projection. Normal and abnormal structures can be more or less visible on one lateral projection than on the other.
2. Ventrodorsal projection. In cats, easier to do than dorsoventral projection and results in a more constant appearance of the heart.
3. Right and left dorsoventral (or ventrodorsal) oblique projections. Assessment of cardiac chamber size is unreliable on oblique projections.

Contrast Radiography

1. Esophagram
   a. Evaluation of mediastinal and heart-based masses
   b. Diagnosis of vascular ring anomalies (e.g., persistent right fourth aortic arch)
   c. Localization of the esophagus before transthoracic biopsy of mediastinal, pulmonary, or heart-based masses
2. Nonselective angiogram
   a. Evaluation of the cranial or vena cava and heart base
   b. Visualizing the anatomy of the right heart, the presence of severe pericardial effusion, and in assessing some cardiac wall masses
   c. Diagnosis and differentiation of some forms of feline cardiomyopathy
   d. Diagnosis of some congenital heart defects (e.g., pulmonic stenosis, Tetralogy of Fallot)
   e. Demonstration of intracardiac or aortic clots
   f. Diagnosis of pulmonary thrombosis (if severe)
3. Selective angiocardiography:
   a. Provides accurate assessment of congenital and acquired heart disease.
   b. A catheter can be directed to a specific chamber or vessel and permits pressures to be measured at specific sites.
   c. Is optimum for assessment of pulmonary arteries.

4. Pneumopericardiography
   a. Permits delineation of the pericardial sac, the epicardial surface of the heart, and the heart base.
   b. Is most often done when a pericardial effusion is present, and gas is infused into the pericardial cavity after the removal of pericardial fluid.
   c. When ultrasound is available, is rarely indicated.

Other Imaging

1. Echocardiography (also refer to Chapter 1)
   a. Two-dimensional (2-D) echocardiography allows real-time imaging of a plane of tissue (both width and depth), and is useful in assessing the cardiac wall and valvular motion during the cardiac cycle, and allows assessment of the cardiac chamber size and wall thickness.
   b. M-mode provides a one-dimensional view of depth and displays echos from various interfaces along the axis of the beam over time. These echos, which move during the cardiac cycle, are swept across the screen as a function of time.
      1) A high sampling rate is used and provides better images of the cardiac borders and valvular edges.
      2) Allows objective measurements of the thickness of the cardiac wall, the size of the cardiac chambers, and valvular motion that occur during systole and diastole.
   c. Contrast echocardiography uses a substance that contains microbubbles (often agitated saline), which is injected into a peripheral vein or selectively into a specific cardiac chamber. These bubbles are reflective and the flow of blood can be observed. When injected into a peripheral vein, a right to left shunt can be demonstrated. Because the bubbles do not pass through the lung, a selective injection in the left heart can be used to evaluate mitral and aortic valvular disease and left-to-right shunts.
2. Doppler echocardiography
   a. Allows evaluation of blood flow quality and velocity
   b. Enables documentation and quantification of valvular regurgitation or stenosis and some intracardiac shunts
   c. Cardiac output can be determined when combined with 2-D measurements
   d. There are different types of Doppler that are complementary and should be combined in each patient for an accurate and complete evaluation.
      1) Pulsed wave Doppler
         a) Uses short bursts of ultrasound transmitted to a designated point, distant to the transducer, and permits calculation of blood flow velocity, direction, and spectral characteristics (turbulent versus laminar) from a specific point in the heart or blood vessel.
         b) Its limitation is in the assessment of high-velocity signals (>1.5 m/second) because the pulse repetition frequency is limited.
      2) Continuous wave Doppler
         a) Uses dual crystals so that ultrasound waves can be sent and received simultaneously.
         b) High velocity flows (>1.5 m/second) can be measured.
         c) Its major disadvantage is that the sampling of blood flow velocity and direction occurs all along the ultrasound beam, not localized to a specific area.
      3) Color Doppler
         a) Is a form of pulsed wave Doppler that combines the M-mode and 2-D modalities with blood flow imaging.
         b) Instead of one sample volume, many volumes are analyzed along multiple scan lines.
         c) The mean frequency shift is color coded for direction and velocity. Using different maps with variations in color and brightness, differences can be seen in relative velocity of flow and the presence of multiple velocities of flow, as that which occurs with turbulence.
         d) Demonstrates turbulent flow and intracardiac shunts.
         e) Differences in relative flow velocity can be accentuated.
         f) Major disadvantages are that high velocity flows are difficult to evaluate and absolute velocity measurements cannot be derived.
      4) CT angiography
      5) MRI angiography

RADIOGRAPHIC ANATOMY OF NORMAL CANINE AND FELINE HEART (Figures 9.1 through 9.4)

Lateral Projection

1. In the dog, the cardiac silhouette appears somewhat oval in shape and its long axis lies approximately 45° with the cardiac apex oriented caudally. The cat's cardiac silhouette is more slender in diameter with the apex more pointed in shape.
2. The dog's cardiac silhouette usually extends from the third to the eighth thoracic vertebrae with the middle of the heart base at the level of the carina near the fifth or sixth intercostal space. In most cats, the heart is located from the fourth to the sixth ribs.
   a. Normal "rule of thumb" for size of a normal cardiac silhouette in the dog varies with the size and shape of the dog's thorax, but usually ranges from 2.5 to 3.5 times the width of the intercostal spaces. The respiratory phase also alters the relative size of the heart to the thorax. The heart appears relatively smaller on inspiration compared to expiration.

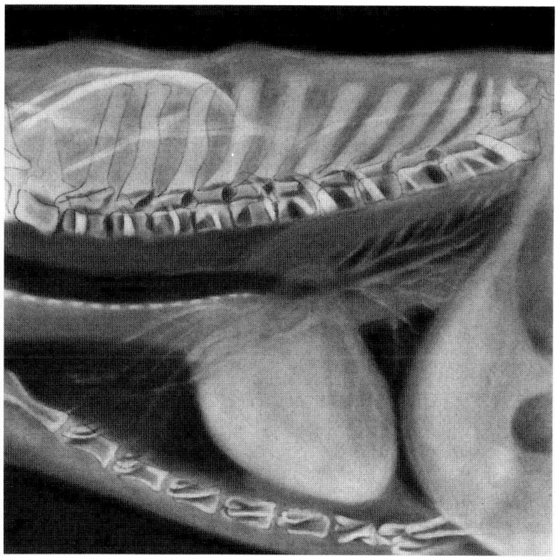

Figure 9.1. Normal canine thorax, lateral projection.

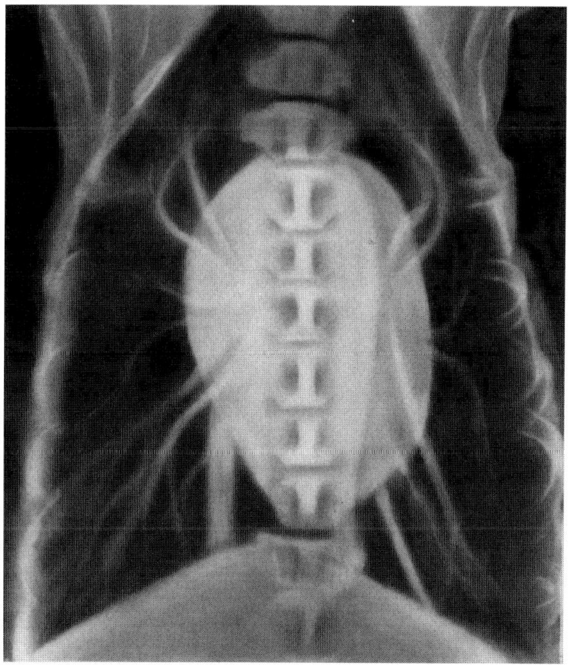

Figure 9.2. Normal canine thorax, dorsoventral projection.

1) A cardiac silhouette the width of 2.5 intercostal spaces is common in deep and narrow-chested dogs, especially if the radiographs are made at the peak of inspiration.
2) Dogs with barrel-shaped chests often have a cardiac silhouette closer to the width of 3.5 intercostal spaces.

b. Normal "rule of thumb" for size of a normal cardiac silhouette in the cat is approximately the width of 2 intercostal spaces.

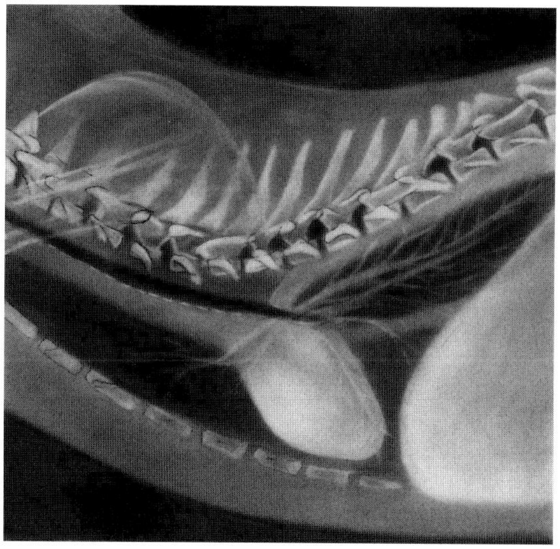

Figure 9.3. Normal feline thorax, lateral projection.

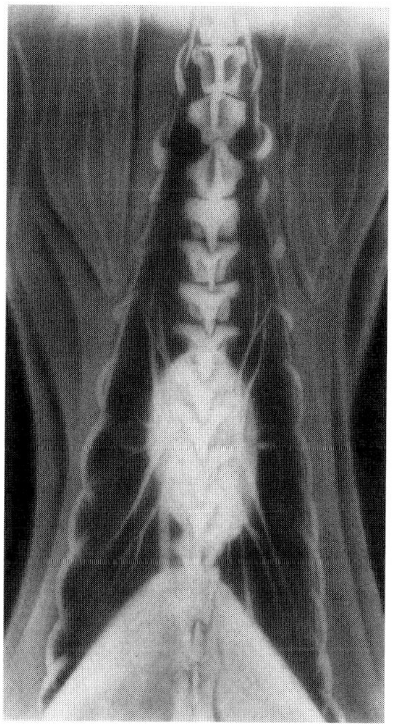

Figure 9.4. Normal feline thorax, dorsoventral projection.

3. The cardiac silhouette usually occupies approximately 70% of the distance from the sternum to the thoracic spine. The long axis of the cat's cardiac silhouette may lie more parallel with the sternum than in the dog.
4. The cranial heart border extends from the ventral surface of the mediastinum, adjacent to the cranial vena cava caudal to the cardiac apex. The dorsal one third of the cranial border is caused by the right auricular appendage and portion of the ascending aorta. The ventral two thirds of the border is caused by the wall of the right ventricle. The cranial "waistline" is the junction of the cranial vena cava and the right ventricular border.

5. The caudal heart border is normally slightly curved. As it extends dorsally from the apex, it forms a small sulcus, the caudal "waistline," corresponding to the junction between the left ventricle and left atrium. The caudal heart border may touch or overlap the cranioventral aspect of the diaphragm near its sternal attachment with the degree of overlap being greater in the expiratory phase.
6. The base of the cardiac silhouette consists of a portion of the aortic arch. Cranially, most of the base is obscured by the trachea and major bronchi.
7. The ascending aorta, present within the mediastinum, is partially superimposed over the right atrium. The aortic arch then extends caudodorsally to form the descending aorta.
8. The main pulmonary artery (pulmonary trunk) cannot be seen on the lateral projection, because of its silhouette with the cardiac base.
   a. The left pulmonary artery can sometimes be seen extending dorsal and caudal to the tracheal bifurcation.
   b. The right pulmonary artery is frequently seen end-on as a spherical shaped soft tissue radiopacity, ventral to the carina as it branches from the main pulmonary artery.
9. The pulmonary arteries and veins can be seen in the hilar and central regions of the lung
   a. The arteries are located dorsal to their respective bronchi and veins.
   b. The cranial lobar vessels can often be seen as two pairs of vessels, cranial to or superimposed over the cardiac silhouette.
      1) On right lateral recumbency, the more ventral pair of vessels are usually the artery and vein to the right cranial lung lobe. The left cranial lobe artery and vein are located more dorsal and usually superimposed on the cranial mediastinum.
      2) The dorsal vessel of each pair is the cranial lobar artery and the ventral vessel of each pair is the cranial lobar vein.
   c. The pulmonary veins from the caudal lobes are seen as they enter the left atrium caudal to the heart base.

Dorsoventral Projection

1. The canine heart is somewhat elliptical in shape with its axis normally oriented approximately 30° to the spine, with the cardiac apex slightly left of the midline.
2. The heart normally extends from the third to the eighth thoracic vertebrae with the caudal border of the heart adjacent to or superimposed on the diaphragm, depending on the phase of respiration.
3. In a dog with mesomorphic conformation, the width of the heart across its widest point is usually 60 to 65% of the thoracic width.
4. In the cat, the heart is more oval and thinner. The cardiac apex is more variable in position, and is usually on or to the left of the midline, but may be to the right of the midline.
5. The borders of the cardiac silhouette are caused by the right atrium and right ventricle on the right side, the aorta and main pulmonary artery on the cranial side, and the left ventricle on the left side.
6. The clock analogy can be used to simplify the radiographic anatomy of the cardiac silhouette (Figure 9.5).
   a. The aortic arch extends from the 11 to 1 o'clock position.
   b. The main pulmonary artery segment is located from the 1 to 2 o'clock position.
   c. In the dog, the normal left atrium does not contribute to the cardiac border; however, when enlarged, the left auricle contributes to the 2 to 3 o'clock position. In the cat, the normal left atrium contributes to the cardiac border from the 2 to 3 o'clock position.
   d. The left ventricle forms the left heart border from the 2 to 6 o'clock position in the dog and the 3 to 6 o'clock position in the cat.
   e. The right ventricle is located from the 6 to 11 o'clock position.
   f. The right atrium is located at the 9 to 11 o'clock position.
7. The pulmonary arteries can usually be seen superimposed over the cardiac silhouette originating from the main pulmonary artery.
   a. The left caudal lobar pulmonary artery extends beyond the left heart border at approximately the 4 o'clock position.

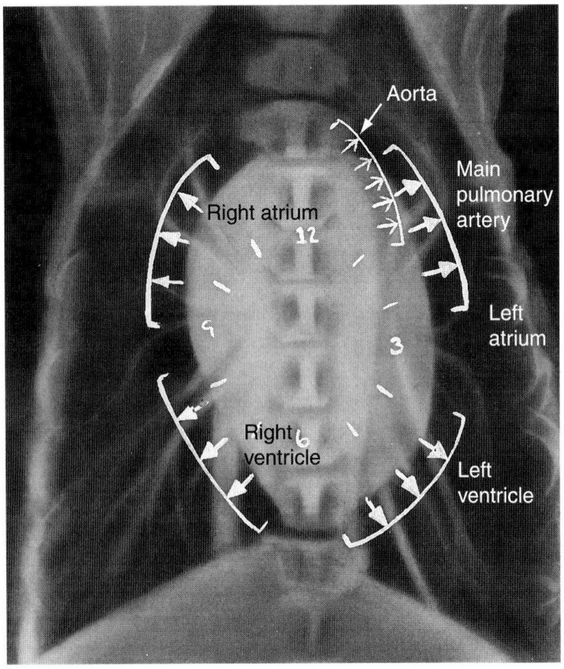

Figure 9.5. Clock analogy of the canine cardiac silhouette.

b. The right caudal lobar pulmonary artery extends beyond the right heart border at approximately the 8 o'clock position.

8. The pulmonary veins can usually be seen as they enter the left atrium.
   a. The left caudal lobar vein is located at approximately the 5 o'clock position.
   b. The right caudal lobar vein is located at approximately the 7 o'clock position.
9. The aortic arch is within the cranial mediastinum at the cranial heart border and is not visible. The descending aorta is seen as a superimposed soft tissue opacity over the heart, extending caudally and medially. The aorta's left lateral border is seen to the left, adjacent to the vertebral column.

RADIOGRAPHIC INTERPRETATION

1. Proper viewing of the radiographs on an x-ray illuminator is essential.
   a. Lateral radiographic projections, both left and right, should be oriented on the illuminator with the animal's head toward the left. The normal heart usually has more sternal contact on a right lateral recumbent projection than on a left lateral recumbent projection. The normal heart on the left lateral recumbent projection can fall away from sternum with less cardiosternal contact and may mimic a pneumothorax.
   b. Dorsoventral and ventrodorsal radiographic projections should be oriented on the illuminator with the animal's left side to the observer's right.
      1) The normal cardiac silhouette is more consistent in its position on the dorsoventral projection. On the ventrodorsal projection, the heart can rotate on its axis and the margin of the normal cardiac silhouette can mimic cardiac disease (e.g., a normal pulmonary artery segment can appear enlarged and mimic heartworm disease or poststenotic enlargement of the main pulmonary artery, especially in deep narrow-chested dogs).
      2) On the ventrodorsal projection, the normal cardiac apex is commonly positioned on the midline. The normal heart is more likely to rotate into the right hemithorax and mimic right heart enlargement (e.g., dextrocardia).
      3) When pleural effusion is present, the heart is usually obscured on a dorsoventral projection. When effusion is present, the cardiac silhouette, lung, and pulmonary vessels are usually more visible on a ventrodorsal view.
2. Evaluate the radiographs for technical quality, positioning, and proper exposure factors.
   a. Positioning:
      1) On the lateral projection, the dorsal portions of the ribs should overlap and be aligned with each other.
      2) On the dorsoventral or ventrodorsal projection, the sternum, vertebral bodies, and dorsal spinous processes should be superimposed.
   b. Proper exposure factors:
      1) Adequate contrast of the lung field and visualization of the pulmonary vessels
      2) Absence of motion artifact (e.g., no blurring of the ribs)
3. Determine whether the radiograph was made at inspiration or expiration by observing the position of the diaphragm relative to the heart.
4. Analyze the extracirculatory structures (spine, sternum, diaphragm, thoracic wall, ribs, and liver).
5. Evaluate the position and diameter of the trachea and the tracheal bifurcation.
6. Evaluate the cranial mediastinum for widening, abnormal radiopacity, or the presence of an abnormal mass.
7. Evaluate the aorta and the aortic arch in terms of size and position.
8. Evaluate the position of the cardiac apex and the caudal mediastinum.
9. Evaluate the size and shape of the main pulmonary artery and the peripheral pulmonary arteries and veins.
10. Evaluate the lung for areas of increased or decreased radiopacity.
11. Evaluate the cardiac borders for enlargement or abnormal position.

NORMAL HEART SIZE AND SHAPE

1. On the radiographs, the cardiac silhouette is a composite of the heart, pericardium, mediastinal fat, and other structures at the hilus of the lung.
   a. The internal chambers of the heart and the coronary arteries are not visible on survey radiographs.
   b. The junctions of the ventricles and atria can be inferred, but are not visible. Estimation of the cardiac chambers on a lateral projection can be done by drawing an imaginary "line" through the middle of the heart from the apex to the carina.
      1) The right side of the heart is located cranial to this line.
      2) The left side of the heart is located caudal to this line.
   c. A second imaginary line drawn perpendicular to the first and approximately two thirds the distance from the apex to the carina roughly divides the atria from the ventricles.
      1) The right and left atria are dorsal to this line.
      2) The ventricles are ventral to this line.

2. Numerous variations of normal exist because of the variations in the shape and size of the thoracic cavity, especially in dogs. There is less variation between breeds of cats.
3. Numerous methods have been proposed for measuring the cardiac silhouette, for identifying abnormalities, and for comparing changes over time. Two of the most useful methods for clinical application include:
   a. Empirical measurement
      1) This measurement uses the lateral and dorsoventral projection in the assessment of heart size.
         a) On the lateral projection, the normal heart in the dog is approximately 2.5 to 3.5 intercostal spaces in width.
         b) On the dorsoventral projection, the normal heart in the dog, at its widest point, is approximately two thirds the width of the thoracic cavity.
         c) On the lateral projection, the normal heart in the cat is approximately the width of 2 intercostal spaces.
      2) On the lateral projection, the relative size of the left and right heart may be a helpful aid for interpretation.
         a) An imaginary line drawn from carina of trachea to the apex, divides the cranial two thirds of the heart into the right heart and the caudal one third of the heart into the left heart for the dog.
         b) The location of carina of heart in the cat should not exceed 70% of the dorsoventral distance, based on a line drawn from the ventral margin of the thoracic vertebra through the long axis of the heart to the apex.
      3) Ranges of normal in the different breeds are largely subjective and based largely on individual experience.
      4) Individual chamber enlargement or overall heart enlargement is more significant if the abnormal changes are seen on both the lateral and dorsoventral projections.
      5) Comparisons of an animal's previous radiographs are helpful for assessing abnormalities and changes in the heart and other structures.
   b. Vertebral heart size (VHS by Buchanan) measures the cardiac dimensions, which are then scaled against the length of specific thoracic vertebra.
      1) In the dog, the sum of the long and short axes of the heart on the lateral projection is measured against the number of vertebrae beginning at T4 and proceeding caudally. The VHS is expressed as a unit of vertebral length. If left heart enlargement is obvious, the short axis measurement is made at the dorsal juncture of the left atrial and caudal vena cava silhouettes. The normal VHS range for the heart in most dogs is 8.5 to 10.5.
      2) In the cat, the short axis of the heart can be measured from the dorsoventral projection, and compared to the number of vertebrae on the lateral view beginning at T4 and proceeding caudally. The normal VHS range for the heart in cats is 3.2 to 3.8.

Normal Variables for Heart Size and Shape

1. Thoracic conformation differences
   a. Deep narrow-chested breeds (e.g., Setters, Collies, and Afghans) (Figures 9.6 and 9.7)

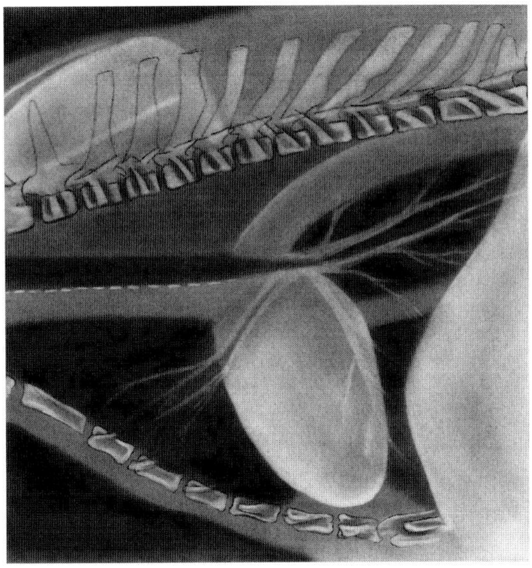

Figure 9.6. Normal thorax of deep narrow-chested breed (e.g., Setter).

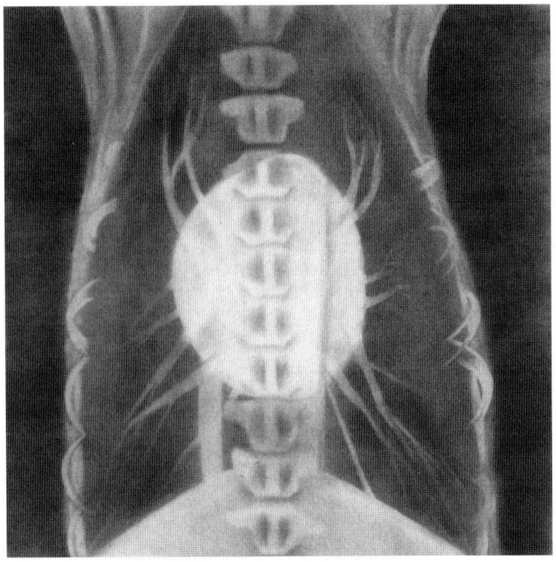

Figure 9.7. Normal thorax of deep narrow-chested breed (e.g., Setter).

1) On the lateral projection, the heart appears more vertical and narrower (approximately 2 ½ intercostal spaces in width).
2) On the dorsoventral projection, the heart appears more rounded and smaller.

b. Shallow wide-chested breeds (e.g., chondrodystrophoid breeds) (Figures 9.8 and 9.9).
   1) On the lateral projection, the heart appears more rounded with increased sternal contact and a more dorsal position of the trachea. The heart also appears larger, often measuring 3 to 3 1/2 intercostal spaces in width.
   2) On the dorsoventral projection, the heart is more rounded.

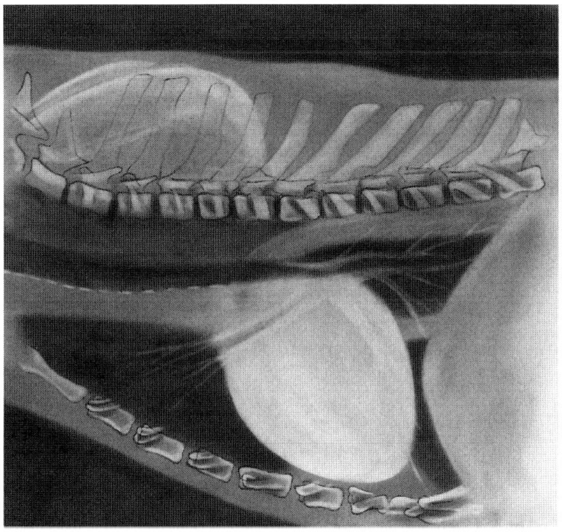

Figure 9.8. Normal thorax of shallow wide-chested breed (e.g., Dachshund).

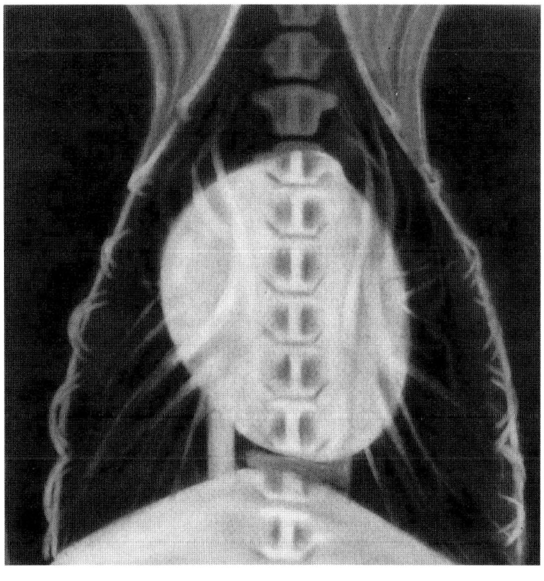

Figure 9.9. Normal thorax of shallow wide-chested breed (e.g., Dachshund).

2. Age differences
   a. Younger animals appear to have larger hearts, relative to the thoracic size, than they do at maturity.
   b. Older cats may have a heart with less inclination on the lateral projection with increased sternal contact, and an arched or kinked appearance to the aortic arch. The aortic arch is seen as a rounded and prominent structure on the dorsoventral/ventrodorsal projection (Figures 9.10 and 9.11).

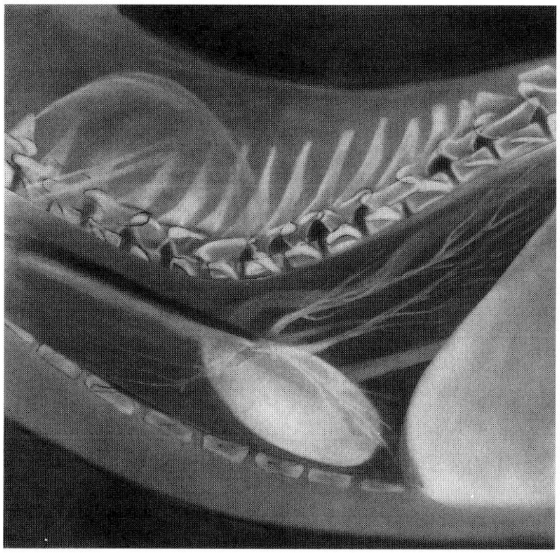

Figure 9.10. Normal thorax of aged cat. Note the more horizontal positon of the heart and the tortuosity of the descending aorta.

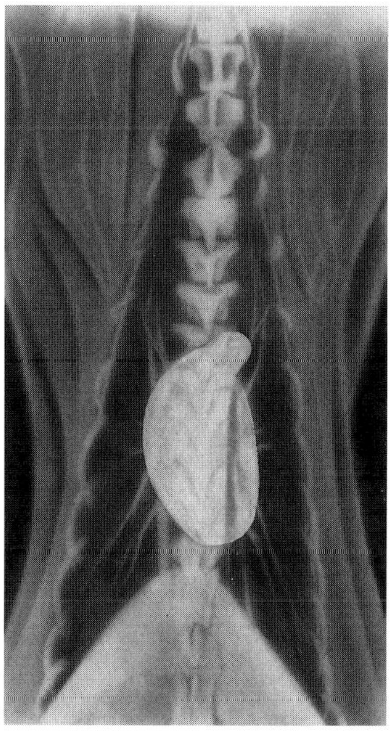

Figure 9.11. Normal aged cat. The aortic arch is more prominent and seen as a round structure.

3. Systole versus diastole. During systole, the heart is slightly smaller than during diastole; however, this difference is difficult to perceive on radiographs.
4. Phase of respiration at time of radiographic exposure
   a. The heart does not change in size or shape, but appears smaller on inspiration than it does on expiration because of the relative size of thoracic cavity.
   b. During expiration, there is increased sternal contact of the right heart and dorsal elevation of the trachea, falsely suggesting right heart enlargement.
5. Positional differences
   a. Slight obliquity on the dorsoventral or ventrodorsal projection will cause significant differences in the cardiac size and shape.
   b. The cardiac shape is more variable on the ventrodorsal than the dorsoventral projection.

EVALUATION OF HEART CHAMBER ENLARGEMENT

1. It is often difficult to recognize individual chamber enlargement because of many factors, including normal variation, and the restriction of the pericardial sac in allowing the protrusion or enlargement of an individual chamber. In many animals with cardiac disease, two or more chambers are usually affected by a volume or pressure load, with dilation and/or hypertrophy.
2. The normal anatomy of the heart is schematically illustrated in Figures 9.12 through 9.14.

The following discussion of individual chamber enlargement is intended to serve as a guideline in the radiographic assessment.

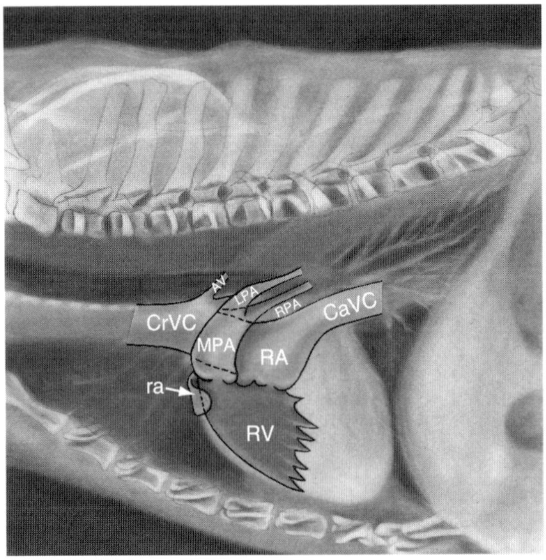

Figure 9.12. Cardiac anatomy of canine right heart: cranial vena cava (**CrVC**), caudal vena cava (**CaCV**), right atrium (**RA**), right ventricle (**RV**), right auricle (**ra**), main pulmonary artery (**MPA**), left pulmonary artery (**LPA**), right pulmonary artery (**RPA**), and azygous vein (**AV**).

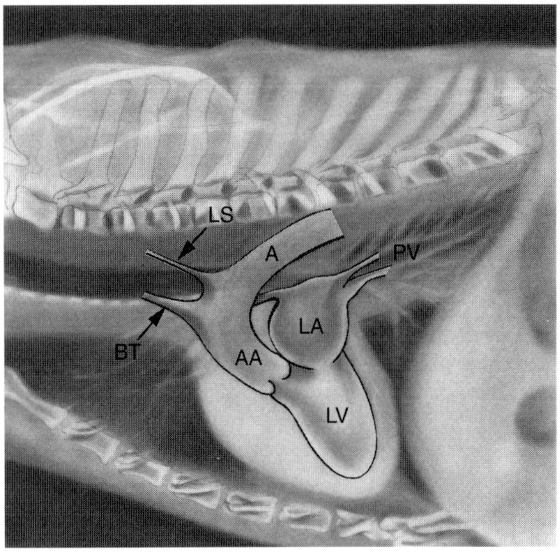

Figure 9.13. Cardiac anatomy of canine left heart. Left atrium, left ventricle (**LV**), aortic arch (**AA**), aorta (**A**), pulmonary veins (**PV**), brachycephalic trunk (**BT**), and left subclavian artery (**LS**).

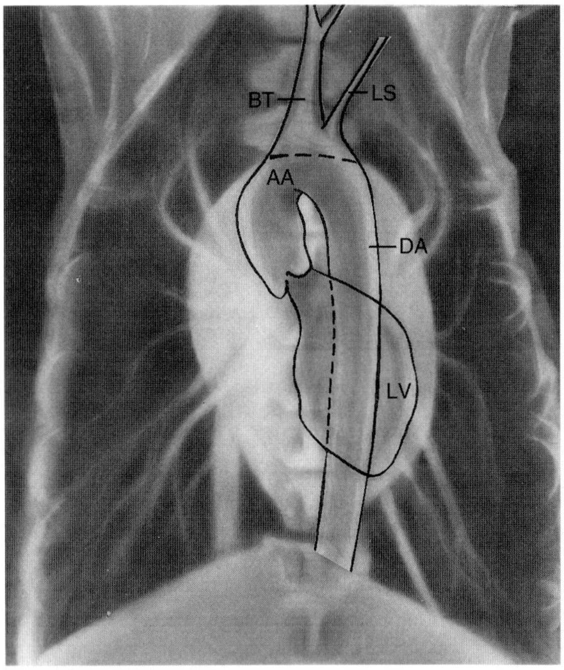

Figure 9.14. Cardiac anatomy: left ventricle and aorta of canine, left ventricle (**LV**), aortic arch (**AA**), descending aorta (**DA**), brachycephalic trunk (**BT**), and left subclavian vein (**LS**).

Right Atrial Enlargement

Radiographic findings

1. Lateral projection
   a. Elevation of the trachea as it courses dorsally over the right atrium
   b. Cranial bulging of the cardiac silhouette with loss of the cranial waist

2. Dorsoventral projection. Enlargement of the cardiac border at the 9 to 11 o'clock position

Causes of right atrial enlargement

1. Tricuspid insufficiency (See Figures 9.31 and 9.32)
2. Cardiomyopathy
3. Right-atrial tumor
4. Cor pulmonale

Differential diagnosis

1. Superimposed enlargement of the main pulmonary artery or aortic arch
2. Hilar lymphadenopathy
3. Heart base tumor (e.g., chemodectoma) (See Figures 9.43 and 9.44)
4. Cranial mediastinal tumor

Right Ventricular Enlargement

Radiographic findings

1. Lateral projection:
   a. Increased sternal contact of the right heart and elevation of the cardiac apex
   b. Dorsal elevation of the trachea relative to the thoracic spine
   c. Rounding of the right heart border
   d. Elevation of the caudal vena cava
2. Dorsoventral projection:
   a. Rounding of the right heart border
   b. Shift of the cardiac apex to the left
   c. In marked enlargement, the right ventricle assumes an inverted "D" sign.

Causes of right ventricular enlargement

1. Tricuspid insufficiency (See Figures 9.31 and 9.32)
2. Cardiomyopathy (See Figures 9.37 and 9.38)
3. Pulmonary hypertension
   a. Cor pulmonale
   b. Heartworm disease (See Figures 9.34 and 9.35)
   c. Pulmonary thromboembolism
4. Congenital heart disease:
   a. Pulmonic stenosis (See Figures 9.21 and 9.22)
   b. Left-to-right shunts (e.g., atrial and ventricular septal defects, aortic pulmonary window)
   c. Tetralogy of Fallot

Left-Atrial Enlargement

Radiographic findings

1. Lateral projection:
   a. Dorsal elevation of the distal portion of the trachea and the carina
   b. Dorsal displacement of the left bronchus
   c. Mild enlargement will cause loss of caudal waist.
   d. Severe enlargement may cause accentuation of the caudal waist with the dilated atrium extending dorsally and caudally.
   e. In the cat, the distal trachea and carina may be elevated, but left bronchial displacement is not seen.
2. Dorsoventral projection
   a. Increased opacity over the heart base is caused by summation of the enlarged left atrium.
   b. Bulging of the left heart border is caused by dilation of the left auricular appendage
      1) In the dog usually at the 2 to 3 o'clock position
      2) In the cat, usually at the 1 to 3 o'clock position

Causes of left atrial enlargement

1. Mitral insufficiency (See Figures 9.27, 9.28, 9.29, 9.30)
2. Cardiomyopathy (See Figures 9.35 and 9.42)
3. Congenital heart disease
   a. Mitral dysplasia
   b. Patent ductus arteriosus (See Figures 9.19 and 9.20)
   c. Ventricular septal defect

Differential Diagnosis

1. Hilar lymphadenopathy
2. Cardiac tumor

Left Ventricular Enlargement

Radiographic findings

1. Lateral projection
   a. Loss of the caudal waist, with the left heart border straighter and more vertical than normal.
   b. Elongation and/or widening of the cardiac silhouette
   c. Elevation of the distal trachea and carina
2. Dorsoventral projection
   a. Rounding of the left ventricular border
   b. Decreased distance between the left heart border and the chest wall
   c. Shift of the cardiac apex to the right (especially in cats)

Causes of left ventricular enlargement

1. Mitral insufficiency (See Figures 9.27 through 9.30)
2. Cardiomyopathy (See Figures 9.35 and 9.42)
3. Congenital heart disease:
   a. Patent ductus arteriosus (See Figures 9.19 and 9.20)
   b. Aortic stenosis (See Figures 9.23 and 9.24)
   c. Ventricular septal defect
4. High output heart disease:
   a. Hypervolemia (e.g., fluid overload)
   b. Chronic anemia
   c. Peripheral arteriovenous fistula
   d. Obesity
5. Hyperthyroidism
6. Systemic hypertension

Generalized Heart Enlargement

Radiographic findings (Figures 9.15 and 9.16)

1. There are variable degrees of enlargement of two or more cardiac chambers.

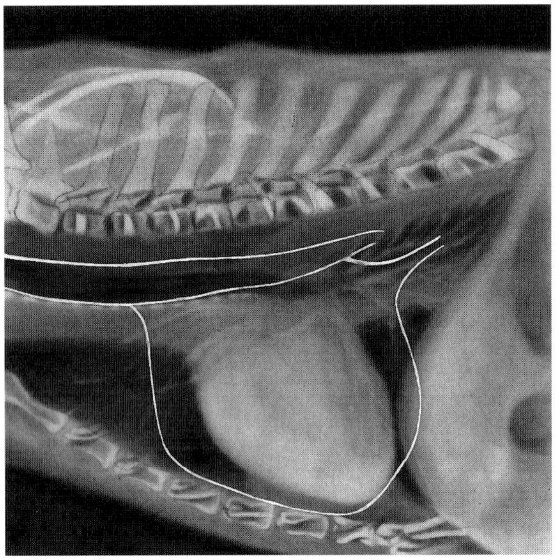

Figure 9.15. Cardiomegaly. Enlargement of the cardiac silhouette is primarily caused by enlargement of the ventricles. Right ventricular enlargement causes increased sternal contact of the cardiac border and elevation of the trachea. The left ventricular border is straighter than normal with caudodorsal displacement of the left atrium.

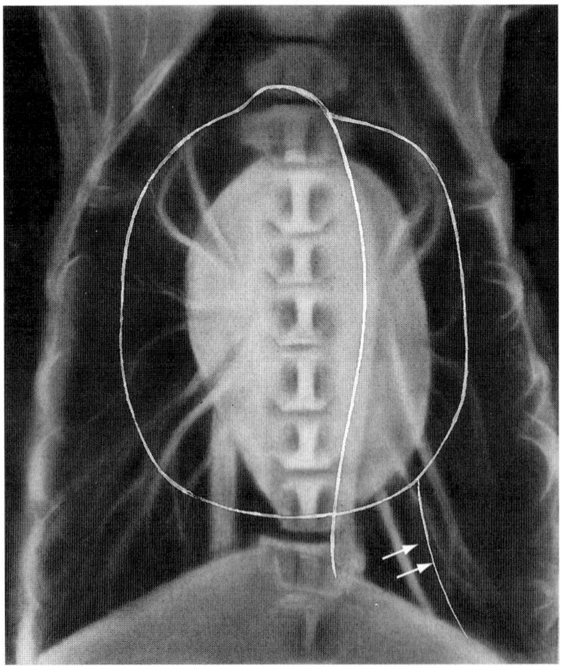

Figure 9.16. Cardiomegaly. Enlargement of the cardiac silhouette is primarily caused by ventricular enlargement. Note that the aortic arch is displaced cranially and the cardiac apex is shifted to the left (arrows).

2. Chamber enlargement implies dilatation, hypertrophy, or both.
3. Enlargement of the cardiac silhouette also includes the pericardium and contents of the pericardial cavity.

Causes of generalized cardiomegaly

1. Chronic mitral and tricuspid insufficiency (See Figures 9.27 through 9.32)
2. Left-sided heart failure
3. Cardiomyopathy (See Figures 9.35 through 9.42)
4. Ventricular septal defect

Differential diagnosis

1. Pericardial effusion (See Figures 9.45 and 9.46)
2. Peritoneal-pericardial diaphragmatic hernia
3. Obesity with increased pericardial fat

EVALUATION OF MAJOR VESSELS

Aortic Arch and Aorta

Radiographic findings

1. Lateral projection
   a. Elongated cardiac silhouette
   b. Enlargement of the craniodorsal heart border
   c. Loss of cranial waist
2. Dorsoventral projection
   a. Widened aortic arch at the cranial heart border (11–1 o'clock position)
   b. Irregular enlargement of the aortic arch or descending aorta

Causes of enlarged aortic arch

1. Aortic stenosis. A poststenotic dilatation is most prominent on the lateral projection, but may also be seen on the dorsoventral or ventrodorsal projection. (See Figures 9.23 and 9.24)
2. Patent ductus arteriosus. An aneurysmal bulge (ductus diverticulum) is best seen on the dorsoventral or ventrodorsal projection as a protrusion on the left side of the descending aorta. (See Figures 9.19 and 9.20)
3. Aortic aneurysm
4. Is a normal variant in aged cats in which aortic arch is seen as being dilated and tortuous. On the dorsoventral or ventrodorsal projection, a knob is often seen to the left of the midline. (See Figures 9.10 and 9.11)
5. Normal anatomic variant in some dogs.

Pulmonary Artery Segment Enlargement

Radiographic findings

1. Lateral projection. Protrusion of the craniodorsal heart border
2. Dorsoventral projection. Lateral bulge of the heart border at the 1 to 2 o'clock position

Causes for enlarged pulmonary artery segment
1. Pulmonic stenosis (See Figures 9.21 and 9.22)
2. Dirofilariasis (See Figures 9.33 and 9.34)
3. Congenital heart disease with left-to-right shunts
   a. Patent ductus arteriosus (See Figures 9.19 and 9.20)
   b. Atrial septal defect
4. Pulmonary hypertension (e.g., pulmonary thromboembolism)

Differential diagnosis
Positional artifact (especially on the ventrodorsal projection of the thorax)

Caudal Vena Cava
Radiographic findings
1. Increased width or narrowed diameter of the caudal vena cava on the lateral or dorsoventral projection.
2. There is no "rule of thumb" measurement for determining the normal diameter.
   a. Diameter is variable depending on the stage of the cardiac cycle and respiratory phase.
   b. Diameter commonly is larger at the height of inspiration when intrathoracic pressure is less.
3. Diameter is not a useful indicator of cardiac disease.
4. The cranial vena cava is not visible on radiographs, but, if enlarged, may contribute to an impression of widening of the cranial mediastinum.

Causes for enlargement
1. Congestive right heart failure (e.g., tricuspid insufficiency, heartworm disease)
2. Pericarditis or pericardial effusion
3. Mass (e.g., tumor, heartworms, embolus) causing partial obstruction, usually located in the caudal vena cava or near the junction of the heart and caudal vena cava.

Causes for small size
1. Hypovolemia, especially if present on several projections
2. Hypoadrenocorticism

EVALUATION OF THE PULMONARY CIRCULATION

Hypovascularity
Radiographic findings
1. Lung is more radiolucent than normal.
2. Pulmonary arteries and veins are smaller than normal.

Causes
1. Right to left shunting (e.g., Tetralogy of Fallot)
2. Pulmonic stenosis (severe)
3. Hypovolemia
4. Hypoadrenocorticism

Differential diagnosis
1. Emphysema
2. Overinflation
3. Overexposure

Hypervascularity
Radiographic findings
1. Arteries and veins are larger than normal.
   a. Arteries and veins of the right cranial lung lobe on the lateral projection are equal in size, but exceed the smallest diameter of the proximal aspect of the right fourth rib.
   b. The lung appears more opaque than normal because of increased vasculature.

Causes
1. Pulmonary arterial hypertension (arteries are larger than veins)
   a. Dirofilariasis (See Figure 9.33)
   b. Pulmonary thromboembolism
2. Left to right shunts (patent ductus arteriosis, ventricular, and atrial septal defects).
3. Pulmonary venous hypertension secondary to left heart failure (veins are larger than corresponding arteries) (See Figure 9.29)
4. Severe anemia
5. Thyrotoxicosis
6. Fluid overload

Differential diagnosis (artifactual causes)
1. Underexposure
2. Expiratory radiograph

DISEASES/DISORDERS

Congestive Heart Failure
Clinical correlations
1. Congestive heart failure exists when the heart is unable to maintain adequate circulation at a normal venous pressure.
2. Heart failure can be subdivided into right heart failure or left heart failure.
   a. Right heart failure occurs when there is an inadequate right ventricular output into the pulmonary arteries and a concomitant reduced acceptance of blood from the systemic venous circulation, or an increase in systemic venous pressure secondary to dysfunction of the right heart. Causes of right heart failure include:
      1) Mechanical causes with pressure or volume overload
      2) Secondary to left heart failure
      3) Cor pulmonale secondary to dirofilariasis or pulmonary thromboembolism

4) Pulmonic stenosis
5) Tricuspid valve dysplasia/tricuspid regurgitation
6) Arteriovenous fistula
7) Myocardial failure
   a) Dilated cardiomyopathy
   b) Myocarditis
8) Interference with cardiac filling
   a) Pericardial effusion with tamponade
   b) Restrictive pericarditis
   c) Triscuspid valve dysplasia (stenosis)
   d) Endocardial fibroelastosis

b. Left heart failure occurs when there is an inadequate left ventricular output into the arterial system and a diminished acceptance of blood from the venous system, or increased pulmonary venous pressure secondary to a cardiac defect. Causes of left heart failure:
   1) Mechanical causes with volume or pressure overload
      a) Mitral insufficiency
      b) Aortic regurgitation
      c) Atrial or ventricular septal defects
      d) Patent ductus arteriosus
      e) Aortic stenosis
      f) Systemic hypertension
   2) Myocardial failure
      a) Dilated cardiomyopathy
      b) Myocarditis
      c) Myocardial ischemia
      d) Myocardial neoplasia
   3) Interference with cardiac filling
      a) Hypertrophic cardiomyopathy
      b) Severe arrhythmia
   4) Increased requirement for cardiac output (high output failure)
      a) Overexercise
      b) Anemia
      c) Hyperthyroidism
      d) Pregnancy

Radiographic findings of congestive right heart failure

1. All radiographic findings of heart failure are extracardiac, and the heart may be normal in size and shape (e.g., arrhythmias).
   a. Distended vena cava
   b. Pleural effusion
   c. Hepatomegaly
   d. Ascites
   e. Depending on the cause of the right heart failure, there may also be right heart enlargement or an enlarged pulmonary artery segment as seen with dirofilariasis, pulmonic stenosis, and pulmonary thromboembolism.

Radiographic findings of congestive left heart failure

1. Distended pulmonary veins (e.g., veins larger in diameter than corresponding arteries) associated with pulmonary venous hypertension.
2. Pulmonary edema
   a. Initially, perivascular interstitial infiltrates cause blurring of the vascular markings.
   b. With progression, a diffuse increased interstitial infiltrate may be seen with prominent peribronchial cuffing, and ultimately, alveolar flooding.
   c. Alveolar edema is characterized by fluffy, coalescing infiltrates, often with air bronchograms.
   d. The edema is often perihilar, dorsal, and bilateral and tends to fade peripherally.
   e. Asymmetric increased opacity of the lung is seen, especially in the dependent lobes if the animal has been laterally recumbent. In a nonrecumbent position, has been reported to occur more asymmetrically in the right lung because of differing lymphatic drainage between the right and left sides.
3. May cause a pleural effusion in cats.
4. If the left heart failure is caused by mitral insufficiency, the left ventricle and left atrium are commonly enlarged.

Microcardia

Clinical correlations

1. A small heart is most often associated with disease conditions in which there is a reduced blood volume, but can also occur with severe cachexia.
2. The most common causes are:
   a. Hypovolemic shock, blood loss, or severe dehydration
   b. Hypoadrenocorticism
   c. Emaciation
   d. Constrictive pericarditis (rare)
3. The heart may be normal in size, but may appear relatively small in relationship to the size of the thorax. The most common causes are:
   a. Overinflation of the thorax, commonly when anesthetized with positive pressure ventilation
   b. Hyperinflation of the thorax or lung related to pneumothorax or other diseases such as emphysema.

Radiographic findings (Figure 9.17 and 9.18)

1. The cardiac silhouette is narrower and smaller than normal.
2. The small heart has less sternal contact and more lung visible between heart and diaphragm.
3. The pulmonary vasculature is less prominent than normal.

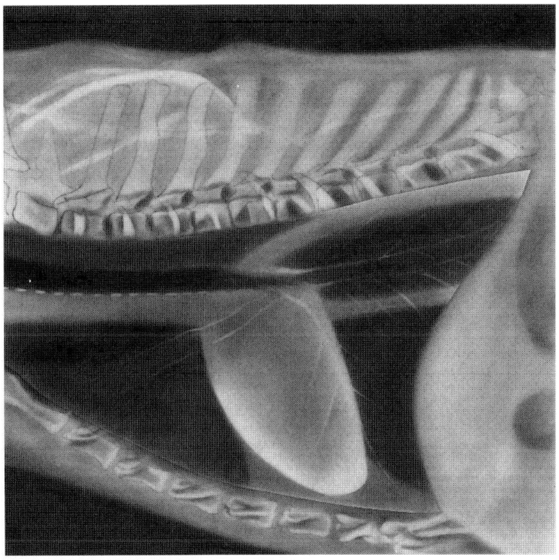

Figure 9.17. Microcardia. The heart is smaller than normal and more vertical in position. The lungs are underperfused and the caudal vena cava is smaller.

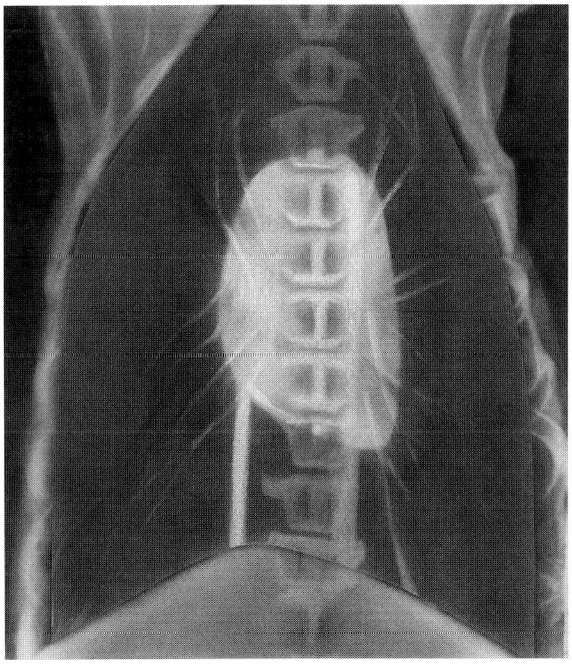

Figure 9.18. Microcardia. The heart is small and rounded. The pulmonary vessels and caudal vena cava are smaller from underperfusion.

Differential diagnosis

1. Pulmonary hyperinflation from asthma, emphysema, or secondary to positive pressure ventilation.
2. Tension pneumothorax

CONGENITAL HEART DISEASE (Tables 9.1 through 9.3)

1. Most congenital heart defects, which can occur in any dog or cat breed, have a suspected genetic basis. The breed and sex predilection for the more common congenital cardiac defects are listed in Table 9.1, 9.2, and 9.3.
2. The clinical signs of congenital heart disease vary depending on the type and severity of the anomaly and the size and age of the dog or cat.
   a. Many affected dogs and cats are asymptomatic.
   b. Stunted growth may be present.
   c. Exercise intolerance is common in moderate to severe congenital heart disease.
   d. Respiratory distress, tachypnea, and fainting are

TABLE 9.1

Congenital Heart Disease in the Dog, Listed by Defect

Defect	Predilection
Patent Ductus Arteriosus	Poodle, Collie, Pomeranian, German Shepherd Dog, Shetland Sheepdog (female : male 2.2 : 1)
Pulmonic Stenosis	Beagle, Bulldog, Fox Terrior, Miniature Schnauzer, Chihuahua, Samoyed, Labrador Retriever
Subaortic Stenosis	Newfoundland, Boxer, German Shepherd Dog, German Shorthair Pointer, Golden Retriever, Rottweiler, Bull Terrier
Ventricular Septal Defect	English Bulldog, English Springer Spaniel
Atrial Septal Defect	Samoyed, Boxer, Doberman Pinscher
Mitral Dysplasia	Great Dane, German Shepherd Dog (male > female), Bull Terrier
Tricuspid Dysplasia	Great Dane, German Shepherd Dog, Weimaraner, Labrador Retriever (male > female)
Tetralogy of Fallot	Keeshond, English Bulldog
Persistent Right Fourth Aortic Arch	German Shepherd Dog, Irish Setter

TABLE 9.2

Breed Predilections in Dogs with Congenital Heart Disease[a]

Airedale Terrier	Pulmonic stenosis (PS)-2
Beagle	PS[b]
Bichon Frise	Patent ductus arteriosus (PDA)-2
Boxer	Aortic stenosis (AS)-3
Boykin Spaniel	PS[b]
Bull Terrier	Mitral dysplasia (MD)[b]
Chihuahua	PS, PDA[b]
Cocker Spaniel	PDA-1, PS-1
Collie	PDA-1
Doberman Pinscher	Atrial septal defect (ASD)[b]
English Bulldog	PS-3, ventricular septal defect (VSD)-3, AS-1 Tetrology of Fallot (TF)[b]
English Springer Spaniel	PDA-2
German Shepherd Dog	Tricuspid dysplasia (TD)-3, AS-1, persistent right aortic arch (PRAA)-2, MD, PDA[b]
German Shorthair Pointer	AS[b]
Golden Retriever	AS-3, TD[b]
Great Dane	AS-1, PRAA-3, MD, TD[b]
Irish Setter	PRAA[b]
Keeshond	PDA-2, TF[b]
Kerry Blue Terrier	PDA-3
Labrador Retriever	TD-3
Maltese	PDA-3
Mastiff	PS-3
Miniature Schnauzer	PS-2
Newfoundland	AS-3
Pomeranian	PDA-3
Poodle	PDA-2
Rottweiler	AS-3
Samoyed	PS-3, AS-1, ASD[b]
Scottish Terrier	PS-2
Shetland Sheepdog	PDA-3
West Highland White Terrier	PS-3
Weimaraner	Td, peritoneopericardial hernia[b]
Yorkshire Terrier	PDA-1

[a]Data from Veterinary Medical Data Base (VMDB) at Purdue University, 1987–1989:1320 dogs with congenital heart disease of 154,233 dogs. Numbers 1–3 identify predisposed breeds represented by four or more affected dogs in which relative risk for the indicated abnormality was significantly elevated in this series ($P < .05$ to $P < .000$).

−1, mildly increased risk (Odds ration 1.5–2.9 times all other dogs).

−2, moderate risk (Odds ration 3–4.9 times others).

−3, marked risk (Odds ration >5 times others).

[b]Breed-associated diseases unconfirmed in this study but suggested or confirmed by others. Sex predominance: PDA (females 3 : 1), PS in English bulldogs (makes 4 : 1), mitral and tricuspid dysplasia (makes 2 : 1).

Source: Buchannan JW. Causes and prevalence of cardiovascular disease. In: Kirk RW, Bonagura JD, eds. *Current Veterinary Therapy XI.* Philadelphia: W.B. Saunders; Philadelphia, 1992, with permission.

TABLE 9.3.

Congenital Defects in Cats

The most common congenital defects in cats are:
1. Atrioventricular valve malformations (mitral and tricuspid valve dysplasias)
2. Ventricular septal defect
3. Endocardial fibroelastosis
4. Patent ductus arteriosus

Less common congenital defects in cats are:
1. Vascular ring anomalies (persistent right fourth aortic arch)
2. Aortic stenosis
3. Tetralogy of Fallot
4. Atrial septal defect
5. Common atrioventricular canal
6. Pulmonic stenosis

common when congestive heart failure or cyanotic heart disease (e.g., Tetralogy of Fallot) is present.

3. The diagnosis of a specific cardiac defect can be made by correlating the data obtained from:
   a. Clinical history
   b. Physical examination
   c. Auscultation
   d. Electrocardiography
   e. Survey thoracic radiographs
   f. Echocardiography (best with Doppler)
   g. Angiocardiography (in selected cases)
   h. Pressure studies of the heart chambers and the major vessels
4. Survey radiographs of the chest enable:
   a. An assessment of cardiac chamber enlargement or presence of generalized cardiomegaly
   b. An assessment of the pulmonary circulation (hypovascularity versus hypervascularity)
   c. An assessment of the degree of cardiac decompensation (left and/or right heart failure)
5. Contrast radiography
   a. Selective angiography
   b. Nonselective angiography
6. Other Imaging
   a. Echocardiography
   b. CT angiography
   c. MRI angiography

Patent Ductus Arteriosus (Left to Right Shunt)

Clinical correlations

1. Is a common congenital heart defect in which there is left-to-right shunting of blood from the aorta through the ductus, into the pulmonary arteries.

2. Continuous systolic and diastolic machinery murmur at the left heart base
3. Mitral regurgitation is a common complication.
4. Signs of left heart failure are common.
5. Dog and cat breed predilections (See Tables 9.1 through 9.3)
6. Is surgically treatable by ligation of the ductus arteriosum.
7. If not surgically treated, most dogs will die within the first few years of life.

Radiographic findings (Figures 9.19 and 9.20)

1. Left ventricular and left atrial enlargement
2. Enlarged ascending aorta with aneurysmal-like dilatation (ductus diverticulum or ductus bump) of the descending aorta
3. Enlarged pulmonary artery segment
4. Pulmonary overcirculation

Reverse Patent Ductus Arteriosus (Right-to-Left Shunt)

Clinical correlations

1. Is also commonly referred to as a reverse patent ductus arteriosus (PDA).
2. An uncommon condition in which right-to-left shunting through the ductus develops secondary to increased pulmonary vascular resistance.
3. A murmur is often absent. If present, is usually a low grade systolic murmur.
4. The affected animal may show clinical signs of shortness of breath, weakness, and collapse, usually of the pelvic limbs. Often a differential cyanosis is present with normal mucous membranes of the head and with cyanotic membranes caudally (e.g., genital mucosa).
5. Dog and cat breed predilections (See Tables 9.1 through 9.3)
6. A secondary polycythemia is common, caused by renal perfusion with hypoxemic blood.
7. No surgical treatment is indicated. Conservative management with rest, limitation of exercise, and phlebotomy, as needed, to keep packed cell volume (PCV) less than 65%.

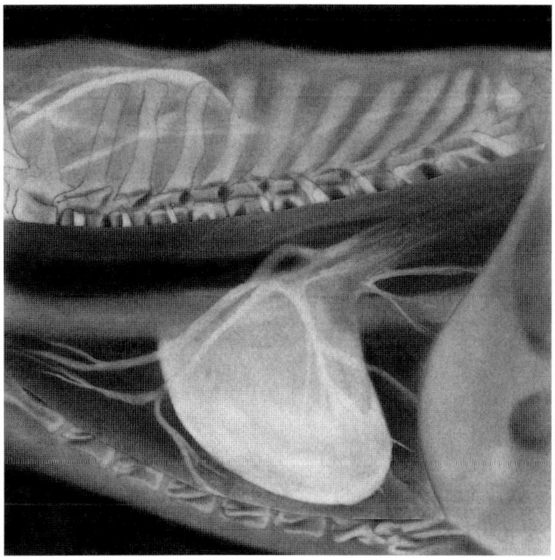

Figure 9.19. Patent ductus arteriosus. There is enlargement of the left ventricle and left atrium. There is overcirculation with the pulmonary arteries and veins appearing larger than normal.

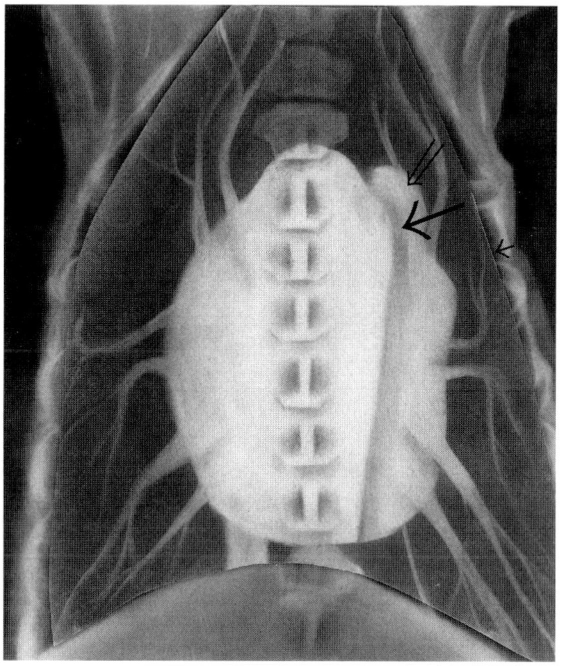

Figure 9.20. Patent ductus arteriosus. There is enlargement of the left ventricle and left auricle (small arrow), an aneurysmal-like dilation of the descending aorta (straight arrow) and prominence of the pulmonary artery segment (open arrow). Overcirculation is present with increased size of the pulmonary vasculature.

Radiographic findings

1. Generalized cardiomegaly
2. Right heart enlargement with increased prominence of the pulmonary artery segment
3. Prominent proximal lobar pulmonary arteries, but peripheral hypoperfusion
4. A "ductus bump" is not usually present on the proximal descending aorta.

Pulmonic Stenosis

Clinical correlations

1. Systolic murmur is heard loudest over the pulmonic valve.
2. Stenosis may be subvalvular, valvular, or supravalvular (rare). In dogs, a combination of valvular and subvalvular is most common.

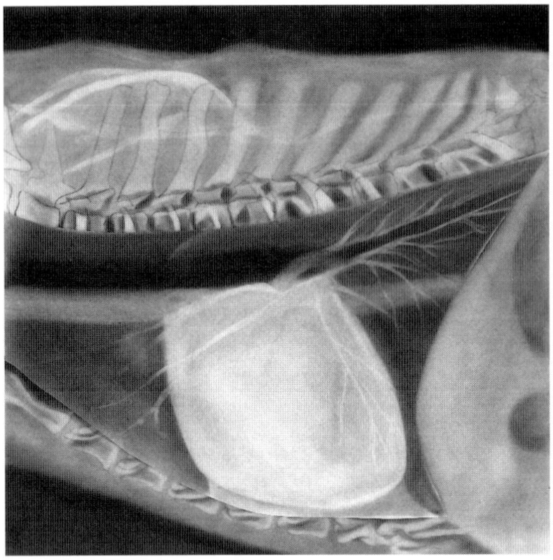

Figure 9.21. Pulmonic stenosis. There is marked enlargement of the right ventricle with increased sternal contact and resultant dorsal displacement of the trachea.

3. Is usually an isolated defect but may occur with other congenital disorders (e.g., Tetralogy of Fallot).
4. Dog breed predilections (See Tables 9.1 and 9.2)
5. Many affected dogs are asymptomatic. If the pressure gradient is high, common clinical signs of progressive exercise intolerance, syncope, and right heart failure may develop.
6. If the pressure gradient is high (greater than 80 mm Hg) surgical therapy or balloon valvuloplasty is recommended.

Radiographic findings (Figures 9.21 and 9.22)

1. Right ventricle is enlarged.
2. Enlargement of the main pulmonary artery caused by poststenotic dilation
3. The peripheral pulmonary arteries may be normal or decreased in size.

Aortic Stenosis

Clinical correlations

1. Dog and cat breed predilections (See Tables 9.1 through 9.3)
2. Systolic murmur is heard loudest over the aortic valve.
3. Most commonly, the stenosis is subvalvular (subaortic). Valvular stenosis is the second most common form. Supravalvular stenosis is rare.
4. The severity of the stenosis as determined by the pressure gradient across the aortic valve is usually directly related to the degree of clinical signs and prognosis.
   a. Dogs with mild stenosis (less than 30 mmHg) are often asymptomatic and have a normal life expectancy.
   b. Dogs with moderate stenosis (30–70 mmHg) often show signs of exercise intolerance and syncope.

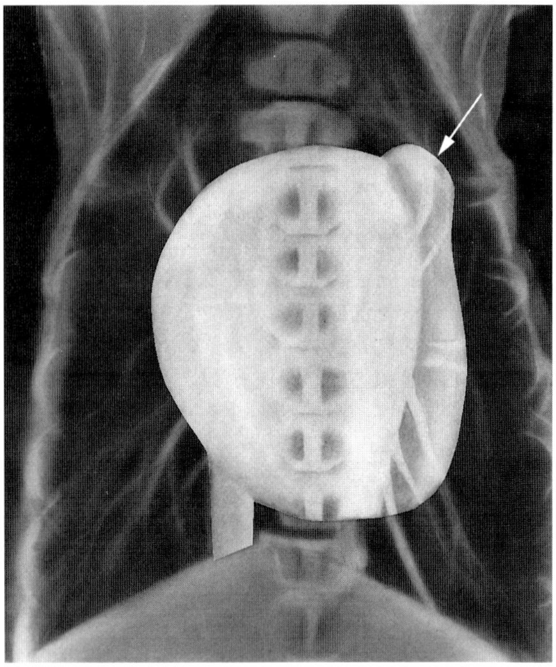

Figure 9.22. Pulmonic stenosis. There is marked rounding of the right ventricle and prominence of the main pulmonary artery (arrow).

   c. Dogs with severe stenosis (greater than 70 mmHg) have a greater risk of syncope, exercise intolerance, and sudden death.
5. Surgical therapy should be considered for dogs with moderate to severe gradients of stenosis.

Radiographic findings (Figures 9.23 and 9.24)

1. Left ventricle enlargement
2. Poststenotic dilatation of the aorta
3. Enlarged aortic arch

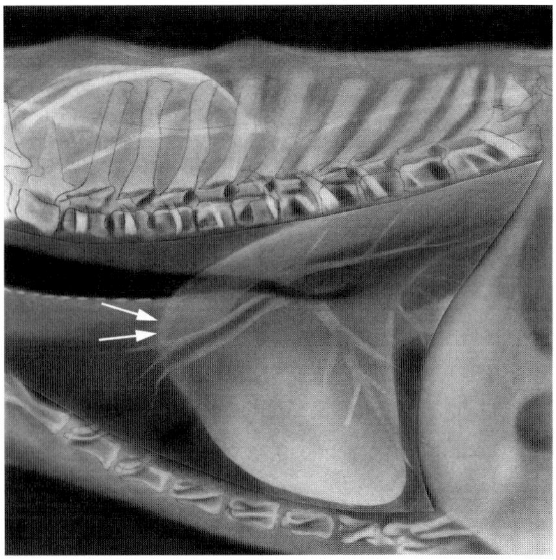

Figure 9.23. Aortic stenosis. There is left ventricular enlargement and accentuation of the craniodorsal heart border as a result of enlargement of the aortic arch (arrows).

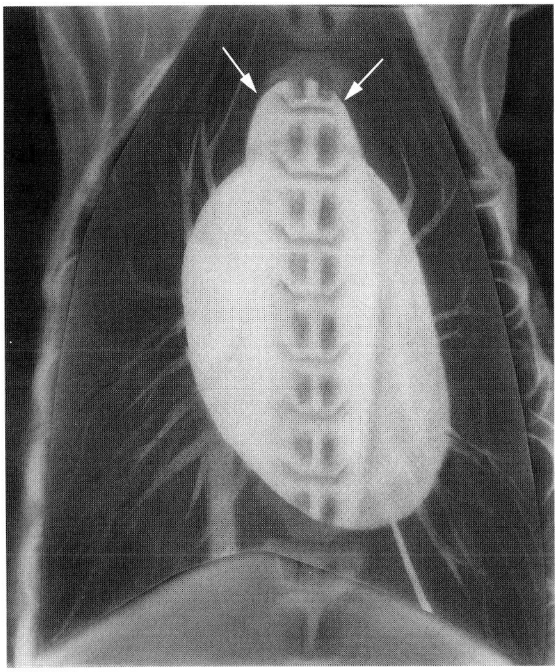

Figure 9.24. Aortic stenosis. There is rounding and enlargement of the left ventricular border with prominence and enlargement of the aortic arch (arrows).

Ventricular Septal Defect (VSD)

Clinical correlations

1. Usually blood is shunted from the left to the right side, unless pulmonary hypertension is present.
2. The size and location of the septal defect varies; most defects are small and in the high septal (perimembranous) region.
3. Is a common defect in cats and may be associated with other congenital defects.
   a. In cats, 33% are associated with tricuspid dysplasia.
   b. Can occur with pulmonic stenosis, aortic insufficiency, atrial septal defects, mitral regurgitation, and others.
4. In a dog or cat with an uncomplicated VSD, a loud holosystolic murmur is present, often bilateral, but usually loudest in the right cranioventral thorax.
5. Dog and cat breed predilections (See Tables 9.1 through 9.3)
6. Is best documented with echocardiography or angiography.

Radiographic findings

1. The appearance of the heart size and degree of pulmonary perfusion will vary, depending on the size of the defect, the amount of blood shunted, and the ratio between the pulmonary and systemic pressures.
2. If the VSD is small, the cardiac size will be normal.
3. With larger defects, right ventricular, left ventricular, and left atrial enlargement is often seen.
4. Enlargement of the pulmonary artery segment and overcirculation to the lungs may be present in large shunts.

Tetralogy of Fallot

Clinical correlations

1. The four features of this anomaly are:
   a. Ventricular septal defect
   b. Pulmonic stenosis (subvalvular or valvular)
   c. Right ventricular hypertrophy
   d. Over-riding of the aorta
2. The severity of the condition depends on the changing degree of pulmonic stenosis relative to systemic vascular resistance.
3. The clinical signs vary, but are usually present during the first year of life including stunted growth, exercise intolerance, and weakness.
4. Cyanosis, polycythemia, and tachycardia are common.
5. A loud high-pitched systolic murmur is usually heard over the pulmonic valve.
6. Dog and cat breed predilection (See Tables 9.1 through 9.3)

Radiographic findings

1. A normal to slightly enlarged cardiac silhouette
2. Enlargement of the right ventricle
3. A normal or enlarged pulmonary artery segment
4. Hyperlucent lung field caused by decreased pulmonary perfusion

Atrioventricular Valve Malformation and Dysplasia

Clinical correlations

1. The most common congenital defect in the cat, uncommon in the dog (See Tables 9.1 through 9.3).
2. The clinical signs vary with the severity of the lesion. Many cats are only mildly affected. Some cats show progressive clinical deterioration with right and/or left heart failure as early as 6 months of age.
3. Tricuspid dysplasia may be associated with a VSD or mitral valve malformation.
4. Acquired myocardial disease may coexist.
5. A loud systolic murmur is often present. A left-sided murmur is more common with mitral dysplasia and a right-sided murmur more common with tricuspid dysplasia.

Radiographic findings

1. Moderate to severe cardiomegaly
2. Atrial dilation is usually pronounced:
   a. Right-atrial dilation with tricuspid dysplasia
   b. Left-atrial dilation with mitral dysplasia
3. Right- or left-sided heart failure may occur, depending on the type of decompensation.
4. The diagnosis is confirmed with echocardiography.

Vascular Ring Anomalies

Clinical correlations

1. Vascular ring anomalies are caused by a disturbance in the normal development of the aortic arch and its branches.
2. The vascular ring lesion encircles the esophagus and trachea. The degree of esophageal compression depends on the vascular structures involved. The encirclement of the trachea rarely causes any clinical signs.
3. The most common defect is persistent right fourth aortic arch. The encirclement of the esophagus is caused by the dextro aorta (right and dorsally), the ligamentum arteriosum (dorsally and to the left), and the pulmonary artery and heart (ventrally).
4. Other vascular ring anomalies include:
   a. Double aortic arch
   b. Dextro aorta with aberrant left subclavian artery
   c. Aberrant right subclavian artery and normal aortic arch
5. Clinical signs of all vascular ring anomalies are secondary to esophageal compression by the vascular anomaly.
   a. Regurgitation, often occurring before 3 months of age
   b. Stunted growth
   c. Coughing, nasal discharge, and respiratory distress caused by aspiration pneumonia
6. Dog and cat breed predilections (See Tables 9.1 through 9.3)

Radiographic findings (Figures 9.25 and 9.26)

1. Cardiac silhouette is normal in size.

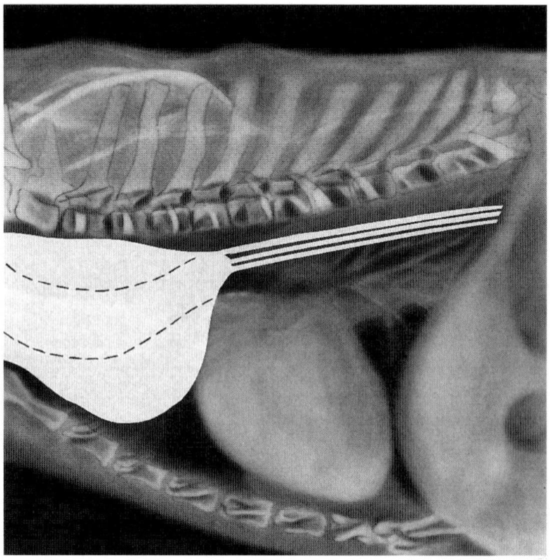

Figure 9.25. Vascular ring anomaly (persistent right fourth aortic arch). A barium swallow shows the saccular dilation of the esophagus within the cranial mediastinum. The trachea is displaced ventrally (dotted line). The esophagus is normal caudal to the anomaly.

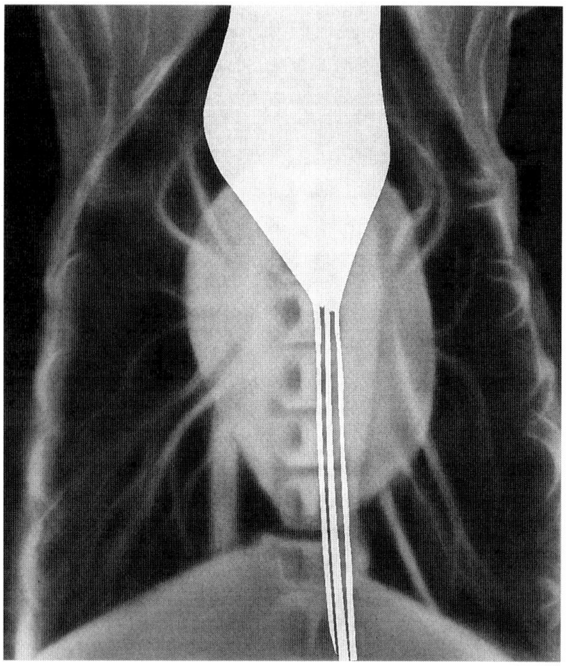

Figure 9.26. Vascular ring anomaly (persistent right fourth aortic arch). A barium swallow shows saccular dilation of the esophagus cranial to the heart base. The mucosal folds of the esophagus are normal caudal to the stricture.

2. There is localized esophageal dilation cranial to the heart base.
3. If the esophageal dilation is large, the trachea and heart may be displaced ventrally.
4. Aspiration pneumonia is common.
5. If dextro aorta is present, the trachea may be seen to the left of the midline.
6. A barium esophagram will demonstrate the esophageal dilation.
   a. The esophageal lumen is usually narrowed near the fourth intercostal space dorsal to the heart.
   b. The cranial thoracic esophagus is commonly greatly distended, often extending into the cervical region.
   c. The caudal thoracic esophagus is normal unless megaesophagus coexists.
7. Differential considerations:
   a. Megaesophagus (entire esophagus is dilated)
   b. Esophageal stricture
   c. Esophageal diverticulae
   d. Esophageal foreign bodies

Situs Inversus

Clinical correlations

1. Congenital malformation in which the thoracic and abdominal viscera are reversed, as mirror images of their normal location.
2. Rare anomaly.
3. Known as Kartagener's syndrome if associated with sinusitis and bronchitis.

4. Can have anomaly in which only the thoracic or abdominal viscera are reversed in position, not both.

Radiographic findings

1. Location of thoracic and abdominal viscera are reversed in position. The anomaly is identified on ventrodorsal or dorsoventral projections.
   a. Cardiac apex is on right side.
   b. Caudal vena cava is on left side.
   c. Accessory lobe originates on left side.
   d. Stomach fundus is on right side and pyloric antrum on the left.
   e. Left kidney is more cranial in position than is right kidney.
2. Must differentiate from:
   a. Mislabeled radiographs that mimic situs inversus
   b. Mediastinal shift of heart caused by lung or pleural diseases.
   c. Dextrocardia, as a variant of normal on ventrodorsal projections, as a result of the heart falling away from the sternum.

ACQUIRED HEART DISEASE

1. The incidence of acquired heart disease increases with age.
2. The degree of clinical severity of heart disease varies.
   a. Type of clinical signs
   b. Progression of cardiac decompensation and failure
3. The diagnosis of heart disease is made by correlating the data obtained from:
   a. History and physical examination
   b. Auscultation
   c. Electrocardiography
   d. Survey thoracic radiography
   e. Echocardiography
   e. Angiocardiography (in some cases)
4. The most common types of acquired heart disease are:
   a. Mitral insufficiency
   b. Tricuspid insufficiency
   c. Cardiomyopathy
   d. Pericardial effusion
   e. Dirofilariasis
5. Contrast radiography
   a. Selective angiography
   b. Nonselective angiography
6. Other imaging:
   a. Echocardiography
   b. CT angiography
   c. MR angiography

Chronic Valvular Disease

Clinical correlations

1. Also referred to as endocardiosis.
2. The most common acquired heart disease in dogs, uncommon in cats.
   a. Small breed dogs are affected more than large breed dogs.
   b. Males are affected more commonly than females.
3. Is a degenerative mitral valvular disease causing mitral insufficiency.
4. Tricuspid insufficiency is usually seen in dogs that also have mitral insufficiency.
5. Degenerative lesions of the aortic and pulmonic valves are uncommonly seen.
6. The etiology of valvular degeneration is unknown.
7. Mitral insufficiency is a progressive disease with volume overload to the left atrium and left ventricle, often with eccentric hypertrophy.
8. The clinical signs of decompensation include weight loss, dyspnea, tiring, restlessness, cough, syncope, or ascites.
9. Arrythmias are common in advanced disease. Atrial tachycardia, atrial premature contractions, and atrial fibrillation are most common, with ventricular tachycardia occurring less commonly.

Mitral Valvular Insufficiency

Clinical correlations

1. Also referred to as mitral regurgitation and is common in aged dogs of all breeds.
2. Systolic murmur is heard loudest over the mitral valve area.
3. A progressive, degenerative disease of the mitral valve leaflets.
4. Many dogs have coexistent tricuspid regurgitation.
5. The severity of the murmur often does not correlate with the severity of the hemodynamic changes.

Radiographic findings (Figures 9.27 through 9.30)

1. Radiographic findings vary depending on the duration and severity of the mitral regurgitation.
2. Early in the disease, only left atrial dilation may be seen.
3. With progression, left atrial and left ventricular enlargement is present.
4. Severe left atrial dilation may be seen in advanced disease, causing elevation and compression of the left bronchus.
5. Left heart failure with venous congestion, as well as interstitial and alveolar edema occur with decompensation. In the dog, the pulmonary edema is usually bilaterally symmetric, and often is more marked in the hilar and central lung fields.
6. Acute, severe mitral regurgitation, as in the rupture of a chordae tendinae, may show minimal left atrial dilation but severe pulmonary edema.
7. In advanced mitral valve disease, splitting of the left atrium may occur, causing hemopericardium. In these dogs the cardiac silhouette is usually globular, because of pericardial effusion and severe left atrial dilation is usually present.

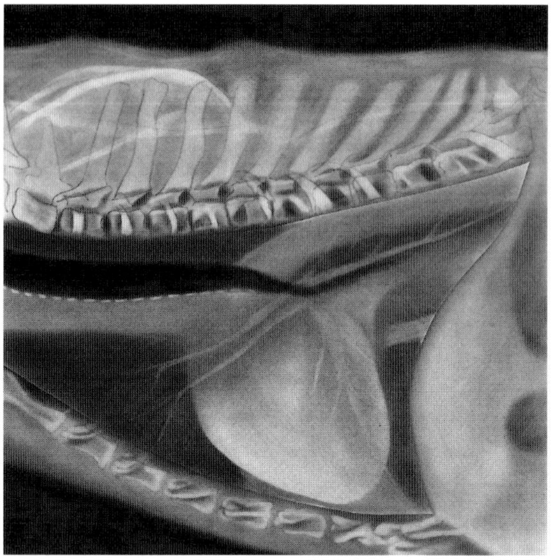

Figure 9.27. Mitral insufficiency with mild decompensation. There is enlargement of the left atrium and blurring of the pulmonary veins in the hilar area.

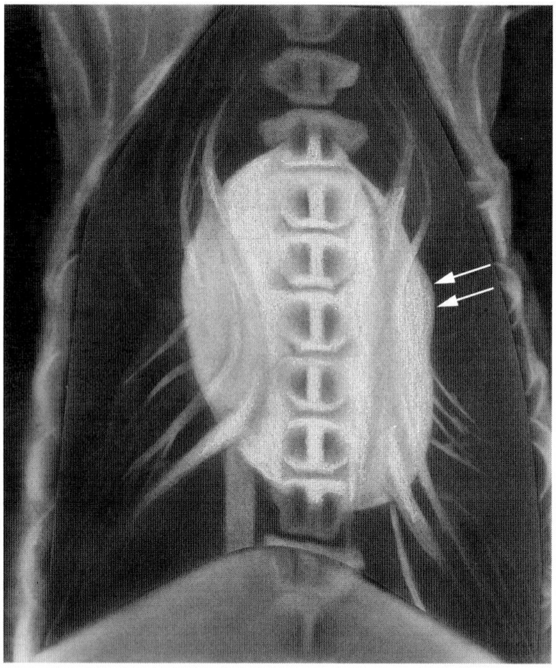

Figure 9.28. Mitral insufficiency with mild decompensation. There is enlargement of the left auricular appendage (arrows) and distension of the caudal lobar pulmonary veins.

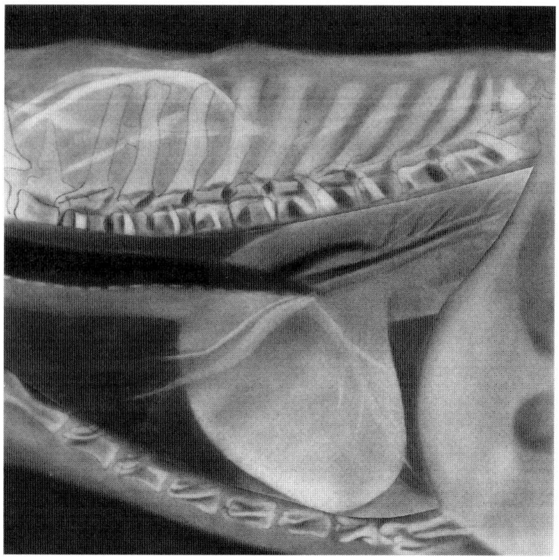

Figure 9.29. Mitral insufficiency with severe decompensation. There is marked enlargement of the left atrium. The cranial lobar veins are distended and there is mixed alveolar infiltrate in the hilar area fading into the peripheral lung field.

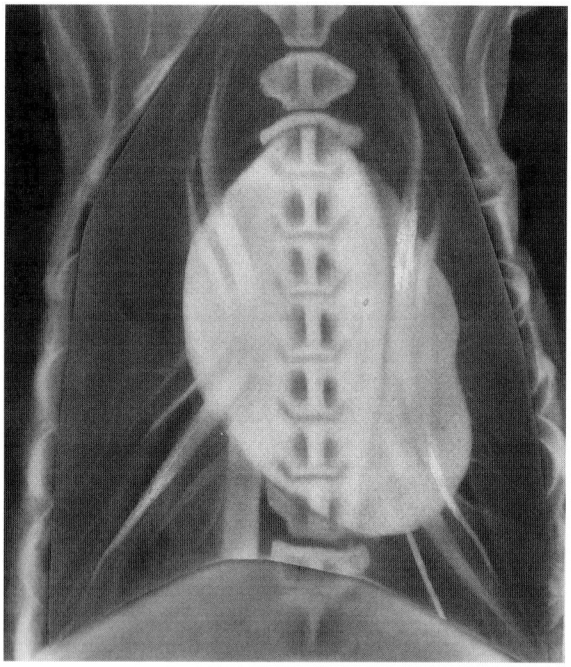

Figure 9.30. Mitral insufficiency with severe decompensation. There is rounding and enlargement of the left ventricular border, marked enlargement of the left auricular appendage and severe enlargement of the pulmonary veins.

Tricuspid Valvular Insufficiency

Clinical correlations

1. Commonly referred to as tricuspid regurgitation.
2. Common in aged dogs, often is present in addition to mitral insufficiency.
3. Systolic murmur is heard loudest in right ventral thorax over tricuspid valve, but is often bilateral because mitral insufficiency is often present concurrently.

Radiographic findings (Figures 9.31 and 9.32)

1. Right atrial and right ventricular enlargement
2. When mitral insufficiency is present concurrently, may also see left atrial and left ventricular enlargement (i.e., generalized cardiomegaly).

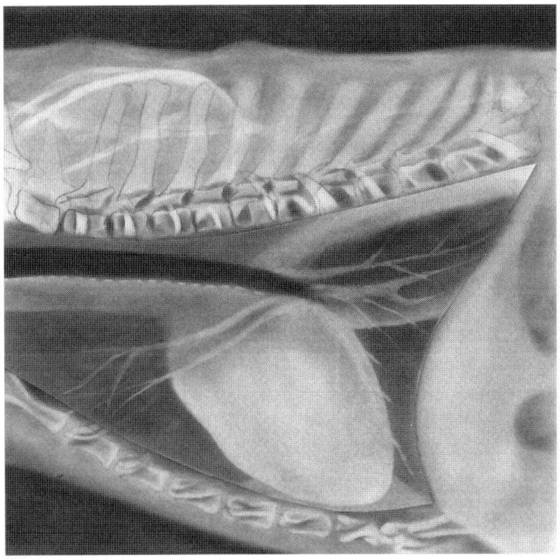

Figure 9.31. Tricuspid insufficiency. There is marked enlargement of the right atrium.

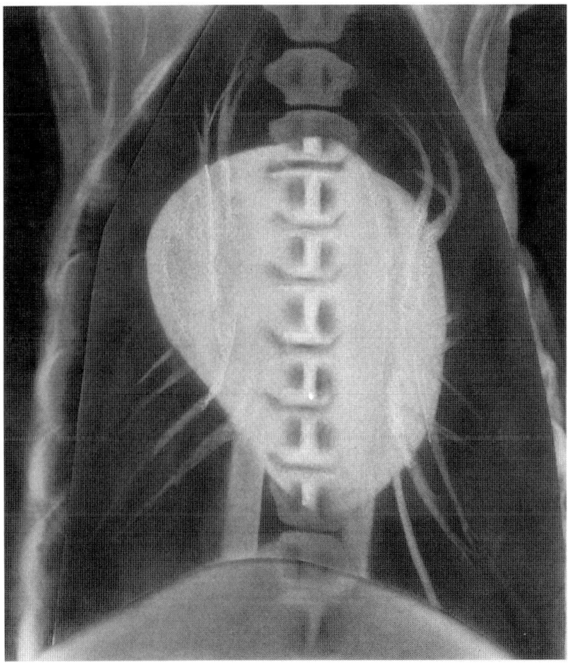

Figure 9.32. Tricuspid insufficiency. There is marked enlargement of the right atrium.

3. Right heart failure may occur with decompensation (e.g., pleural effusion, hepatomegaly, ascites).

Infectious Endocarditis

Clinical correlations

1. Caused by a bacterial infection involving the valves or myocardium and may be acute, subacute, or chronic.
2. More common in dogs, rare in cats.
3. Most often affects the mitral and aortic valves.
4. Most infections are caused by gram-positive bacteria (e.g., B- hemolytic *Streptococci* and *S. aureus*).
5. Degenerative valves are more susceptible to endocarditis, but normal valves can also be infected.
6. Congestive heart failure may develop from valvular regurgitation, with or without valvular stenosis.
7. Clinical signs are variable usually relating to valvular regurgitation or stenosis, bacteremia, infection in other body systems, congestive heart failure, or thromboembolism.

Radiographic findings

1. Thoracic radiographs are normal with acute infection.
2. With a chronic infection, variable degrees of cardiac enlargement will be present.
3. Pulmonary edema may be seen if left heart failure develops.

Dirofilariasis

1. Also known as heartworm disease and is caused by adult worms of *Dirofilaria immitis*.
2. The incidence of heartworm disease is associated with the population of various species of mosquitoes that transmit the infection.
3. Life cycle:
   a. A mosquito ingests a microfilariae or first stage larvae (L1) from an infected host animal.
   b. The L1 stage undergoes two molts within the mosquito (usually takes 2 to 2-1/2 weeks) to become stage three larvae (L3).
   c. Stage three larvae (L3) are deposited into an animal during mosquito feeding.
   d. The larvae travel within the subcutis, molting into the L4 stage (in 9–12 days) and then into the L5 stage as young worms.
   e. The young worms enter the vascular system (at approximately 100 days after infection) and migrate to the pulmonary arterial system.
   f. It usually takes 5 to 6 months before a patent infection, when the female worms release the microfilariae into the circulation system.
4. Pathophysiology
   a. The adult worms live primarily within the pulmonary arteries, but can migrate to the right ventricle or right atrium.
   b. Arteritis develops within the pulmonary arteries, characterized by villous myointimal proliferation and endothelial swelling.
   c. Pulmonary hypertension may develop secondary to vascular occlusion.
   d. Thrombosis and infarction may occur secondary to the arteritis and vascular occlusion.
   e. Secondary to the pulmonary hypertension, right ventricular hypertrophy occurs.
   f. Right heart failure occurs with severe infections (hepatomegaly and ascites).

g. Chronic hepatic congestion may cause hepatic fibrosis.
h. Glomerulonephritis may develop secondary to the circulating immune complexes.
i. Rarely, embolization of the eye, brain, or other systemic arteries may occur.

5. Serologic diagnosis
   a. In the infected dog, circulating microfilaria are usually present. In the infected cat, circulating microfilaria are rare.
   b. Occult infections may be diagnosed with enzyme-linked immunosorbent assay (ELISA) or immunofluorescent antibody (IFA) tests that detect antibodies to the adult worms or the microfilariae.

Canine Heartworm Disease

Clinical correlations

1. Occurs in dogs older than 6 months of age.
2. Dogs living outdoors are at greater risk than those that live indoors because the disease is associated with mosquito exposure.
3. Many infected dogs are asymptomatic.
4. With severe infections, clinical signs of exercise intolerance, dyspnea, cough, weight loss, and congestive heart failure may be present.
5. Severe thromboembolism may cause disseminated intravascular coagulation (DIC), thrombocytopenia, or hemoglobinuria.
6. Eosinophilia, basophilia, and/or monocytosis is common.
7. The electrocardiogram (ECG) may be normal or show evidence of right axis deviation.

Radiographic findings (Figures 9.33 and 9.34)

1. The radiographs may be normal with mild infections.
2. With more severe infections, the radiographic changes are best identified on the lateral and dorsoventral projections, which include:
   a. Right ventricular enlargement
   b. Increased prominence of the pulmonary artery segment
   c. Enlarged, tortuous, and blunted pulmonary arteries
      1) Usually is most evident in the caudal lobar arteries.
      2) The diameter of the right and left caudal pulmonary arteries is usually larger than the ninth rib at the point of intersection of the rib with its corresponding artery.
   d. Localized or generalized interstitial and/or alveolar infiltrates are often present, either associated with eosinophilic pneumonia, thromboembolism, or infarction.
3. If right heart failure ocurrs, hepatomegaly, splenomegaly, and ascites are usually present.

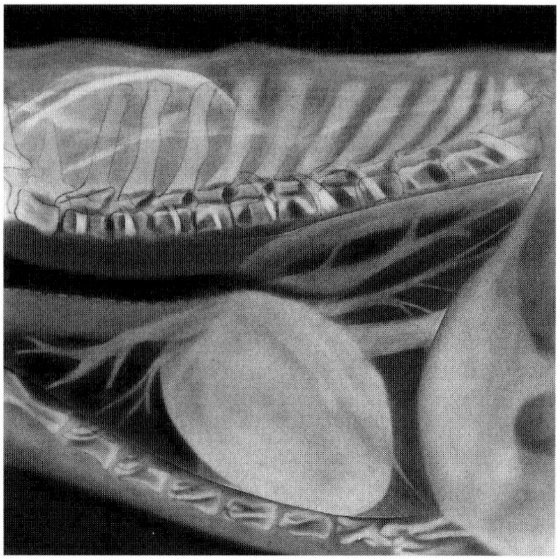

Figure 9.33. Heartworm disease. There is marked right heart enlargement and enlargement of the pulmonary arteries.

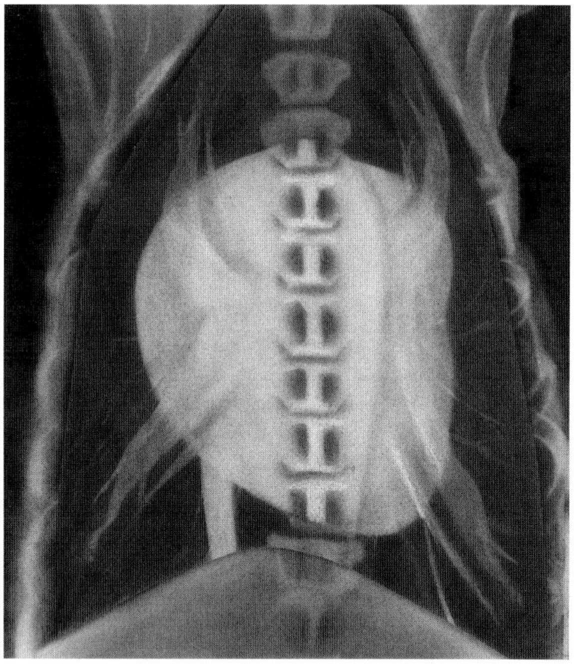

Figure 9.34. Heartworm disease. There is marked right heart enlargement with displacement of the cardiac apex to the left. The pulmonary artery segment is enlarged and the main pulmonary arteries are enlarged, tortuous, and pruned.

Feline Heartworm Disease

Clinical correlations

1. The occurrence of heartworm disease in cats is similar to the dog in geographic area, but the incidence is lower in the cat.
2. Infected cats have fewer adult worms than dogs, probably because the worms mature more slowly, have

fewer number of infective larvae that mature to adults, and the adult worm life span is shorter.
3. In most cats, circulating microfilariae do not occur or last for only a short period of time
4. The pathophysiologic changes in the heart and lungs are similar to those in the dog.
5. The arterial changes are most severe in the caudal lobes.
6. Many infections are self-limiting.
7. The most common clinical signs include lethargy, cough, and vomiting. Syncope, right heart failure, and sudden death may occur. With aberrant worm migration, neurologic signs including seizures, ataxia, and circling may be seen.
8. Aberrant worm migration, often to the brain, occurs more often than in the dog.
9. Microfilaria concentration test results are usually negative; the occult serologic tests of ELISA or IFA (antibodies to the adult antigen) usually are positive.
10. Eosinophilia occurs in approximately one third of infected cats.

Radiographic findings
1. Thoracic radiographs are useful as a screening test.
2. An unstructued interstitial pulmonary infiltrate is nonspecific, and most commonly present.
3. Enlarged, torturous pulmonary arteries may be present, and are usually best identified on the dorsoventral projection.
3. Mild to moderate right ventricular enlargement may be present.
4. Variable degrees of alveolar infiltrates, usually most commonly seen in the caudal lung lobes.
5. Right heart failure is rare, but if present, causes hepatomegaly and ascites.

Cardiomyopathy
Clinical correlations
1. Cardiomyopathy is a disease of the heart muscle. It is exclusive of acquired valvular disease, congenital heart defects, coronary arterial disease, and pulmonary vascular or parenchymal disorders.
2. Myocardial diseases that occur in the dog and cat may be primary or secondary, exhibit varied clinical presentations, and have variable prognosis depending on the form of disease present.
3. Types of myocardial disease include:
   a. Primary myocardial disease
      1) Dilated (congestive) cardiomyopathy
      2) Hypertrophic cardiomyopathy
         a) Obstructive form
         b) Nonobstructive form
      3) Restrictive cardiomyopathy
      4) Indeterminate (unclassified) cardiomyopathy
   b. Secondary myocardial disease
      1) Drugs (e.g., doxorubricin)
      2) Genetic
      3) Infiltrative (e.g., mucopolysaccharidosis, neoplasia)
      4) Metabolic (e.g., diabetes, hyperthyroidism)
      5) Hypertension (renal disease, idiopathic)
      6) Nutritional (e.g., tarurine deficiency, L-carnitine deficiency)
      7) Inflammatory (myocarditis)
         a) Infectious viral, bacterial, fungal, protozoal (parvovirus, distemper, Lyme disease)
         b) Noninfectious
4. The diagnosis of cardiomyopathy is made by correlating information derived from the clinical history, physical examination, thoracic radiography, electrocardiography, and echocardiography.
5. With disease progression, depending on the pattern of morphologic changes within the myocardium, heart failure develops with systolic and/or diastolic dysfunction. Therapy is directed toward relieving congestion, treating clinical and related hemodynamic abnormalities, and correcting arrhythmias.

Other imaging
1. Echocardiography

Canine Dilated Cardiomyopathy
Clinical correlations
1. The etiology is unknown, but may represent the end stage of severe myocardial injury from various metabolic, toxic, nutritional, or infectious causes.
2. In the classic form of disease, all four cardiac chambers are dilated, with reduced cardiac output associated with systolic dysfunction.
3. Affects animals of any age (6 months to 14 years, mean 4–6 years), predominately male and large or giant dog breeds.
   a. The large and giant dog breeds most commonly affected are:
      1) Great Dane
      2) Doberman Pinscher
      3) Saint Bernard
      4) Irish Wolfhound
      5) Old English Sheepdog
   b. Occasionally occurs in other dog breeds
      1) Cocker Spaniel
      2) English bulldog
      3) Miniature Schnauzer
      4) Portuguese Water Dog
4. Common clinical signs include dyspnea, cough, syncope, exercise intolerance, or abdominal distension.
5. On auscultation, a left or right apical murmur is commonly present.
6. An electrocardiogram may show left heart enlargement, conduction disturbances (e.g., premature contractions) or tachyarrhythmias (e.g., atrial fibrillation).

Radiographic findings (Figures 9.35 and 9.36)

1. Generalized cardiomegaly is usually present.
2. Left atrial dilation may be present.
3. Pulmonary edema may be present if left heart failure predominates.
4. Pleural effusion, hepatomegaly, and ascites may be present if right heart failure predominates.
5. Globular cardiac silhouette is caused by cardiomegaly and/or pericardial effusion.

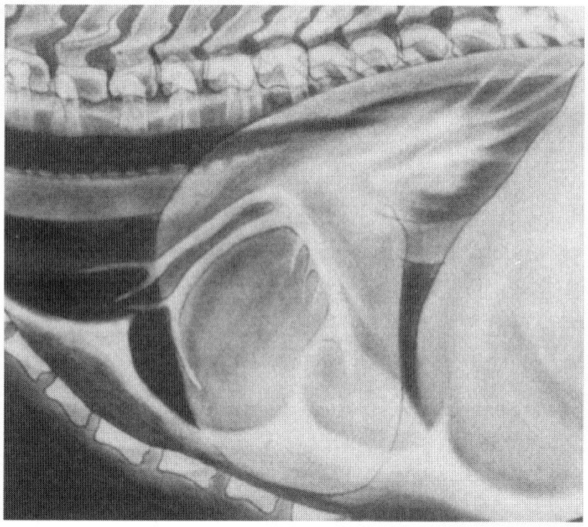

Figure 9.35. Canine dilated cardiomyopathy. There is generalized heart enlargement with marked left atrial dilation. Hilar edema and pleural effusion are present, indicative of combined left and right heart failure.

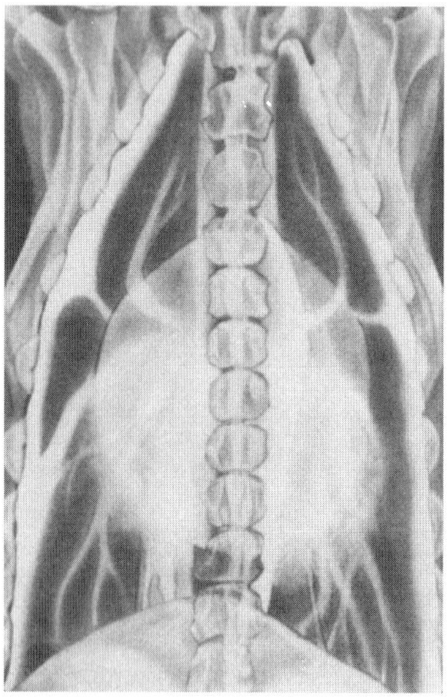

Figure 9.36. Canine dilated cardiomyopathy. There is generalized heart enlargement. The caudal heart borders are partially obscured because of pulmonary edema. Bilateral pleural effusion is present with visualization of pleural fissures and retraction of the lung border from the chest wall.

Other imaging

1. Echocardiography

Doberman Pinscher Cardiomyopathy

Clinical correlations

1. Most often affects middle-aged dogs, more often in the male.
2. Affected dogs often have ventricular arrhythmias (e.g., ventricular premature contractions [VPCs]).
3. Many dogs exhibit acute clinical signs of coughing or dyspnea secondary to pulmonary edema.
4. A systolic murmur resulting from mitral regurgitation is common.
5. The prognosis is poor; most dogs die within 6 to 12 months.

Radiographic findings

1. Mild cardiomegaly with marked left atrial dilation is common.
2. Occasionally, severe generalized cardiomegaly will be present.
3. Variable degrees of pulmonary edema will be present, often with prominent peribronchial cuffing, distended pulmonary veins, and symmetrical mixed alveolar infiltrates.
4. If acute and fulminate, severe diffuse alveolar edema may be present.

Other imaging

1. Echocardiography

Boxer Cardiomyopathy

Clinical correlations

1. Predilections:
   a. Males more common than females
   b. Mean age of onset is 8.5 years
   c. More prevalent in some breed lines, suggesting a familial component
2. Three categories of disease have been described
   a. Asymptomatic with arrythmias
   b. Episodic weakness or syncope without congestive heart failure
   c. Arrythmias and congestive heart failure
3. Ventricular arrythmias commonly include unifocal premature contractions and paroxysmal or sustained ventricular tachycardia.
4. L-Carnitine deficiency has been seen in some dogs.
5. 50% of dogs have a systolic murmur caused by mitral regurgitation.
6. Variable prognosis:
   a. Dogs with congestive heart failure often die within 6 months following diagnosis.
   b. Dogs with mild arrhythmias may be effectively treated and may live for 2 or more years. The dis-

ease, however, is often progressive, ultimately resulting in congestive heart failure and death.

c. Some dogs die of sudden death due to ventricular arrhythmias.

Radiographic findings

1. The heart size and shape are often normal.
2. Mild-to-moderate cardiomegaly is common.
3. With congestive heart failure, pulmonary edema is most commonly seen.
4. Biventricular failure with pulmonary edema, pleural effusion, and ascites are uncommon.

Other imaging

1. Echocardiography

English Cocker Spaniel Cardiomyopathy

Clinical correlations

1. Predilections:
   a. No sex predilection
   b. Age of onset 2 to 9 years (mean 5.8 years)
   c. A familial predisposition is suspected.
2. Common clinical signs include cough, exercise intolerance, acute dyspnea, and sudden death.
3. Murmurs are common, usually mitral regurgitation.
4. Affected dogs may have concurrent atrioventricular endocardiosis.

Radiographic findings

1. Mild to moderate cardiac enlargement, often biventricular
2. Pulmonary edema may be seen if left heart failure is present.

Other imaging

1. Echocardiography

Canine Hypertrophic Cardiomyopathy

Clinical correlations

1. Characterized by severe hypertrophy of the left ventricular wall and interventricular septum. Asymmetric hypertrophy with severe septal hypertrophy may cause partial outflow obstruction.
2. Increased stiffness of the left heart causing diastolic dysfunction.
3. A rare disease in the dog, is most often reported in the German Shepherd.
4. Clinical signs range from weakness, syncope, and coughing to sudden death.
5. A murmur may be present, caused by aortic outflow obstruction or mitral regurgitation.

Radiographic findings

1. Mild-to-moderate generalized heart enlargement
2. Pulmonary edema may be present if left heart failure predominates.
3. Pleural effusion, hepatomegaly, and ascites may be present if right heart failure predominates.

Other imaging

1. Echocardiography

Feline Hypertrophic Cardiomyopathy

Clinical correlations

1. Characterized by severe hypertrophy of the left ventricular wall, and is often associated with septal hypertrophy, which causes a severe reduction in the size of the left ventricular chamber. If failure ensues, it is a result of diastolic dysfunction.
2. Predilections:
   a. Wide age range of 5 months to 17 years (mean 4.8 to 7 years)
   b. More common in the domestic short hair cat
   c. More common in males
3. Common clinical signs include anorexia, vomiting, and acute dyspnea. Paresis or paralysis caused by thromboembolic disease may be the only clinical sign.
4. On auscultation, common findings include a gallop rhythm, a low grade systolic murmur, and arrythmias.
5. Electrocardiographic abnormalities are seen in 35 to 70% of cats. Left ventricular enlargement patterns are most common.

Radiographic findings (Figures 9.37 through 9.40)

1. Mild to moderate left ventricular enlargement with moderate to severe left atrial enlargement is the most common finding.
2. A "valentine" cardiac shape is often seen.
3. The cardiac size may be normal.
4. The pulmonary veins may be engorged or tortuous.
5. If left heart failure is present, variable degrees of mixed

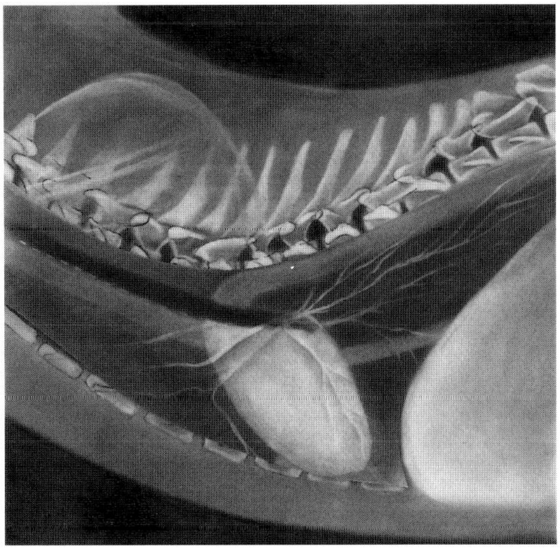

Figure 9.37. Feline cardiomyopathy with mild hypertrophy. There is mild enlargement of the cardiac silhouette.

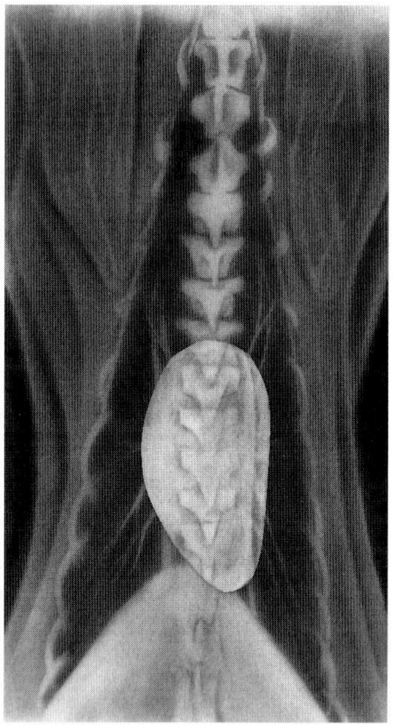

Figure 9.38. Feline cardiomyopathy with mild hypertrophy. The cardiac silhouette appears elongated and slightly enlarged.

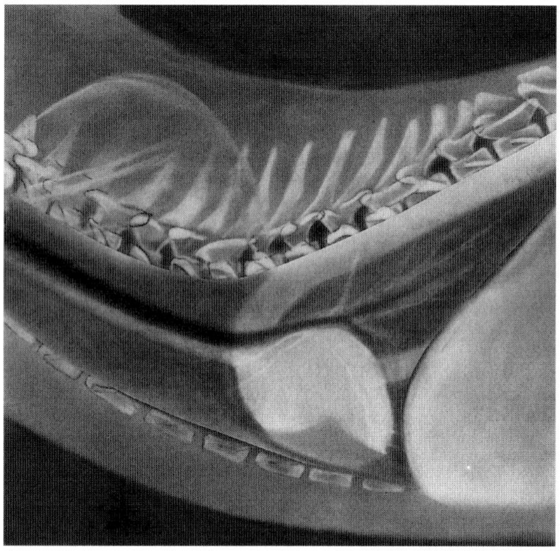

Figure 9.39. Feline cardiomyopathy with moderate hypertrophy. The cardiac silhouette is enlarged and the pulmonary vessels are enlarged and ill defined. Increased interstitial pulmonary infiltrate is present because of edema.

interstitial and alveolar infiltrate may be seen. A diffuse edema is more common; perihilar edema is less common.

6. Pleural effusion is uncommon, but if present, it usually indicates biventricular failure.

Contrast radiography

1. Selective angiography
2. Nonselective angiography

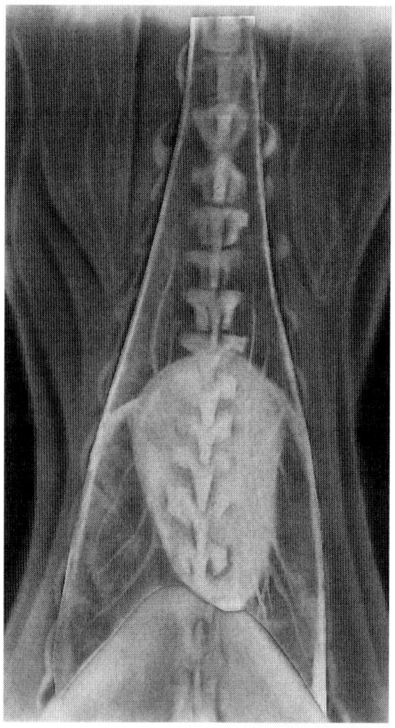

Figure 9.40. Feline cardiomyopathy with moderate hypertrophy. There is moderate enlargement of the cardiac silhouette. There is patchy mixed infiltrate in both lungs, indicative of edema and mild pleural effusion.

Other imaging

1. Echocardiography

Feline Restrictive Cardiomyopathy

Clinical correlations

1. Is a variant of hypertrophic cardiomyopathy in which diastolic function is impaired as a result of endocardial, subendocardial, or myocardial fibrosis or because infiltrative disease is present.
2. Is less common than hypertrophic or dilative cardiomyopathy.
3. Predilections:
   a. Wide age variation (8 months to 19 years)
   b. No breed or sex predilection
4. Clinical signs are often acute and associated with left or right heart failure. Dyspnea, lethargy, and abdominal distension are most commonly seen.
5. Electrocardiography may be normal or show varied arrhythmias. Premature ventricular contractions and atrial fibrillation are common.
6. Prognosis is guarded to poor for long-term survival.

Radiographic findings

1. Mild to moderate generalized cardiomegaly, usually with marked left atrial dilation
2. Pulmonary edema and/or pleural effusion is common.

Other imaging

1. Echocardiography
2. Nonselective angiography

Feline Congestive Cardiomyopathy

Clinical correlations

1. The etiology is unknown. Taurine deficiency has been associated with dilated cardiomyopathy with a reversible myocardial failure.
2. In the classic form of the disease, all four cardiac chambers are dilated, severe reduced contractility is present, and failure is caused by systolic dysfunction.
3. Predilections:
   a. Age range 5 months to 16 years (mean 7.5 years)
   b. More common in Siamese, Abyssinian, and Burmese breeds
   c. No sex predilection
4. The clinical signs vary and are often vague. Anorexia, dyspnea, lethargy, and vomiting are common. Syncope is rare.
5. The electrocardiogram is normal in 50% of cats. A bradycardia is seen in less than 25% of cats. Left ventricular enlargement and premature complexes are common.

Radiographic findings (Figures 9.41 and 9.42)

1. Generalized cardiac enlargement is most common.
2. Pleural effusion, hepatomegaly, and ascites are commonly seen when right heart failure predominates.
3. Pulmonary venous congestion or edema, if present, is usually mild.
4. Differential diagnosis:
   a. Pericardial effusion
   b. Peritoneal-pericardial diaphragmatic hernia
   c. Congenital heart disease (e.g., VSD, AV valve dysplasia, common AV canal)

Contrast radiography

1. Selective angiography
2. Nonselective angiography

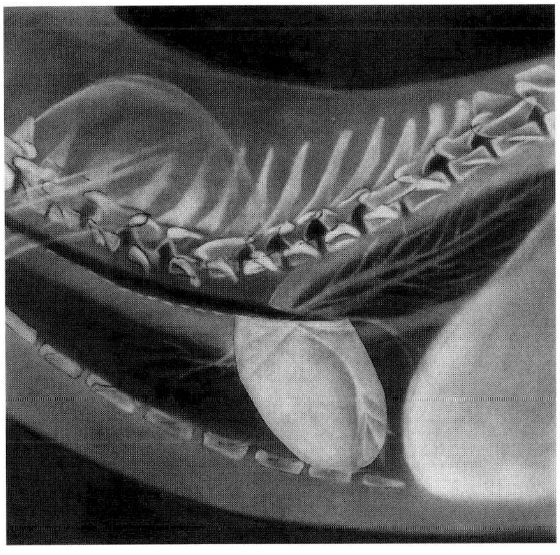

Figure 9.41. Feline dilated cardiomyopathy. The cardiac silhouette is enlarged and rounded.

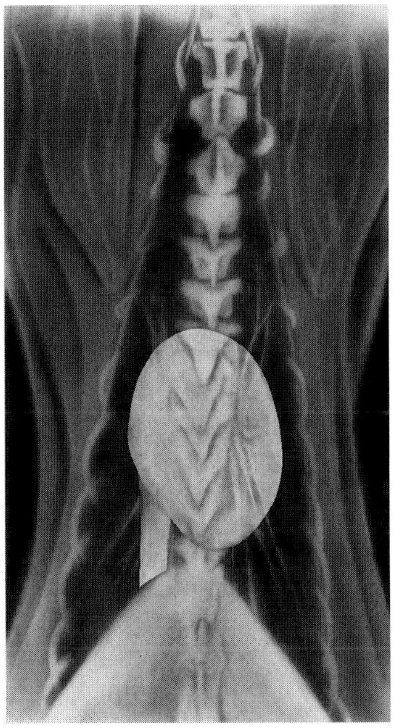

Figure 9.42. Feline dilated cardiomyopathy. There is moderate enlargement of the cardiac silhouette with enlargement of the caudal vena cava.

Other imaging

1. Echocardiography

Intermediate (Indeterminate) Cardiomyopathy

Clinical correlations

1. Is an unclassified form of myocardial disease in the cat, which does not fit the typical criteria of other feline myocardial diseases.
2. Can affect cat of any age.
3. Has variable clinical signs depending on the type and severity of congestive heart failure. Clinical signs may be nonspecific, including lethargy, dyspnea, abdominal distension, or collapse.
4. Electrocardiographic changes are variable, ranging from normal to ventricular or atrial arrhythmias.
5. Prognosis is poor for long-term survival.

Radiographic findings

1. Mild to severe cardiac enlargement
2. Pulmonary edema and/or pleural effusion depends on whether left- or right-sided heart failure predominates.

Contrast radiography

1. Selective angiography
2. Nonselective angiography

Other imaging

1. Echocardiography

Hyperthyroid Myocardial Disease

Clinical correlations

1. In the cat, left ventricular hypertrophy can develop secondary to hyperthyroidism as a result of the combined effects of chronic volume overload, high sympathetic tone, systemic hypertension, and the direct effect of thyroid hormone on the myocardium.
2. Clinical signs are variable; tachypnea and dyspnea are most common.
3. Electrocardiography may show a mild tachycardia, left ventricular enlargement, and a variety of ventricular arrhythmias.
4. The myocardial disease may resolve after medical or surgical treatment of the hyperthyroidism.

Radiographic findings

1. Radiographic findings are normal in 50% of cats.
2. Mild to moderate cardiomegaly is present in 50% of cats.
3. If failure occurs, pulmonary edema is seen in approximately 25% of cats and pleural effusion in approximately 75% of cats.

Other imaging

1. Echocardiography

Systemic Hypertension

Clinical correlations

1. Diseases that can cause hypertension include:
   a. Hyperthyroidism
   b. Chronic renal disease
   c. Diabetes mellitus
   d. Acromegaly
   e. Primary aldosteronism
2. Bilateral ocular hemorrhage and/or retinal detachments are common.
3. Pathologic changes within the heart are indistinguishable from hypertrophic cardiomyopathy.

Radiographic findings

1. Mild to severe generalized cardiomegaly
2. Pulmonary edema and/or pleural effusion, if heart failure is present
3. Cannot differentiate from other causes of myocardial disease.

Other imaging

1. Echocardiography

Myocardial Neoplasia

Clinical correlations

1. Malignant tumors are most common.
   a. Hemangiosarcoma (most common)
   b. Chemodectoma
   c. Fibrosarcoma
   d. Lymphosarcoma
   e. Metastatic tumors (e.g., adenocarcinoma of the lung or mammary gland, melanoma)
2. Benign tumors include:
   a. Fibroma
   b. Myoma
   c. Rhabdomyoma
3. Tumors may cause cardiac arrhythmias, or obstruct chamber filling or emptying. Pericardial involvement may occur from local extension, usually with pericardial effusion.
4. Clinical signs vary depending on the location and extent of disease.
   a. Weakness, collapse, or seizures
   b. Signs associated with left heart failure (e.g., coughing)
   c. Signs associated with right heart failure (e.g., pleural effusion, ascites.)

Radiographic findings

1. Mild to severe cardiomegaly
2. Globular cardiac enlargement, if pericardial effusion is present
3. Alteration of cardiac contour
4. Pulmonary edema and/or pleural effusion depending on whether left and/or right heart failure predominates

Contrast radiography

1. Pneumopericardiography
2. Selective angiography

Other imaging

1. Echocardiography
2. CT angiography
3. MR angiography

Heart Base Tumors

Clinical correlations

1. The most common heart-based tumor is the chemodectoma, which arises from nonchromaffin paraganglia of the aortic bodies.
2. Other less common tumors:
   a. Lymphosarcoma
   b. Ectopic thyroid carcinoma
   c. Ectopic parathyroid carcinoma
3. Chemodectomas occur more commonly in dogs, especially in the Boxer, Boston Terrier, German Shepherd, and Collie.
4. More commonly seen in male dogs older than 8 years of age.
5. Commonly causes pericardial effusion
6. Clinical signs vary, but commonly include:
   a. Weakness or collapse
   b. Abdominal distension secondary to cardiac tamponade

Radiographic findings (Figures 9.43 and 9.44)

1. Globular cardiac enlargement, if severe pericardial effusion is present.
2. Dorsal displacement of the trachea over the heart base (as seen from the lateral projection).
3. Displacement of the trachea to the right over the heart base (as seen from the dorsoventral projection).

Contrast radiography

1. Cranial vena cava venography
2. Selective angiography

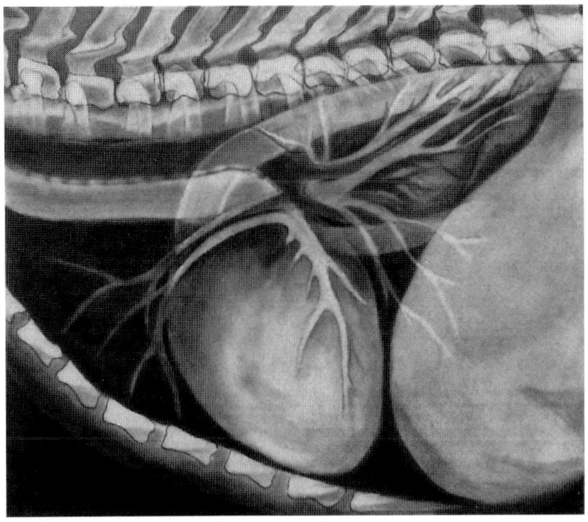

Figure 9.43. Heart base tumor. There is elevation of the trachea over the heart base. The tumor mass is unidentified because of its direct anatomic association with the heart (silhouette sign).

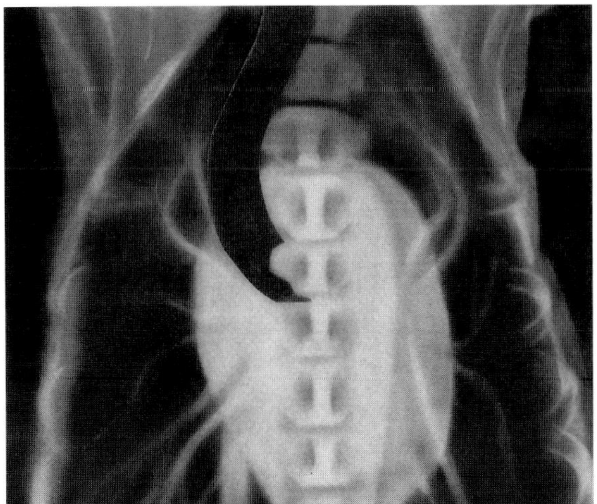

Figure 9.44. Heart base tumor. Large tumors in the heart base often displace the trachea to the right.

Other imaging

1. Echocardiography
2. CT angiography
3. MRI angiography

Aortic Thromboembolism

Clinical correlations

1. Is most often seen in cats with hypertrophic or restrictive cardiomyopathy; is rare in dilated cardiomyopathy.
2. Clot formation is thought to be precipitated by a combination of endothelial damage, sluggish blood flow, and increased blood coagulability.
3. The clinical consequences of systemic arterial embolization depend on the site of embolization, the completeness of obstruction, the functional patency of collateral circulation, and the duration of the obstruction.
4. The most common site for thromboembolism is the aortic trifurcation including the iliac arteries. Other sites include the abdominal aorta (renal, mesenteric arteries) and the brachial, coronary, and cerebral arteries.

Radiographic findings

1. Moderate-to-severe cardiomegaly on thoracic radiographs.
2. Pulmonary edema and/or pleural effusion depends on whether left or right heart failure predominates.
3. Survey abdominal radiographs are normal, or may show hepatomegaly and ascites if right heart failure is present.

Contrast radiography

1. Nonselective angiography
2. Selective angiography

Other imaging

1. Echocardiography
2. CT angiography
3. MRI angiography

PERICARDIAL DISEASES

Anatomy and Physiology

1. The pericardium envelops the heart with attachments to the base of the heart, enclosing the origins of the aorta, pulmonary artery, and the vena cavae. It is composed of two layers. An inner serous layer is contiguous with the epicardium (the visceral pericardium) and reflects back on itself lining the outer fibrous layer (the parietal pericardium). The fibrous layer has strong attachments from the heart base and forms the pericardiophrenic ligament, which is attached to the diaphragm. The pericardial cavity is between the two layers of serous pericardium.

2. A small amount of fluid is within the pericardial cavity, ranging in volume from 1 to 15 mL in normal dogs.
3. The functions of the pericardium include myocardial surface lubrication, protection of the heart from infections or adhesions, maintenance of the heart in a fixed position within the chest, regulation of stroke volume between the two ventricles, and prevention of cardiac dilatation.
4. Diseases of the pericardium result in increased pericardial fluid, abnormal pericardial contents (e.g., tumors or other mass lesions), or from thickening of the pericardium (e.g., constrictive pericarditis).
5. Cardiac tamponade and right heart failure occur if pericardial pressures are significantly increased. Increased pericardial pressure is a function of the rate of fluid accumulation, the absolute fluid volume, and the physical characteristics of the pericardium.

Peritoneopericardial Diaphragmatic Hernia

Clinical correlations

1. Is the most common congenital diaphragmatic defect in the dog and cat.
2. Is caused by faulty development of the ventral portion of the diaphragm, allowing a continuation of the peritoneum through the defect contiguous with the serosal surface of the pericardial sac.
3. Is often associated with sternal anomalies (e.g., absent sternabra or xyphoid).
4. Herniated abdominal viscera most often include liver, falciform fat, or bowel.
5. May be an incidental finding, and animals commonly are asymptomatic.
6. Dog breed predilections (See Table 9.2)

Radiographic findings

1. Globular enlargement of the cardiac silhouette
2. Inhomogeneous radiopacity of the cardiac silhouette is caused by fat, gas, or soft tissue and fat opacities (depending on herniated viscera).
3. Inability to identify the cranioventral diaphragm clearly on both projections.
4. Differential considerations:
   a. Pericardial effusion
   b. Cardiomegaly

Contrast radiography

1. Celiography
2. Pneumoperitoneography
3. Barium upper gastrointestinal study
4. Selective or nonselective angiocardiography

Other imaging modalities to confirm diagnosis

1. Ultrasound
2. Radiographic tomography
3. CT
4. MRI

Pericardial Cysts

Clinical correlations

1. Is rare in the dog and cat.
2. Cause is unknown but theorized to be incarcerated omentum or falciform fat from a peritoneal pericardial diaphragmatic hernia or abnormal development of mesenchymal tissues within the pericardium.
3. May prevent normal cardiac movement within the pericardial cavity.

Radiographic findings

1. Globular enlargement of the cardiac silhouette
2. If tamponade or restricted cardiac function is present, right heart failure may occur (hepatomegaly and ascites).

Other imaging

1. Echocardiography

Pericardial Effusion

Clinical correlations

1. Types of pericardial effusion are commonly based on fluid characteristics.
   a. Transudative effusions
      1) Congestive heart failure (e.g., cardiomyopathy, right heart failure)
      2) Hypoproteinemia
      3) Peritoneopericardial diaphragmatic hernia
      4) Uremia
   b. Hemorrhagic effusions
      1) Neoplasia
         a) Secondary to right atrial or auricular hemangiosarcoma
         b) Heart base tumor (e.g., chemodectoma)
         c) Mesothelioma
         d) Lymphosarcoma
      2) Secondary to left atrial rupture (usually in small dogs with severe left atrial dilation from mitral regurgitation)
      3) Idiopathic (most common)
      4) Trauma
      5) Coagulopathy (e.g., rodentacide)
   c. Exudative effusions
      1) Infections (bacterial or fungal, actinomycosis, tuberculosis)
      2) Feline infectious peritonitis
2. The clinical signs of pericardial effusion depend on the volume, type, and rate of fluid accumulation.
   a. With mild pericardial effusion, no clinical signs will be present.
   b. With moderate cardiac compression in which the pericardial effusion has accumulated gradually, signs of right heart failure are often seen, including:
      1) Lethargy, weakness, and fatigue
      2) Dyspnea and cough

3) Syncope with exertion
4) Abdominal distension caused by hepatomegaly and ascites

c. With severe cardiac compression or rapid development, signs of low cardiac output are seen, including:
1) Marked weakness and collapse
2) Dyspnea and tachypnea
3) Sudden death

3. Other common clinical findings of moderate to severe effusion include:
   a. Systemic venous hypertension (e.g., jugular pulse)
   b. Muffled heart sounds on auscultation
   c. Electrocardiography often shows diminished amplitudes of the QRS complexes and electrical alternans.

Radiographic findings (Figures 9.45 and 9.46)

1. The degree of cardiac silhouette enlargement is proportional to the volume of pericardial effusion.
2. With small effusions, the cardiac silhouette shape may appear normal or mildly enlarged.
3. With severe effusions, the cardiac silhouette will appear round and globular in shape on lateral and dorsoventral projections.
4. If right heart failure is present, other findings include:
   a. Distension of the caudal vena cava
   b. Pleural effusion
   c. Hepatomegaly
   d. Ascites
5. Abnormalities of the shape of the cardiac silhouette may reflect the underlying cause of the effusion.
   a. Severe left atrial dilation, in addition to globular shaped cardiac silhouette, may be caused by left-atrial rupture in the dog.

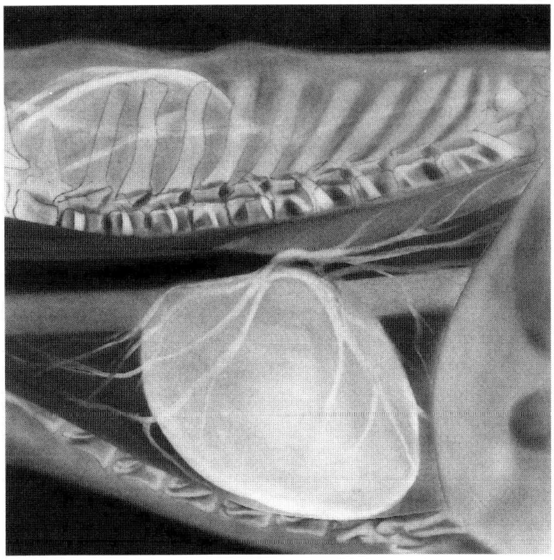

Figure 9.45. Pericardial effusion. There is globular enlargement of the cardiac silhouette.

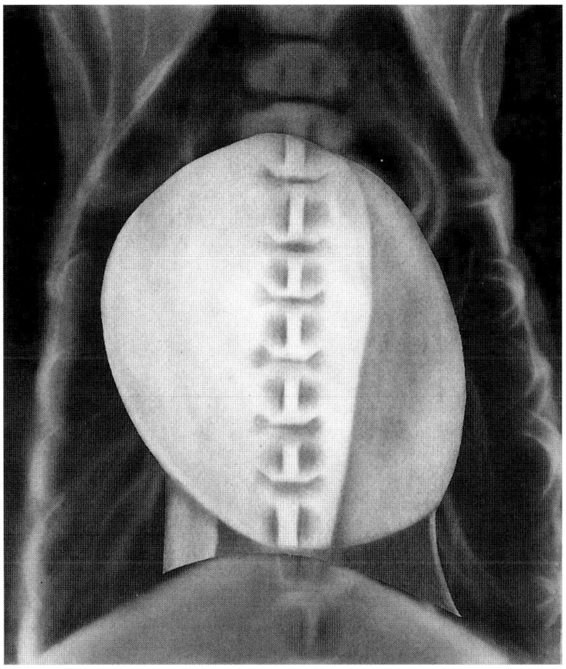

Figure 9.46. Pericardial effusion. There is globular enlargement of the cardiac silhouette.

   b. Elevation of the trachea at the heart base or a soft tissue mass seen in the heart base area may be caused by a heart base tumor.
   c. Protrusion of the right cranial heart border may be seen in tumors of the right atrium.
   d. Irregular outline of the cardiac silhouette may occur with a pericardial cyst, granuloma, or abscess.

Contrast radiography

1. Fluoroscopy may show absent or diminished cardiac motion.
2. Nonselective venography/angiography
3. Pneumopericardiography

Other imaging

1. Echocardiography
2. CT angiography
3. MR angiography

Constrictive Pericarditis

Clinical correlations

1. Associated with chronic fibrosis of the pericardium, in which the volume of pericardial effusion is usually small, and the clinical effects are secondary to the constrictive effects on cardiac function.
2. Causes that have been reported include:
   a. Infections
   b. Foreign bodies
   c. Neoplasia (heart base tumor, mesothelioma)
   d. Recurrent hemorrhagic pericardial effusion
   e. Idiopathic (most common)

3. Clinical signs associated with right heart failure
   a. Weakness, lethargy, and dyspnea
   b. Venous hypertension (e.g., jugular pulse)
   c. Abdominal distension (hepatomegaly and ascites)

Radiographic findings
1. Mild to moderate cardiac enlargement
2. Rounding of the cardiac silhouette in the lateral and/or dorsoventral projections
3. Distension of caudal vena cava
4. Pleural effusion
5. Hepatomegaly and ascites

Contrast radiography
1. Nonselective angiocardiography
2. Selective angiocardiography

Other imaging
1. Echocardiography

Pericardial Masses
Clinical correlations
1. Pericardial masses may include:
   a. Neoplasms (e.g., mesothelioma, heart base tumor)
   b. Granuloma
   c. Cyst
   d. Abscess
2. Pericardial effusion is often present concurrently.
3. Clinical signs may include:
   a. Muffled heart sounds
   b. Depressed QRS complexes on electrocardiogram
   c. Weakness, lethargy, and collapse depending on the severity of right heart failure

Radiographic findings
1. Radiographs may be normal if the pericardial mass is small and the degree of pericardial effusion is minimal.
2. Enlargement of the cardiac silhouette is variable depending on the volume of pericardial effusion; with severe effusion the heart will appear round and globular in shape on lateral and dorsoventral projections.
3. The border of the silhouette may be irregular with some pericardial mass lesions.
4. If right heart failure is present other findings include:
   a. Distension of the caudal vena cava
   b. Pleural effusion
   c. Hepatomegaly
   d. Ascites

Contrast radiography
Pneumopericardiography

Other imaging
1. Echocardiography
2. CT angiography
3. MR angiography

chapter ten

10

Abdomen: Peritoneal and Retroperitoneal Cavities

ANATOMY (Figure 10.1)

1. The abdominal cavity consists of peritoneal and retroperitoneal spaces.
2. The peritoneum is a thin serous membrane that, as parietal, visceral, or connecting layers, covers all structures within the peritoneal cavity.
   a. The parietal peritoneum lines the diaphragm and abdominal wall, and separates the peritoneal from the retroperitoneal compartments.
   b. The visceral peritoneum covers the abdominal organs and the connecting peritoneum covers the mesentery, omentum, and intraabdominal ligaments.
3. The retroperitoneal space is demarcated ventrally by the parietal peritoneum and dorsally by the sublumbar musculature (psoas muscles) and extends caudally to the pelvic inlet.
4. Within the retroperitoneal space are the kidneys, ureters, adrenal glands, major blood vessels (e.g., abdominal aorta, caudal vena cava, cisterna chyli), and certain lymph nodes (e.g., renal, medial iliac, and sacral).

RADIOGRAPHIC INTERPRETATION (Figures 10.2 and 10.3)

1. Each radiograph should be systematically evaluated with emphasis on assessing the size, shape, radiopacity, position, and external architecture of all abdominal viscera, including margins of the diaphragm, the abdominal wall, and the dorsal and caudal limits of the peritoneal and retroperitoneal spaces.
2. The normal abdominal viscera assume known positions within the abdomen; however, their known position may be altered by many normal situations or disease processes. Common causes for organ displacement include:
   a. Amount of ingesta and gas within the stomach and bowel
   b. Diaphragmatic or abdominal wall hernia
   c. Pregnancy
   d. Masses arising from peritoneal, retroperitoneal, or abdominal wall structures
   e. Localized or generalized abdominal effusion
3. Abdominal organs and adjacent structures are visible because of differences in radiopacity (e.g., thickness of tissue and type of tissue). The inherent contrast of gas within the stomach and bowel, as well as intraabdominal fat, provides radiographic contrast. For example, abdominal viscera are not visible when there is an absence of fat within the abdomen, as in emaciation.
4. When two structures of similar radiopacity touch, their margins are obscured. This is called the silhouette sign. When two structures of similar radiopacity are physically separated, their margins are each visible and no silhouette sign is seen.
5. Abdominal detail may be enhanced by free gas within the peritoneal or retroperitoneal space, or obscured by effusion, carcinomatosis, or other disease processes.
6. Enlargement of an organ or part of an organ may cause displacement of adjacent abdominal structures. This finding commonly aids in the recognition of the organ responsible for the displacement.

Loss of Abdominal Detail

Clinical correlations

1. Decreased intraabdominal fat
   a. Immaturity
   b. Emaciation

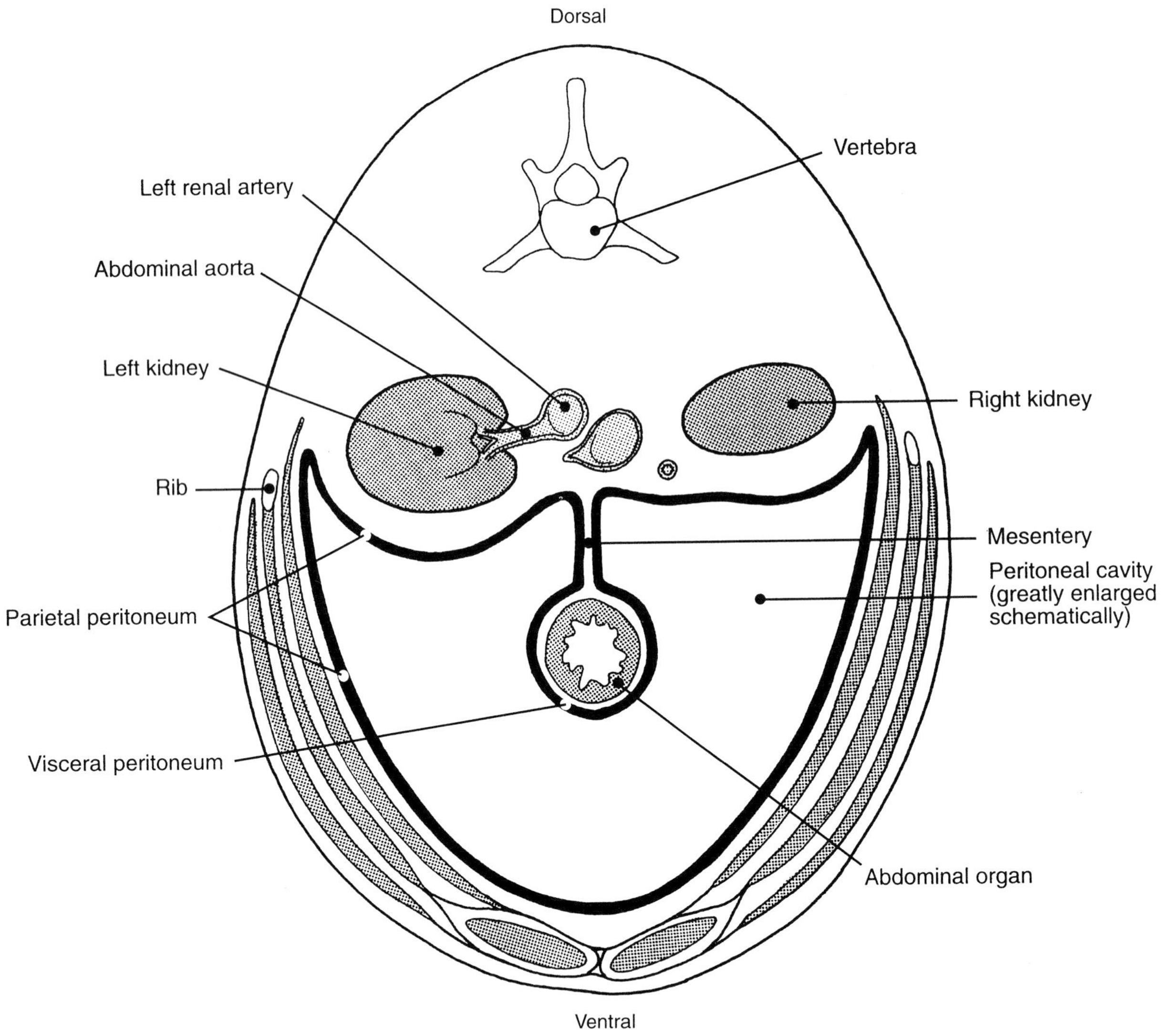

Figure 10.1. Schematic representation of the abdominal cavity, mesentery, peritoneum, and peritoneal cavity. (From Anderson WD, Anderson BG. Atlas of Canine Anatomy. Philadelphia: Lea & Febiger; 1994:608. With permission of Williams & Wilkins, Baltimore.)

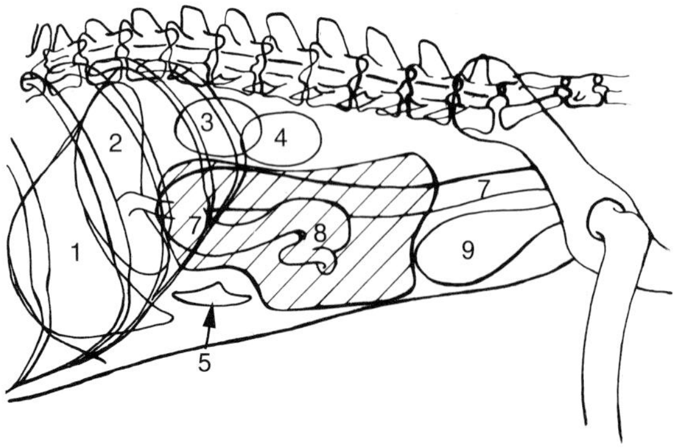

Figure 10.2. Normal lateral projection: **1**) liver, **2**) stomach, **3**) right kidney, **4**) left kidney, **5**) spleen, **6**) small intestine, **7**) large intestine, **8**) cecum, **9**) urinary bladder.

2. Abdominal effusion
   a. Transudate (e.g., ascites)
      1) Right heart failure
      2) Hypoproteinemia
      3) Portal hypertension
   b. Exudate (Peritonitis)
      1) Bowel perforation
      2) Abdominal abscess
      3) Feline infectious peritonitis (FIP)
      4) Pancreatitis
   c. Hemorrhage
      1) Neoplasia
      2) Trauma
   d. Chyle
   e. Urine (e.g., ruptured urinary bladder)
   f. Bile (biliary rupture)

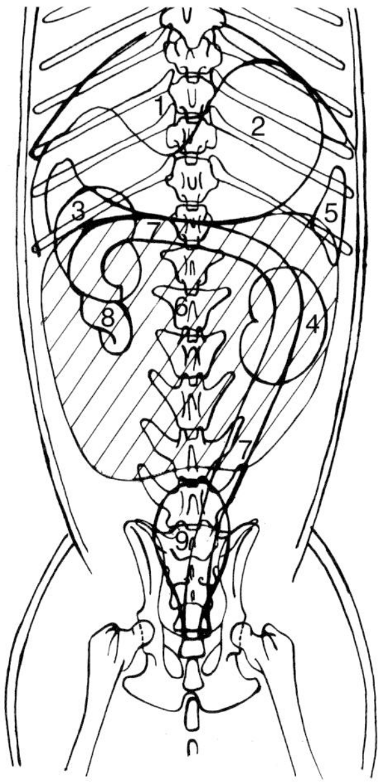

Figure 10.3. Normal ventrodorsal projection: **1**) liver, **2**) stomach, **3**) right kidney, **4**) left kidney, **5**) spleen, **6**) small intestine, **7**) large intestine, **8**) cecum, **9**) urinary bladder.

3. Carcinomatosis
   a. Pancreatic carcinoma
   b. Adenocarcinoma of bowel
   c. Ovarian carcinoma
   d. Hemangiosarcoma
4. Lack of sufficient fat for contrast in abdomen (e.g., thin)
5. Normal young animal (e.g., Brown fat)

Radiographic findings

1. Small amounts of peritoneal effusion
   a. Hazy or mottled appearance in localized area
   b. Blurring or indistinctness of the serosal borders
   c. Soft tissue nodules with the omentum
2. Large amounts of peritoneal effusion
   a. Homogeneous opacity throughout the abdomen obscuring the serosal margins of all abdominal viscera (ground glass-like appearance)
   b. Abdominal distension
   c. Cranial displacement of the diaphragm
   d. Renal contour is seen if no retroperitoneal effusion and if adequate retroperitoneal fat is present.
   e. Gas-filled bowel loops tend to float to the top and central portion of abdomen on the lateral and ventrodorsal projections.

Intraabdominal Gas Accumulation

Clinical correlations

1. Free peritoneal gas
   a. Postlaparotomy
      1) Immediately postoperatively, a small to moderate amount of free abdominal gas will be evident. This gas is resorbed over time and is usually not visualized after 3 to 7 days.
      2) It is difficult to differentiate normal postoperative gas in the abdomen from the postoperative complication of gastrointestinal perforation.
   b. Ruptured hollow viscus as a result of perforated ulcer, ingested foreign body, or projectile missile
      1) Stomach
      2) Small bowel
      3) Large bowel
   c. Secondary to emphysematous infection and rupture of the urinary bladder, gall bladder or uterus
   d. Iatrogenic
      1) Ruptured urinary bladder during pneumocystography
      2) Pneumoperitoneogram
   e. Penetrating wounds of the abdomen
2. Abnormal localized gas accumulation within abdominal organs
   a. Gas ileus of a bowel loop
   b. Gas mixed with ingesta or fecal material within stomach and bowel
   c. Abdominal abscess (e.g., spleen, liver, mesentery)
   d. Emphysematous cholecystitis
   e. Emphysematous cystitis
   f. Pneumatosis coli
   g. Physometra (emphysematous metritis)
3. Gas accumulation in the retroperitoneal space
   a. Secondary to pneumomediastinum
   b. Penetrating wound
   c. Sublumbar abscess

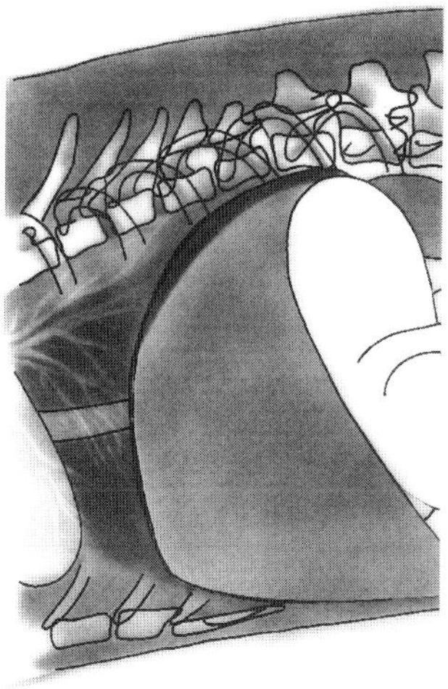

Figure 10.4. Free abdominal gas: the gas is seen between the diaphragm, liver, and body wall.

Radiographic findings (Figures 10.4 and 10.5)

1. Peritoneal gas
   a. A small volume of gas may be difficult to recognize because gas bubbles are small and irregular in shape.
   b. Large gas volumes may coalesce into larger gas bubbles and are seen usually in the highest point (least dependent) area of the abdomen.

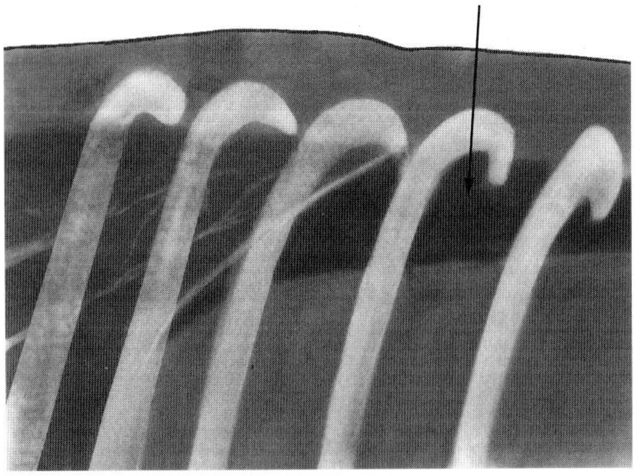

Figure 10.5. Free abdominal gas: in a left lateral recumbent projection (using horizontal x-ray beam), there is gas (arrow) between the diaphragm and the liver.

1) Lateral view: caudal to the diaphragm and below the cranial lumbar muscles
2) Ventrodorsal projection: caudal to the diaphragm
3) There is increased visualization of the serosal surfaces of the stomach, urinary bladder, bowel walls, or liver lobes

c. Use of horizontal x-ray beam allows detection of a small amount of peritoneal gas. Method to follow:
   1) Position the animal in left lateral recumbency for 5 minutes.
   2) Expose a ventrodorsal projection with a horizontal beam directed at the cranial right abdomen.
   3) Free peritoneal gas will be seen between the diaphragm and lobes of the right lateral liver.

2. Localized gas accumulation
   a. Small or large radiolucent gas bubbles are seen within the wall, lumen, or parenchyma of an organ (e.g., splenic abscess, hepatic abscess, emphysematous metritis, pneumatosis coli, emphysematous cholecystitis, emphysematous cystitis).
   b. Oblique projections or horizontal beam radiographs may aid in the recognition of abnormal intraperitoneal gas.
3. Retroperitoneal gas accumulation
   a. There is increased radiolucency of the retroperitoneal space.
   b. The kidneys are delineated by the retroperitoneal gas, and this is especially prominent on the lateral projection of the abdomen.
   c. The descending colon may be displaced ventrally with a large volume of retroperitoneal gas accumulation.

Intraabdominal Focal Opacities

Clinical correlations

1. Calcific or opaque material in the stomach or bowel
   a. Food
   b. Bone chips
   c. Medication (e.g., bismuth compounds, some antibiotics such as ampicillin, amoxicillin, sulfa drugs)
   d. Opaque foreign bodies (e.g., pebbles, glass fragments)
   e. Lead or other heavy metal
2. Calculi
   a. Gall bladder and bile ducts (intrahepatic and extrahepatic)
   b. Renal, ureteral, or urinary bladder
   c. Prostate
3. Mineralization: calcium or other mineral salts are deposited in body tissues. Different causes include:
   a. Dystrophic mineralization secondary to tissue necrosis may occur with:
      1) Renal infarct, tumor, or abscess
      2) Chronic cystitis or neoplasia
      3) Hepatic abscess, cyst, or tumor
      4) Splenic abscess or tumor
      5) Mesenteric or omental cyst (in the cat)
      6) Ossified hematoma
      7) Fat mineralization (e.g., chronic steatitis)
   b. Metastatic mineralization
      1) Disorder of calcium and phosphorus metabolism as can occur in:
         a) Hypervitaminosis D
         b) Primary hyperparathyroidism
         c) Secondary hyperparathyroidism
         d) Hyperadrenocorticism
      2) Examples include:
         a) Nephrocalcinosis
         b) Calcinosis cutis
         c) Gastric wall calcification (usually with secondary renal hyperparathyroidism and renal failure)
         d) Vascular calcification (aorta, iliac, celiac and mesenteric arteries)
            (1) Idiopathic
            (2) Atherosclerosis
            (3) Secondary renal hyperparathyroidism
            (4) Hyperthyroidism
   c. Benign osseous metaplasia (e.g., liver, kidney, pancreas, mesentery)
   d. Extra skeletal osteosarcoma (e.g., liver, spleen, kidney)
   e. Normal pregnancy with fetal ossification

Radiographic findings

1. Focal areas of mineralization
2. May appear punctate, linear, amorphous, or cystic
3. If focal mineralized opacity is perceived as possibly within the lumen of the stomach or bowel, consider repeating the abdominal radiographs after an enema or fast.
4. Mesenteric or omental cysts in cats are usually round with an "egg shell" like mineralized rim.

5. If an organ is ruptured, calculi may be visible in the cranial abdomen (e.g., calculi from ruptured urinary bladder).
6. Ossified fetus may be in the uterus, free in abdominal cavity (e.g., ectopic pregnancy) or within the gastrointestinal tract (e.g., after ingestion of the fetus).

Contrast radiography

1. Upper GI study
2. Intravenous urography
3. Cystography
4. Pneumoperitoneography

Other imaging

1. Ultrasound
2. CT
3. MRI

Abdominal Lymph Nodes

Clinical correlations

1. The abdominal lymph nodes are grouped anatomically according to their drainage patterns.
   a. Visceral lymph nodes
      1) Hepatic
      2) Splenic
      3) Cranial mesenteric
      4) Colic
      5) Pancreatoduodenal
      6) Gastric
   b. Parietal
      1) Lumbar aortic
      2) Medial iliac
      3) Hypogastric
      4) Sacral
      5) Deep inguinal
2. Enlargement of the lymph nodes can be caused by inflammatory or neoplastic disease.
3. Enlargement of the medial iliac lymph nodes (formerly called external iliac and internal iliac lymph nodes) is usually caused by neoplastic disease.
   a. Lymphosarcoma
   b. Metastasis from perianal carcinoma or other neoplasms of the pelvic region (e.g., bladder, urethra, cervix, prostate, testicle, or rectum), caudoventral abdominal wall or rear legs.
   c. Occasionally as a result of inflammatory disease from pelvic, caudal abdominal, or perianal infections.
   d. May cause edema of the rear limbs because of lymphatic obstruction or compression of the caudal vena cava or iliac veins.

Radiographic findings (Figure 10.6)

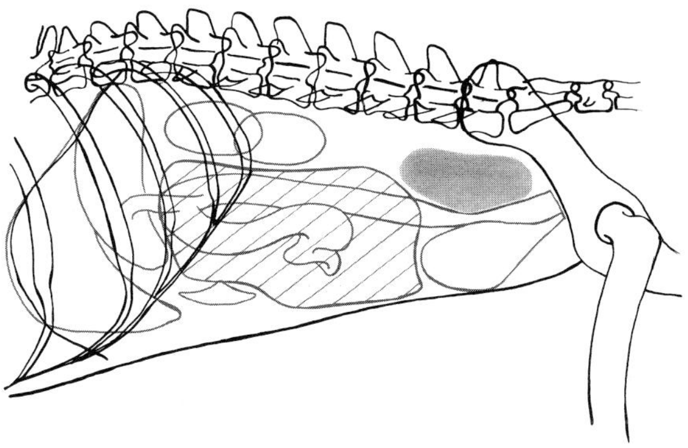

Figure 10.6. Enlarged medial iliac lymph nodes: there is ventral displacement of the descending colon.

1. The normal lymph nodes in the peritoneal or retroperitoneal spaces are not seen on survey radiographs because their small size and degree of their soft tissue radiopacity is similar to adjacent structures.
2. Enlarged medial iliac lymph nodes will cause increased soft tissue opacity in the retroperitoneal space, usually ventral to L6 and L7. Ventral displacement of the caudal portion of the descending colon may be seen.
3. Enlarged mesenteric or colic lymph nodes may cause a mass effect or increased soft tissue opacity in the mid abdomen with displacement of the adjacent bowel.
4. Dystrophic mineralization secondary to necrosis, occasionally may be visible within a lymph node.
5. Some oily contrast agents used for lymphangiography may be retained within a lymph node and visible as a radiopacity.

Contrast radiography

Lymphangiography

Other imaging

1. Ultrasound
2. Scintigraphy
3. CT
4. MRI

Peritoneal Hernias

Clinical correlations

1. As a result of congenital or acquired weakness in the muscular or tendinons portions of the peritoneal lining
2. Common congenital hernia include:
   a. Umbilical hernia
   b. Femoral or inguinal hernia
   c. Peritoneal-pericardial diaphragmatic hernia
   d. Scrotal hernia
3. Usually, acquired hernias are traumatic.
   a. Diaphragmatic hernia
   b. Ventral or lateral abdominal hernia
   c. Mesenteric hernia
4. Clinical signs will vary, depending on the organ present within the hernia and the degree of incarceration and dysfunction of the organ.

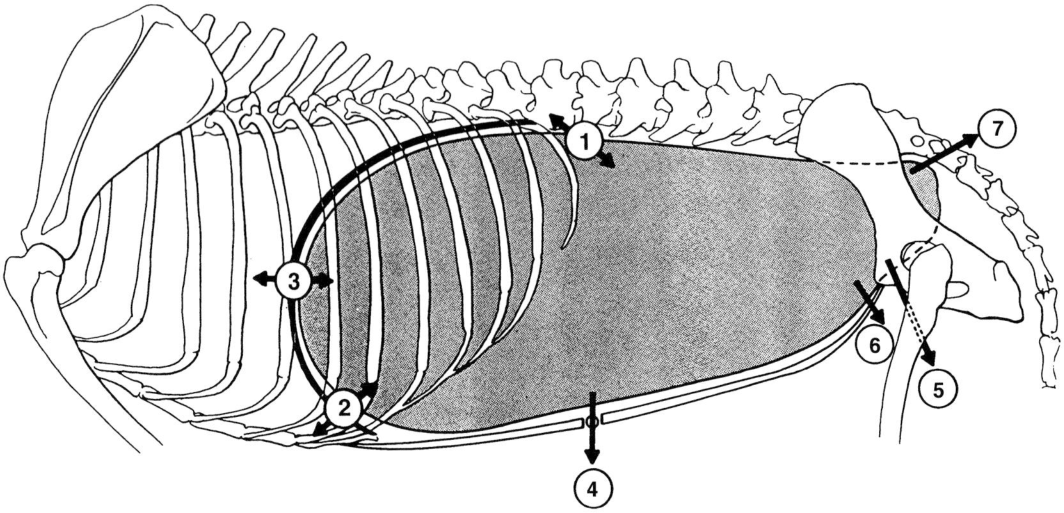

Figure 10.7. Common locations for hernias: **1**) dorsal diaphragm, **2**) ventral diaphragm, **3**) normal openings in diaphragm between the thorax and abdomen at aortic hiatus, esophageal hiatus, and vena cava foramen, **4**) umbilicus, **5**) femoral, **6**) inguinal, **7**) perineal. (Adapted from Anderson WD, Anderson BG. Atlas of Canine Anatomy. Philadelphia: Lea & Febiger; 1994:583. With permission of Williams & Wilkins, Baltimore.)

Radiographic findings (Figure 10.7)

1. If a loop of bowel is contained within the hernia, the gas-filled loop may be seen to extend beyond the confines of the peritoneal cavity.
2. If the organ within the hernia is solid or fluid-filled (e.g., uterus, liver, bladder), a soft tissue mass will be seen outside the confines of the peritoneal cavity.
3. If the hernia is internal (e.g., mesenteric hernia), the affected loop of bowel will be dilated and filled with gas or fluid as part of an obstructive ileus.

Contrast radiography

1. Depending on the location of the hernia and the organ(s) contained within the hernia, one or more of the following contrast procedures may aid in the visualization of the hernia.
2. Types of contrast studies
   a. Barium or iodinated upper GI study
   b. Pneumoperitoneography
   c. Positive contrast peritoneography
   d. Urethrocystography
   e. Intravenous urography

Other imaging

1. Ultrasound
2. CT

chapter eleven

11

Gastrointestinal System

RADIOGRAPHIC ANATOMY (Figure 11.1)

1. The soft tissue structures of the pharynx, oropharynx, nasopharynx, and larynx are visualized because of adjacent air within these structures.
2. The pharynx is bordered by the base of the tongue (ventrally) and the pharyngeal wall (dorsally and caudally). The normal epiglottis may be located dorsal, end-on, or ventral to the soft palate.
3. The nasopharynx is separated from the oropharynx by the soft palate, which extends to the epiglottis.
4. The larynx, hyoid bones, and trachea are readily identified. The larynx usually is ventral to the first two cervical vertebrae on a lateral projection with the neck in a normal position.
5. Variants of normal anatomy exist, especially with different breeds of dogs. Examples include:
   a. Size and shape of pharynx and larynx vary
   b. Obese or brachycephalic dogs usually have more soft tissues and fat within the cranial, cervical, and pharyngeal region, which may partially obscure visualization of the pharynx.
   c. Focal and diffuse mineralization of the laryngeal cartilages commonly is present in chondrodystrophoid dog breeds and in older animals. The absence of laryngeal cartilage mineralization may prevent identification of the laryngeal structures, especially in immature animals.
   d. Variation in the position of the head, tongue, and neck will cause variations in the position and angles between the hyoid bones.
6. Radiographically, the normal pharyngeal structures are visualized best on the lateral projection with the neck extended.
   a. The retropharyngeal space is of soft tissue radiopacity. A "rule of thumb" for normal width on the lateral projection is equal to two thirds to one time the length of the third cervical vertebra. The lateral projection should be symmetrical with an approximate 135° angulation between the vertebral canal and horizontal rami of the mandibles.
   b. A flexed lateral or oblique projection will artifactually increase the radiopacity or size of the retropharyngeal space.

DISEASES/DISORDERS

Pharyngeal Inflammation

Clinical correlations

1. Pharyngeal inflammation commonly is associated with oral or systemic illness. The tonsils and the pharyngeal soft tissues are often affected.
2. Edema is often secondary to trauma from ingested foreign bodies, insect bites, or infection.
3. Edema and swelling of the pharyngeal soft tissues may impair respiration.
4. An examination of the oral areas provides the most direct assessment of the pharynx and tonsils.

Radiographic findings (Figure 11.2)

1. In many instances, no radiographic abnormality is seen. Occasionally soft tissue swelling or a mass is visible.
2. Radiopaque foreign bodies are readily identified.
3. Subcutaneous gas within the fascial planes may occur with penetrating wounds, foreign bodies, or from gas-forming infections.
4. Occasionally, an elongated soft palate is visible. This finding is commonly associated with other airway abnormalities, such as stenotic nares and hypoplastic trachea.

Pharyngeal and Retropharyngeal Masses

Clinical correlations

1. Masses may arise inside or outside the airway of the nasopharynx or oropharynx, and may be associated

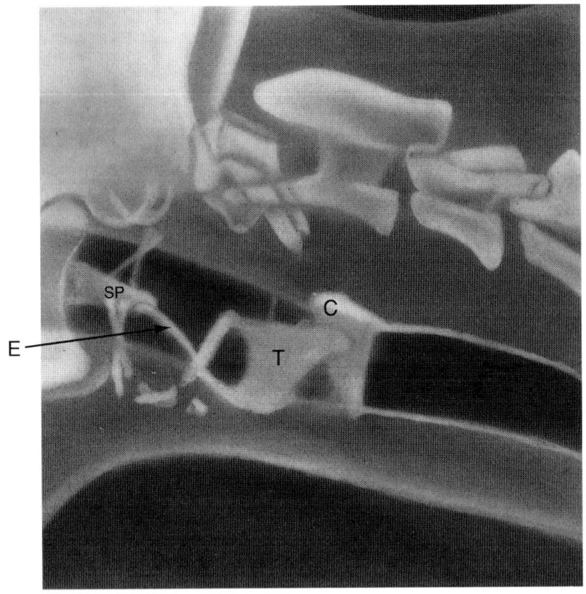

Figure 11.1. Normal canine pharynx. Radiographic landmarks of pharynx include: nasopharynx (**n**), oropharynx (**or**), pharynx (**p**), soft palate (**sp**), and the base of the tongue (**t**). Radiographic landmarks of the larynx are: epiglottis (**E**), thyroid cartilage (**T**), and the cricoid cartilage (**C**).

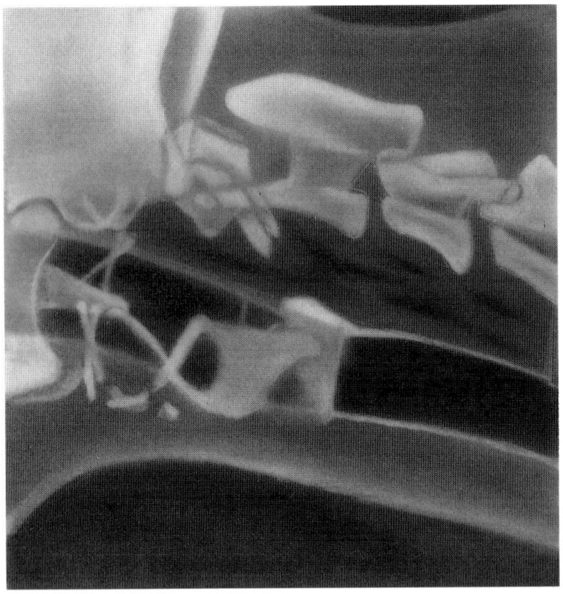

Figure 11.2. Retropharyngeal gas.

with the tonsils, the retropharyngeal lymph nodes, the mandibular or parotid salivary glands, the epiglottis, or the soft palate.

2. Clinical signs vary depending on the cause, location, and severity of the mass lesion. Common clinical signs include dysphagia, respiratory distress, and hypersalivation.
3. Neoplasms of the pharynx include the following:
   a. Soft palate: melanoma, fibrosarcoma
   b. Pharyngeal wall: sarcoma, extension of tonsilar carcinoma
   c. Tonsil: squamous cell carcinoma, lymphosarcoma
4. Pharyngeal polyps can occur within the nasopharynx or from the middle ear (more common in cats) and commonly with concurrent clinical and radiographic evidence of middle ear disease.
5. Mucous gland retention cysts occur within the oropharynx near the base of the epiglottis.
6. Abscessation of the pharynx, salivary glands, and adjacent lymph nodes may result from local or systemic infections or secondary to foreign bodies.
7. Enlargement of the retropharyngeal space commonly is caused by lymphadenopathy associated with inflammatory or neoplastic disease. Common neoplasms that spread to the retropharyngeal lymph nodes include malignant oral tumors, thyroid carcinoma, lymphosarcoma, and occasionally nasal tumors.
8. Endoscopy is often helpful for diagnosis of pharyngeal masses.

Radiographic findings (Figures 11.3 and 11.4 A,B)

1. There is diminished size of the pharyngeal air space, which varies with displacement of normal adjacent soft tissue structures or hyoid bones.
2. Obstruction of the nasopharynx or oropharynx may be identified depending on the origination and size of the mass lesion. A mass may be seen impinging on or protruding into the nasopharynx or oropharynx.
3. Enlarged retropharyngeal lymph nodes cause an increased retropharyngeal space, dorsal compression of the pharyngeal walls, or decreased size of the pharynx. If the node enlargement is asymmetrical, lateral displacement may be present.

Contrast radiography

1. A barium study with fluoroscopy is necessary to evaluate the oropharynx and nasopharynx.
2. May identify an abnormal mass as displacement of normal structures.

Other imaging

1. Ultrasound
2. CT
3. MRI

Dysphagia and Cricopharyngeal Achalasia

Clinical correlations

1. Functional disorders of oropharyngeal stages of swallowing.
2. Difficulty swallowing and hypersalivation are common clinical signs. Gagging, excessive mandibular and head

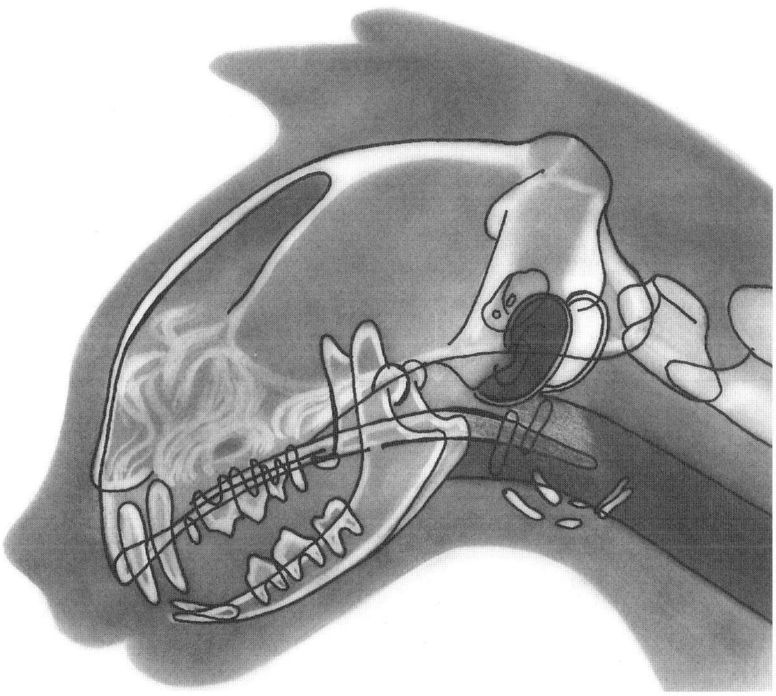

Figure 11.3. Nasopharyngeal polyp is visible in nasopharynx (arrow). Increased opacity to one tympanic bulla also present.

motion, and dropping food from mouth may also be present.

3. Most often results from neuromuscular diseases (e.g., polymyositis, hypothyroidism, myasthenia gravis, brain stem disease), but also may be caused by stricture, foreign body, trauma, neoplasia, or inflammatory diseases.
4. Dysphagia occurs more commonly in middle-aged to older animals, whereas most cases of cricopharyngeal achalasia occur in young dogs.
5. Electromyography may aid in diagnosis.

Radiographic findings

1. Usually no radiographic abnormality is seen unless there is a radiopaque foreign body, or mass lesion within the pharynx or retropharyngeal region.
2. A barium swallow study with fluoroscopy usually is required to make a diagnosis.
   a. One (or more) of the oropharyngeal phases of swallowing is absent or incoordinated.
   b. It may be difficult to differentiate pharyngeal dysfunction from cricopharyngeal achalasia, which is characterized by an inadequate relaxation of the cricopharyngeal muscle during swallowing.
   c. During attempts to swallow, barium may also be aspirated into the larynx or refluxed into the nasopharynx
3. Bronchopneumonia may be present secondary to aspiration.

Esophagus

RADIOGRAPHIC ANATOMY (Figures 11.5 and 11.6)

1. The esophagus extends from the cricopharyngeal muscle to the cardia of the stomach.
2. The esophagus lies dorsal to the trachea in the neck, to the left of the midline at the thoracic inlet and dorsal to the trachea and carina in the thorax.
3. The distal thoracic esophagus lies slightly to the left of the midline and passes through the left crus of the diaphragm to the cardia of the stomach.
4. The normal esophagus is a collapsed tube within the mediastinum and is not usually visible radiographically.
   a. In the dog, the full length of the esophagus is composed of striated muscle.
   b. In the cat, the proximal portion of the esophagus is composed of striated muscle, but the distal one third is composed of smooth muscle.
5. Occasionally, a small amount of gas can be seen within the normal esophageal lumen because of aerophagia or neuromuscular relaxation, secondary to sedation or anesthesia. Small amounts of gas related to normal swallowing are most often visible in the cranial cervical or midthoracic regions of the esophagus.

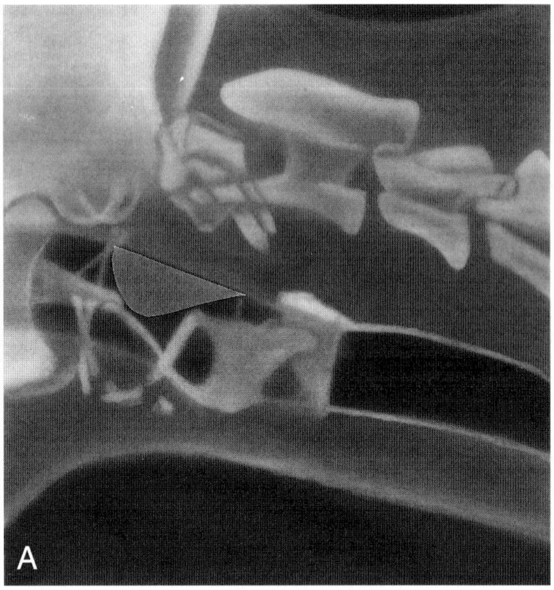

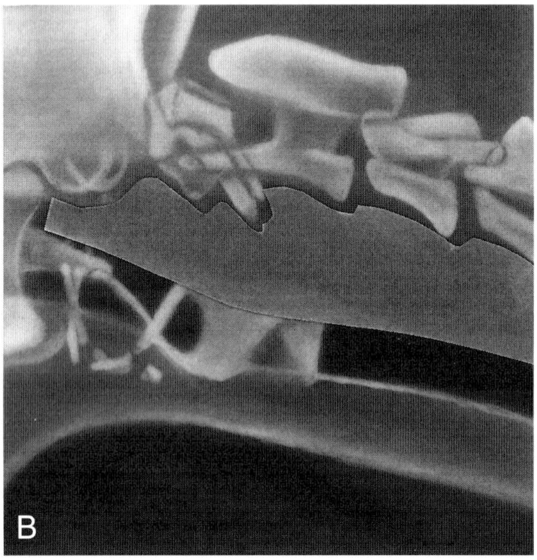

Figure 11.4. **A.,** Pharyngeal mass. There is a mass originating from the caudal dorsal pharyngeal wall, extending into the pharynx. **B.,** Retropharyngeal swelling. There is enlargement of the retropharyngeal soft tissues with ventral displacement of the pharynx and larynx and occlusion of the nasopharynx.

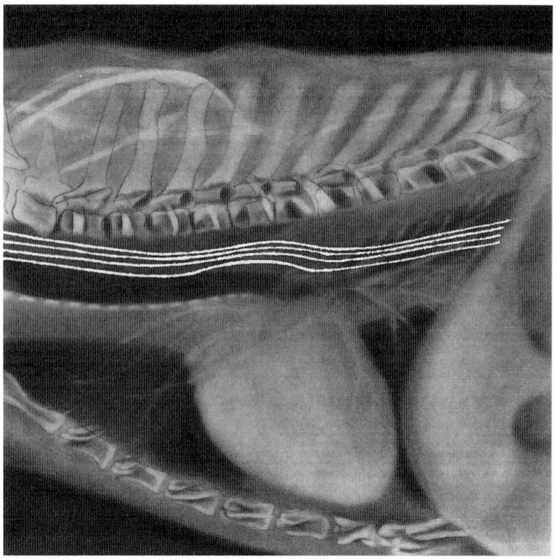

Figure 11.5. Normal canine esophagus.

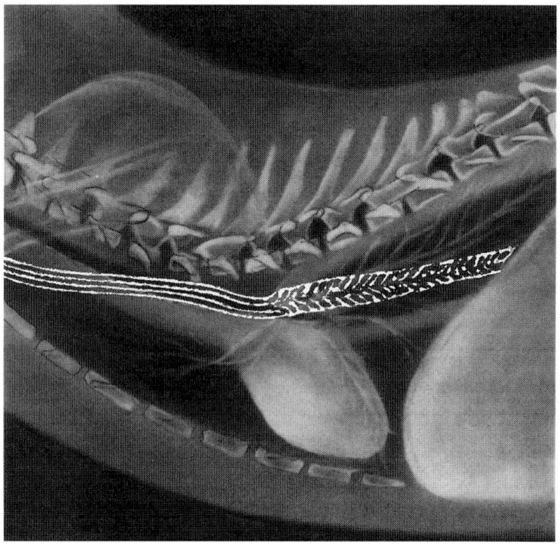

Figure 11.6. Normal feline esophagus.

6. Abnormal gas, fluid, retained food, mass, or other luminal content is often indicative of esophageal disease. Differential considerations include:
   a. Megaesophagus, both congenital and acquired
   b. Esophagitis
   c. Foreign body
   d. Tumor
   e. Granuloma or abscess
   f. Stricture
   g. Vascular ring anomalies
   h. Gastroesophageal intussusception
   i. Hiatal hernia
7. If abnormal gas is seen around the esophagus, this may be a result of:
   a. Pneumothorax
   b. Pneumomediastinum
   c. Esophageal perforation

CONTRAST RADIOGRAPHY (see Chapter 3)

1. A barium esophagram is frequently necessary to evaluate the location, position, lumen, and function of the esophagus.

2. The normal canine esophagus appears as parallel longitudinal mucosal folds, which are barium coated, that extend the entire length of the esophagus. In many normal dogs, slight irregularity of the mucosal folds may be seen at the thoracic inlet. In some dogs, usually brachiocephalic breeds, the normal esophagus may have a diverticulum-like ventral deviation located cranial to the heart, near the thoracic inlet.
3. The normal feline esophagus has parallel longitudinal mucosal folds in the proximal two thirds of the esophagus. The caudal third of the esophagus, from the heart base to the cardia, has mucosal folds that appear more transverse and spiral (referred to as a "herringbone" pattern).

DISEASES/DISORDERS

Esophagitis

Clinical correlations

1. Primary esophagitis usually occurs secondary to trauma from swallowed foreign bodies, as a sequel from the ingestion of caustic materials or from gastroesophageal reflux.
2. Esophagitis may include inflammation, erosion, and ulceration of the mucosa.
3. Chronic esophagitis can cause scar and stricture formation.
4. Clinical signs vary with the extent and severity of the disease, but commonly include dysphagia, regurgitation, excessive salivation, extension of the head and neck during swallowing, and avoidance of food.
5. The presence and severity of esophagitis is best assessed by endoscopy and biopsy.

Radiographic findings

1. Survey radiographs of chest and neck are usually normal.
2. Increased soft tissue opacity of the caudal thoracic esophagus may be seen in some cases (most often with reflux esophagitis).
3. Other disease, such as pneumonia, may be present.

Contrast radiography

1. On a barium esophagram, irregular mucosa, mucosal ulceration, segmental narrowing, esophageal dilation, strictures, and diffuse esophageal hypomotility may be seen.
2. The esophageal wall may appear thickened and, if significant mucosal erosion or ulceration is present, barium may adhere to the mucosa.
3. A normal appearing esophagus does not exclude esophagitis.
4. Differential considerations:
   a. Esophageal stricture
   b. Esophageal neoplasm

Esophageal Foreign Bodies

Clinical correlations

1. Foreign bodies that lodge in the esophagus are usually bones or objects with irregular or sharp edges (e.g., wood fragments, sewing needles, fish hooks).
2. The most common locations for foreign bodies to lodge are at the level of the thoracic inlet, the heart base, and cranial to the cardia.
3. Esophageal perforation and mediastinitis may occur.
4. Other potential sequel include esophageal stricture, diverticulum, or esophageal-bronchial fistula.
5. Common clinical signs vary depending on the size and shape of the foreign body and duration of obstruction, and include anorexia, dysphagia, ptylalism, and regurgitation.

Radiographic findings

1. Metallic, bony, and other radiopaque foreign bodies are readily identified.
2. Foreign bodies having a soft tissue radiopacity may mimic a cervical or mediastinal mass.
3. If complete esophageal obstruction is present, the esophagus cranial to the foreign body may be distended with gas, fluid, or ingesta.
4. If perforation has occurred, the mediastinum may be widened with fluid accumulation (mediastinitis), or gas dissection may be seen adjacent to the esophageal wall in the neck or mediastinum (pneumomediastinum).

Contrast radiography

Esophagram

1. If the obstruction is complete, the esophagus proximal to the obstruction will be dilated and barium-filled on an esophagram.
2. If the obstruction is incomplete, a filling defect caused by the foreign body will be seen.

Vascular Ring Anomalies

Clinical correlations

1. Congenital malformations of the aortic arches that anatomically entrap the esophagus.
2. The most common vascular ring anomaly is persistence of the right fourth aortic arch (PRAA).
3. Other less common vascular ring anomalies include:
   a. Aberrant left or right subclavian arteries (second most common anomaly in dog and cat)
   b. Double aortic arch
   c. Persistent right aortic arch
   d. Left aortic arch and right ligamentous arteriosum
   e. Aberrant intercostal arteries
4. As a result of the vascular ring anomaly, the esophagus is compressed between the aorta and the trachea, and a stenosis occurs. There is secondary dilation of the esophagus cranial to the site of stenosis.
5. The most common clinical sign is that of regurgitation of solid food usually seen after weaning. Coughing associated with aspiration pneumonia is also frequent.

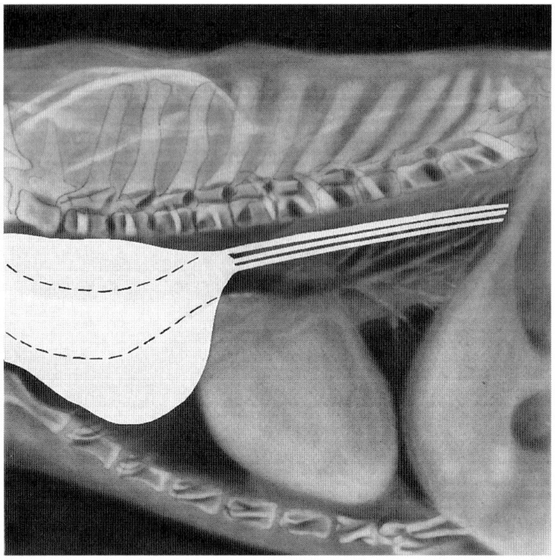

Figure 11.7. Persistent right fourth aortic arch. The trachea (dotted line) is usually displaced ventrally.

Radiographic findings (Figures 11.7 and 11.8)

1. Dilation of the esophagus cranial to the heart base, usually with fluid, gas, or ingesta.
2. On the lateral projection the dilated esophagus often displaces the trachea ventrally.
3. On the ventrodorsal projection the distended esophagus is seen as a widening within the cranial mediastinum.
4. The caudal thoracic esophagus is usually not dilated. However, in some dogs and cats, the esophagus may be dilated as a result of interference with normal esophageal motility or concurrent congenital megaesophagus.
5. Aspiration pneumonia is a common associated finding, usually visible as alveolar infiltrate in the dependent portions of the cranial and middle lung lobes.

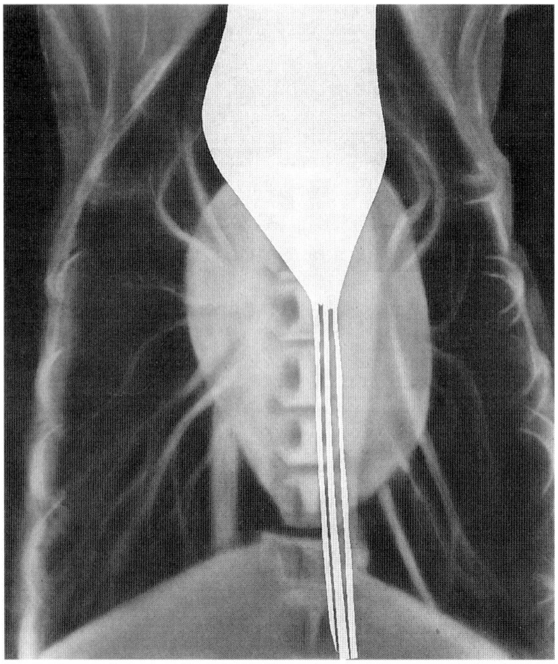

Figure 11.8. Persistent right fourth aortic arch.

Contrast radiography

Esophagram

1. A barium swallow study readily identifies the dilated esophagus and the site of luminal narrowing.
2. The esophagus distal to the stricture may or may not be identified, if the stricture is severe.
3. Must differentiate vascular ring anomalies from generalized megaesophagus. The entire esophagus should be visualized with barium because some cases of generalized megaesophagus can mimic esophageal dilation resulting from a vascular ring anomaly.
4. Also differentiate from anomalous "pseudodiverticulum" and mural stricture caused by trauma, chemical irritant, or tumor.

Esophageal Stricture

Clinical correlations

1. Esophageal stricture is an abnormal narrowing of the lumen as a result of a periesophageal masses or mural or intraluminal diseases.
2. Periesophageal masses include: cervical and thoracic masses (e.g., thyroid carcinoma, lymphosarcoma, heart base tumor, abscess, foreign body, or lymphadenopathy).
3. Esophageal stricture occurs with most vascular ring anomalies at the heart base.
4. May occur secondary to severe esophagitis, foreign body, or neoplasia.
5. Common clinical signs include dysphagia and regurgitation, but vary with the severity and extent of the stricture. Liquid meals often are better tolerated than solid meals.
6. Associated bronchopneumonia may be present.
7. Intraluminal strictures are often best diagnosed by endoscopy.

Radiographic findings

1. Survey radiographs are usually normal, especially if the lumen diameter is not significantly compromised.
2. If the stricture is severe, the esophagus cranial to the stricture may be distended with fluid, gas, or ingesta.

Contrast radiographs

Esophagram

1. The esophageal lumen is narrowed at the site of stricture.
2. Small strictures may be missed with liquid barium, barium mixed with food, or iodinated oral contrast media.
3. Small luminal structures are often diagnosed best by

administering different sizes of boluses (e.g., variable sizes of gelatin capsules filled with barium, or barium impregnated marshmallows).

Esophageal Neoplasia

Clinical correlations

1. Primary, paraesophageal, and metastatic esophageal neoplasms are uncommon in the dog and cat.
2. Primary tumors include:
   a. Squamous cell carcinoma
   b. Fibrosarcoma
   c. Osteosarcoma
   d. Leiomyoma
   e. Leiomyosarcoma
   f. Adenocarcinoma
3. Secondary tumors include:
   a. Bronchogenic adenocarcinoma
   b. Gastric carcinoma
   c. Thyroid carcinoma
   d. Mammary adenocarcinoma
   e. Squamous cell carcinoma
   f. Thymic tumors
   g. Heart base tumors
4. *Spiricerca lupi* granulomas can transform into fibrosarcoma or osteosarcoma.
5. Common clinical signs include progressive regurgitation, dysphagia, weight loss, and anorexia.
6. A specific diagnosis usually is made with endoscopy and biopsy.

Radiographic findings

1. An abnormal soft tissue mass may be seen within the cervical or mediastinal regions.
2. A tumor may cause a stricture with secondary dilation of the esophagus cranial to the site of stricture and esophageal mass.
3. Esophageal masses can be intraluminal, mural, or extraluminal.

Contrast radiography

Esophagram

1. The location of the esophagus is readily determined.
2. Ulceration of the esophageal mucosa or alteration of the esophageal wall may be observed.
3. If a partial obstruction has occurred, the esophagus is usually dilated cranial to the obstruction.

Esophageal Diverticuli

Clinical correlations

1. Diverticuli can be congenital or acquired.
2. Congenital diverticuli are thought to be caused by abnormal separation of the tracheal and esophageal embryonic buds, which causes a congenital weakness of the esophageal wall.
   a. Esophageal diverticuli is recognized most often at the thoracic inlet.

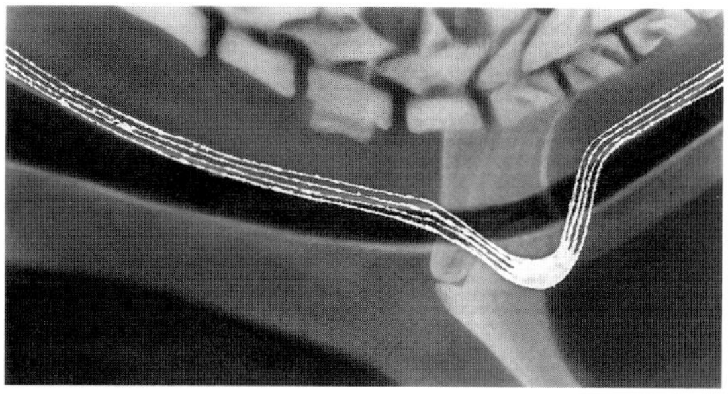

Figure 11.9. Pseudodiverticulum of esophagus.

   b. Is considered a normal variant, "pseudodiverticulum," in some bachycephalic dogs (e.g., English Bulldog).
   c. Most diverticuli do not cause any clinical signs.
3. Acquired diverticuli can be traction or pulsion.
   a. Pulsion diverticuli usually occur secondary to esophageal stenosis or severe esophagitis. There is herniation of the mucous membrane through the muscular coat of the esophagus.
   b. Traction diverticuli occur secondary to adhesions of the wall of the esophagus, which creates a diverticulum in which all esophageal layers remain intact.
4. Common clinical signs include dysphagia, regurgitation, intermittent anorexia, and lethargy.
5. May prevent easy passage of an orogastric tube.

Radiographic findings (Figures 11.9 and 11.10)

1. Survey radiographs commonly appear normal.
2. Pulsion diverticuli are seen in the distal thoracic esophagus (called epiphrenic diverticuli).
3. Congenital are usually seen in the cranial thoracic esophagus.
4. Differentiate from pseudodiverticulum.

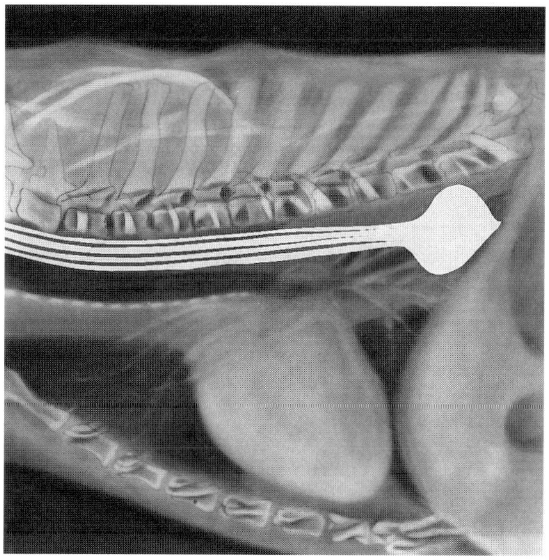

Figure 11.10. Epiphrenic esophageal diverticulum. There is saccular enlargement of the distal thoracic esophagus.

Contrast radiography

Esophagram

1. The normal and abnormal portions of the esophagus will be identified.
2. Barium readily outlines the diverticulum as a pouch or deviation away from the esophageal lumen. Most congenital diverticuli have a normal size lumen, but the lumen is deviated ventrally or laterally.

Megaesophagus

Clinical correlations

1. Esophageal dilation can be congenital or acquired.
2. Congenital megaesophagus is more common in dogs and considered inheritable in the Miniature Schnauzer and Fox Terrier. There is an increased breed incidence in German Shepherd Dog, Irish Setter, Labrador Retriever, Chinese Shar Pei, and Great Dane.
3. Most causes of adult onset megaesophagus have no known etiology and are referred to as idiopathic.
4. Commonly, the drug effects of sedation and anesthesia cause a dilated esophagus, which mimics megaesophagus.
5. Some acquired cases may be associated with:
   a. Hypoadrenocorticism
   b. Hypothyroidism
   c. Myasthenia gravis
   d. Lead poisoning
   e. Polyneuritis
   f. Polymyositis
   g. Chronic esophagitis
   h. Obstruction (e.g., gastric volvulus)
   i. Hiatal hernia
   j. Pyloric canal dysfunction in cats
   k. Dysautonomia in cats (Key-Gaskell syndrome)
6. Common clinical signs include regurgitation of water, food, and/or foamy saliva and weight loss. Coughing and fever are common if aspiration pneumonia occurs as a sequel.

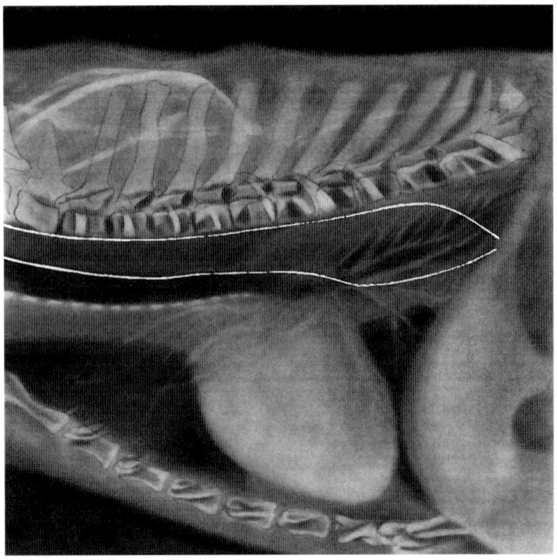

Figure 11.11. Megaesophagus on a survey radiograph.

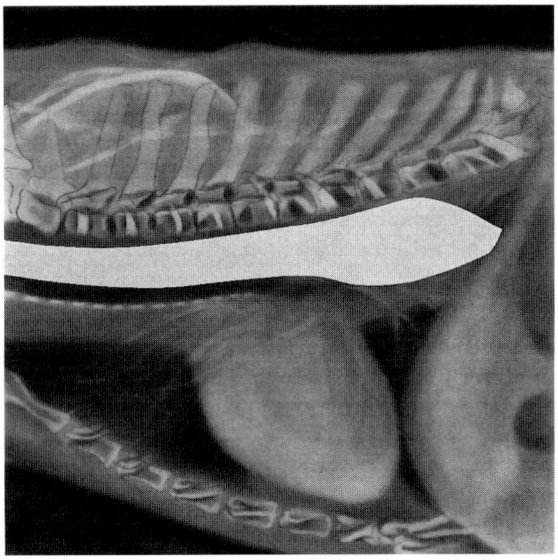

Figure 11.12. Megaesophagus on an esophagram.

Radiographic findings (Figures 11.11 through 11.13)

1. Distension of the esophagus with air, fluid, or ingesta.
2. Esophageal distension is usually generalized but may be seen only in the cervical or the thoracic regions.
3. A tracheoesophageal stripe sign is present. This stripe sign is a soft tissue line, combining the radiopacity of the ventral wall of the esophagus and the trachea, and is usually seen extending from the bifurcation to the thoracic inlet.

Contrast radiography

Esophagram

1. Dilation of the esophagus with barium usually involves the cervical and thoracic portions.
2. Sufficient barium must be administered to visualize the entire esophagus. Partial filling of a generalized megaesophagus can mimic a vascular ring anomaly or other localized esophageal disease.

Gastroesophageal Intussusception

Clinical correlations

1. Results from invagination of the stomach into the esophagus, with or without other abdominal organs (e.g., spleen, pancreas, omentum).
2. Reported in young dogs, usually younger than 3 months of age, and is more common in males.
3. Gastroesophageal intussusception may be inheritable, with the highest prevalence reported in German Shepherd Dogs.
4. May be associated with megaesophagus; the dilated esophagus may accommodate the invagination.

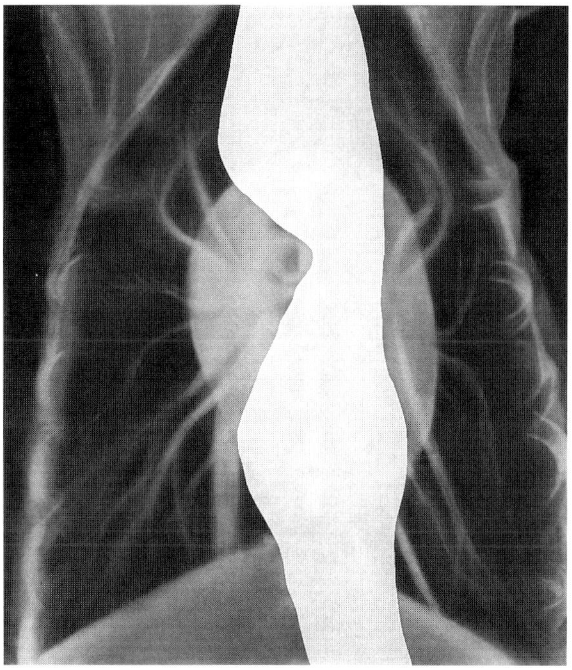

Figure 11.13. Megaesophagus on an esophagram.

5. Common clinical signs include regurgitation and vomiting.

Radiographic findings (Figure 11.14)

1. The esophagus is dilated with gas cranial to the intussusception.
2. Well-demarcated and increased soft tissue radiopacity within the caudal esophagus adjacent to the esophageal hiatus.

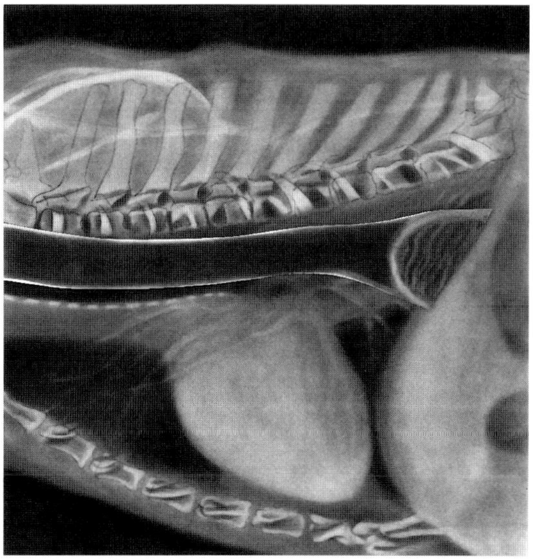

Figure 11.14. Gastroesophageal intussusception. The esophagus is dilated with gas. The gas-filled stomach is intussuscepted into the lumen of the distal esophagus.

3. The rugal folds of stomach may be identified within the intussuscepted portion of the stomach if sufficient gas is present within the gastric lumen.

Contrast radiography

1. The esophagus cranial to the intussusception will be dilated and filled with barium.
2. If barium is present within the gastric lumen, the rugal folds may be seen within the intussusceptum.

LIVER

RADIOGRAPHIC ANATOMY (Figure 11.15)

1. The liver in the dog and cat consists of six lobes: left medial, left lateral, right medial, right lateral, caudate, and quadrate lobes. The caudate lobe has caudate and papillary processes.
2. The diaphragmatic surface or cranial margin of the liver conforms to the shape of the diaphragm.
3. The left lobes are to the left of the spine. The left medial lobe is located cranioventrally and the left lateral lobe forms most of the caudal liver silhouette. The stomach is in contact with the gastric impression of the left lateral lobe.
4. The right lateral and right middle lobes are located to the right of the midline and to the right of the caudal vena cava. The right lateral lobe is located more dorsally and the right medial lobe more cranioventrally.
5. The caudate lobe is located on the midline dorsally, and the quadrate lobe is located near the midline ventrally.
6. The proximal duodenum is located in the duodenal impression at the junction of the right lateral and quadrate lobes.
7. The right kidney is in contact with the renal fossa of the caudate process of the caudate lobe.
8. The gall bladder is a pear-shaped structure that lies between the quadrate lobe medially and the right medial lobe laterally. In the cat, the right medial (or "cystic") lobe contains the gall bladder.

NORMAL RADIOGRAPHIC APPEARANCE (Figures 11.16 and 11.17)

1. The appearance of the normal liver varies with body conformation, age, overall body condition, stage of respiration, and posture. The normal liver usually has sharp margins and usually does not extend caudal to the costal arch.

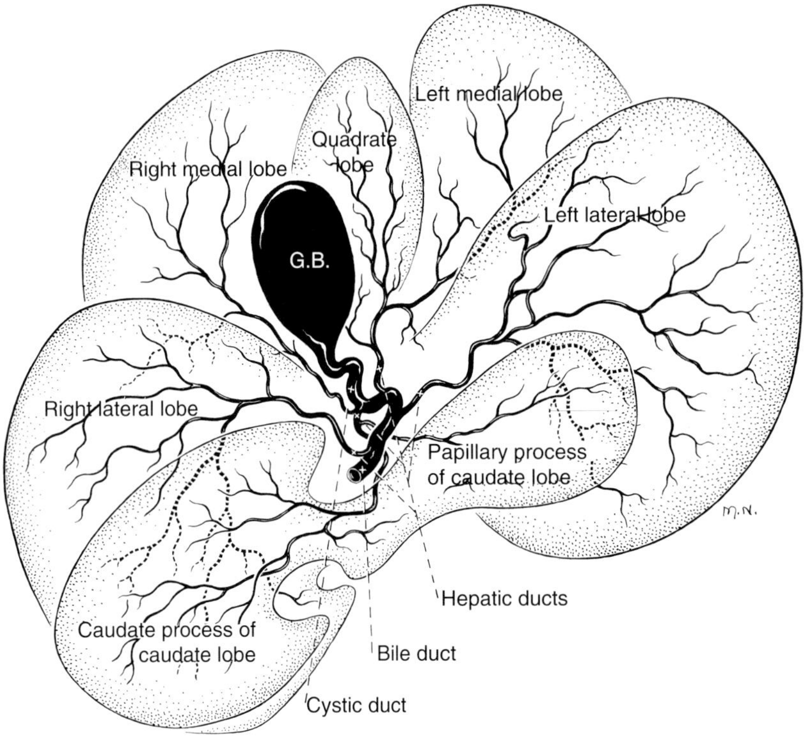

Figure 11.15. Scheme of the gall bladder and hepatic ducts: visceral aspect. (From Evans HE. The digestive apparatus and abdomen. In: Evans HE, ed. Miller's Anatomy of the Dog. 3rd ed, Philadelphia: W.B. Saunders; 1993:456. Courtesy of and with permission of Dr. Howard E. Evans.)

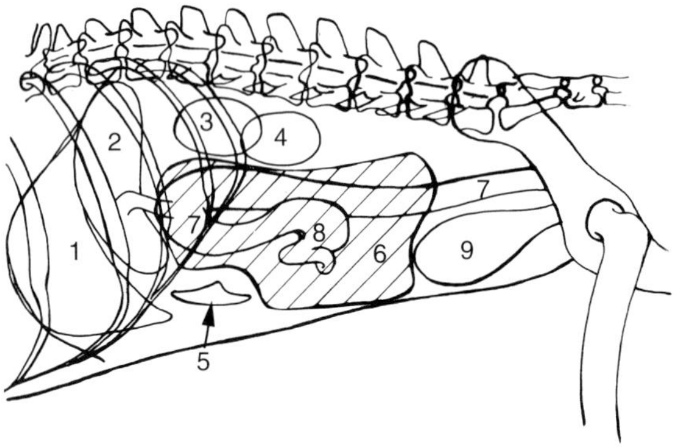

Figure 11.16. Normal lateral projection: liver (**1**), stomach (**2**), right kidney (**3**), left kidney (**4**), spleen (**5**), small intestine (**6**), large intestine (7), cecum (**8**), and urinary bladder (**9**).

2. The position of the stomach axis (line drawn from fundus to antrum) is a good indicator of liver size. The "rule of thumb" for the normal stomach axis is: perpendicular to the spine, or parallel with the plane of the ribs, on the lateral projection and either parallel or slightly angulated caudally on the ventrodorsal projection. The normal antrum of the cat is near the midline on the ventrodorsal projection, and in the right cranial quadrant for the dog.

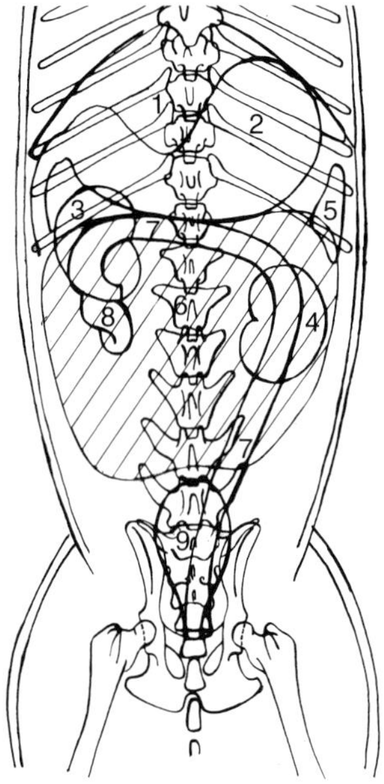

Figure 11.17. Normal ventrodorsal projection: liver (**1**), stomach (**2**), right kidney (**3**), left kidney (**4**), spleen (**5**), small intestine (**6**), large intestine (**7**), cecum (**8**), and urinary bladder (**9**).

a. In deep-chested dogs, the liver may appear subjectively smaller on the lateral projection because the liver may not extend caudal to the costal arch. The gastric axis will often appear more vertical and may be angulated cranially. Barrel-chested dogs may seem to have an enlarged liver because the liver may extend caudal to the costal arch.
b. Young or immature animals appear to have enlarged livers because the liver mass is larger in terms of percentage of body weight as compared to normal adult dogs and cats.
c. The liver appears smaller on expiration than on inspiration because of the normal different positions of the diaphragm.
d. The normal liver commonly appears larger on a right lateral recumbent projection than on the left lateral projection.

3. The lateral projection:
   a. The cranial surface of the liver is in contact with the diaphragm.
   b. The caudoventral margin usually projects slightly beyond the margin of the costal arch, and the border of the liver, as seen, is triangular in shape and sharply pointed.
   c. In right lateral recumbency, the right liver moves cranially and the caudal border of the liver is usually the left lateral lobe.
   d. In left lateral recumbency, the left liver moves cranially and the caudal border of the liver is usually the right medial lobe.
   e. The liver may be seen in contact with the ventral abdominal wall or separated from the abdominal wall by the falciform ligament.
   f. The caudate process of the caudate lobe is the most dorsal caudal limit of the liver. The right kidney is located within the renal fossa of this lobe, which may be identified in some obese dogs and cats.
4. The ventrodorsal projection:
   a. The liver is in contact with the diaphragm.
   b. The only visible liver margins are the caudolateral margins of the right and left lateral lobes.

DISEASES/DISORDERS

Liver Enlargement

Clinical correlations

1. Enlargement may be localized or diffuse.
2. Common causes of generalized enlargement include:
   a. Passive venous congestion (e.g., right heart failure)
   b. Acute hepatitis
   c. Fat or glycogen infiltration (e.g., vacuolar hepatopathy, lipidosis) is often associated with other diseases (e.g., diabetes mellitus, hyperadrenocorticism, steroid therapy).

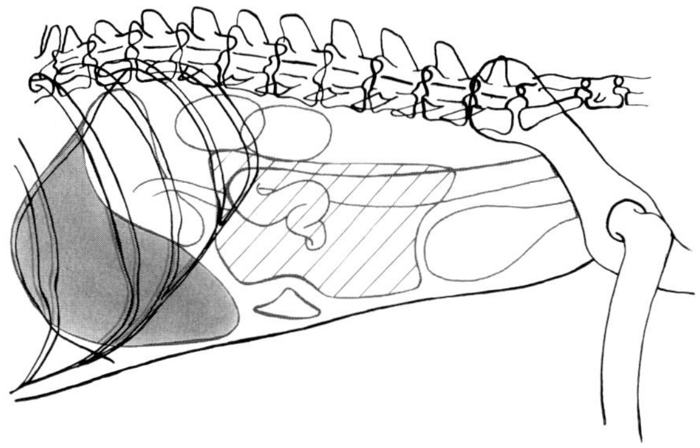

Figure 11.18. Generalized hepatomegaly. The stomach is displaced caudally by the enlarged liver. The caudal margin of the liver is rounded.

   d. Primary neoplasia (e.g., hepatocellular carcinoma, bile duct carcinoma)
   e. Metastatic neoplasia (sarcoma, carcinoma, or lymphoma)
   f. Chronic hepatitis with nodular hyperplasia
3. Common causes of localized enlargement:
   a. Primary neoplasia (e.g., hepatocellular carcinoma, bile duct carcinoma, hepatoma, adenoma)
   b. Metastatic neoplasia
   c. Hepatic or biliary cyst
   d. Abscess
   e. Nodular hyperplasia

Radiographic findings

Generalized hepatomegaly (Figures 11.18 and 11.19)

1. Lateral projection
   a. Caudal displacement of the stomach axis
   b. Caudal extension of the ventral portion of the hepatic border, usually caudal to the costal arch
   c. Rounding of the caudal hepatic border
2. Ventrodorsal projection
   a. Caudal displacement of the stomach axis
   b. Displacement of the pylorus toward the midline
   c. Displacement of the stomach fundus toward the right side
   d. Caudal displacement of the stomach, head of the spleen, small intestine, and right kidney

Localized Hepatomegaly (Figures 11.20 through 11.22)

1. Variable visceral displacement will occur, depending on the lobe involved and size of the mass.
2. Enlargement of the left lateral lobe will cause:
   a. Displacement of the cardia and fundus of the stomach to right on the ventrodorsal projection
   b. Displacement of the stomach caudally, and dorsally on the lateral projection

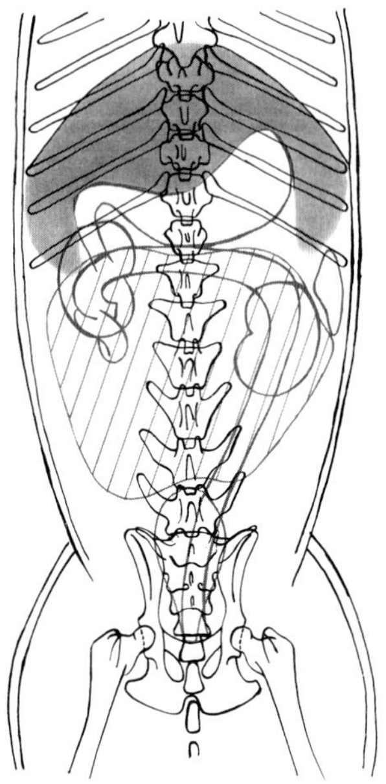

Figure 11.19. Generalized hepatomegaly. The stomach is displaced caudally. The caudal margins of the liver are rounded.

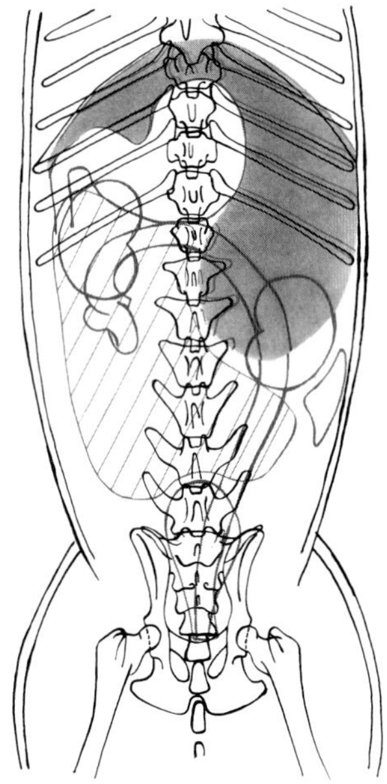

Figure 11.20. Localized liver enlargement involving the left side of the liver. The stomach and the bowel are displaced medially. The left kidney and spleen are displaced caudally.

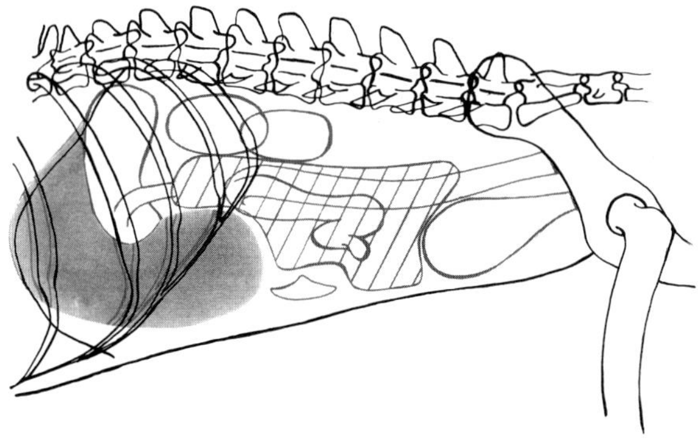

Figure 11.21. Localized liver enlargement involving the right or left sides of the liver. The stomach is displaced dorsally, and the bowel and spleen are displaced caudally.

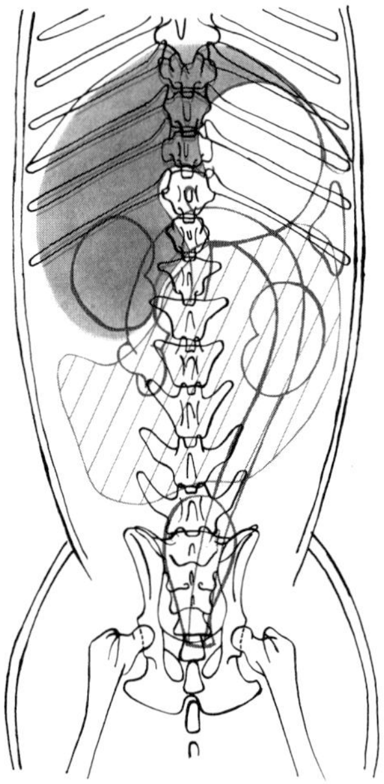

Figure 11.22. Localized liver enlargement involving the right side of the liver. The pylorus and duodenum are displaced medially, and the right kidney is displaced caudally.

   c. The small intestine and spleen are often displaced caudally on both projections.
3. Enlargement of the right lateral lobe will cause medial displacement of the duodenum, as seen on the ventrodorsal projection, and dorsal displacement of the duodenum as seen on the lateral projection.
4. Enlargement of the caudate lobe (especially the caudate process) will often displace the right kidney caudally, as seen on the lateral and ventrodorsal projections.

Decreased Liver Size

Clinical correlations

1. Decreased liver size is usually associated with chronic diseases or congenital abnormalities of the liver
   a. Portosystemic vascular shunts
   b. Cirrhosis or fibrosis
   c. Hernia with part or all of the liver displaced into the thorax (e.g., peritoneopericardial diaphragmatic hernia or diaphragmatic hernia).

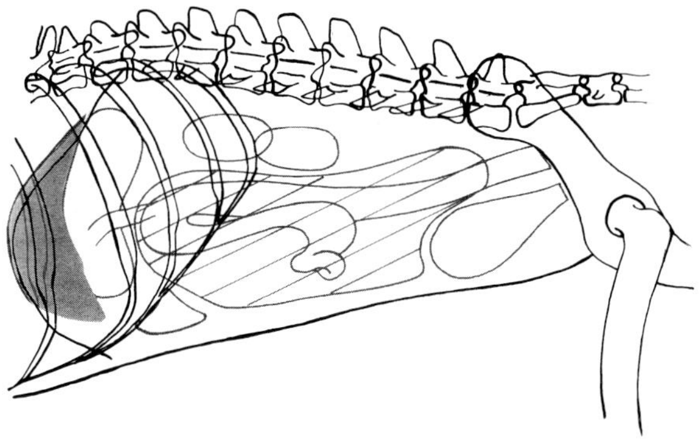

Figure 11.23. Small liver. There is cranial displacement of the gastric axis.

Radiographic findings (Figures 11.23 and 11.24)

1. Cranial displacement of the pyloric antrum and axis of the stomach.
2. The stomach appears closer to the diaphragm.
3. The impression of a small liver is more accurate if the entire liver is small, rather than when only a portion of the liver is small.

Contrast radiography

1. Angiography
   a. Mesenteric angiography
   b. Venous portography
   c. Hepatic angiography
2. Pneumoperitoneography

Other imaging

1. Ultrasound
2. Scintigraphy
3. CT
4. MRI

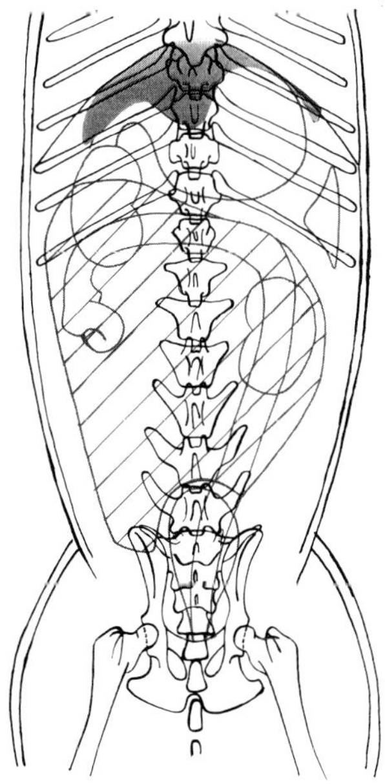

Figure 11.24. Small liver. There is cranial displacement of the pylorus and duodenum.

GALL BLADDER

ANATOMY (Figure 11.25)

1. The biliary system consists of the gall bladder, common bile duct, hepatic ducts, cystic duct, and the small bile ductules and canaliculi.
2. The gall bladder is a pear-shaped, fluid-filled structure. It lies between the quadrate lobe of the liver medially, and the right medial lobe of the liver laterally.
3. The gall bladder consists of a body, a rounded end (or fundus), and a neck that tapers into the cystic duct. The cystic duct leads to the common bile duct, which is joined by the hepatic ducts from the individual liver lobes.
4. A bifid gall bladder is a congenital anomaly in the cat.

RADIOGRAPHIC ANATOMY

1. The gall bladder is not seen as a separate structure from the liver.
2. In some anorectic cats, a distended gall bladder may be identified as a rounded soft tissue mass extending from the right cranioventral liver margin.

DISEASES/DISORDERS

Cholecystitis

Clinical correlations

1. Cholecystitis is an inflammatory disease of the gall bladder, which usually involves the associated bile ducts.

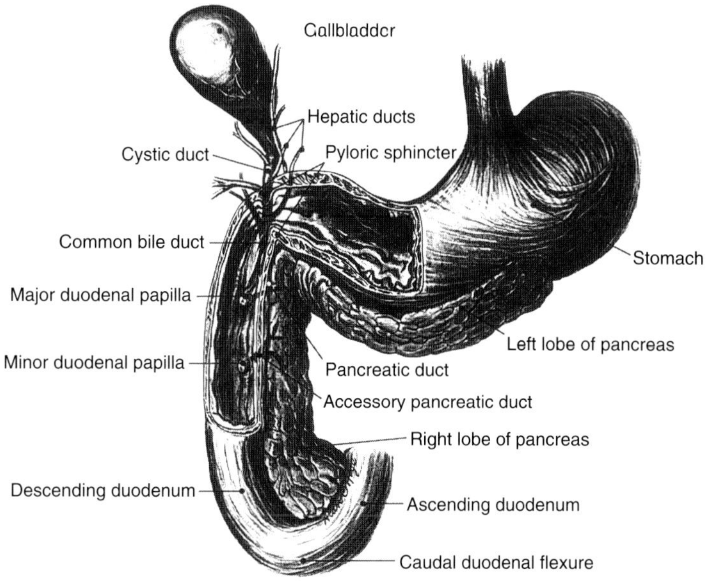

Figure 11.25. The duodenum, pancreas, gallbladder, and associated ducts (ventral view). (From Anderson WD, Anderson BG. Atlas of canine anatomy. Philadelphia: Lea & Febiger; 1994:647. With permission of Williams & Wilkins, Baltimore.)

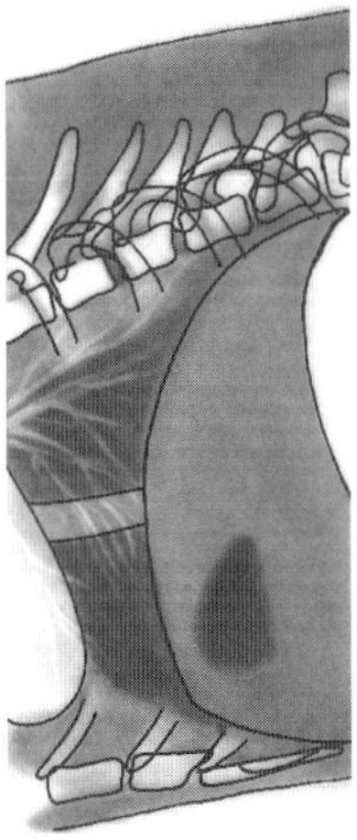

Figure 11.26. Emphysematous cholecystitis. There is gas within the lumen of the gall bladder.

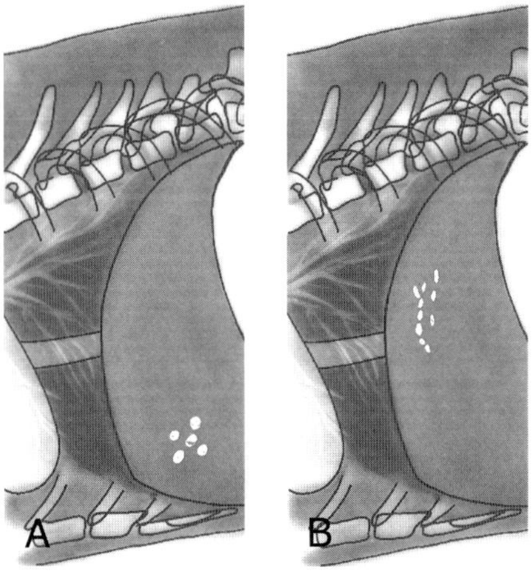

Figure 11.27. **A.**, Cholelithiasis. Opaque calculi are seen in the gall bladder. **B.**, Choledocholithiasis. Small opaque calculi are seen within the intrahepatic bile ducts.

2. Can be caused by reflux of bacteria from the intestine through the common bile duct or through a hematogenous infection.
3. Necrotizing cholecystitis can cause injury to the wall of the gall bladder resulting in peritonitis.
4. Emphysematous cholecystitis occurs when the gall bladder is infected with gas forming bacteria, most commonly *Escherichia coli* and *Clostridium perfringens.*

Radiographic findings (Figure 11.26)
1. The survey radiographs are normal in most instances.
2. If the gall bladder is severely enlarged, a mass may be seen projecting from the liver, most often identified on the lateral projection.
3. In emphysematous cholecystitis, gas bubbles may be seen in the wall or the lumen of the gall bladder. Differentiate from a focal liver abscess.

Cholelithiasis
Clinical correlations
1. Often seen incidentally.
2. Clinical signs of illness usually are not present unless calculi are in the common bile duct (choledocholelithiasis) and causing biliary obstruction or infection.
3. Can be associated with cholecystitis with clinical signs of vomiting, fever, abdominal pain, and icterus.
4. The chemical composition of the calculi can be cholesterol, bilirubin, and mixed stones.
5. Rarely causes erosion of the duct wall of the gall bladder.

Radiographic findings (Figure 11.27 A,B)
1. Most calculi in the dog and cat are radiopaque.
2. Calculi vary in size and shape.
3. Calculi also may be seen within the hepatic ducts, cystic duct, or common bile duct.

Contrast radiography
1. Cholecystography

Other imaging
1. Ultrasound
2. CT
3. MRI

Parasitic Disease of the Gall Bladder and/or Bile Ducts
Clinical correlations
1. Caused by a liver fluke, *Platynosomum concinnum,* that is found principally in Hawaii, Florida, and the Caribbean.
2. The fluke infects cats after the cat eats a lizard or toad, which acts as an intermediate host.
3. The fluke migrates to the gall bladder or bile ducts and can cause fibrosis or obstructive disease.
4. The infection may be asymptomatic or may cause signs of cholecystitis.
5. Diagnosis is made by finding ova on a fecal examination.

Radiographic findings
1. Survey radiographs are usually normal.
2. A distended gall bladder may be seen.

Other imaging
1. Ultrasound

SPLEEN

RADIOGRAPHIC ANATOMY

1. The spleen is a flat, elongated, radiopaque soft tissue organ located in the cranial left abdomen and caudal to the stomach.
2. The spleen consists of a dorsal extremity (the head), a midsection (the body), and a ventral extremity (the tail). The dorsal extremity is less variable in position because of the fixed position of the short gastrosplenic ligament.
   a. On the ventrodorsal projection, the dorsal extremity is usually triangular and located adjacent to the left body wall of the gastric fundus and the cranial pole of the left kidney.
   b. The ventral extremity is more variable in position and may be seen extending across the midline on the lateral projection or lying along the left abdominal wall on the ventrodorsal projection.

RADIOGRAPHIC INTERPRETATION

1. The splenic margins are normally smooth and sharp.
2. The normal size of the spleen is variable.
3. The spleen may vary in location depending on the animal's position and size of adjacent viscera.
   a. If the stomach is empty, the spleen is usually located in the left cranial abdomen.
   b. If the stomach is distended with fluid, gas, or ingesta, the spleen is usually located more caudally within the central midabdomen.
4. On the ventrodorsal projection, the head of the spleen is usually seen as a triangular soft tissue opacity caudal and lateral to the gastric fundus.
5. On the lateral projection, the tail of the spleen is usually seen adjacent to the ventral abdominal wall caudal to the liver margin especially on the right lateral projection. On the left lateral projection, the spleen often is superimposed over other viscera in the central midabdomen. In some animals, the head of the spleen can be seen as a triangular soft tissue opacity in the dorsal abdomen, caudal to the stomach and superimposed over the kidneys.

DISEASES/DISORDERS

Splenomegaly

Clinical correlations

1. Splenic enlargement may be generalized or localized.
2. Causes for diffuse splenomegaly include:
   a. Physiologic response to some drugs (e.g., phenothiazene tranquilizers or general anesthetics)
   b. Neoplasia (e.g., lymphosarcoma, mast cell, hemangiosarcoma, metastatic tumors)
   c. Vascular congestion (e.g., splenic torsion, gastric volvulus, or right heart failure)
   d. Hemolytic anemia
   e. Infections (bacterial, mycotic)
3. Causes for localized splenic enlargement include:
   a. Hematoma
   b. Nodular hyperplasia
   c. Neoplasia (e.g., hemangiosarcoma, primary and secondary sarcomas and carcinomas)

Radiographic findings (Figures 11.28 and 11.29)

1. Generalized splenic enlargement, a subjective determination: the spleen appears wider, thicker and longer than normal.

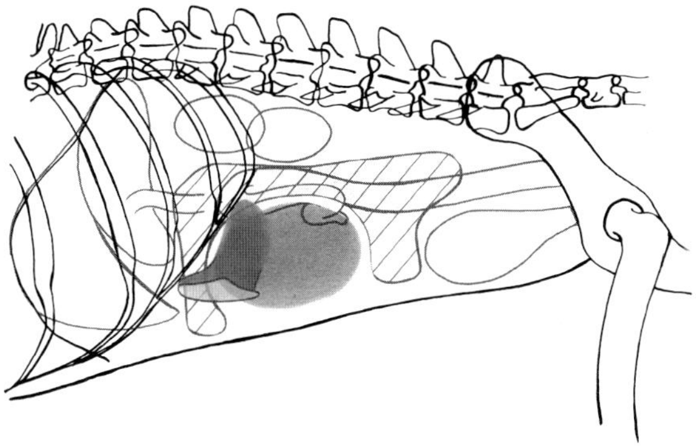

Figure 11.28. Splenomegaly.

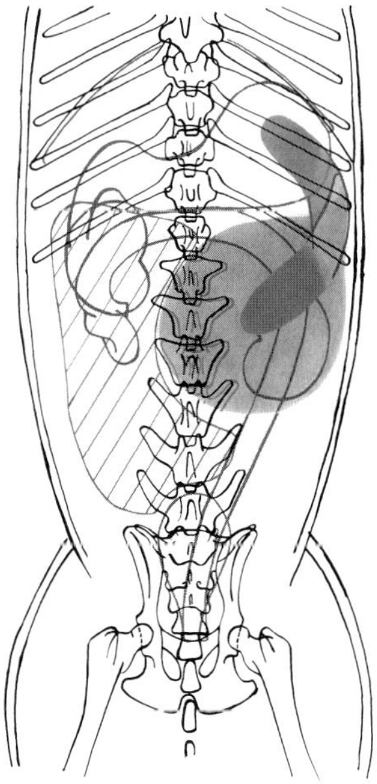

Figure 11.29. Splenomegaly.

2. With localized splenic enlargement, a splenic mass may be well-defined or ill-defined and is identified by its close association with the spleen on one or both projections and by displacement of adjacent abdominal organs.

Other imaging
1. Ultrasound
2. CT
3. MRI

Splenic Torsion
Clinical correlations
1. Occurs most commonly in large, deep-chested dogs.
2. Is often in association with gastric dilation and volvulus.
3. May occur as a separate entity.
4. The spleen is usually markedly enlarged and readily palpable.
5. Common clinical signs of splenic torsion without gastric dilation and volvulus are anorexia, vomiting and abdominal pain, and anemia.

Radiographic findings (Figure 11.30)
1. The spleen is often displaced from its normal location, commonly in the right lateral midabdomen (e.g., the triangular head may be seen on the right side rather than in the left cranial quadrant).
2. The spleen is usually moderately to severely enlarged.
3. On either the lateral or ventrodorsal projection, the tail and head of the enlarged spleen may be seen as triangular soft tissue opacities in the ventral midabdomen.

Splenic Neoplasia
Clinical correlations
1. Common in dogs and cats.
2. Primary splenic neoplasms include:
   a. Lymphoreticular tumors (e.g., lymphoma, myeloma)
   b. Vascular tumors (e.g., hemangiosarcoma, hemangioma)
   c. Connective tissue tumors (e.g., fibrosarcoma, leiomyosarcoma)
3. Secondary tumors include:
   a. Carcinoma
   b. Sarcoma (hemangiosarcoma, lymphoma, or mast cell tumor)
4. Hemangiosarcoma, both primary and metastatic, most often affects large-breed dogs (e.g., German Shepherd Dog, Golden Retriever, Great Dane, Boxer).
   a. Vascular cystic tumors often rupture, causing hemoperitoneum
   b. Regenerative anemia is common.
   c. Acute or chronic disseminated intravascular coagulation is common.
   d. Common metastatic sites include the liver, lung, and the heart.
5. Common clinical signs include:
   a. Abdominal distension
   b. Palpable abdominal mass
   c. Weakness and anemia (if internal hemorrhage has occurred)
   d. Right heart failure (if pericardial tamponade has occurred, secondary to right atrial neoplasia)

Radiographic findings (Figures 11.31 and 11.32)
1. Localized or generalized splenic enlargement is apparent.
2. There is abdominal effusion, if splenic rupture has occurred or if right heart failure is present secondary to pericardial effusion.

Other imaging
1. Ultrasound
2. CT
3. MRI

Splenic Abscess
Clinical correlations
1. Uncommon in the dog and cat.
2. May be associated with localized or systemic infections.

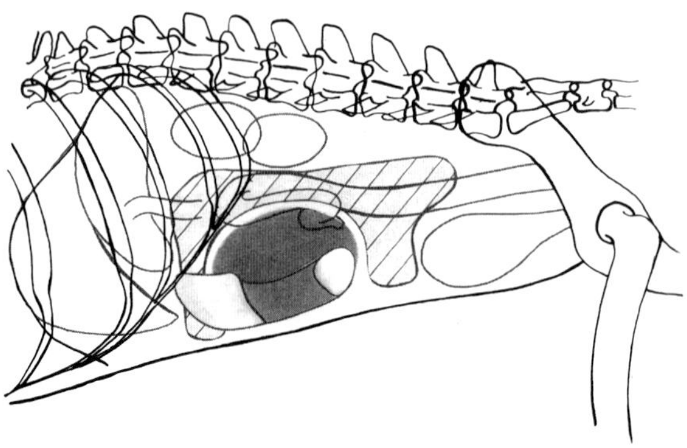

Figure 11.30. Splenic torsion.

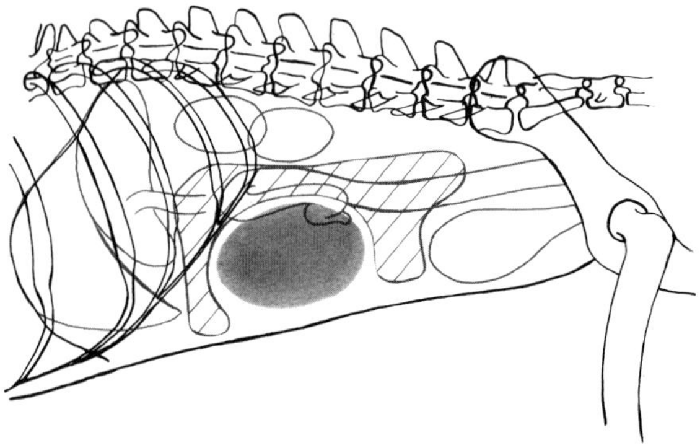

Figure 11.31. Splenic mass.

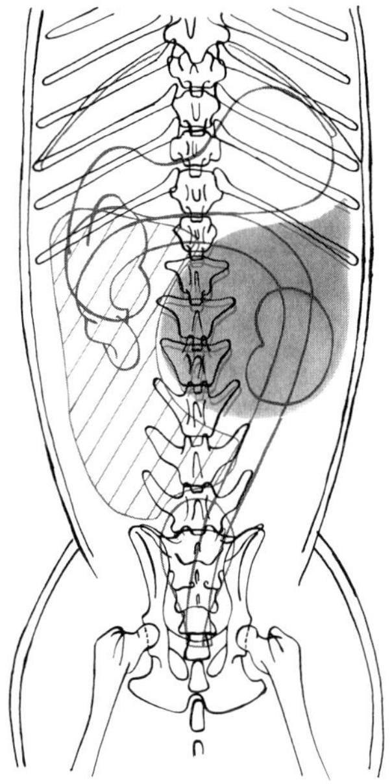

Figure 11.32. Splenic mass.

3. May be associated with splenic torsion or gastric dilation and volvulus.

Radiographic findings (Figure 11.33)
1. Splenic enlargement may be generalized or localized.
2. Gas bubbles within the splenic parenchyma may be seen if a gas-forming infection is present.

Other imaging
1. Ultrasound

Splenic Rupture
Clinical correlations
1. May occur associated with abdominal trauma or secondary to rupture of a splenic tumor.
2. Common clinical signs may include abdominal distension with effusion, weakness, anemia, and a palpable abdominal mass.

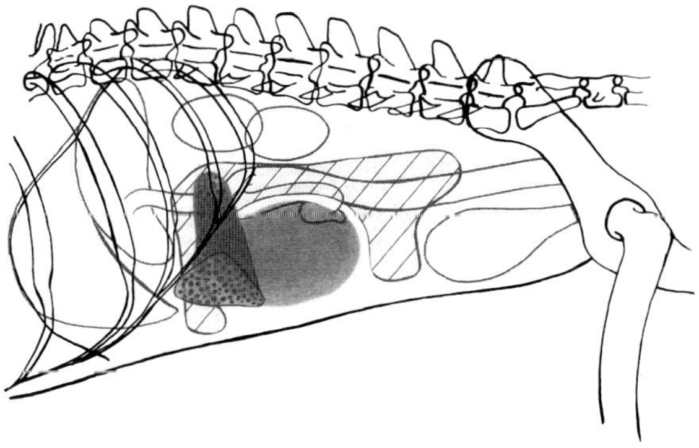

Figure 11.33. Splenic abscess.

Radiographic findings
1. Localized abdominal detail is lost adjacent to the spleen.
2. Peritoneal effusion is observed, especially if hemorrhage is extensive.
3. A splenic mass may be visible.

Other imaging
1. Ultrasound
2. CT
3. MRI

PANCREAS

RADIOGRAPHIC ANATOMY
1. The pancreas is a small, dense, soft tissue organ. It consists of the left limb, adjacent to the caudal border of the gastric body, and the right limb medial to the descending duodenum.
2. The pancreas is adjacent to the cranial border of the transverse colon.
3. The normal pancreas is not visible because of its small size and positive silhouette with other adjacent viscera.

DISEASES/DISORDERS
Pancreatitis
Clinical correlations
1. Pancreatitis may be acute or chronic.
2. The clinical signs of acute pancreatitis are variable, but most commonly include vomiting, abdominal pain, and fever.
3. Differential considerations include:
   a. Gastroenteritis
   b. Bowel obstruction
   c. Peritonitis
   d. Renal failure
4. The diagnosis often is made on correlation of history, clinical signs, and the results of selected laboratory tests.

Radiographic findings (Figure 11.34)
1. No single sign or group of signs are pathognomonic for pancreatitis.
2. Common signs may include:
   a. Increased soft tissue radiopacity and diminished contrast in the right cranial abdomen.
   b. Displacement of the gastric antrum to the left.
   c. Displacement of the proximal duodenum to the right

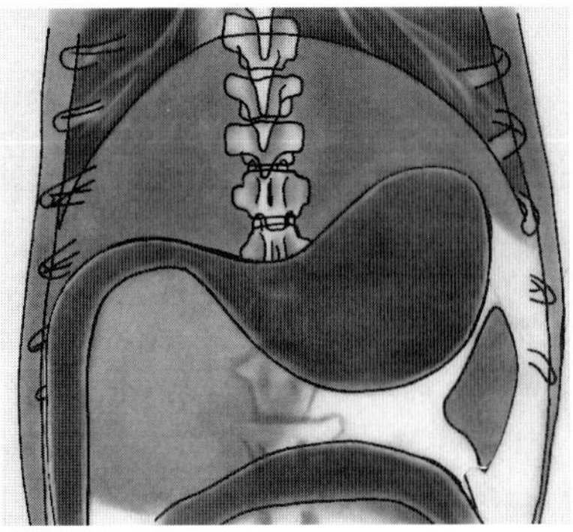

Figure 11.34. Pancreatitis. On ventrodorsal projection, there is an ill-defined mass in region of pancreas with displacement of the duodenum to the right, and displacement of the pyloric antrum to the left. There is gas in the proximal duodenum and transverse colon as a result of localized ileus.

   d. Displacement of the transverse colon caudally
   e. Static gas pattern (localized ileus) of the duodenum
   f. Static gas pattern of the transverse colon
3. Focal mineralization in the pancreas may be seen with chronic pancreatitis from fat saponification.
4. Differential considerations:
   a. Pancreatic mass
   b. Localized peritonitis
   c. Other abdominal mass

Contrast radiography
1. Barium upper gastrointestinal (UGI) study
   a. The UGI study demonstrates the abnormal location of the stomach and duodenum (e.g., right lateral displacement of the proximal duodenum and displacement of the pylorus toward the left side.
   b. Fixed position and shape of the duodenum are usually seen.

Other imaging
1. Ultrasound
2. CT
3. MRI

Pancreatic Masses
Clinical correlations
1. Pancreatic masses may be associated with pancreatitis, pseudocyst, abscess, or tumor.
2. Pancreatic tumors can be benign or malignant.
   a. Nodular hyperplasia and adenoma
   b. Adenocarcinoma
   c. Insulinoma
   d. Metastatic neoplasms are rare.
3. Pancreatic adenocarcinoma often is aggressive.
   a. Early metastasis to regional lymph nodes, stomach, duodenum, and liver.
   b. May cause gastric outflow obstruction and obstruction of the common bile duct and icterus.
   c. May cause carcinomatosis and peritoneal effusion.
4. Pancreatic abscess may be a sequel to chronic pancreatitis.
5. Clinical signs are variable depending on the location and extent of disease.
   a. Signs often include vomiting, anorexia, depression, weight loss, and fever.
   b. Abdominal distension caused by effusion may be present.
   c. A cranial abdominal mass may be palpated.

Radiographic findings
1. Radiographic findings are similar to acute pancreatitis.
2. A localized loss of detail (with a mass effect) may be identified in the cranial midabdomen with displacement of the stomach to the left and the duodenum to the right.
3. Abdominal effusion may be present as a result of ascites, peritonitis, or carcinomatosis.

Contrast radiography
Barium UGI study
1. Outline of the pancreatic mass may be seen.
2. Infiltration into the duodenum or gastric wall may be identified.

Other imaging
1. Ultrasound
2. CT
3. MRI

STOMACH

RADIOGRAPHIC ANATOMY (Figures 11.35 through 11.37 A,B,C,D)

1. The major areas of the stomach are the cardia, fundus, body, pyloric antrum, and pyloric canal. These regions are illustrated in Figures 11.38 and 11.39.
2. The appearance of the stomach depends on the volume and type of gastric contents and on the radiographic position of the animal.
3. If fluid and gas are within the gastric lumen, the gas tends to move to the nondependent area (up side) and the fluid to the dependent area (down side) because of gravity.
   a. Ventrodorsal projection: gas usually is present in the pyloric antrum in the right cranial quadrant of the abdomen; fluid is usually in the fundus in the left cranial quadrant.

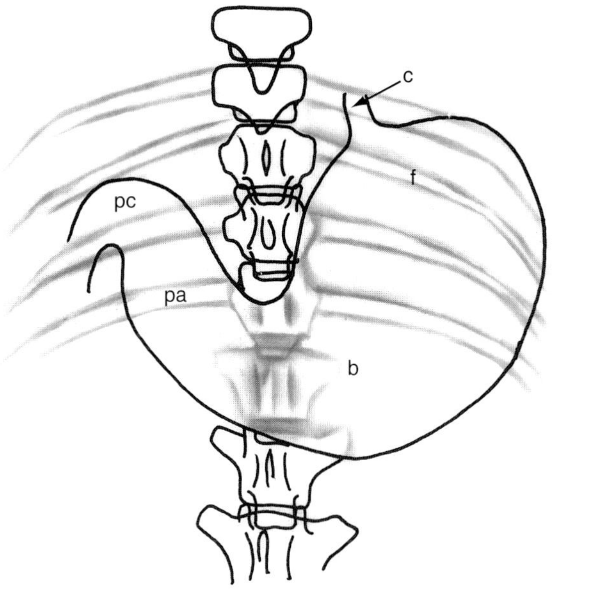

Figure 11.35. Normal canine stomach. Normal regions of the canine stomach include the cardia (**c**), fundus (**f**), body (**b**), pyloric antrum (**pa**), and pyloric canal (**pc**).

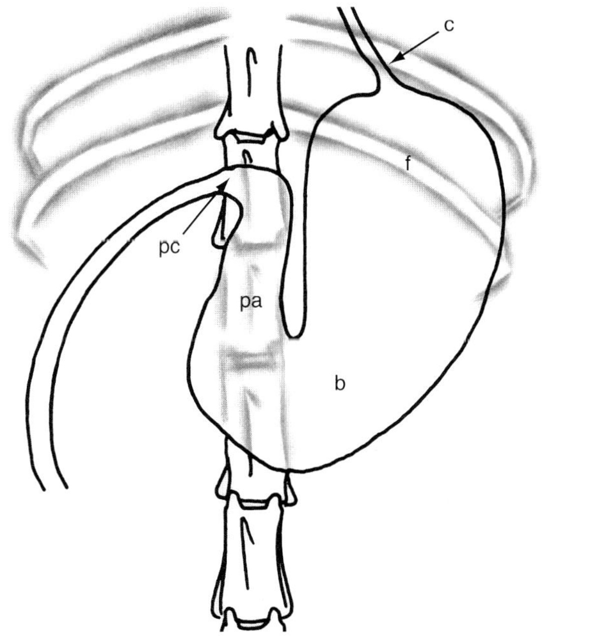

Figure 11.36. Normal feline stomach. Normal regions of the feline stomach include the cardia (**c**), fundus (**f**), body (**b**), pyloric antrum (**pa**), and pyloric canal (**pc**).

b. Dorsoventral projection: gas usually is present in the fundic portion of the stomach in the left cranial quadrant adjacent to the left crus of the diaphragm.
c. Right lateral projection: gas usually is present in the fundus of the stomach in the dorsocranial quadrant of the abdomen. Fluid usually is present in the pyloric antrum in the ventral abdomen. The normal fluid-distended antrum commonly appears as a spherical soft tissue opacity caudal to the liver.
d. Left lateral projection: gas usually is present in the pyloric portion of the stomach in the ventrocranial abdomen caudal to the liver; fluid usually would be located in the body and fundic portions of the stomach.

4. The stomach, unless distended, is normally within the rib cage margin and does not project caudal to the last rib.
5. The gastric axis can be estimated by drawing a line from the fundus to the pyloric region. This subjective judgement of stomach axis can vary, depending on the size of the stomach and stage of gastric contractions.
   a. On the lateral projection, the axis normally is vertical to the spine or parallel to the ribs.
   b. On the ventrodorsal projection, the axis usually is perpendicular to the spine.
6. The stomach of the cat is similar in its position to that of the dog on the lateral projection. On a ventrodorsal or dorsoventral projection, the pyloric antrum of a cat usually is seen on the midline or slightly to the right of the midline.

Radiographic Interpretation

1. On survey radiographs, assessment includes the location, size, and shape of the stomach, as well as the type of gastric contents and the appearance of the gastric rugae and wall.
2. The position and shape of the stomach varies with the amount of intragastric contents (fluid, gas, and ingesta) and the animal's positioning and body conformation.
3. Caudal displacement of the stomach is usually caused by hepatic enlargement or caudal displacement of the diaphragm, secondary to thoracic disease (e.g., pneumothorax, pleural effusion, or hyperinflation).
   a. Generalized hepatomegaly usually causes caudal and dorsal displacement of the stomach, especially of the body and antral portions.
   b. Enlargement of the right liver lobes usually causes the pylorus to be displaced caudally and dorsally.
   c. Enlargement of the left liver lobes usually causes medial displacement of the fundus and body of the stomach.
4. Cranial displacement of the stomach may occur if the liver size is decreased (e.g., cirrhosis from chronic liver disease, portosystemic shunts, or secondary to diaphragmatic hernia in which the liver is herniated into the chest).
5. Displacement of the stomach and reduction in gastric size can occur, secondary to masses that are caudal to or involving the gastric wall.
   a. Splenic or left liver enlargement can distort the lesser or greater curvature of the fundus and body regions.

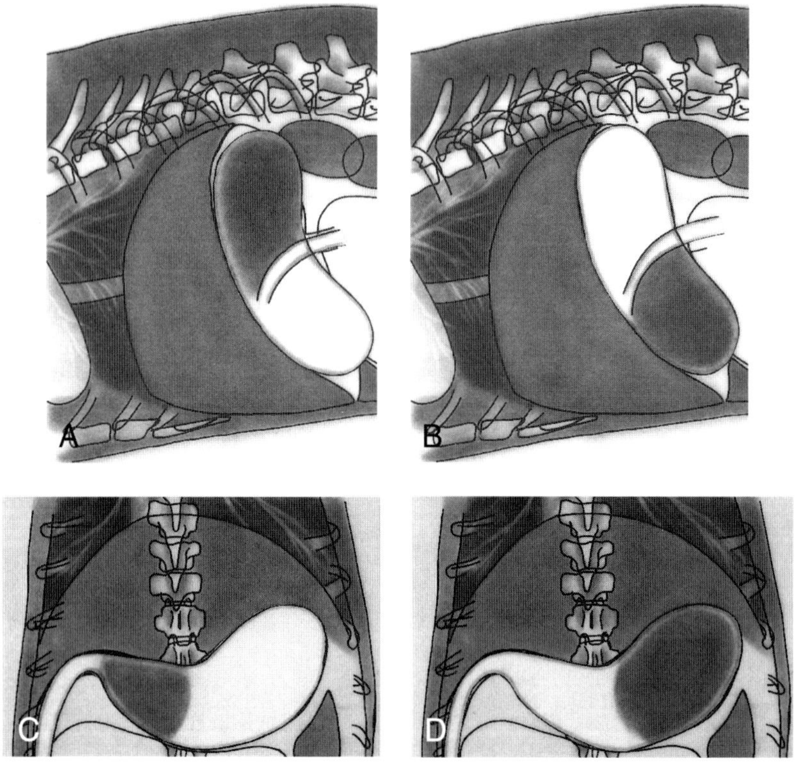

Figure 11.37. The location of gas and fluid in the gastric lumen as observed in different radiographic projections. The location of the gas/fluid correlates with position of an animal's body during different projections. **A.,** Right recumbent lateral. Fluid is present in the pyloric antrum and gas is in the body and fundus. **B.,** Left recumbent lateral. Gas is present in the pyloric antrum and fluid in the body and fundus. **C.,** Ventrodorsal projection. Gas is present in the pyloric antrum and fluid in the body and fundus. **D.,** Dorsoventral projection. Fluid is present in the pyloric antrum and gas is present in the body and fundus.

   b. A pancreatic, bowel, or mesenteric mass can distort the pyloric or body region of the stomach.
   c. Gastric wall masses can cause local distortion of the gastric silhouette depending on size of mass.
6. The thickness of the gastric wall and the rugal folds are difficult to assess on survey radiographs because of the variable degrees of gastric distension and the type and volume of gastric contents. If visible, rugae are larger and more numerous in the dog than in the cat. The rugae also are more numerous in the fundus and body than in the pyloric antrum. Increased rugal thickness or mineralization is usually associated with specific diseases, such as gastritis and renal failure.
7. A UGI contrast study can provide further assessment of the stomach wall and rugae.

DISEASES/DISORDERS

Gastric Enlargement

Clinical correlations

1. Fluid or ingesta distention of the stomach can be caused by:
   a. Recent meal
   b. Pyloric outflow obstruction:
      1) Pyloric hypertrophy
      2) Hypertrophic gastritis
      3) Pyloric neoplasia
      4) Foreign body
   c. Gastric atony
   d. Gastric foreign matter
2. Gas-filled distention of the stomach could be caused by:
   a. Aerophagia associated with normal swallowing of air, or secondary to stress, pharyngeal or esophageal disease
   b. Passage of orogastric tube and infusion of air
   c. Gastric dilatation/volvulus (GDV)

Radiographic findings

1. Increased fundic diameter, a convex caudal margin of greater curvature, caudal displacement of the fundus and body, and an increased diameter and length of the pyloric antrum may be observed.
2. In the normal stomach, the diameter of the pylorus should be approximately half that of the gastric body. When the pylorus is larger than this relationship, it may suggest disease in the pyloric canal.
3. The spleen and bowel are displaced caudally.

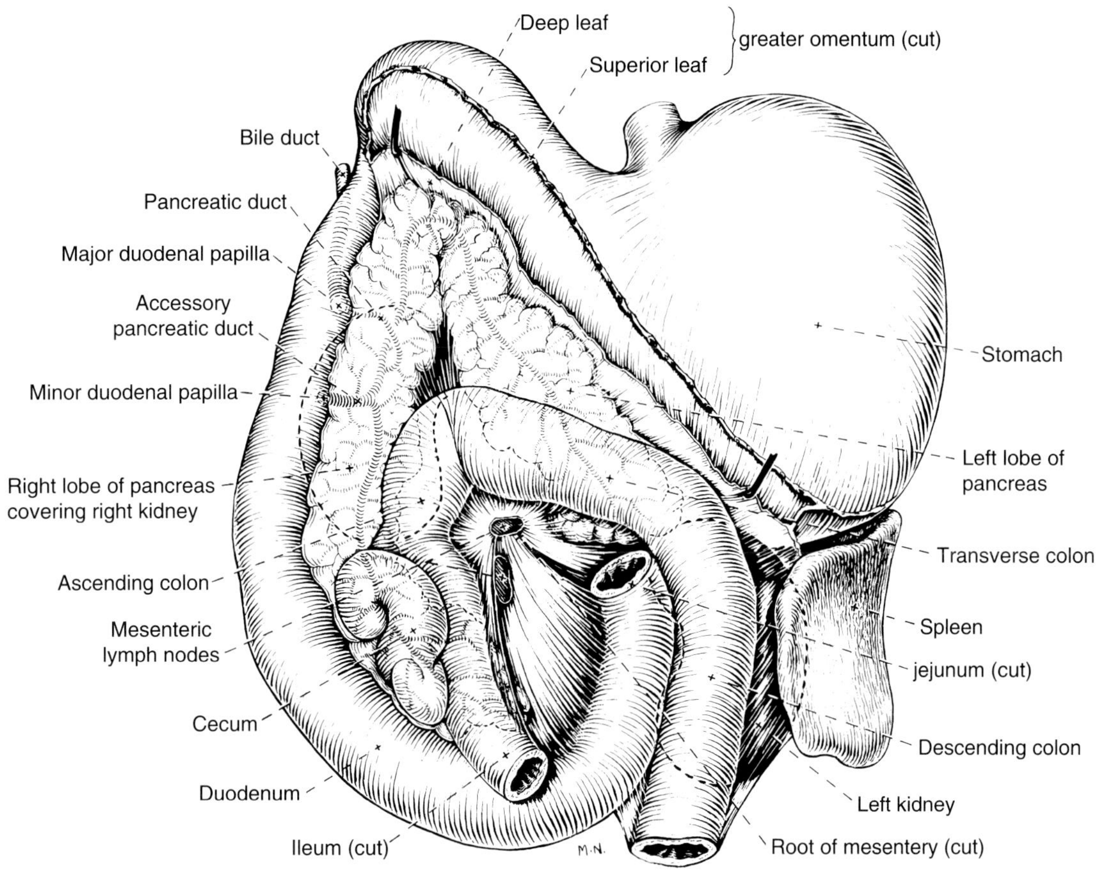

Figure 11.38. Abdominal viscera: ventral aspect. (From Evans HE. The digestive apparatus and abdomen. In: Evans HE, ed. Miller's Anatomy of the Dog. 3rd ed, Philadelphia: W.B. Saunders, 1993:435. Courtesy of and with permission of Dr. Howard E. Evans.)

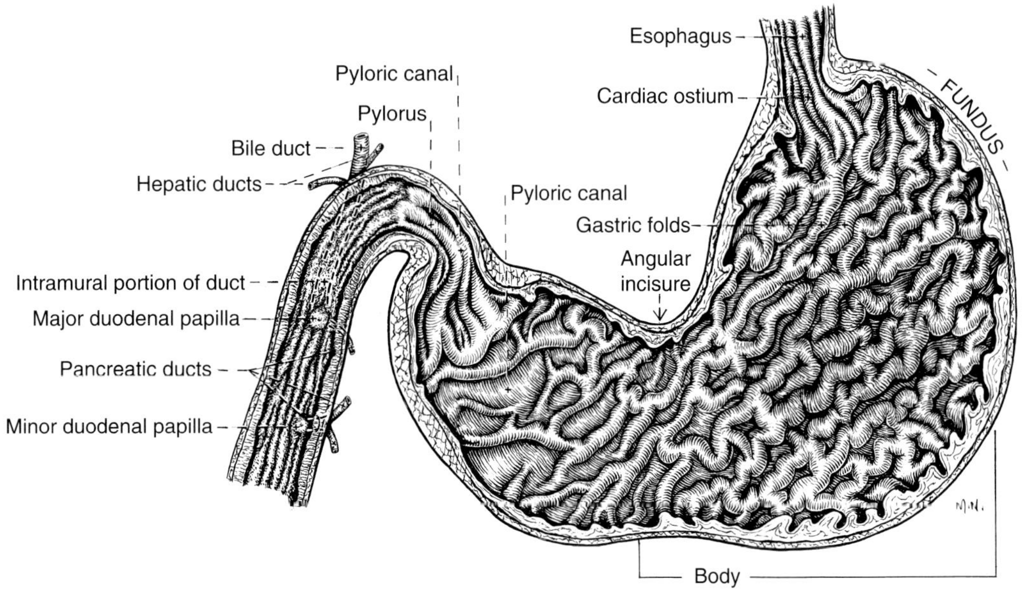

Figure 11.39. Longitudinal section of stomach and proximal portion of duodenum. (From Evans HE. The digestive apparatus and abdomen. In: Evans HE, ed. Miller's Anatomy of the Dog. 3rd ed, Philadelphia: W.B. Saunders; 1993:437. Courtesy of and with permission of Dr. Howard E. Evans.)

Gastric Wall Abnormalities

Clinical correlations

1. Lesions can involve the mucosa and submucosa including the rugal folds or affect the serosa and muscularis portions of the gastric wall.
2. The location and extent of disease can vary from localized to diffuse.
3. Thickened and less distensible gastric wall lesions can occur because of:
   a. Edema or hemorrhage
   b. Cellular infiltrates (e.g., lymphosarcoma, eosinophilic gastritis)
   c. Muscular infiltration (e.g., neoplasia, scar formation)
4. Mucosal and submucosal lesions can be associated with irregularity and thickening of the rugal folds as a result of chronic inflammation, ulceration, or neoplasia.
5. Ulceration can vary from mild to severe and may be associated with benign or malignant disease.
6. Endosopy best assesses the presence and severity of gastric ulceration.

Radiographic findings

1. Variable appearance of the gastric wall and rugal folds depending on the degree of gastric distention and the volume and type of gastric contents.
2. A localized mass lesion may alter the serosal contour of the stomach.
3. A mucosal or mural mass may be seen if surrounded by gas.
4. Nonchanging (fixed) appearance to the stomach shape, size, or position.

Contrast radiography

Upper gastrointestinal study

1. Localized mucosal lesions are identified by alteration in the appearance of the rugae. The rugae may appear irregular or thickened.
2. Ulcer craters are seen as outpouchings from the gastric lumen. Although difficult to visualize, ulcers usually are most visible when the radiographic beam is tangential to the lesion.

Other imaging

1. Ultrasound
2. CT
3. MRI

Gastric Emptying

1. The rate of gastric emptying during a UGI contrast study, can be altered by a variety of factors:
   a. Volume and type of gastric contents
   b. Various reflex mechanisms
   c. Some medications (e.g., sedatives, atropine)
   d. Patient variables (e.g., anxiety, fear, or pain)
   e. Type, temperature, and consistency of the contrast media
2. Barium is more likely to demonstrate a gastric lesion than is iodinated contrast media.
   a. With an empty stomach, the stomach is usually empty of barium by 1 to 2 hours. If barium is mixed with food, gastric emptying takes longer, up to 12 to 15 hours in some normal dogs.
   b. The stomach of normal cats empties more rapidly, usually within 15 to 30 minutes.
   c. More rapid gastric emptying usually has no significance.
   d. Delayed gastric emptying (more than 3 hours) usually implies a pathologic condition.
3. Causes of delayed gastric emptying:
   a. Motility disorder
   b. Pyloric outflow obstruction
      1) Pyloric stenosis
      2) Pyloric neoplasia
      3) Pyloric or proximal duodenal foreign body
      4) Parvovirus infection
      5) Hypertrophic gastritis
   c. Chronic gastritis
   d. Gastric neoplasia
4. Iodinated contrast media, although less sensitive for detecting lesions, empty more rapidly from the stomach and have a faster transit time through the bowel than does barium.
5. Fluoroscopic observation during a barium contrast study is helpful for assessment of stomach contractions and emptying.
6. Scintigraphy is the most sensitive imaging modality for evaluation of gastric emptying and gastroduodenal reflux.

DISEASES/DISORDERS

Acute Gastritis

Clinical correlations

1. Defined as inflammation resulting from an insult to the gastric mucosa.
2. Common causes include:
   a. Ingestion of rancid food or foreign bodies.
   b. Chemical intoxication (e.g., cleaning agents, petroleum products).
   c. Drugs (e.g., aspirin, corticosteroids, nonsteroidal anti-inflammatory drugs [NSAIDS]).
3. Common clinical signs are frequent vomiting, lethargy, dehydration, and abdominal pain.
4. Clinical diagnosis is based on history, physical examination, and exclusion of other causes of vomiting.
5. Best diagnosed with endoscopy and biopsy.

Radiographic findings (Figure 11.40 A,B)

1. Survey radiographs are usually normal.
2. Opaque or dense soft tissue foreign bodies may be seen.

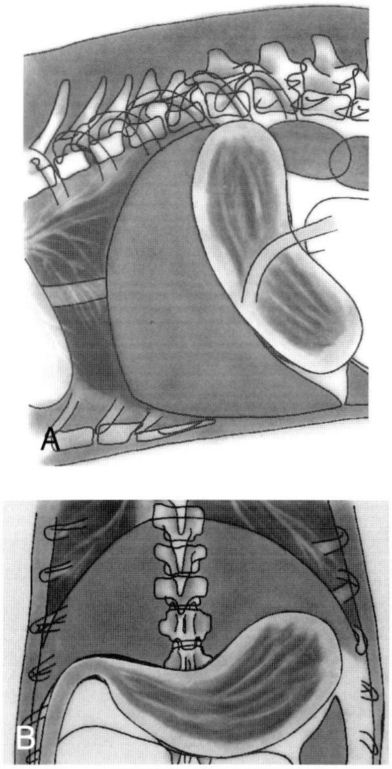

Figure 11.40. **A.,** Gastritis. The rugal folds are prominent and the gastric wall appears thickened. **B.,** Gastritis. The rugal folds are prominent and the gastric wall appears thickened.

3. Rugal folds may appear (subjectively) enlarged and thickened.

Chronic Gastritis

Clinical correlations

1. By definition, chronic gastritis occurs after repeated insult to the gastric mucosa with chronic inflammation.
2. In most cases, a definite etiology is never determined.
3. Atrophic gastritis usually is a result of chronic superficial gastritis in which the gastric glands atrophy and the mucosa becomes thinned. It may result in achlorhydria, gastric ulceration, and small bowel bacterial overgrowth.
4. Hypertrophic gastritis may result form chronic inflammation or from the trophic action of histamine or gastrin on the gastric mucosa.
5. Eosinophilic gastritis can occur from allergic, parasitic, or immune-mediated disease.
6. Common clinical signs include:
   a. Chronic intermittent vomiting
   b. Hematemesis or melena if ulceration has occurred
   c. Weight loss and anorexia are common
7. Best diagnosed with endoscopy and biopsy.

Radiographic findings

1. Survey radiographs usually appear normal.
2. Rugal folds may be enlarged, irregular, and thickened, often with gastric wall thickening.

Contrast radiography

Gastrogram

1. Decreased rugal folds are observed with atrophic gastritis.
2. Large, irregular, and thickened rugal folds are observed with hypertrophic gastritis.
3. Mucosal nodules or masses with gastric wall thickening is commonly noted with eosinophilic gastritis.
4. Gastric emptying is often delayed.
5. Fluoroscopic observation during barium study is useful.

Gastric Ulcers

Clinical correlations

1. Gastric ulcers may be small superficial erosions or deep indurated ulcers of the gastric mucosa.
2. Causes include:
   a. Agents that cause acute or chronic gastritis
      1) Foreign body
      2) Rancid food
      3) Toxic chemicals
   b. Exogenous factors:
      1) Corticosteroids
      2) Phenylbutazone
      3) Aspirin
      4) Other NSAIDS
   c. Altered gastric blood flow
      1) Hypotension or shock
      2) Sepsis
      3) Thromboembolism
   d. Metabolic disease
      1) Renal failure
      2) Liver disease
   e. Neoplasia
      1) Adenocarcinoma
      2) Lymphosarcoma
      3) Systemic mastocytosis
3. Common clinical signs include:
   a. Chronic vomiting
   b. Hematemesis
   c. Melena
   d. Abdominal pain
   e. Anorexia and weight loss
4. Best diagnosed with endoscopy.

Radiographic findings (Figure 11.41 A)

1. Survey radiographs commonly appear normal.
2. If perforation has occurred, free abdominal fluid or free abdominal gas may be seen.

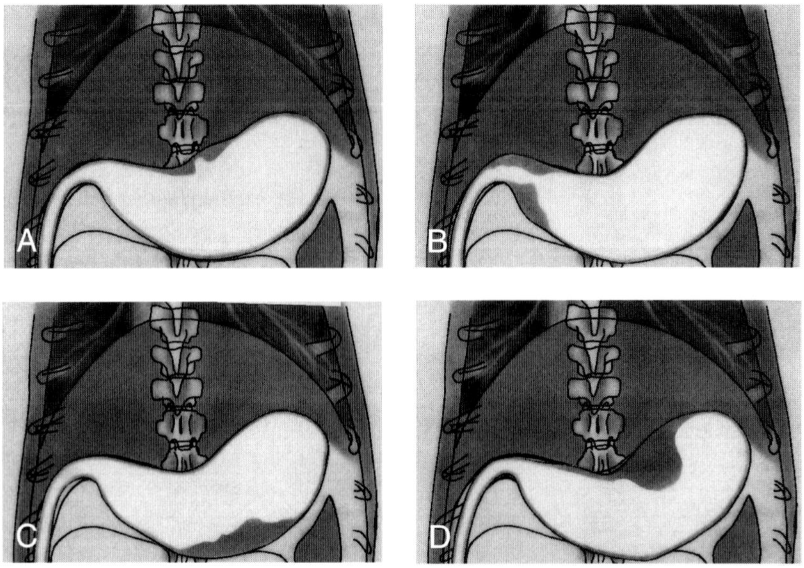

Figure 11.41. **A.,** Gastric neoplasia with ulceration (barium gastrogram). There is thickening of the lesser curvature with a well-defined ulcer. **B.,** Gastric neoplasia (barium gastrogram). Localized thickening of the wall of the antrum. **C.,** Gastric neoplasia (barium gastrogram). Thickening of the wall of the greater curvature. **D.,** Gastric neoplasia (barium gastrogram). There is severe thickening of the lesser curvature of the stomach.

Contrast radiography

Gastrogram

1. The ability to recognize an ulcer depends on its size, location, contrast study chosen, and direction of the x-ray beam (relative to patient's position). A double contrast gastrogram is more sensitive than a barium contrast study.
2. Ulcers range in size and shape from small indentations to irregular or square defects within the mucosa.
3. Large chronic ulcers may have thickened mucosa adjacent to the crater.
4. Ulcers appear different depending on the alignment of the ulcer with the x-ray beam.
   a. If seen en face and dependent, the ulcer may contain barium with a radiolucent border as a result of the localized thickening of the gastric wall.
   b. If seen en face and nondependent, the ulcer may contain gas rather than barium, especially in a double contrast gastrogram.
   c. If seen tangentially, the crater may be seen projecting from the gastric lumen with the irregular mucosa projecting into the lumen.

Gastric Neoplasia

Clinical correlations

1. Benign tumors include:
   a. Adenomatous polyps
      1) Peduculated nodules of mucosal proliferation
      2) Occur secondarily to inflammation
   b. Leiomyoma
      1) Usually in older dogs
      2) Vary in size and distribution
      3) May cause obstruction at the cardia or pyloric canal
2. Malignant tumors include:
   a. Adenocarcinoma
      1) The most common malignant tumor in the dog.
      2) Average age is 8 years.
      3) Tumor is usually raised and ulcerated
      4) Is most often in the pyloric or antral region, but may be diffuse.
      5) Metastasis is common.
   b. Lymphosarcoma
      1) The most common malignant tumor in cats.
      2) Can be diffuse or localized.
   c. Leiomyosarcoma
   d. Fibrosarcoma
   e. Other metastatic tumors
3. Tumors exert their effect by altering normal motility, by causing pyloric outflow obstruction or mucosal ulceration.
4. Common clinical signs include vomiting, anorexia, and weight loss.

Radiographic findings (Figure 11.41 A,B,C,D)

1. Survey radiographs may be normal.
2. Localized or generalized gastric wall thickening may be observed.
3. Mass lesion involving the gastric wall.

Contrast radiography

Gastrogram

1. There is localized or generalized area of gastric wall thickening and abnormal fixation to the gastric wall (stiffness), which is reproducible on multiple radiographs.
2. Distortion of gastric lumen and derangement of the rugal folds
3. Mucosal mass lesion with filling defects
4. Ulceration
5. Gastric emptying is delayed, especially if pyloric outflow obstruction is present.
6. Differential diagnosis:
   a. Chronic hypertrophic gastritis
   b. Eosinophilic gastritis
   c. Phycomycosis

Gastric Foreign Bodies

Clinical correlations

1. Gastric foreign bodies are common.
2. Foreign bodies vary in size, type, shape, and radiopacity. If a foreign body appears metallic, the possibility of lead or zinc should be considered.
3. May cause acute or chronic clinical signs. Vomiting is the most common sign.

Radiographic findings (Figure 11.42 A,B)

1. Radiopaque foreign bodies are easily identified (e.g., bone, metallic objects)

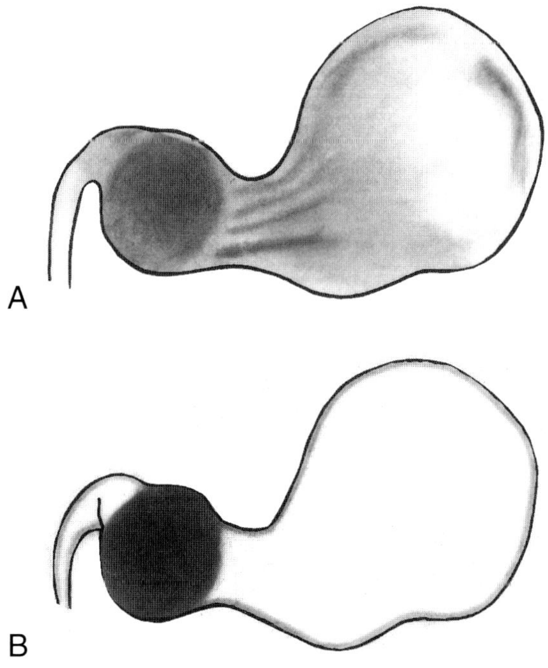

Figure 11.42. **A.,** Radiolucent or nonopaque gastric foreign body on a survey radiograph a radiolucent foreign body may not be seen. **B.,** On a barium gastrogram, the foreign body is visualized contrasted with the barium.

2. Soft tissue or more radiolucent foreign bodies may be visible if surrounded by gastric gas (e.g., wood, plastic)
3. Follow-up radiographs may aid in determining whether the gastric contents is ingesta or foreign matter.

Contrast radiography

1. Survey radiographs should always be made first because positive contrast media (e.g., barium) can obscure a foreign body.
2. Many foreign bodies will be visible (as a relative radiolucency) within the radiopaque contrast media.
3. Fabric or other porous (e.g., hair) foreign bodies may retain barium and be most visible after the stomach is empty.

Gastric Dilation and Volvulus

Clinical correlations

1. Acute gastric dilation is characterized by an acute distension of the stomach with fluid, gas, or food.
2. Many factors contribute to dilation and potential volvulus.
   a. Aerophagia
   b. Bacterial fermentation of carbohydrates
   c. Excessive ingestion of food and water
   d. Alteration or abnormalities of gastric motor activity
      1) Hypotonia
      2) Pyloric dysfunction
   e. Inability to eructate associated with dysfunction of lower gastroesophageal sphincter.
   f. Mechanical pyloric obstruction caused by foreign body, stenosis, or tumor.
3. May result in dilation only or dilation and volvulus.
4. Most affected animals have acute disease; chronic disease is less common.
5. Most common in large deep-chested dogs (e.g., Great Dane, Irish Setter, and German Shepherd Dog), and is rare in cats and small dogs.

Radiographic findings (Figures 11.43 through 11.46)

1. Gastric dilation
   a. There is abnormal distension of the stomach with gas, fluid, or ingesta with caudal displacement of the intestines.
   b. The pylorus and fundus are in a normal position.
2. Gastric volvulus
   a. There is distension of the stomach with gas and fluid (primarily gas) with the pylorus and fundus in an abnormal position.
   b. The most common volvulus is a 180° volvulus in which the pylorus is displaced dorsally and to the left side of the abdomen. The right and left lateral projections are useful for differentiation of a volvulus versus dilation.
      1) The abnormal position of the pylorus can be seen best on the right lateral projection, in which the gas fills the left displaced pylorus, and fluid shifts

into the dependent gastric body or fundus. The pylorus appears narrower and more tubular than the rest of the stomach.

2) In left lateral positioning, the displaced pylorus usually is dependent and fills with fluid, and the gas in the stomach moves dorsally into the nondependent fundus of the stomach.

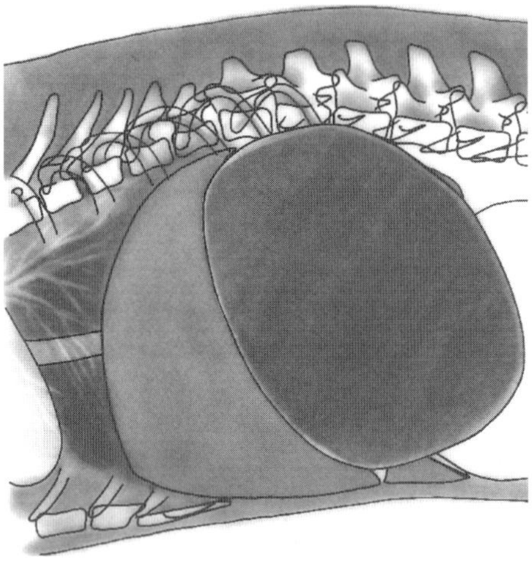

Figure 11.43. Gastric dilation: lateral abdomen.

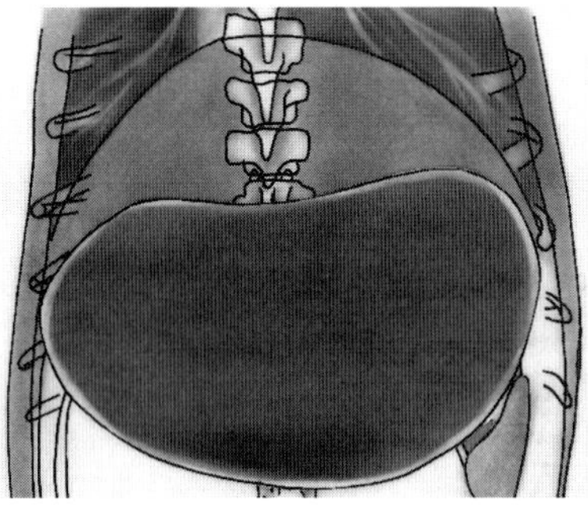

Figure 11.44. Gastric dilation: ventrodorsal abdomen.

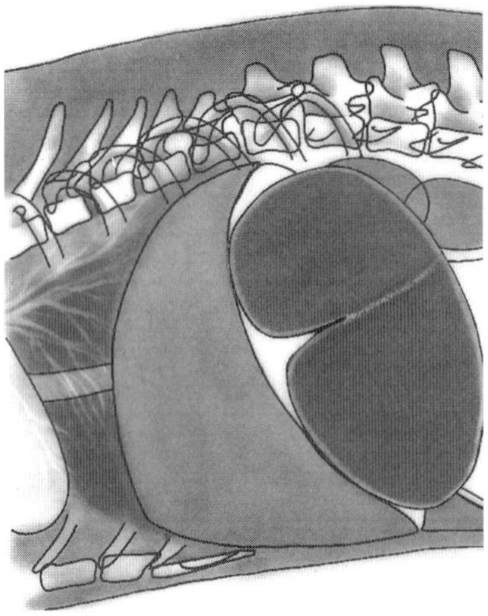

Figure 11.45. Gastric volvulus: lateral abdomen.

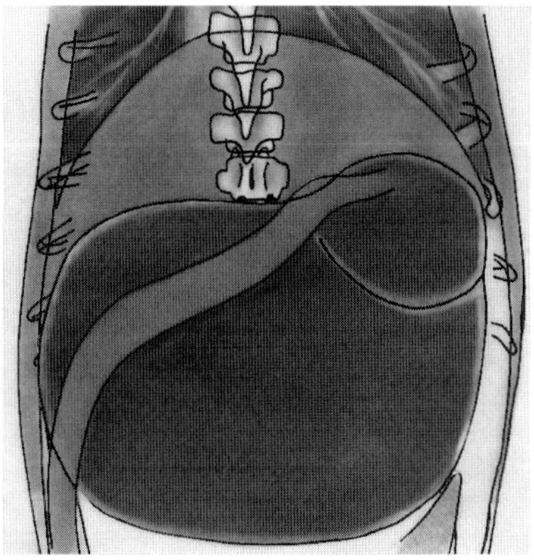

Figure 11.46. Gastric volvulus: ventrodorsal abdomen.

3. Compartmentalization of the stomach is an abnormal appearance of the stomach, in which soft tissue radiodense bands project into or across the lumen of the gas-filled stomach as a result of the stomach folding in on itself.
4. If pyloric and fundus positions are indeterminate on survey radiographs, a barium GI contrast study can be done. Right and left lateral and ventrodorsal or dorsoventral projections should be obtained.
5. Splenomegaly is commonly present as a result of passive congestion, infarction, or concomitant splenic torsion.
6. Other radiographic findings that may be present include:
   a. Megaesophagus
   b. Microcardia caused by hypovolemia
   c. Bronchopneumonia secondary to aspiration

Pyloric Outflow Obstruction

Clinical correlations

1. Partial pyloric outflow obstructive disease, either congenital or acquired, is caused by pyloric muscular stenosis, mucosal hypertrophy, foreign bodies, or infiltrative lesions, both benign and neoplastic.
2. Congenital disease is caused by hypertrophy of the circular smooth muscle fibers within the pyloric canal. It is reported most commonly in brachycephalic dogs (e.g., Boston Terriers, Bulldogs, Boxers) and in Siamese cats.
3. Acquired lesions can be focal, multifocal, or diffuse, and are most commonly seen in small-breed dogs of middle age. Potential causes include:
   a. Chronic hypertrophic gastritis
   b. Excessive gastrin secretion secondary to chronic gastric distension
   c. Immune-mediated inflammation
4. Gastric retention with fluid, gas, and ingesta can cause gastric distension and atony.

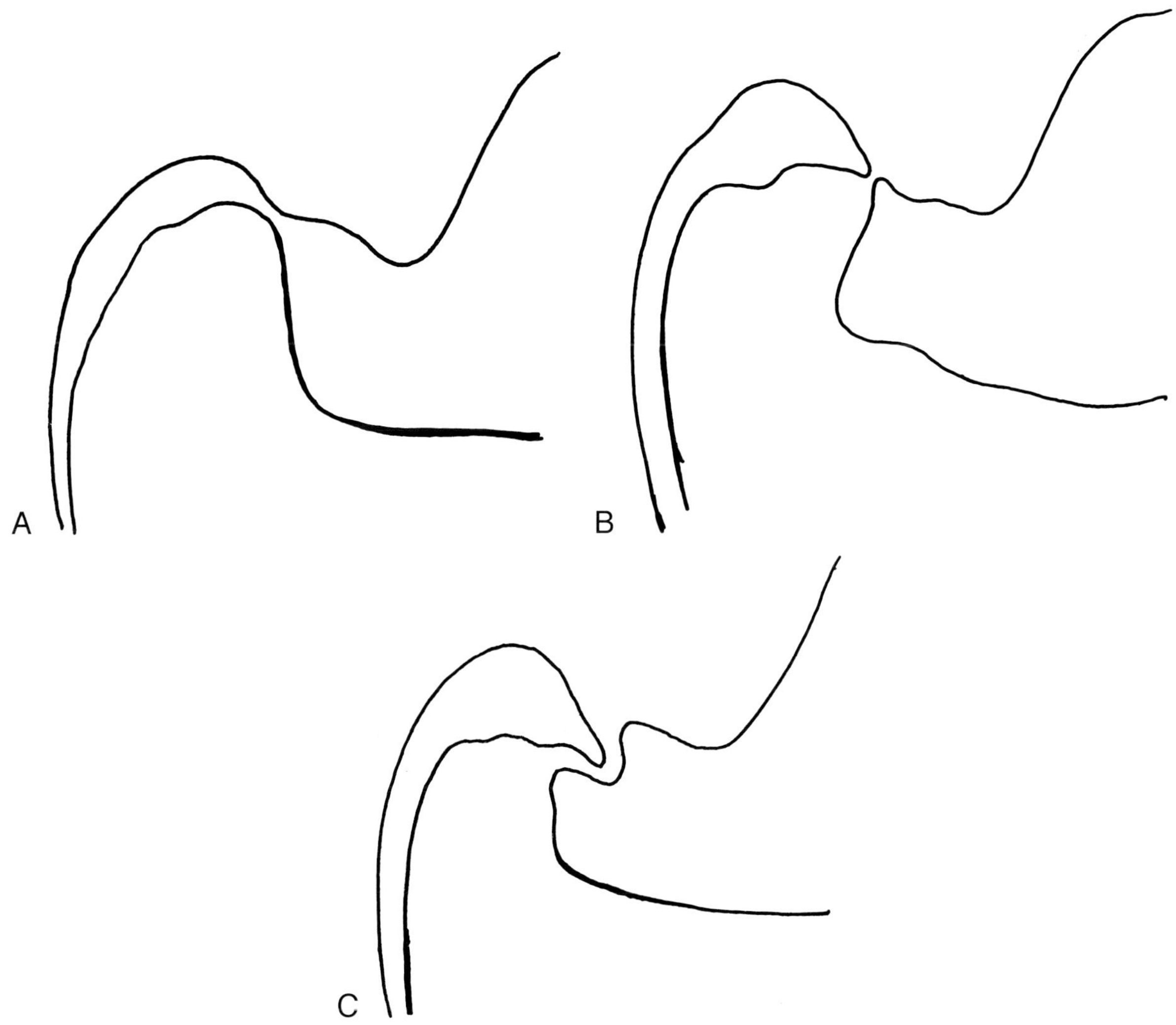

Figure 11.47. Pyloric canal. The normal pyloric canal is depicted in **A**. With pyloric outflow obstructive disease, the pyloric canal may appear "beak like" as in **B** or inverted as in **C**.

5. Common clinical signs include vomiting undigested food, weight loss, and abdominal distension. Chronic vomiting (often projectile and of undigested food) occurs at variable intervals after a meal. In congenital disease, vomiting is first observed shortly after weaning.

Radiographic findings (Figure 11.47 A,B,C)

1. Survey radiographs often show a fluid distended stomach and lesser amounts of gas.
2. Enlargement of the stomach is variable, depending on the severity and duration of the stenosis.

Contrast radiography

1. Gastric distension and delayed gastric emptying are observed.
2. A narrowed "beak" of contrast at the pyloric canal is commonly seen. It is caused by bulging of antrum around a narrowed pyloric canal during gastric contraction.
3. Circumferential narrowing of the pyloric canal may be seen ("String" or "Tram track" sign)
4. Fluoroscopy often is helpful in differentiating pyloric muscular hypertrophy from pyloric foreign body and pyloric neoplasia.
5. In some animals, liquid barium may pass through the pyloric canal readily, whereas barium mixed with food may demonstrate abnormal gastric retention.

SMALL BOWEL

RADIOGRAPHIC ANATOMY

1. The small intestine includes the duodenum, jejunum, and ileum. The distribution of the small bowel within the abdomen varies depending on the animal's confor-

mation, its nutritional status, and the size, shape, and position of adjacent abdominal viscera (e.g., distended versus empty urinary bladder). In thin dogs and cats, the small bowel can extend from the liver to the pelvic cavity. In obese dogs and cats, intraabdominal fat tends to displace the small bowel into the central midabdomen between the stomach and bladder.

2. The proximal duodenum lies adjacent to the caudal surface of the right side of the liver. It is relatively fixed in position by the hepatoduodenal ligament. The descending duodenum lies parallel to the right abdominal wall (as the caudal duodenal flexure), and the ascending duodenum extends cranially toward the caudal border of the stomach.
3. The position of the jejunum and ileum is variable in the midabdomen.

RADIOGRAPHIC INTERPRETATION

On survey abdominal radiographs, the position, contour, size, and margination of the small intestine can usually be identified. The gas pattern and type of intraluminal contents also are visible. Contrast studies are needed to assess mucosal irregularities, peristalsis, segmentation, and contrast media transit times. The serosal border of the small intestine is usually seen in animals with adequate intraabdominal fat. In immature or emaciated animals, or if peritoneal effusion is present, the serosal borders of the bowel walls may not be clearly visualized.

Change in position of the small bowel can occur:

1. Relative to body conformation and degree of intraabdominal fat
2. Because of changes in the size, shape, or position of other abdominal organs (e.g., full urinary bladder) or abnormal abdominal masses
3. Secondary to peritoneal and body wall diseases or disorder (e.g., diaphragmatic and abdominal wall hernia)

Change in size and shape can occur:

1. Variability depends on intraluminal contents and motility.
2. The normal proximal duodenum is often slightly larger in diameter than the jejunum and ileum.
3. Abnormal dilation of the small bowel with fluid or gas is associated with the inability of intestinal contents to pass normally, and is called ileus.
   a. Rules of thumb for normal diameter in the dog include:
      1) Diameter should not exceed 2 to 3 times the width of a rib, less than the width of an intercostal space.
      2) Diameter should not exceed height of the central part of a lumbar vertebra.
      3) All of the small bowel should have a similar diameter. A segment of small bowel is abnormal if it is more than 50% larger than other small bowel loops.
   b. Rules of thumb for normal diameter in the cat include:
      1) Diameter should not exceed twice the height of the central portion of the L4 vertebral body.
      2) Diameter should not exceed 12 mm.
4. The degree of ileus varies depending on the etiology, location and extent of disease. The ileus can be further evaluated as mild or severe, and localized or generalized.

Types of ileus include mechanical and paralytic:

1. Mechanical (obstructive or dynamic) ileus:
   a. Partial or complete obstruction of the bowel
   b. Causes include:
      1) Intraluminal obstruction (foreign body, enterolith, or parasites)
      2) Mural thickening (neoplasia, granuloma, or stricture)
      3) Internal hernia
      4) Volvulus of the small bowel
      5) Intussusception
2. Paralytic (functional, adynamic) ileus is:
   a. A decreased or absent peristalsis
   b. Bowel lumen usually patent
   c. Causes of paralytic ileus include:
      1) Mesenteric thrombosis
      2) Parasympatholytic stimulation (e.g., atropine)
      3) Peritonitis
      4) Bowel infarction
      5) Severe viral enteritis (e.g., parvovirus)
      6) Postoperative
      7) Neurologic injury (e.g., spinal cord trauma)
      8) Electrolyte imbalance (e.g., hypokalemia)

CONTRAST RADIOGRAPHS

Use an upper gastrointestinal study (UGI) barium contrast study (using positive contrast media [See Chapter 3 for method]). The barium contrast media is administered orally and a series of radiographs are obtained at varying time intervals for assessment of the stomach, the small bowel, and the colon.

General Indications for a UGI Study

1. Must assess the GI tract for lesions that alter the size, shape, or position of the stomach and small bowel that cannot be adequately characterized from the survey radiographs.
2. Need to evaluate an animal with a suspected partial or complete bowel obstruction.
3. Need to evaluate the mucosa of the small bowel.
4. Need to differentiate abdominal masses of GI tract origin from lymph nodes and other organs.

CONTRAST MEDIA

The choice of contrast media depends on suspected disease.

1. Barium sulfate suspension of 30% wt/wt provides adequate mucosal coating and contrast for radiographic visualization.
2. Iodinated gastrointestinal contrast media can be used in those animals with suspected perforation. However, ionic and nonionic iodinated media are less sensitive for the detection of many mucosal lesions and may not demonstrate a perforation or a fistula.

DISEASES/DISORDERS

1. Diseases of the small intestine can be localized or generalized and may be either primary diseases or associated with systemic illness.
2. Abdominal radiographs are often helpful when GI disease is suspected.
3. Common clinical signs of intestinal disease include vomiting, diarrhea, weight loss, and abdominal pain.
4. Many diseases of the small bowel have nonspecific radiographic findings or show no abnormality. Many of the abnormal radiographic findings can be associated with a multitude of different diseases.

Enteritis and Inflammatory Bowel Disease

Clinical correlations

1. This is nonspecific terminology to denote many inflammatory diseases of the small intestine that may be acute or chronic and be ulcerative or nonulcerative.
2. Many causes include:
   a. Intestinal parasitism
   b. Dietary indiscretion
   c. Infiltrative disease
   d. Immune-mediated disease
   e. Hemorrhagic gastroenteritis
   f. Infectious disease (bacterial, viral, mycotic, or protozoal)
   g. Food allergy
3. Diseases often are subclassified histiologically by type of cellular infiltrate.
   a. Eosinophilic enteritis
   b. Neutrophilic enteritis
   c. Plasmacytic and lymphocytic enteritis
4. Clinical signs vary depending on etiology, but most common signs are vomiting, diarrhea, and weight loss.

Radiographic findings

1. Survey radiographs are usually normal
2. Often, the GI tract will be devoid of ingesta with a slightly increased amount of fluid or gas within the small bowel loops

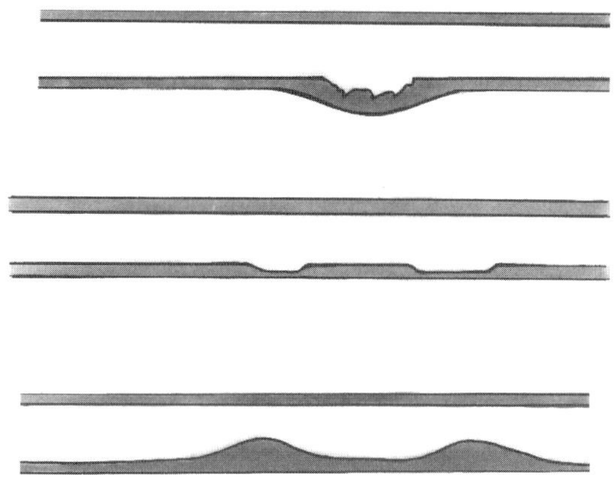

Figure 11.48. Small bowel mucosal defects. On a barium study, mucosal defects can be seen, they include: **A)** ulceration with localized wall thickening; **B)** pseudoulcers without wall thickening, and **C)** localized smooth mucosal thickening.

3. Increased thickness of small bowel wall. This must be differentiated from normal wall where fluid/gas interface can mimic wall thickening.
4. Ileus is not usually present.

Contrast radiography (Figure 11.48 A,B,C)

Upper gastrointestinal study

1. Usually not indicated
2. Used to rule out obstructive disease
3. Nonspecific findings:
   a. Rapid gastric emptying and small bowel transit time of contrast media
   b. Prominent peristalsis (requires fluoroscopic observation)
   c. Irregular mucosal surface (e.g., thumb printing)
4. Differential diagnosis:
   a. Pseudoulcers; normal outpouchings of mucosal between aggregates of lymphoid tissue.
   b. Neoplasia (e.g., lymphosarcoma)

Intestinal Obstruction

Clinical correlations

1. Obstruction most often results from ingestion of foreign bodies.
2. Other causes include:
   a. Mural masses (tumor, granuloma, abscess, scar tissue, or hematoma)
   b. Intussusception
   c. Hernia (e.g., mesenteric, abdominal wall, or diaphragmatic)
   d. Adhesions
3. Clinical signs can be acute or chronic, depending on the etiology, location, and severity of the obstruction.

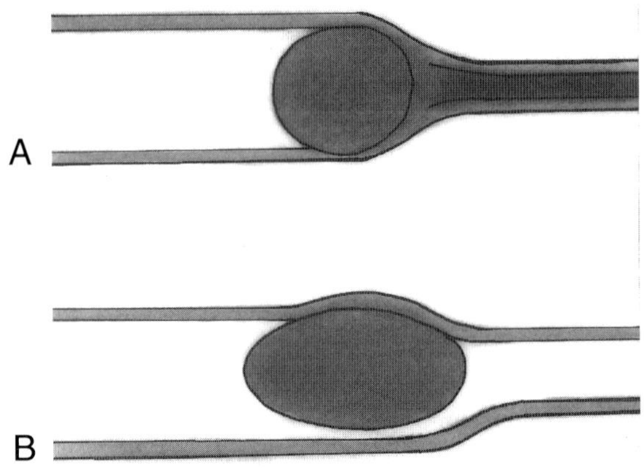

Figure 11.49. **A.,** Small bowel obstruction caused by foreign body on a barium study, with a complete obstruction. There is dilation of the bowel lumen cranial to the radiolucent foreign body. **B.,** The bowel distal to the site of obstruction is of normal diameter. When partially obstructioned, there is often dilation of the bowel lumen cranial to the radiolucent foreign body. The foreign body may be recognized when contrasted against the barium, and when the bowel lumen distal to the foreign body is of normal diameter and contains barium.

Radiographic findings (Figures 11.49 A,B and 11.50)

1. There is variation in the radiographic changes depending on the cause, location, and duration of the obstruction.
2. Radiopaque foreign bodies are easily identified.
3. Nonradiopaque foreign bodies may be visible if they contain gas, are surrounded by gas, or have an uneven texture.
4. Bowel dilation with gas and fluid is usually present with a complete obstruction. The degree of dilation depends on the location and duration of the obstruction. The bowel caudal to the obstruction usually is normal in diameter unless there is a concurrent paralytic ileus.
5. If the obstruction is partial, incomplete, or caused by a linear foreign body, the bowel may not be dilated.
6. Commonly, if the obstruction is at the pyloric canal or in proximal duodenum, the stomach is distended with fluid and gas.
7. In mid or distal small bowel obstructions, the degree and character of dilated bowel will vary depending on the cause (foreign body, tumor, or granuloma) and whether the foreign body is moving through the bowel (e.g., foreign body, bezoar). The bowel distal to the site of obstruction is usually normal in size.
8. When a linear foreign body is anchored proximal to the small bowel (e.g., stomach, base of tongue), the partially obstructed loops of small bowel commonly have a "pleated" or "plicated" appearance and small, often comma-like in shape.
9. Other associated findings, such as free gas in peritoneal cavity secondary to perforation and peritonitis, may be present.

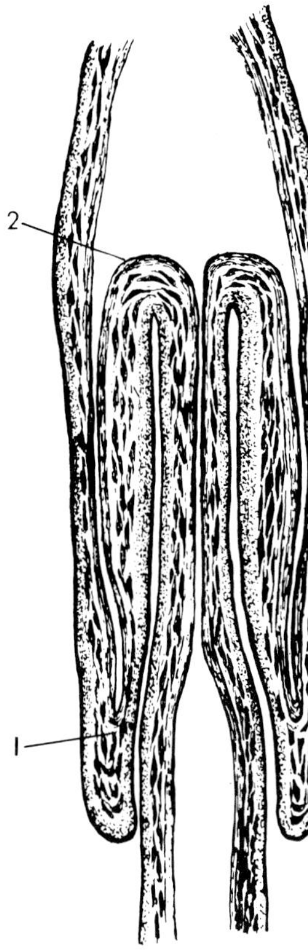

Figure 11.50. Intussusception. The invaginated segment called the intussusceptum (**2**) is within the receiving segment, the intussuscipiens (**1**). (Courtesy of and with the permission of O'Brien, TR, as originally published in: O'Brien TR. Radiographic Diagnosis of Abdominal Disorders in the Dog and Cat. Philadelphia: W.B. Saunders; 1978:314.)

Contrast radiography

Upper gastrointestinal study

1. Contrast material accumulates within the dilated bowel lumen proximal to the obstruction. The severity of the ileus and the motility of the bowel depends on the duration and degree of the obstruction.
2. Intraluminal foreign bodies appear as radiolucent defects surrounded by the positive contrast media
3. Focal intramural lesions may be characterized by:
   a. Filling defect causing narrowing of the lumen
   b. Focal enlargement of the bowel lumen because of ulceration of the bowel segment
   c. Localized thickening of the affected bowel segment
   d. Combination of two or more of the above signs
4. When a linear foreign body is present, the affected bowel segment will appear plicated and the bowel obstruction frequently is partial.

Other imaging

1. Ultrasound
2. CT
3. MRI

Linear Foreign Bodies

Clinical correlations

1. Linear foreign bodies are common in dogs and cats.
2. Types of linear foreign bodies often encountered include thread, string, nylon fishing line, recording tape, and dental floss.
3. Usually are fixed in position proximal to the small intestine (e.g., wrapped around base of tongue or in stomach). The linear material enters the small bowel and the bowel attempts to propel the foreign body aborally through normal peristalsis. The intestines then become pleated or plicated in appearance.
4. May cause partial or complete obstruction.
5. May perforate and cause peritonitis.
6. Clinical signs vary in severity depending on the duration and the severity of the foreign body obstruction. Vomiting and abdominal discomfort are most common.

Radiographic findings (Figure 11.51)

1. Abnormal localized pockets of gas within the bowel lumen may be observed.
2. Bunching of the small bowel is seen, usually pleated or plicated in appearance.
3. Dilation of bowel is variable with amounts of gas and fluid.
4. Foreign body is occasionally visible.
5. Free gas or fluid is observed in the abdomen if peritonitis is present.

Contrast radiography

Upper gastrointestinal study

1. Plication (pleating) of the affected bowel loop is observed.
2. Foreign body may be seen as a relative radiolucency when contrasted against the radiopacity of barium
3. In the cat, a normal mucosal fold in the proximal duodenum may produce a linear filling defect and mimic a linear foreign body, the "pseudo-string" sign.

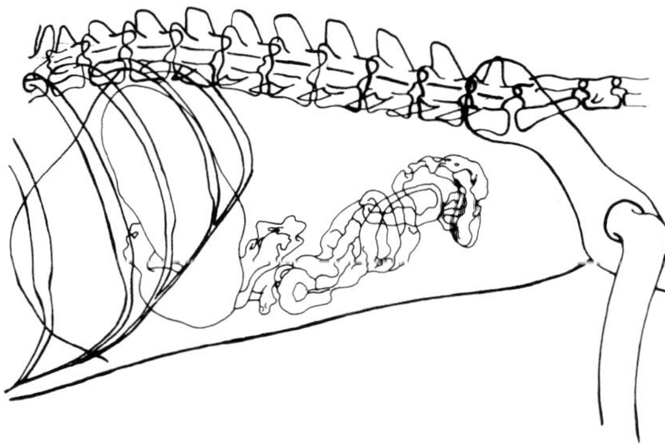

Figure 11.51. Linear foreign body (feline). There is plication of the proximal small intestine.

Intussusception

Clinical correlations

1. Is characterized by the invagination of a segment of the intestine into an adjacent portion of the intestine. The invaginated segment is called the intussusceptum and the receiving segment is called the intussusception.
2. In the dog and cat, a common site of intussusception is the ileum invaginating into the colon (ileocolic). Less common sites include the more proximal small bowel and descending colon.
3. Common clinical signs include vomiting, abdominal pain, and a palpable tubular abdominal mass. Some animals will have diarrhea that often contains blood and mucus.
4. The severity of the clinical signs depends on the degree and duration of vascular compromise from the obstruction.
5. This often is seen in young dogs and cats with intestinal parasitism or severe enteritis. It may occur in older dogs and cats associated with localized or generalized bowel disease.

Radiographic findings (Figure 5.52)

1. There are variable degrees of gas and fluid ileus depending on the location, duration, and severity of the obstruction.
2. A soft tissue mass may be seen associated with the intussusception.
3. If the intussusception is ileocolic, the ascending colon and cecum will usually not contain gas, whereas the normal cecum commonly contains gas.
4. If peritonitis is present, there may be gas or fluid in the peritoneal cavity.

Contrast radiography

1. UGI study
   a. The study will demonstrate the presence of the obstructed segment with marked ileus proximal to the site of obstruction.
   b. If the obstruction is partial, a thin line of contrast may be seen through the affected segment of bowel.
2. Barium enema
   a. Study is more sensitive for ileocolic or colocolic intussusception.

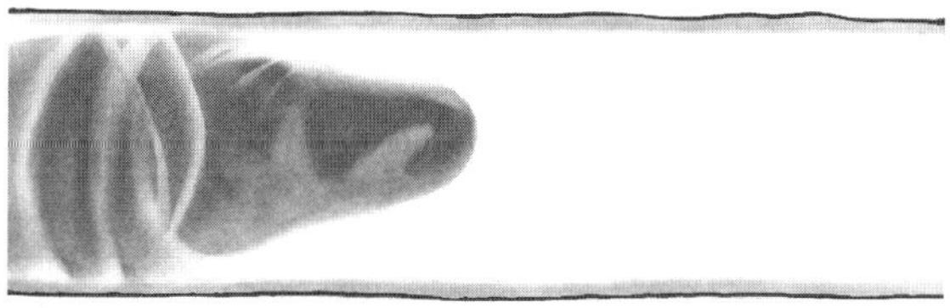

Figure 11.52. Intussusception. On a barium study, the intussuscepted segment of bowel is seen as a radiolucent defect within the colonic lumen. A "coiled spring" pattern is often present surrounding the intussuscepted segment of bowel.

b. Filling defect within colon is associated with the invaginated segment of bowel.
c. A "coiled spring" appearance may be seen as a result of the accumulation of a small amount of barium between the intussusceptum and the intussuscipiens.

Other imaging
1. Ultrasound
2. CT
3. MRI

Small Bowel Neoplasia
Clinical correlations
1. Common in the dog and cat.
2. Most common tumors are adenocarcinoma and lymphosarcoma.
3. Other tumors include leiomyosarcoma and leiomyoma.
4. Common clinical signs are referable and variable, depending on the location and degree of bowel obstruction, and include vomiting, weight loss, and diarrhea.
5. Tumor may be intraluminal, mural, or extraluminal and cause partial to complete obstruction.

Radiographic findings (Figures 11.53 A,B and 11.54 A,B)
1. Survey radiographs may be normal, especially if the tumor is small and only partial obstruction is present.
2. A soft tissue mass or fluid or gas ileus may be seen, depending on the size of the tumor and the location and degree of obstruction.

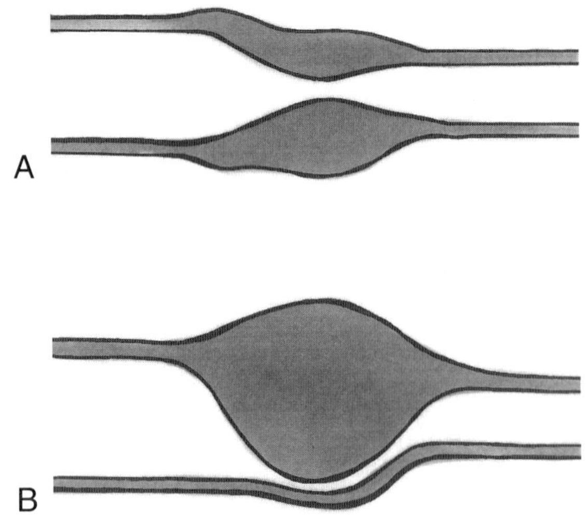

Figure 11.53. Small bowel neoplasia. On a barium study, bowel tumors are often **A)** annular or **B)** eccentric with variable degrees of luminal obstruction.

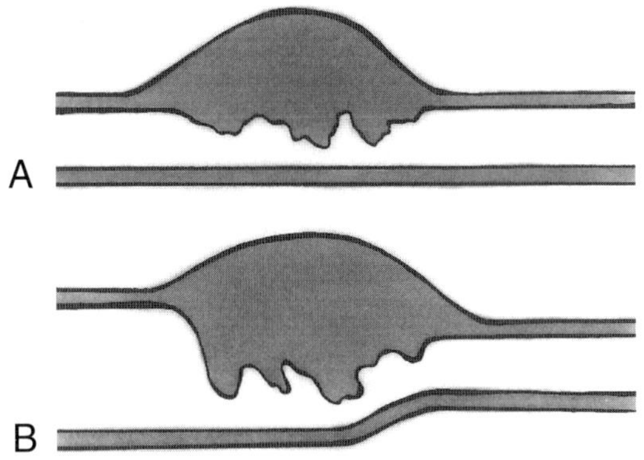

Figure 11.54. Small bowel neoplasia. On a barium study, eccentric mucosal and mural tumors cause bowel wall thickenings, which are often **A)** nonobstructive or **B)** partially obstructive.

Contrast radiography
Upper gastrointestinal study
1. Dilation of the bowel loops proximal to the site of obstruction may be observed.
2. Mural masses may be annular constrictions (common with adenocarcinoma) or eccentric mural lesions.
3. Ulceration of mucosa may be present

Other imaging
1. Ultrasound
2. CT
3. MRI

Mesenteric Volvulus
Clinical correlations
1. With volvulus of the bowel, the intestines twist about the root of the mesentery, causing vascular compromise.
2. More common in large breed dogs.
3. Common clinical signs include nausea, retching, vomiting, abdominal pain, and depression.
4. Is often fatal because of bowel divitalization associated with the vascular compromise.

Radiographic findings
1. Severe uniform gas ileus of the small bowel.
2. Peritoneal effusion or free gas caused by peritonitis may be present.

Mesenteric Thrombosis
Clinical correlations
1. Mesenteric thrombosis is an infrequent sequel of blunt abdominal trauma in which the mesenteric blood supply is avulsed from the bowel.
2. Common clinical signs are fever and abdominal pain.

Radiographic findings
1. Localized gas ileus of the affected portion of the small bowel.

2. There is usually localized or generalized loss of peritoneal detail caused by effusion.

Intestinal Perforation

Clinical correlations

1. Intestinal perforation can result from an intestinal foreign body, abdominal trauma (e.g., stab wound, bullet), or bowel tumor.
2. Clinical signs are variable, depending on the severity and location of the perforation and the degree of peritonitis present.

Radiographic findings

1. There is localized or generalized loss of peritoneal detail as a result of effusion associated with peritonitis.
2. Free abdominal gas in peritoneal cavity is often observed.
   a. A small amount of gas may be difficult to detect, but if present, may be seen between the liver margins and the diaphragm.
   b. With large amounts of gas, the bowel loops or other viscera will be more visible and distinct than normal (e.g., gas outlining the serosal surface).
   c. Using a horizontal x-ray beam and with the animal in left or right lateral recumbency, the free gas moves upward and may be easily identified.

LARGE BOWEL (Figures 11.55 through 11.57)

RADIOGRAPHIC ANATOMY

1. The large bowel of the dog and cat is composed of the cecum, colon, rectum, and anal canal.
2. The cecum in the dog and cat vary in anatomy and size.
   a. In the dog, the cecum is a corkscrew or "C" shaped structure with ileocolic and cecocolic sphincters.
   b. In the cat, the cecum is a small cone-like structure and lacks a distinct cecocolic sphincter.
3. The colon is divided into ascending, transverse, and descending parts that are recognized by their shape, size, and location.
   a. The distal ileum enters the ascending colon from a medial direction.
   b. The ascending colon extends cranially to the right of the midline turning leftward as the transverse colon. This juncture of the ascending and transverse colon is called the hepatic or right colic flexure.
   c. The transverse colon passes from right to left across the midline. This juncture of the transverse and descending colon is called the splenic or left colic flexure.
   d. The descending colon extends caudally and moves toward the midline entering the pelvic canal and becoming the rectum.
   e. The rectum terminates at the anal canal.
4. Relationships of the colon to other abdominal viscera.
   a. The ascending colon lies adjacent to the descending colon, right limb of the pancreas, right kidney, mesentery, and small bowel.
   b. The transverse colon lies adjacent to the greater curvature of the stomach, left limb of the pancreas, liver, small bowel, and mesentery.
   c. The descending colon usually lies along the left side of the abdomen adjacent to the small bowel, left kidney, urinary bladder, and uterus.
   d. The most distal portion of the descending colon, anal canal, and rectum are closely associated with the urinary bladder, urethra, cervix, vagina, prostate and the medial iliac and sacral lymph nodes.

RADIOGRAPHIC FINDINGS

1. On survey radiographs the normal large bowel usually is identified by the presence of gas, fluid, or fecal material within its lumen. Commonly, gas also is present in the normal cecum of dogs.
2. Variable amounts of colonic contents may be present, affecting the position, size, and shape of the colon.
3. The lumen diameter of the colon varies with the amount of fecal material and defecation habits. A rule of thumb for the normal diameter of the colon is less than the length of the seventh lumbar vertebra and no larger than three times the diameter of the small bowel.
   a. Abnormal dilation of the colon is called megacolon. Causes include:
      1) Chronic constipation or obstipation
      2) Secondary to stricture, tumor, or healed pelvic fracture
      3) Spinal disease (e.g., cauda equina syndrome, dysautonomia, or sacrococcygeal agenesis in the Manx cat)
      4) Aganglionosis (e.g., Hirschsprung's disease)
      5) Idiopathic megacolon
   b. Increased colonic gas with colonic dilation may be caused by:
      1) Severe aerophagia or from rectal examination preceding radiographs
      2) Viral enterocolitis (e.g., Parvovirus)
      3) Severe Trichuris vulpis (whipworm) infection
4. Abnormal shape of the colon may be difficult to determine from the survey radiographs.
   a. Displacement from adjacent viscera or abnormal masses or secondary to adhesions (e.g., chronic pancreatitis) may be present.
   b. Shortening of the colon can be associated with chronic colitis.

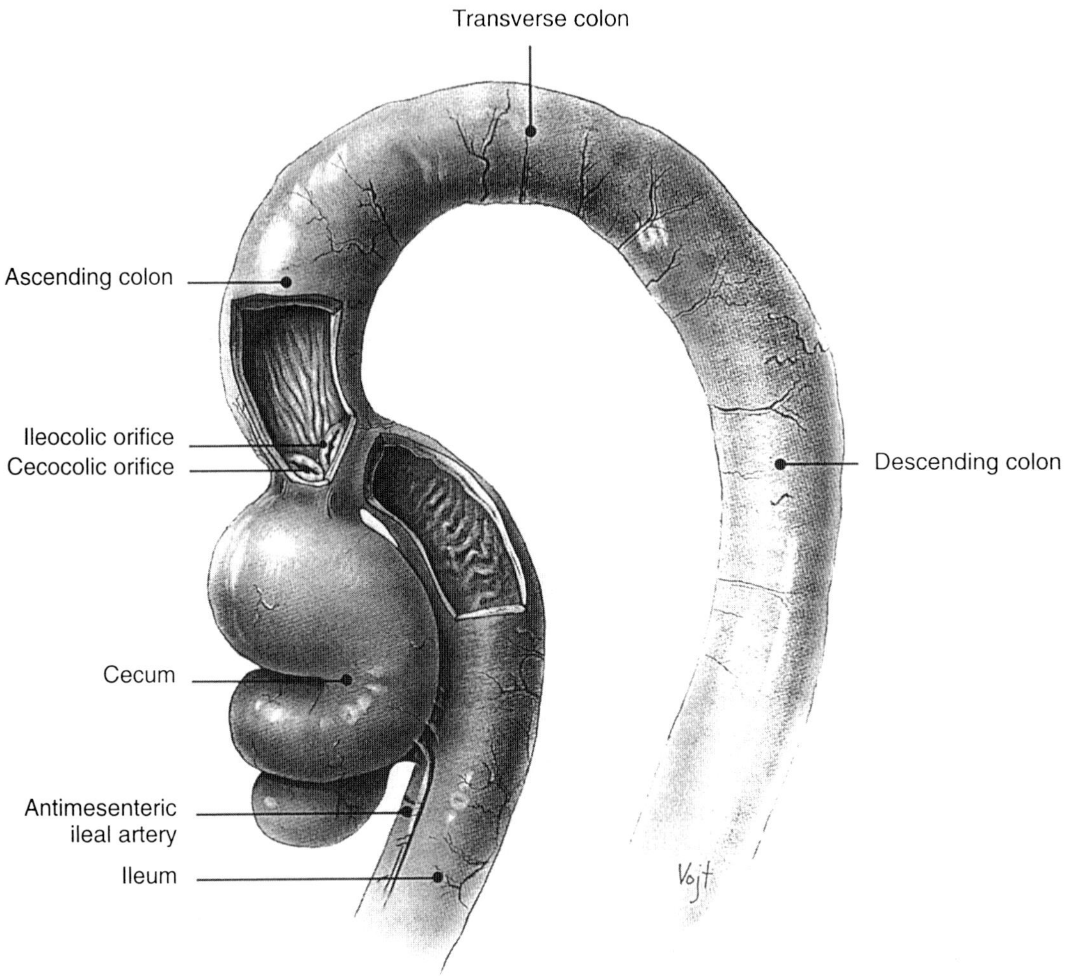

Figure 11.55. The ileum and its relation to the large intestine. (From Anderson WD, Anderson BG. Atlas of Canine Anatomy. Philadelphia: Lea & Febiger; 1994:660. With permission of Williams & Wilkins, Baltimore.)

c. Narrowing of the colonic lumen can be caused by stricture, neoplasm, spasm, or compression by an adjacent mass (e.g., prostatomegaly).

5. Abnormal position of the colon is secondary to displacement by extrinsic masses or enlargement of organs as a result of other diseases (e.g., gastric dilation/volvulus, splenomegaly, pyometra, or pregnancy). Common causes for colonic displacement are:
   a. Lateral projection:
      1) Ventral displacement of colon may be caused by:
         a) Renal mass (e.g., tumor, cyst)
         b) Sublumbar mass (e.g., lymph node, tumor, abscess)
         c) Retroperitoneal effusion (e.g., hemorrhage, ruptured ureter, or infection)
      2) Dorsal displacement of the colon may be caused by:
         a) Splenic mass
         b) Distended urinary bladder
         c) Uterine enlargement (e.g., pregnancy, pyometra)
   b. Ventrodorsal projection:
      1) Right lateral displacement of the colon may be caused by:
         a) Left renal mass
         b) Left ovarian or uterine mass
         c) Distended urinary bladder
         d) Left sublumbar mass
      2) Left lateral displacement of the colon may be caused by:
         a) Distended urinary bladder
         b) Small bowel or mesenteric mass
      3) Caudal displacement of the transverse colon may be caused by:
         a) Gastric distension
         b) Hepatomegaly
         c) Pancreatic mass

6. In the pelvic and antepubic regions, the descending

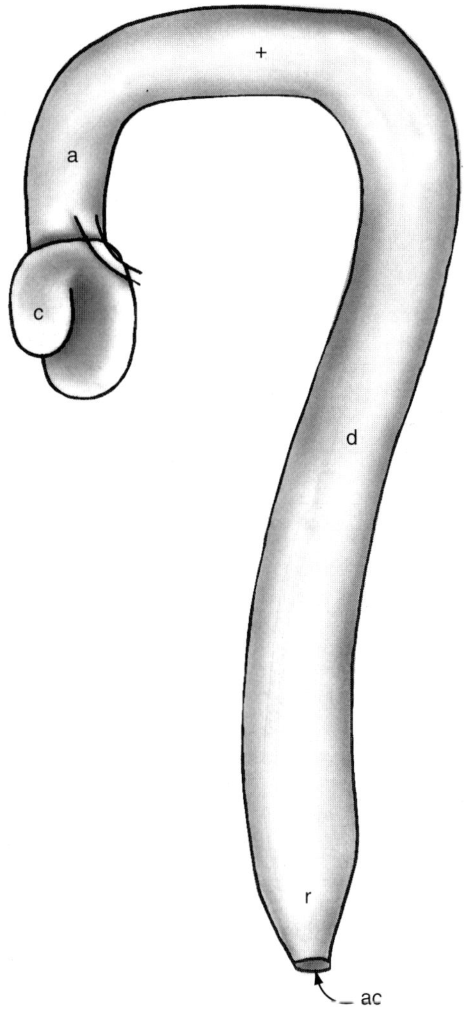

Figure 11.56. The canine large intestine. Anatomic landmarks include: the cecum (**c**), the ascending colon (**a**), the transverse colon (**t**), the descending colon (**d**), the rectum (**r**), and the anal canal (**ac**).

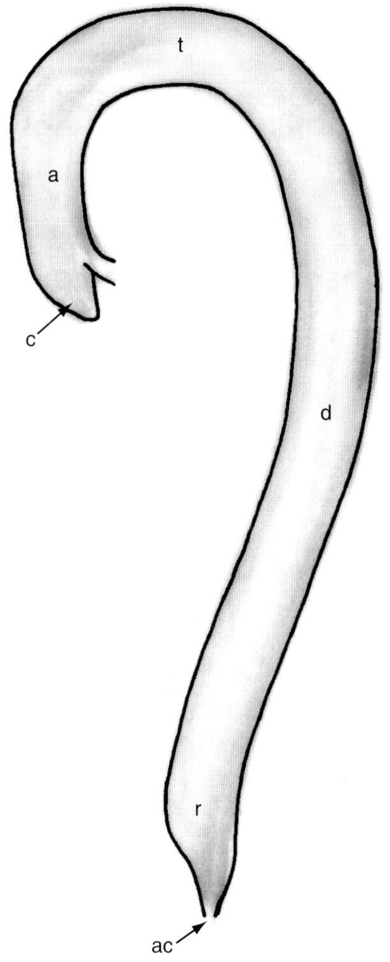

Figure 11.57. The feline large intestine. Anatomic landmarks include: the cecum (**c**), the ascending colon (**a**), the transverse colon (**t**), the descending colon (**d**), the rectum (**r**), and the anal canal (**ac**).

colon and rectum are commonly displaced laterally, dorsally, or ventrally by enlargement or masses of the urinary bladder, iliosacral lymph nodes, prostate, vagina, cervix, and urethra.

7. Abnormal radiopacity of the colon may be caused by:
   a. Intraluminal opaque foreign bodies
   b. Intramural gas associated with severe colitis (pneumotosis coli) associated with gas-producing bacteria.
8. Abnormal radiolucency of the colon may be result from:
   a. Aerophagia or previous rectal examination or cleansing enema
   b. Colitis

CONTRAST RADIOGRAPHS

1. Compression radiography. Compression with a plastic or wooden spoon can be helpful by displacing adjacent bowel or masses for improved radiographic visualization.
2. Pneumocolon. Infusion of a small amount of gas into the descending colon with syringe or enema catheter is a rapid method to assess:
   a. Location of the descending colon
   b. Identification of large intraluminal or mural masses
   c. Aid in differentiation of the colon from adjacent organs or masses
3. UGI contrast study does not provide a complete evaluation of the large bowel. The colon is incompletely distended with contrast material, and fecal material in the colon often creates intraluminal filling defects that may mimic mural and intraluminal lesions.

4. Barium enema (done with animal under general anesthesia) is the best radiographic contrast study for evaluating the large bowel. (See Chapter 3 for method.)
   a. Indications include:
      1) Common clinical signs of large bowel disease include diarrhea (often with red blood or mucus), tenesmus or dyschezia, and abnormally shaped feces (e.g., small diameter).
      2) A need to determine position of the colon because of a caudal abdominal or pelvic mass.
      3) Need to determine whether gas-filled bowel loops are attributable to small bowel or colonic origin.
      4) Clinical conditions are suspected in which a barium enema would be helpful to diagnosis, such as:
         a) Ileocolic intussusception or cecal inversion
         b) Mechanical or functional large bowel obstruction
         c) Mucosal lesion of the colon (colitis, tumor)
         d) A mass extrinsic to the large bowel
   b. Interpretation. The normal colon should have a smooth mucosal surface and the colon should have a uniform diameter. Lesions seen with a barium enema include:
      1) Irregularity of the barium-mucosal interface
      2) Spasm, stricture, or occlusion of the bowel lumen
      3) Outpouching of the bowel wall caused by deep ulcer, diverticulum, or perforation
      4) Filling defects (e.g., tumor, granuloma, or polyp)
      5) Thickening of the colonic wall
      6) Displacement of the large bowel
      7) Shortening of the colon (e.g., chronic colitis)

DISEASES/DISORDERS

Acute Colitis

Clinical correlations

1. An acute inflammatory disease primarily affecting the colonic mucosa.
2. Multiple factors may contribute to colitis.
   a. Dietary indiscretion (e.g., abrasive foreign material)
   b. Bacterial infection secondary to abrasive damage, or debilitative or immunosuppressive disease
   c. Parasitic infection (e.g., Trichuris vulpis)
   d. Food hypersensitivity
3. Common clinical signs include:
   a. Diarrhea with mucus or fresh blood
   b. Abdominal pain
   c. Fever and depression
   d. Vomiting may be present concurrently

Radiographic findings

Barium enema

1. Survey radiographs usually show no abnormality.
2. Colonic contents vary, ranging from fluid and gas only to granular or opaque foreign material and fecal matter.

Contrast radiography

1. Usually, no abnormality is visible.
2. Thickened mucosal folds or small ulcers may be observed.

Chronic Colitis

Clinical correlations

1. Chronic colitis is a chronic inflammatory disease of the colon characterized by a variable infiltration of the colonic wall with lymphocytes, plasma cells, eosinophils, and neutrophils. Often involves structures deeper than the mucosa and may be ulcerative or granulomatous.
2. There are many different types of chronic colitis, including:
   a. Inflammatory bowel disease
   b. Eosinophilic colitis
   c. Histiocytic ulcerative colitis
3. Chronic colitis is most common in purebred dogs, especially German Shepherd Dog.
4. Histiocytic colitis is most commonly reported in the Boxer.
5. Many proposed factors including:
   a. Immune mediated disease
   b. Bacterial infection
   c. Mycotic infection (e.g., histoplasmosis)
   d. Dietary hypersensitivity
   e. Psychologic (stress) factors
   f. Foreign bodies
6. Common clinical signs include:
   a. Increased frequency of defecation
   b. Diarrhea, usually with fresh blood and mucus
   c. Tenesmus and painful defecation
   d. Variable abdominal pain, weight loss, or dehydration
7. Diagnosis is based on clinical signs, biopsy, and exclusion of specific diseases.
8. Differential diagnosis:
   a. Cecal inversion
   b. Neoplasia
   c. Small bowel disease

Radiographic findings

1. Survey radiographs usually show no abnormality.
2. Colonic narrowing and shortening may be suspected.
3. Thickening of the colonic wall
4. There may be other organ abnormalities (e.g., lymphadenopathy, splenomegaly).

Contrast radiography (Figure 11.58 A,B)

Barium enema

1. There may be an irregular mucosal surface, thickened mucosal folds, or ulcers.
2. Strictures or shortening of colon may occur.

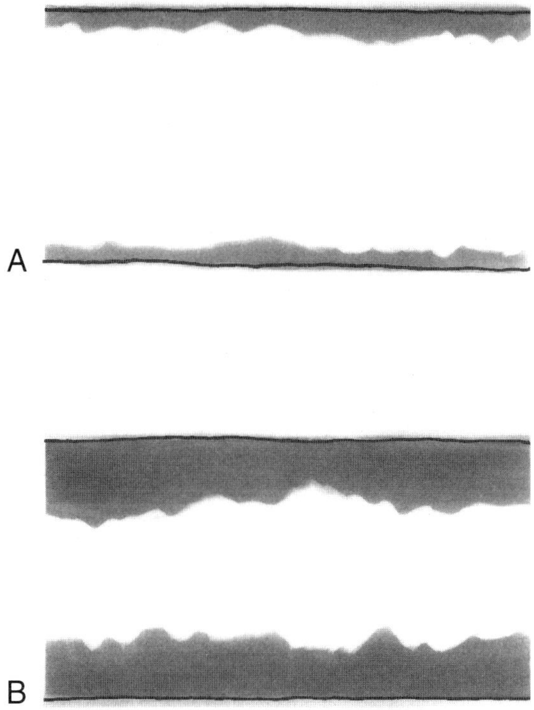

Figure 11.58. Colitis. On a barium enema examination, the irregularity and degree of wall thickening in the colonic mucosa may be **A)** mild or **B)** severe.

Cecal Inversion

Clinical correlations

1. The cecum inverts into the ascending colon causing a partial or complete obstruction. The inverted cecum becomes edematous and congested, bleeds, and may become necrotic and adherent to the colonic wall
2. Is an infrequent occurrence in the dog.
3. Predisposing factors may include:
   a. Trichuris vulpis infection
   b. Inflammatory bowel disease
   c. Weak ileocecocolic ligament
4. Common clinical signs:
   a. Intermittent hematochezia with normal to soft stools
   b. Weight loss
   c. Palpable, often painful, abdominal mass

Radiographic findings

1. Survey radiographs usually show no abnormality.
2. Soft tissue mass in right cranial abdomen may be observed.
3. Absence of gas-filled cecum is noted.

Contrast radiography (Figure 11.59)

Barium enema

1. The cecum is not visible in its normal position.
2. The inverted cecum is seen as a filling defect in the ascending colon.

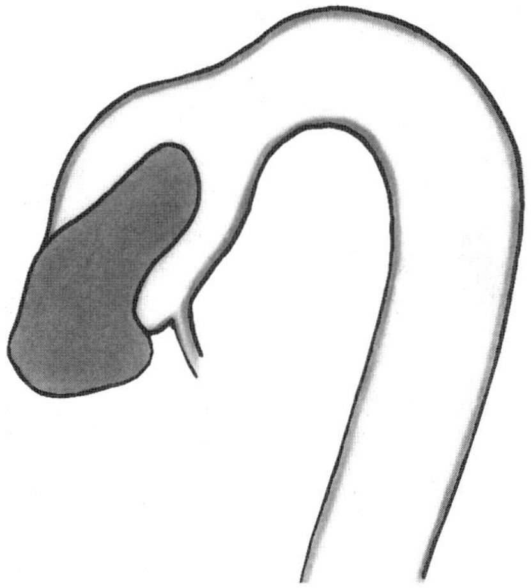

Figure 11.59. Cecal inversion. The inverted cecum is radiolucent on a barium enema examination, and is seen as a filling defect within the lumen of the ascending colon.

Neoplasia

Clinical correlations

1. Most neoplasms are malignant.
   a. Adenocarcinoma and lymphosarcoma are most common.
      1) Adenocarcinomas are usually solitary and often cause an annular constriction of the colon.
      2) Lymphosarcoma can be solitary or diffuse.
   b. Leiomyosarcoma, anaplastic sarcomas, and carcinoid tumors also occur.
2. Benign tumors occur most frequently in the rectum.
   a. Polyps
   b. Leiomyoma
3. Clinical signs vary depending on the tumor type, location, and duration of the lesion.
   a. Tenesmus, hematochezia, and dyschezia are frequent.
   b. Partial rectal prolapse may occur with rectal tumor.
   c. Progressive obstruction may cause frequent defecation with small amount of fecal material, constipation, intermittent bloody diarrhea, or megacolon.
4. Can be diagnosed more easily by endoscopy than with survey or contrast radiography.
5. Differential diagnosis:
   a. Chronic colitis
   b. Granulomatous colitis
   c. Cecal inversion
   d. Colonic stricture
   e. Histoplasmosis

Radiographic findings

1. Survey radiographs may show a soft tissue mass involving a portion of the colon.
2. If obstructive, distension of the bowel proximal to the lesion may be present.

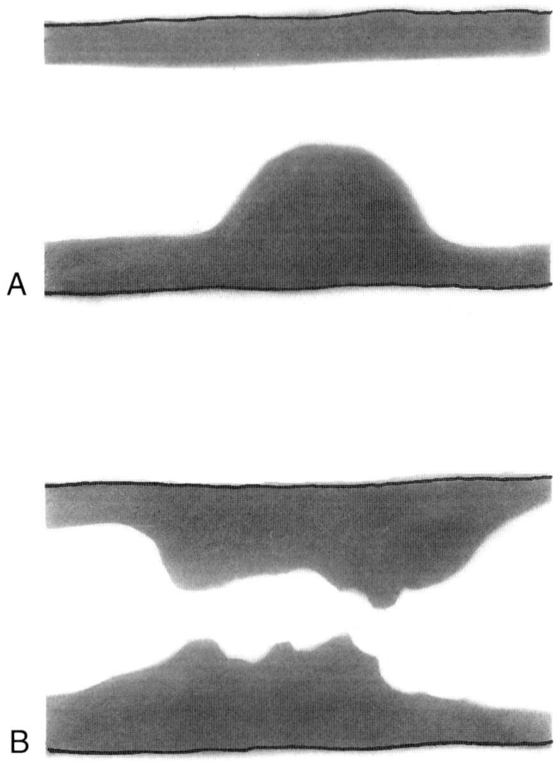

Figure 11.60. Colonic neoplasia. On a barium enema examination colonic tumors vary in their appearance and are often **A)** smooth or **B)** irregular with wall thickening.

3. If regional metastasis is present, the iliac and sacral lymph nodes are usually enlarged.
4. If partial obstruction is present, the colon will often be dilated proximal to the mass.

Contrast radiography (Figure 11.60)
1. Localized stricture of colon
2. Focal ulceration or irregular mucosal mass
3. Localized bowel wall thickening or mass

Other imaging
1. Ultrasound
2. CT
3. MRI

Perineal Hernia and Perineal Diverticuli/ Rectal Diverticuli
Clinical correlations
1. Occurs when the pelvic diaphragm does not support the rectum and the rectal canal deviates laterally.
2. A diverticulum develops when the rectal mucosa protrudes through the muscular wall of the rectum.
3. Occurs most often in older male dogs; is rare in cats.
4. Common clinical signs include dyschezia, constipation, or perineal swelling.
5. Retroflexion of the urinary bladder into the hernia may occur and cause urethral obstruction.
6. On rectal examination, there is rectal deviation and a diverticulum or laxity in the perineal region.

Radiographic findings
1. Survey radiographs usually show fecal impaction of the rectum.
2. A soft tissue mass in the perineal region, ventral and lateral to the tail, usually is seen best on the lateral projection.
3. Lateral deviation of the feces within the anal canal or rectum may be seen on the ventrodorsal projection.

Contrast radiography
1. Barium enema may demonstrate the rectal deviation or diverticulum; however, the inflated bulb of the catheter may obscure some lesions.
2. A retrograde urethrogram will document displacement of the urethra or urinary bladder

Imperforate Anus
Clinical correlations
1. Is a congenital defect resulting from simple failure of perforation of the anal membrane, or a complex anorectal agenesis.
2. May be associated with other malformations, especially of the genitourinary tract, with the distal bowel opening into the urinary bladder, vagina, or urethra.
3. Clinical signs vary, depending on the defect present, but usually, signs are seen in the first few weeks of life.
   a. Failure to defecate when anal atresia is present.
   b. Defecation occurs through an abnormal orifice (e.g., vagina, urethra).

Radiographic findings
1. Moderate to severe fecal distension of the large bowel will be present if the rectum or anus is stenotic or imperforate.

Contrast radiograph
1. Infusion of iodinated contrast media into the urethra, vagina, or rectum may demonstrate a congenital fistula or malformation.

chapter twelve

12

Urinary System and Adrenal Glands

RADIOGRAPHIC TECHNIQUE

1. Standard projections:
   a. Right or left lateral recumbent projection of the abdomen
   b. Ventrodorsal projection of the abdomen
2. Supplemental projections:
   a. Dorsoventral projection
   b. Right and left ventrodorsal (or dorsoventral) oblique projections of the caudal abdomen
   c. Flexed lateral projection of the caudal abdomen and ischial area to visualize the canine male urethra
3. Contrast procedures (See chapter 3 for method)
   a. Intravenous urogram
   b. Cystogram
   c. Pneumocystogram
   d. Double contrast cystogram
   d. Urethrogram
      1) Voiding
      2) Retrograde
   e. Vaginogram
4. Other imaging:
   a. Ultrasound
   b. Nuclear scintigraphy
   c. Computed tomography (CT)
   d. Magnetic resonance imaging (MRI)

KIDNEYS AND URETERS

RADIOGRAPHIC ANATOMY (Figures 12.1 and 12.2)

1. In the normal dog and cat the kidneys are located in the dorsal cranial retroperitoneal space of the abdomen.
2. Both kidneys should have a smooth margin and be of similar size and shape.
   a. The normal canine kidney is "bean shaped."
   b. The normal feline kidney is more "rounded" than bean shaped.
3. Visualization of the renal borders is relative to the amount of perirenal and retroperitoneal fat present.
   a. The kidneys are most readily visualized in cats and obese dogs.
   b. Poor renal visualization is common in young normal dogs and cats, in emaciated animals, and in animals with retroperitoneal disease (e.g., effusion).
4. The right kidney is normally located more cranial than the left and is partially obscured within the rib cage on both lateral and ventrodorsal projections.
   a. In the dog, the right kidney is usually located at the level of T13 to L1.
   b. In the cat, the right kidney is usually located at the level of L1 to L4.
5. The left kidney is more variable in position than the right and is usually more readily seen on survey radiographs.
   a. In the dog, the left kidney is usually located at the level of L2 to L4.
   b. In the cat, the left kidney is usually located at the level of L2 to L5.
6. Quantification of renal size is based on the perceived length of the kidney as seen on the ventrodorsal projection
   a. The normal canine kidney is approximately 2.5 to 3.5 times the length of the second lumbar vertebra.
   b. The normal feline kidney is approximately 2.4 to 3.0 times the length of the second lumbar vertebra.
   c. Normal dogs and cats may have one or both kidneys measuring outside this normal range.
   d. Conversely, normal-sized kidneys do not exclude the presence of renal disease.

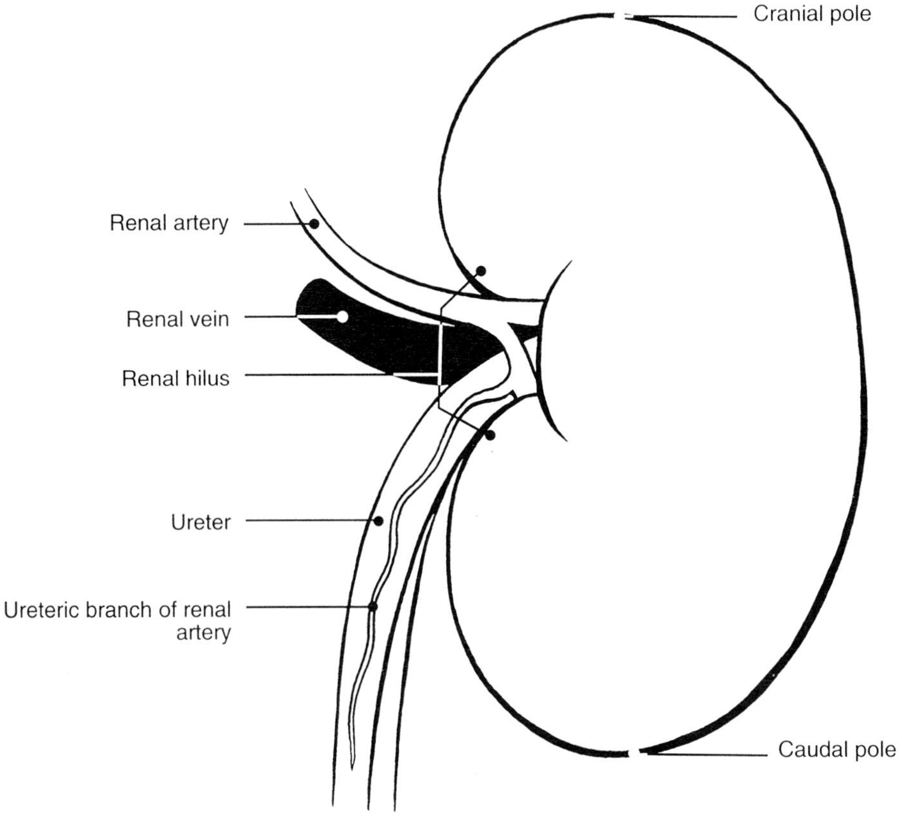

Figure 12.1. Anatomy of kidney. (From Anderson WD, Anderson BG. Atlas of Canine Anatomy. Philadelphia: Lea & Febiger; 1994:734. Used with permission of Williams & Wilkins, Baltimore.)

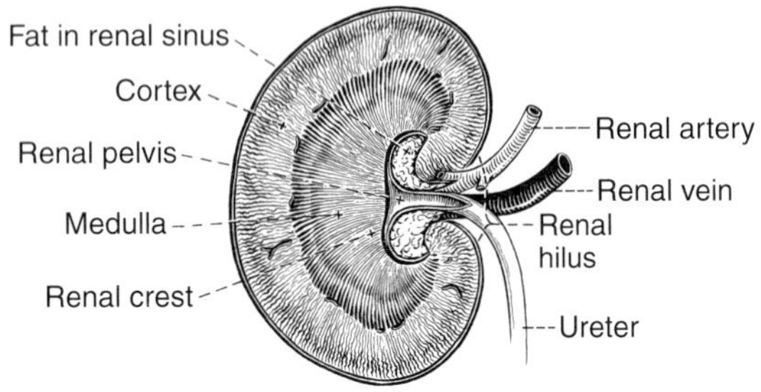

Figure 12.2. Kidney structures. (From Evans HE, Christensen GC. The urogenital system. In: Evans HE, ed. Miller's Anatomy of the Dog. 3rd ed. Philadelphia: W.B. Saunders; 1993:497. Courtesy of and with permission of Dr. Howard E. Evans.)

7. The ureters, located within the retroperitoneal space, transport urine from the renal pelvis to the urinary bladder.
   a. The ureters are not normally visualized on survey radiographs because of their small size and their similar radiopacity to the adjacent retroperitoneal tissues.

RADIOGRAPHIC INTERPRETATION

Survey Radiographs

Ventrodorsal and lateral projections are made to assess the number, size, shape, position, and radiopacity of the kidneys.

Causes of Observed Variations

Causes for alteration in renal number

1. Absence of one kidney: usually a result of congenital renal aplasia
   a. Compensatory hypertrophy of the single kidney commonly occurs.
2. Extra kidney: renal duplication is rare.

Causes for alteration in renal size and shape (Figures 12.3 A,B through 12.7)

1. Bilateral large and smooth margination
   a. Acute nephritis or pyelonephritis
   b. Hydronephrosis (uncommon), usually unilateral
   c. Polycystic disease
   d. Lymphosarcoma
   e. Feline infectious peritonitis (FIP)

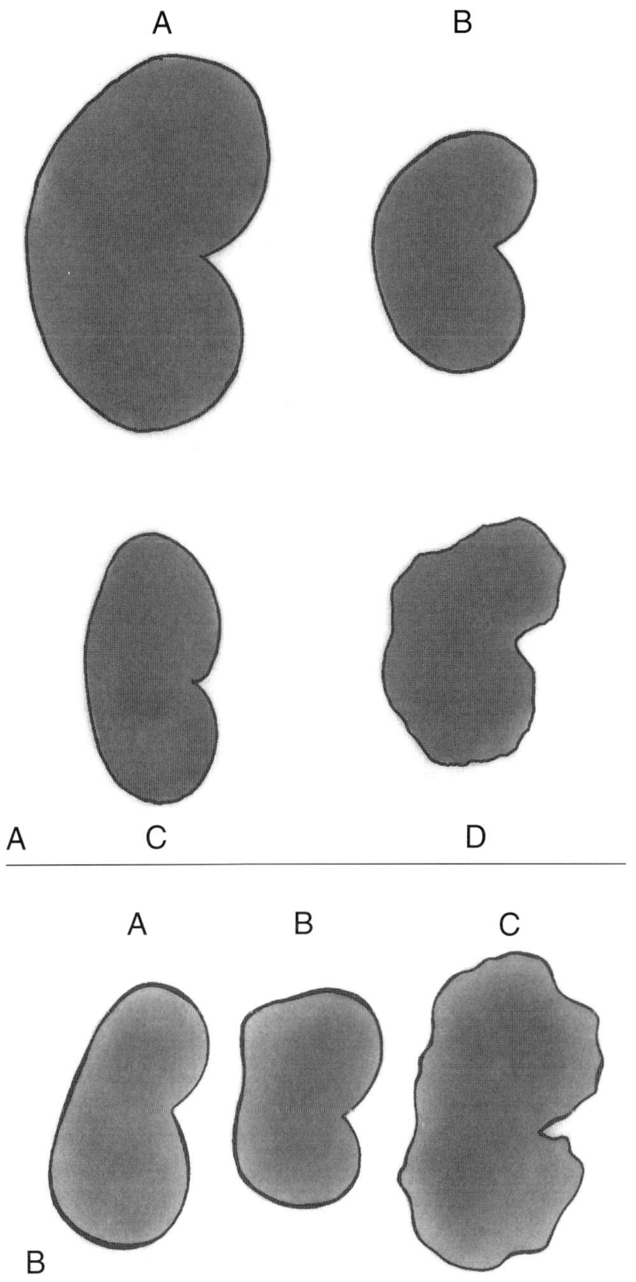

Figure 12.3. **A.** Variations in kidney shape (**A**) normal, (**B**) small and smooth, (**C**) small and narrowed, and (**D**) small and irregular. **B.** Variations in kidney contour (**A**) enlarged caudal pole, (**B**) focal enlargement of cranial pole, and (**C**) enlarged and irregular.

   f. Subcapsular hematoma (rare)
   g. Perirenal cyst or pseudocyst (feline)
   h. Amyloidosis
   i. Primary or secondary neoplasia
2. Bilateral large and irregular margination
   a. Lymphosarcoma
   b. Feline infectious peritonitis (FIP)
   c. Polycystic disease
   d. Primary or metastatic neoplasms (e.g., cystadenocarcinoma in German Shepherd Dog)

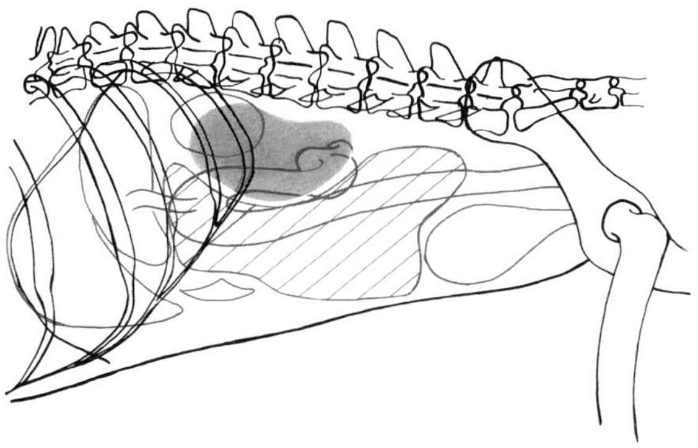

Figure 12.4. Enlargement of the left kidney commonly causes ventral displacement of the descending colon and the small intestine.

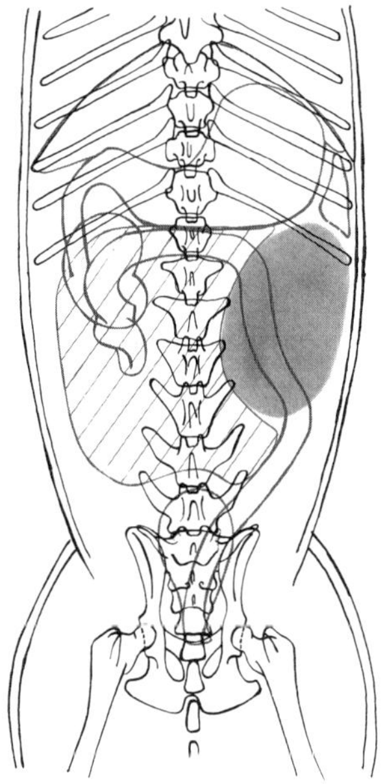

Figure 12.5. Enlargement of the left kidney commonly causes medial displacement of the small intestine and descending colon.

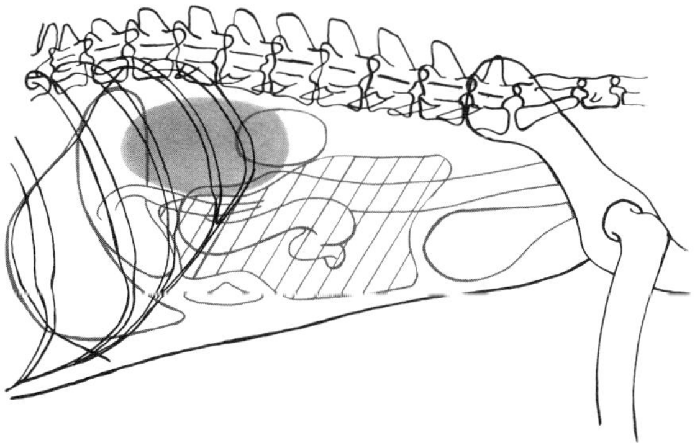

Figure 12.6. Enlargement of the right kidney commonly causes ventral displacement of the proximal duodenum, ascending colon, and small intestine.

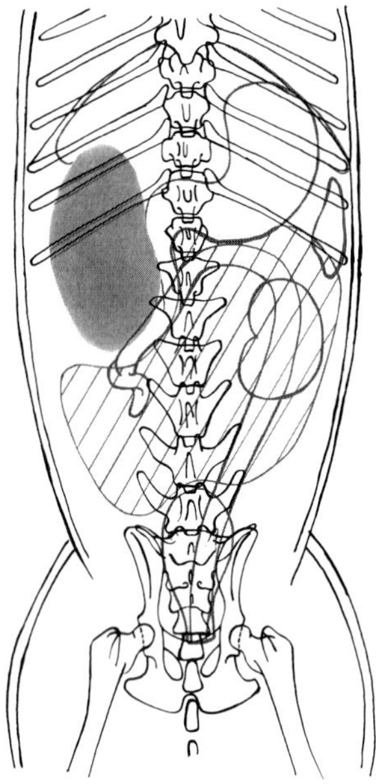

Figure 12.7. Enlargement of the right kidney commonly causes medial displacement of the proximal duodenum, ascending colon, and small intestine.

3. Unilaterally large and smoothly marginated
   a. Compensatory hypertrophy
   b. Hydronephrosis
   c. Primary or secondary neoplasia
   d. Acute nephritis or pyelonephritis
   e. Perirenal cyst or pseudocyst (feline)
   f. Subcapsular hematoma
4. Unilateral large and irregular margination
   a. Cyst or perirenal cyst
   b. Abscess
   c. Primary or metastatic neoplasm
5. Unilateral or bilateral decreased renal size
   a. End stage inflammatory kidney disease
   b. Renal infarction
   c. Congenital renal hypoplasia or dysplasia.

Causes for alteration in renal position

1. Enlargement of the left kidney may cause displacement of the adjacent viscera (e.g., small bowel, proximal descending colon) to the right, caudally, or ventrally.
2. Enlargement of the right kidney may cause displacement of the adjacent viscera (e.g., proximal duodenum, ascending colon) cranially, ventrally, or to the left.
3. Developmental anomaly: one or both kidneys may be normal in size, but vary in location within the retroperitoneal space.

Causes for increased renal radiopacity

1. Nephrocalcinosis (diffuse mineralization of the renal parenchyma, usually bilateral)
   a. Hyperadrenocorticism
   b. Hyperparathyroidism
   c. Hypercalcemia
   d. Ethylene glycol poisoning
   e. Renal tubular defects
   f. Hypervitaminosis D
   g. Chronic renal failure
   h. Idiopathic
2. Renal calculi
   a. Often associated with chronic renal bacterial infection.
   b. May be unilateral or bilateral.
   c. May have concurrent ureteral, cystic, and urethral calculi.
3. Dystrophic mineralization
   a. Neoplasm
   b. Abscess
   c. Chronic infarction and infection

CONTRAST RADIOGRAPHS

Intravenous Urography (See also chapter 3)

Indications for Intravenous Urography

1. Abnormal kidney size or shape
2. Poor visualization of one or both kidneys on survey radiographs
3. Abnormal urine (e.g., hematuria, pyuria)
4. Renal calculi
5. Suspected trauma to kidneys or ureters
6. Abdominal masses that involve or displace the kidneys
7. Suspected ectopic ureters
8. Inability to catheterize the bladder for cystography

Interpretation of the Intravenous Urogram

The arteriographic phase

The aorta, renal artery, and interlobar arterial branches may be visible if the first radiograph is made early in the bolus infusion of contrast media.

The nephrogram phase

1. Is the initial opacification of the renal parenchyma caused by contrast within the renal tubules.
2. The degree of radiopacity is proportional to the dose of contrast medium (plasma concentration), glomerular filtration rate, and the renal tubular osmolarity.
3. Normal kidneys should immediately opacify and be of equal homogeneous density; the degree of opacity should diminish over time.
4. Absence of nephrogram:
   a. Absent kidney
   b. Renal artery obstruction or avulsion
   c. Insufficient dose of contrast medium
   d. Severe parenchymal disease
   e. Severe hydronephrosis
5. Normal or poor nephrogram radiopacity followed by increased radiopacity or persistent radiopacity with no

contrast media visible in renal collecting system or ureters or bladder:
   a. Systemic hypotension
   b. Acute renal failure
      1) Acute tubular necrosis
      2) Contrast media reaction
   c. Acute postrenal obstruction
6. Poor nephrogram radiopacity with decreasing radiopacity over time:
   a. Polyuric renal failure
   b. Normal kidneys with inadequate dose of contrast medium
7. Heterogenous nephrogram radiopacity
   a. Hydronephrosis
   b. Renal tumor
   c. Polycystic disease
   d. Renal cyst or abscess
   e. Renal infarction

The pyelogram phase

1. Is the opacification of the renal collecting system (renal diverticuli and pelvis) and the ureters
2. The radiopacity of the pyelogram depends on the concentration and volume of the contrast medium in the collecting system and ureter.
3. Poor contrast visualization is not always associated with abnormal renal function, nor is normal contrast visualization always associated with normal renal function.
4. Both renal pelves should appear equal in size, shape, and degree of radiopacity. Abdominal compression techniques can aid in filling and visualizing the renal collecting system and proximal ureter.
5. The diverticuli should appear as thin radiating parallel lines from the renal pelvis.
6. Distortion or filling defects of the renal pelvis
   a. Pyelitis or pyelonephritis
   b. Compression caused by cyst, abscess, or tumor
   c. Hydronephrosis
   d. Renal calculi
   e. Blood clot

The ureteral phase

1. Normal rapid ureteral peristalsis usually prevents the entire ureter from being fully distended and visualized with contrast media. Abdominal compression and/or concurrent pneumocystography can enhance ureteral visualization.
2. As the normal ureters enter the urinary bladder, they commonly extend slightly caudal to the ureterovesicular junction and curve back cranially before entering the trigone of the bladder. Normal ureters have the shape of a "shepherd-like crook" at the trigone region.
3. Ureteral dilation
   a. Is most often caused by obstruction.
   b. Localized ureteral dilation may be caused by:
      1) Ureteral calculi
      2) Periureteral masses
      3) Retroperitoneal fibrosis
      4) Ureteral tumor
      5) Localized inflammation
   c. Generalized ureteral dilation may be caused by:
      1) Obstruction of ureterovesicular junction caused by tumor, calculus, inflammation, or ureterocele
      2) Ureteritis
      3) Ectopic ureter
5. Lack of ureteral opacification
   a. Renal pelvic obstruction caused by tumor, calculus, or blood clot
   b. Nonfunctional kidney
   c. Renal failure
   d. Ureteral rupture, usually from trauma

DISEASES/DISORDERS

Congenital Renal Disease

Clinical correlations

1. Defects present at birth.
2. May be genetically predetermined or may represent a developmental abnormality.
3. Types of congenital anomalies include:
   a. Renal aplasia
   b. Renal hypoplasia
   c. Renal dysplasia
   d. Renal dysgenesis
   e. Vascular anomalies
4. Many familial renal disorders have been identified including:
   a. Tubulointerstitial fibrosis (renal dysplasia)
      1) Cocker Spaniel
      2) Norwegian Elkhound
      3) Lhaso Apso
      4) Shih Tzu
      5) Wheaten Terrier
   b. Renal tubular dysfunction (Fanconi syndrome)
      1) Basenji
   c. Glomerular atrophy
      1) Samoyed
      2) Standard poodle
   d. Glomerular sclerosis
      1) Doberman Pinscher
   e. Polycystic disease
      1) Persian cat
      2) Domestic long haired cat
      3) Cairn Terrier
   f. Amyloidosis
      1) Abyssinian cat
   g. Telangiectasia
      1) Pembroke Welsh Corgi
   h. Cystadenocarcinoma
      1) German Shepherd Dog

4. Chronic generalized progressive functional loss usually results in chronic renal failure.

Radiographic findings

1. If one kidney is absent, the opposite kidney is usually enlarged on survey radiographs as a result of compensatory hypertrophy.
2. In renal dysplasia or hypoplasia, both kidneys are frequently small and irregular.
3. In polycystic renal disease, both kidneys are usually enlarged and irregular.

Contrast radiographs (intravenous urogram)

1. The urogram will document the size, shape, and number of functional kidneys, and will also allow visualization of the collecting system (diverticuli, pelves, and ureters).
2. Kidneys that are cystic or scarred usually have a heterogenous opacity to the nephrogram. The renal pelvis may be distorted and irregularly shaped.
3. Most dysplastic kidneys have a homogenous radiopacity to the nephrogram, but are small or irregularly shaped. The renal pelves are usually normal.

Other imaging

1. Ultrasound
2. CT
3. MRI

Ectopic Ureter

Clinical correlations

1. Congenital defect of one or both ureters usually emptying abnormally into the vagina or urethra.
2. May be inheritable.
3. More common in female dogs.
4. Animals often dribble urine or are incontinent.

Radiographic findings

1. Survey radiographs are usually normal.
2. If bilateral ureteral ectopia is present, the urinary bladder may be small because of disuse or hypoplasia.

Contrast radiographs (See chapter 3 for methods) (Figure 12.8 A–C)

1. Visualization of one or both ureters abnormally emptying, partially or completely, into a structure other than the urinary bladder.
2. Dilated ureter(s) as an additional congenital anomaly or caused by ureteritis
   a. Intravenous urography combined with pneumocystography
      1) The presence of an air-filled distended urinary bladder followed by an intravenous urogram can enhance identification and evaluation of the distal ureters, compared to other contrast techniques.

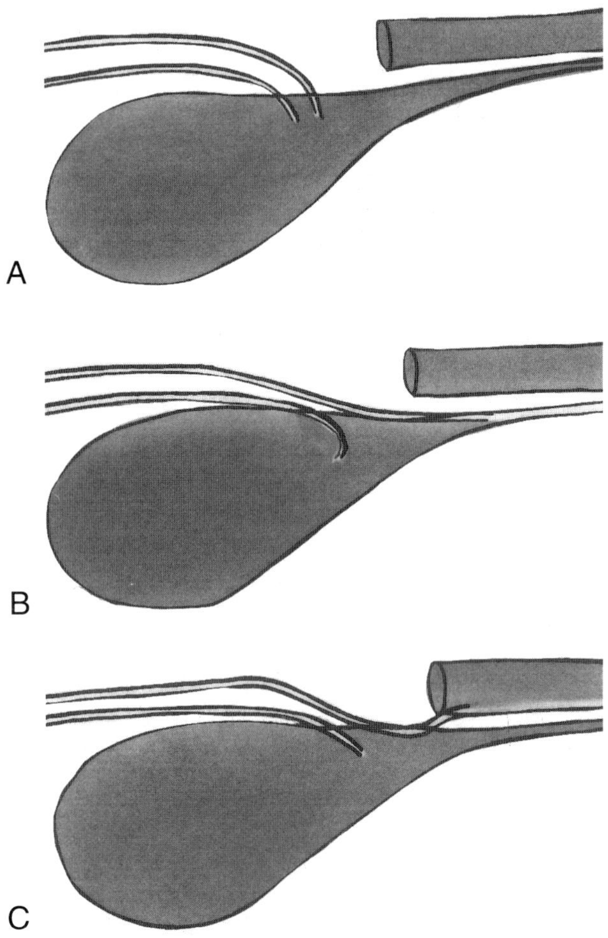

Figure 12.8. Ectopic ureters: **A**) normal ureters, **B**) ectopic ureter into urethra, and **C**) ectopic ureter into vagina.

      2) Oblique right and left ventrodorsal oblique projections will aid in evaluating the distal ureters.
      3) A horizontal beam radiograph made with the animal standing or in ventral recumbency may be helpful.

3. Vaginogram or retrograde urethrogram. An ectopic ureter may be visualized entering the urethra or vagina. Technique does not enable assessment of kidneys and ascending infection to kidney, which can occur if retrograde reflux occurs.

Other imaging

1. Ultrasound

Nephritis and Pyelonephritis

Clinical correlations

1. Is usually caused by an ascending infection from the lower urinary tract.
2. Is best evaluated by nonradiographic methods (e.g., blood chemistry and urine examinations).

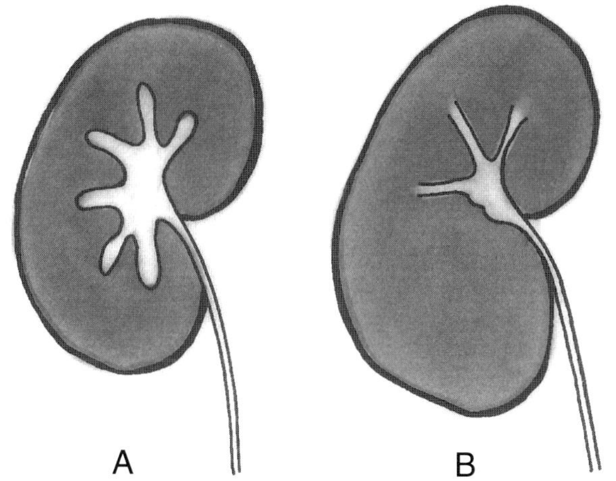

Figure 12.9. Deformed renal pelvis: **A**) irregular dilation (e.g. pyelonephritis) and **B**) compression of renal pelvis from renal tumor.

3. May be associated with nephrolithiasis.
4. May result in chronic renal failure.

Radiographic findings (See Figure 12.3 A,B)

1. In acute nephritis, the kidneys usually appear normal in survey radiographs, but occasionally there is slight enlargement of one or both kidneys.
2. In chronic nephritis, one or both kidneys are commonly smaller and irregularly shaped.
3. Radiopaque renal calculi may be present, commonly visible in the renal pelvis.

Contrast radiographs (intravenous urography) (Figure 12.9 A,B)

1. In acute nephritis or pyelonephritis, the urogram may appear normal.
2. In chronic nephritis or pyelonephritis, a heterogenous opacity in the renal parenchyma may be present or the renal pelvis may appear distorted and irregular.
3. If one kidney has significantly reduced function, the opposite kidney may appear larger than normal because of compensatory hypertrophy.
4. In pyelonephritis, radiographic abnormalities may include:
   a. Normal appearing renal pelvis
   b. Distortion of the renal pelvis
   c. Widened or irregular renal diverticuli
   d. Localized or generalized hydroureter

Other imaging

1. Ultrasound
2. CT
3. MRI

Renal Cysts

Clinical correlations

1. Can be congenital or acquired.
2. Cysts can be single or multiple and unilateral or bilateral.

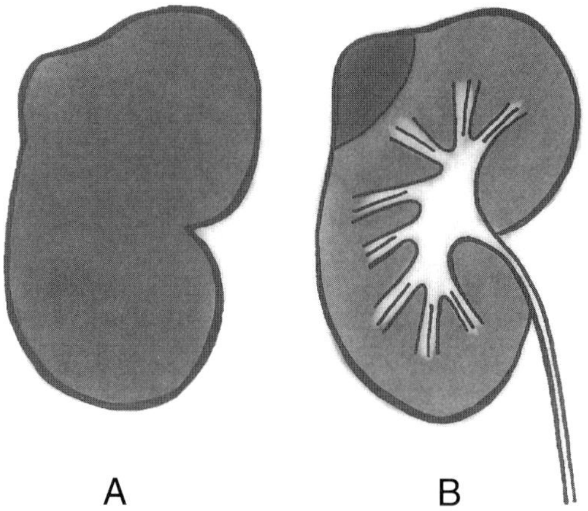

Figure 12.10. Renal cyst: **A**) irregular contour as seen on survey radiograph and **B**) intravenous urogram with cyst appearance less opaque than the renal parenchyma.

3. Can cause progressive renal failure.
4. Cysts can be sterile or infected.
5. Inheritable in Persian cat.

Radiographic findings (Figure 12.10 A,B)

1. If cysts are small, the kidneys commonly appear normal on survey radiographs.
2. Both kidneys may be enlarged and irregular if polycystic disease is present.
3. Localized enlargement of affected kidney if solitary cyst is large.
4. Differential considerations:
   a. Abscess
   b. Hematoma
   c. Tumor

Contrast radiographs (intravenous urography)

1. During the nephrogram phase, cysts are usually seen as radiolucent filling defects within the renal cortex.
2. The renal pelvis may appear normal or distorted depending on the size and location of the cysts.

Other imaging

1. Ultrasound
2. CT
3. MRI

Feline Perirenal Cysts (Perinephric pseudocyst)

Clinical correlations

1. Unknown etiology, may involve one or both kidneys.
2. Most often occurs in male cats older than 8 years.
3. Chronic renal disease may be coexistent.
4. Transudative fluid accumulates between the cortex and the renal capsule (subcapsular) or outside the renal capsule (extracapsular).

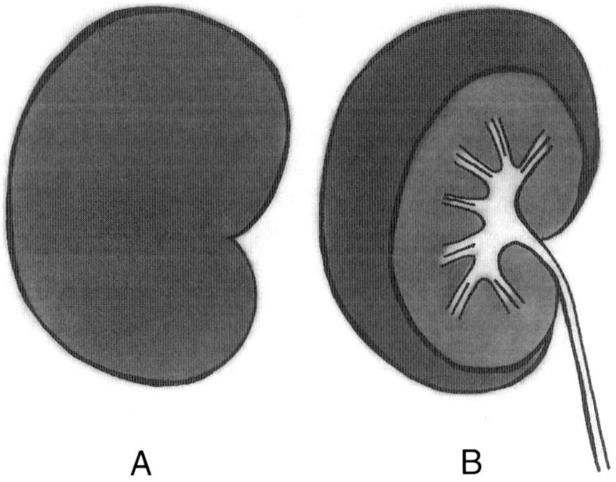

Figure 12.11. Feline perirenal pseudocyst: **A**) enlarged kidney as seen on survey radiograph, and **B**) intravenous urogram with perirenal pseudocyst appearing less opaque than the renal parenchyma.

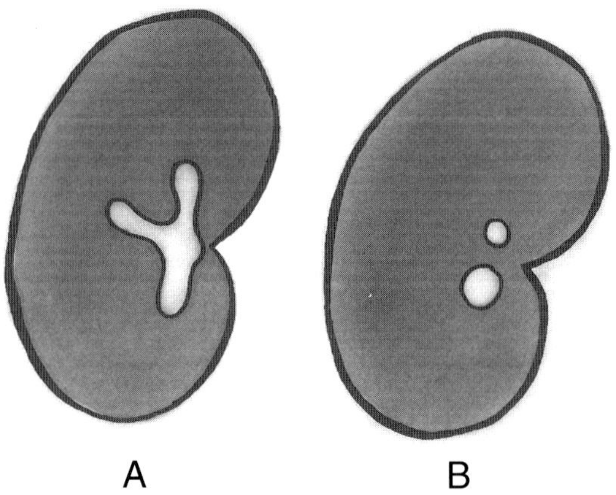

Figure 12.12. Renal calculi: **A**) Staghorn calculus and **B**) small round opaque calculi

5. Affected kidney is usually enlarged and nonpainful.
6. Differential considerations:
   a. Neoplasia
   b. Hydronephrosis
   c. Feline infectious peritonitis
   d. Polycystic disease

Radiographic findings (Figure 12.11 A,B)

1. Affected kidney is enlarged on survey radiographs and usually is smooth.

Contrast radiographs (intravenous urography)

1. The contrast opacified kidney is normal or slightly small, and surrounded by the less radiopaque nonopacified fluid-filled cyst.
2. If chronic renal disease is also present, the kidney may be small and irregularly shaped.

Other imaging

1. Ultrasound
2. CT
3. MRI

Renal and Ureteral Calculi

Clinical correlations

1. Usually caused by current or previous renal infection.
2. In the cat, calculi often occur secondary to ingestion of calculogenic diet (diet high in magnesium).
3. May cause hydronephrosis or hydroureter secondary to obstruction.

Radiographic findings (Figure 12.12 A,B)

1. Many calculi are radiopaque on survey radiographs.
2. Renal calculi may be solitary or multiple and unilateral or bilateral.
3. Differential considerations:
   a. Nephrocalcinosis
   b. Dystrophic mineralization
   c. Osseous metaplasia

Contrast radiographs (intravenous urography)

1. May be normal if calculi are small.
2. Large calculi may be seen as radiolucent filling defects within the contrast filled renal pelvis.
3. Variable degree of hydronephrosis may be present depending on the severity and duration of obstruction.
4. Ureteral calculi may cause localized or generalized ureteral dilation depending on the location and severity of the obstruction.

Other imaging

1. Ultrasound
2. CT
3. MRI

Hydronephrosis

Clinical correlations

1. Is usually caused by obstruction of the ureter or renal pelvis.
   a. Calculus
   b. Stricture (e.g., from spay suture)
   c. Neoplasm, usually of the bladder trigone or distal ureter
   d. Retroperitoneal mass
2. May occur secondary to chronic inflammation, infection, or adhesions.
   a. Pyelonephritis
   b. Parasitic disease (*Dioctophyma renale* infection)
   c. Sequel from previous trauma or surgery
3. Congenital anomaly (rare)

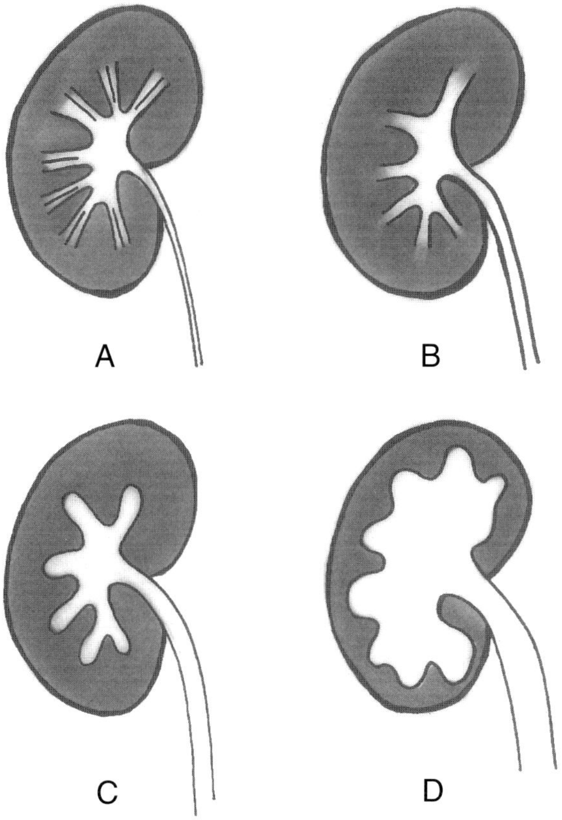

Figure 12.13. Hydronephrosis: **A**) normal renal pelvis, **B**) mild hydronephrosis, **C)** moderate hydronephrosis, and **D**) severe hydronephrosis.

Radiographic findings (Figure 12.13 A–D)

1. If hydronephrosis is not severe, the renal size and shape may be normal on survey radiographs.
2. If severe, the affected kidney is usually enlarged and smoothly marginated; the contralateral kidney is usually normal.

Contrast radiographs (intravenous urography)

1. Renal pelvis dilatation may vary from slight to marked with a normal nephrogram phase.
2. With severe pelvic dilatation only a thin cortical rim of functional renal tissue may be visualized during the nephrogram phase. The renal pelvis and ureter are usually not visualized.
3. If the obstruction is partial, intermittent, or chronic, renal atrophy with hydronephrosis may occur, resulting in the affected kidney being smaller than normal and irregular in contour.

Other imaging

1. Ultrasound
2. CT
3. MRI

Renal Neoplasia

Clinical correlations

1. Metastatic tumors are more common than primary tumors.
   a. Osteosarcoma
   b. Hemangiosarcoma
   c. Lymphosarcoma
   d. Melanoma
   e. Mast cell tumor
2. Most primary tumors are malignant.
   a. Adenocarcinoma is the most common tumor in the dog.
   b. Lymphosarcoma is the most common tumor in the cat.
   c. Transitional cell carcinoma in the renal pelvis is rare.
3. Benign tumors are less common.
   a. Adenoma
   b. Papilloma
   c. Lipoma
   d. Hemangioma
   e. Embryonal nephroblastoma
4. Primary or metastatic tumors can involve one or both kidneys.
5. Clinical signs variable and nonspecific including weight loss, anorexia, abdominal distension, or an abdominal mass.
6. Polycythemia may be present with primary renal carcinoma.
7. Renal failure may be present if both kidneys are involved.
8. Differential considerations:
   a. Cystic disease
   b. Abscess
   c. Hematoma

Radiographic findings (See Figure 12.9 B)

1. On survey radiographs the affected kidney is usually enlarged and irregularly shaped.
2. One or both kidneys may be involved.
3. Mineralization may be present, usually caused by tumor necrosis or osseous metaplasia.

Contrast radiographs (intravenous urography)

1. Absent or heterogenous nephrogram
2. Abnormal renal margination
2. Distorted renal pelvis and diverticuli

Other imaging

1. Ultrasound
2. CT
3. MRI

Renal and Ureteral Rupture

Clinical correlations

1. Usually associated with blunt abdominal trauma.
2. May be associated with rupture of a renal neoplasm.

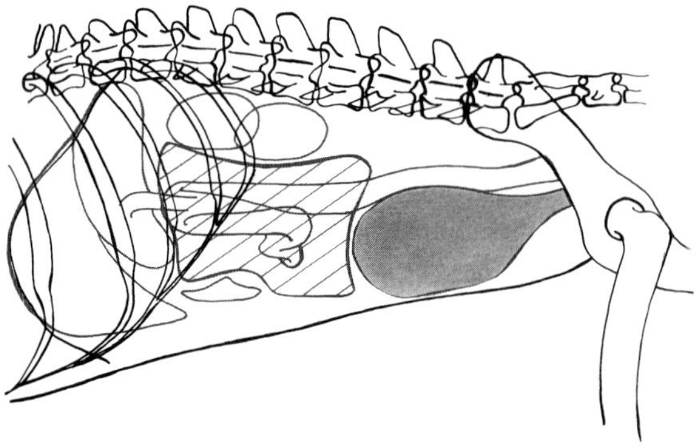

Figure 12.14. Distended urinary bladder. An enlarged urinary bladder commonly displaces the small bowel cranially and the descending colon dorsally.

Radiographic findings

1. Asymmetry, displacement, or poor visualization of the renal contour on survey radiographs.
2. Loss of detail in retroperitoneal space caused by hemorrhage or urine
3. Ventral displacement of the descending colon
4. Fractures of the ribs or spine may be present.

Contrast radiographs (intravenous urogram)

1. If the kidney is avulsed from the aorta, no renal outline or nephrogram will be seen.
2. If the kidney is ruptured, an irregular renal shadow may be seen with a heterogeneous nephrogram.
3. Contrast may accumulate beneath the renal capsule if there is parenchymal injury, but an intact capsule (subcapsular hematoma).
4. If the renal pelvis or ureter is ruptured, extravasation of contrast will be seen in the retroperitoneal space.
5. The renal pelvis may be distorted because of hematoma or blood clot

Other imaging

1. Ultrasound
2. CT
3. MRI

URINARY BLADDER AND URETHRA

RADIOGRAPHIC ANATOMY (Figures 12.14 and 12.15)

1. The urinary bladder is a round or "tear drop shaped" organ in the caudal ventral abdomen cranial to the pubis of the pelvis and ventral to the rectum and descending colon.

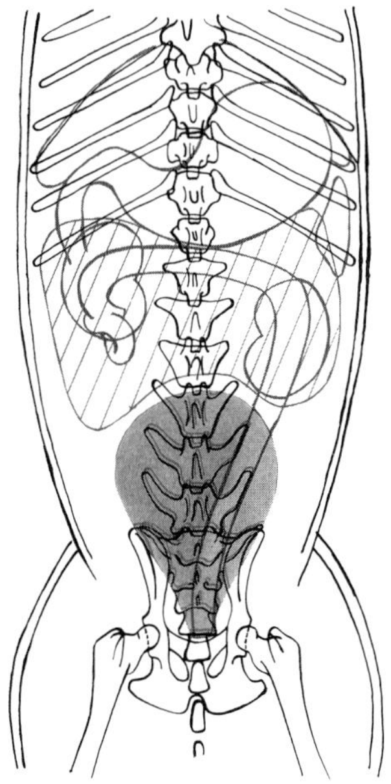

Figure 12.15. Distended urinary bladder. An enlarged urinary bladder commonly displaces the small bowel cranially.

2. The size of the bladder varies and when fully distended displaces the small bowel cranially. Usually the descending colon is more to the left (most common) or to the right.
3. The urethra is not normally seen on survey radiographs.

RADIOGRAPHIC INTERPRETATION

Survey Radiographs

Poor or no visualization of the urinary bladder

1. The bladder is not seen, but peritoneal and retroperitoneal serosal detail is normal.
   a. Normal empty bladder caused by voiding before radiography
   b. Displaced bladder (e.g., perineal or inguinal hernia, pelvic bladder)
   c. Hypoplastic bladder caused by disuse (e.g., associated with bilateral ectopic ureters)
2. Bladder not seen, and poor peritoneal and retroperitoneal serosal detail is present
   a. Ruptured urinary bladder
   b. Abdominal effusion (hemorrhage, ascites, peritonitis)
   c. Emaciation
   d. Normal immature dogs and cats

Displacement of the urinary bladder

1. Ventral displacement
   a. Inguinal hernia
   b. Abdominal wall hernia

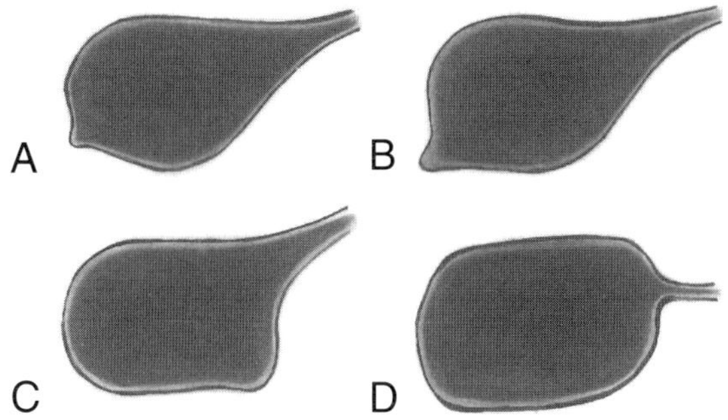

Figure 12.16. Abnormal shape of the urinary bladder: **A**) small urachal diverticulum, **B**) large urachal diverticulum, **C**) mucosal hernia, and **D**) rounded shape.

2. Dorsal displacement
   a. Abdominal masses
3. Cranial displacement
   a. Prostatic enlargement caused by tumor, cyst, infection, or hypertrophy
   b. Urethral mass
4. Cranioventral displacement
   a. Enlarged uterus (pregnancy, mass, pyometra)
   b. Sublumbar mass, usually iliosacral lymphadenopathy
   c. Colonic distension, megacolon, or colonic mass
   d. Uterine stump or cervical mass
5. Caudal displacement
   a. Abdominal mass
   b. Perineal hernia
   c. Pelvic bladder
   d. Congenital shortening of urethra

Abnormally shaped urinary bladder (Figure 12.16 A–D)

1. Indentation by adjacent abdominal masses
2. Neoplasm involving wall or serosa of the bladder
3. Urachal diverticulum
4. Traumatic hernia of the muscular portion of the wall of the urinary bladder
5. Previous bladder surgery with scar formation and adhesions

Abnormal size of the urinary bladder

1. Increased size
   a. Urethral or bladder neck obstruction caused by tumor, stricture, or calculus
   b. Neurogenic atony
   c. Secondary to chronic urine retention
2. Decreased size
   a. Congenital anomalies
      1) Disuse (e.g., ectopic ureter)
      2) Fistulas (e.g., urethrorectal or urethrovaginal fistula)
      3) Pelvic bladder

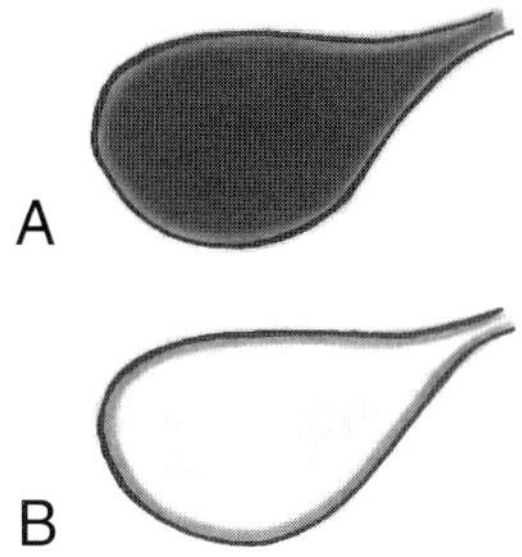

Figure 12.17. Normal urinary bladder: **A**) pneumocystogram and **B**) cystogram.

   b. Recent voiding
   c. Diffuse bladder wall disease (e.g., cystitis, tumor)

Radiopacity changes of urinary bladder

1. Increased radiopacity
   a. Calculi
   b. Mineralization of the bladder wall caused by chronic inflammation or neoplasia
2. Decreased radiopacity
   a. Air in bladder lumen from recent cystocentesis or bladder catheterization
   b. Emphysematous cystitis (gas-forming infection)

Contrast Radiographs (See chapter 3 for method)

Indications for cystography (Figures 12.17 A,B and 12.18 A–D)

1. Nonvisualized or abnormal appearing urinary bladder on survey radiographs
2. Suspected rupture of urinary bladder
3. Abnormal urine (pyruria, hematuria, crystalluria)
4. Clinical signs of stranguria, incontinence, or inappropriate urination
5. Suspected calculi, chronic infection, or neoplasia

Interpretation of cystography

1. Irregular mucosal border
   a. Incomplete distension of the normal urinary bladder

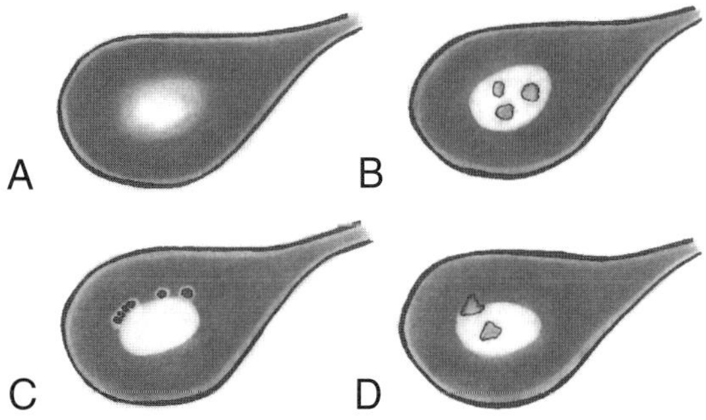

Figure 12.18. Double contrast cystogram: **A**) normal, **B**) calculi, **C**) air bubbles, and **D**) blood clots.

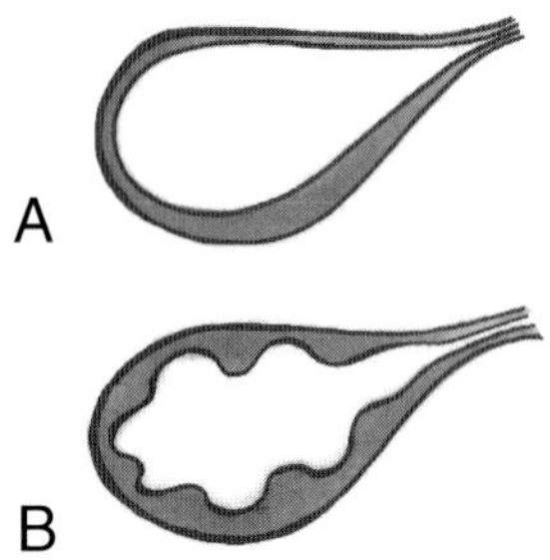

Figure 12.19. Cystitis: **A**) diffuse smooth wall thickening and **B**) diffuse irregular wall thickening.

can mimic bladder wall thickening and mucosal lesions.
   b. May be focal or diffuse
   c. Ulcer crater may contain contrast media.
   d. Differential considerations:
      1) Ulcerative or nonulcerative cystitis
      2) Neoplasia
2. Thickening of the bladder wall (Figure 12.19 A,B)
   a. Normal fully distended bladder wall is approximately 1 mm thick
   b. Best evaluated with double contrast cystography
   c. May be focal or diffuse
   d. Differential considerations:
      1) Cystitis
      2) Trauma
      3) Neoplasia
3. Filling defects (See Figure 12.18 B–D)
   a. Any lesion that alters filling of the bladder lumen
   b. Is usually more radiolucent relative to the radiopacity of the positive contrast media or more radiopaque relative to the radiopacity of negative contrast media.
   c. Freely movable filling defects
      1) Air bubbles
      2) Calculi
      3) Foreign bodies
      4) Blood clots
      5) Cellular debris (e.g., mucous plugs, sediment)
   d. Attached filling defects
      1) Neoplasia
      2) Polyps
      3) Blood clots
      4) Mural hematomas
      5) Ureterocoele
4. Extravasation of contrast media outside the normal bladder lumen can be caused by:
   a. Vesicoureteral reflux
   b. Patent urachus
   c. Diverticuli (urachal or traumatic)
   d. Submucosal dissection (trauma or iatrogenic)
   e. Ruptured urinary bladder
   f. Fistulas (e.g., rectal or vaginal)
5. Pseudo lesions or artifacts associated with cystography:
   a. Intraluminal air bubbles simulating calculi or blood clots
   b. Intraluminal large air bubble simulating bladder wall thickening
   c. Filling defects involving wall of urinary bladder as a result of incomplete distension of bladder wall or compression by adjacent abdominal organs (e.g., colon, prostate, uterus).

DISEASES/DISORDERS

Cystitis

Clinical correlations

1. Can be acute or chronic.
2. Common clinical signs include hematuria, dysuria, and increased frequency of urination.
3. May be associated with prostatic disease or cystic calculi.
4. Nephritis or pyelonephritis may be present concurrently.

Radiographic findings

1. On the survey radiographs, the bladder may appear small or normal in size.

Contrast radiographs

Double contrast cystography (See Figure 12.19)
1. In acute cystitis, the bladder may appear normal.
2. In chronic cystitis, the bladder wall is frequently thickened and irregular.
   a. The thickening may be generalized or localized. Localized thickening is often present in the cranioventral aspect of the bladder wall.
   b. Polypoid cystitis is usually characterized by diffuse thickening of the bladder wall and multiple filling defects involving the mucosa.
   c. May also have cystic calculi or intraluminal blood clots.
3. May have concurrent other abnormalities (e.g., urachal diverticulum).
4. Differential considerations:
   a. Foreign body (e.g., catheter or plant awn)
   b. Neoplasia

Other imaging

1. Ultrasound

Cystic Calculi

Clinical correlations

1. Most calculi are struvite and composed of magnesium ammonium phosphate.
   a. In the dog, usually results from urinary tract infections, commonly *Staphylococcus aureus*.
   b. Usually occurs in the cat without urinary tract infection.

2. Urate calculi
   a. Can occur in dogs and cats
   b. Is common in the Dalmatian.
   c. Increased incidence in animals with portal vascular anomalies or chronic hepatic insufficiency.
3. Cystine calculi are associated with inborn error of metabolism.
   a. Is more common in male dogs.
   b. More common in the Dachshund and English Bull Dog
4. Other calculi include:
   a. Silica
   b. Calcium phosphate (apatite)
   c. Calcium oxalate
   d. Mixed calculi
5. Common clinical signs include hematuria, dysuria, or inappropriate urination; however, many animals have no clinical signs.

Radiographic findings (see Figure 12.18 B)

1. Many calculi, especially struvite, are radiopaque in survey radiographs.
2. Calculi may be singular or multiple and vary in size.
3. Calculi may also be visible in the kidneys, ureters, or urethra.

Contrast radiographs (cystography) (see chapter 3)

1. Calculi are usually visible in the central dependent portion of the bladder within the iodinated contrast puddle.
2. Thickening of the bladder wall may be present if chronic cystitis is also present.
3. Urachal diverticuli may be present concurrently.
4. Differential considerations:
   a. Air bubbles are usually round and located at the peripheral border of the contrast puddle.
   b. Blood clots are usually irregular in shape and may be located in the dependent or peripheral portion of the contrast puddle.

Other imaging

1. Ultrasound

Ruptured Bladder

Clinical correlations

1. Is usually a sequela of abdominal trauma or penetrating wounds.
2. May occur secondary to abdominal palpation or faulty catheterization.
3. Clinical signs vary depending on the severity of bladder trauma.
   a. Hematuria may be present.
   b. Abdominal distension and discomfort are frequent.

Radiographic findings

1. There is loss of peritoneal detail in the caudal abdomen.
2. Depending on the duration and extent of bladder rupture, varying degrees of ascites or bowel ileus may be present.
3. If the rupture involves the bladder neck or urethra, the bladder may appear intact but be displaced cranially.

Contrast radiographs

Cystography

1. A positive contrast cystogram or retrograde cystogram is preferred to a pneumocystogram, because of the greater contrast and accuracy provided by the iodinated contrast medium.
2. The contrast material will be seen extravasated into the peritoneal cavity.
3. If a small rupture is present, local extravasation of contrast may be seen adjacent to the tear in the bladder wall.

Emphysematous Cystitis

Clinical correlations

1. Gas accumulation within the bladder lumen or bladder wall secondary to infection by gas-forming bacteria, most often *Escherichia coli*.
2. May occur more often in animals that have diabetes mellitus.

Radiographic findings (Figure 12.20 A,B)

1. Gas can be seen within the wall or lumen of the urinary bladder.
2. Occasionally the gas will dissect through the bladder wall and locate within the adjacent perivesicular fat.
3. Must differentiate from the more common cause of intraluminal gas, which is previous catheterization or cystocentesis.

Neoplasms of the Urinary Bladder

Clinical correlations

1. Is most common in aged female dogs.
2. Most malignant tumors are transitional cell carcinomas.
3. Less common malignant tumors are:
   a. Rhabdomyosarcoma
   b. Squamous cell carcinoma

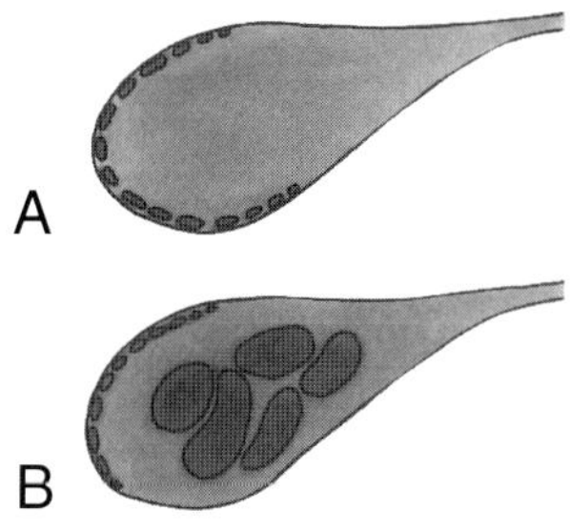

Figure 12.20. Emphysematous cystitis: **A**) air bubbles in bladder wall, **B**) air bubbles in bladder wall and lumen.

c. Metastatic prostatic adenocarcinoma
d. Lymphosarcoma
e. Leiomyosarcoma
4. Benign tumors are uncommon
a. Papilloma
b. Leiomyoma
5. Tumors within the bladder may cause obstruction of the ureterovesicular junction or the urethra.
6. Common clinical signs include hematuria, stranguria, or inappropriate urination.
7. Metastasis of transitional cell carcinoma can occur to the iliosacral lymph nodes, spine, pelvis, or lungs.

Radiographic findings
1. Commonly the survey radiographs are normal.
2. The bladder may be enlarged if urethral obstruction is present.
3. The bladder may appear irregular in outline if a mesenchymal mass is present.
4. Iliosacral lymphadenopathy or aggressive bony lesions of the lumbar vertebra and pelvis may be present if regional metastasis has occurred.

Contrast radiographs
Cystography or double contrast cystography (Figures 12.21 A,B and 12.22 A,B)
1. Filling defect associated with the mucosa or bladder wall

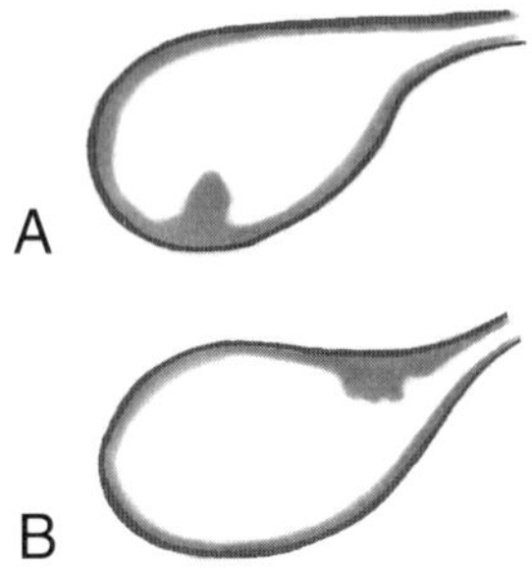

Figure 12.21. Localized mucosal lesion (cystogram): **A**) polyp and **B**) tumor.

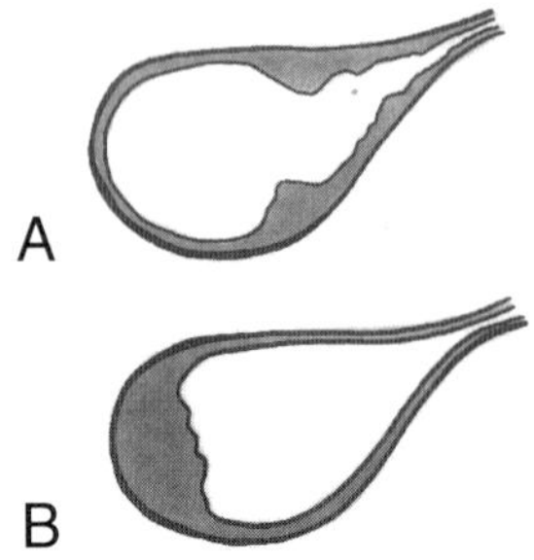

Figure 12.22. Bladder neoplasia (cystogram): **A**) neck of urinary bladder and **B**) apex of urinary bladder.

2. Localized or diffuse bladder wall thickening, often with ulceration
3. Most carcinomas occur in the trigone region of the bladder.
4. Differential considerations:
a. Chronic cystitis
b. Polypoid cystitis

Other imaging
1. Ultrasound

URETHRA

ANATOMY

1. The male urethra is divided into three portions.
a. The prostatic urethra extends from the neck of the bladder to the caudal border of the prostate gland.
b. The membranous urethra extends from the caudal border of the prostate gland to the ischial arch in the dog and the bulbourethral gland in the cat.
c. The penile urethra extends from the ischial arch to the tip of the penis.
2. The female urethra is shorter and wider than the male urethra and extends from the neck of the bladder to the external urethral orifice.

RADIOGRAPHIC INTERPRETATIONS

1. The normal urethra is not visualized on survey radiographs because of its small size and similar opacity of adjacent soft tissue structures.
2. Radiopaque calculi may be identified.
3. Rupture of the urethra may be suspected if there is loss of detail in the caudal abdomen.

Contrast Radiographs
Retrograde urethrography, voiding cystourethrography (Figure 12.23 A)
1. Filling defects within positive contrast-filled urethra may represent:
a. Intraluminal defects caused by:
1) Air bubbles
2) Calculi
3) Blood clots
b. Mural defects caused by:
1) Inflammatory disease
2) Granulomatous disease
3) Neoplasia
4) Fibrous tissue from previous surgery or trauma

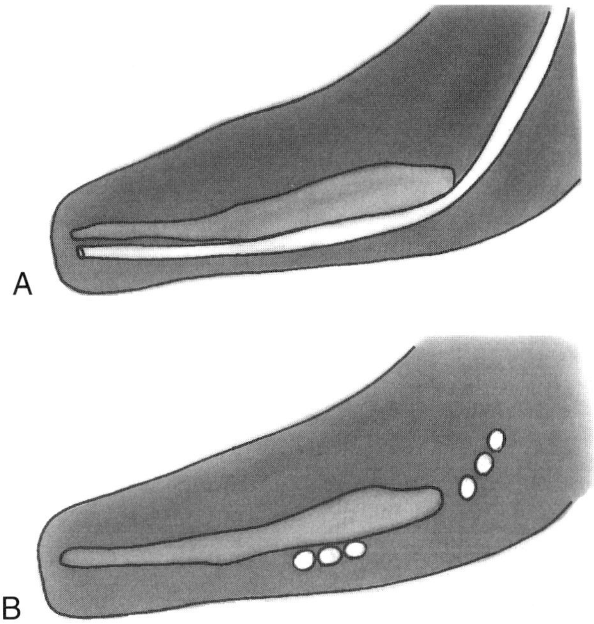

Figure 12.23. Penile urethra: **A**) normal urethrogram and **B**) urethral calculi within the penile urethra and proximal to the os penis bone.

   c. Extramural defects caused by:
      1) Prostatic neoplasia or hypertrophy
      2) Periurethral mass
2. Extravasation defects may be caused by:
   a. Soft tissue extravasation associated with urethral rupture.
   b. Vascular extravasation if urethrocavernous reflux occurs.
   c. Fistulas (e.g., urethrorectal, urethrovaginal) caused by congenital or acquired disease.
   d. Prostatic reflux
   e. Ectopic ureter

DISEASES/DISORDERS

Urethritis

Clinical correlations

1. Noninfectious urethritis
   a. Commonly caused by faulty catheterization
   b. May be associated with strictures, trauma, calculi, or neoplasia of the urethra
2. Infectious urethritis is most often associated with cystitis, prostatitis, or vaginitis.
3. Granulomatous urethritis is a rare condition that mimics urethral neoplasia.
4. Common clinical signs are dysuria, stranguria, and dribbling.

Radiographic findings

Usually no abnormality is seen on the survey radiographs.

Contrast radiographs (retrograde urethrography)

1. May see irregular mucosa, narrowed lumen, or strictures
2. Differential considerations:
   a. Neoplasia
   b. Calculi

Urethral Calculi

Clinical correlations

1. Commonly have concurrent cystitis and cystic calculi
2. Common clinical signs are hematuria, dysuria, stranguria, or anuria.

Radiographic findings

Survey radiographs (Figure 12.23 B)

1. In male dogs, calculi frequently lodge in the urethra proximal to the os penis bone.
2. Calculi in the pelvic urethra are best visualized with a ventrodorsal or lateral oblique projection.

Contrast radiographs

Retrograde urethrogram

1. Calculi will appear as radiolucent filling defects relative to the iodinated contrast media.
2. Calculi are usually round to slightly irregular in shape.
3. Urethritis may also be present with irregular mucosa.
4. Differential considerations:
   a. Air bubbles
   b. Blood clots

Ruptured Urethra

Clinical correlations

1. Usually caused by blunt trauma from motor vehicle accidents and often is associated with pelvic fractures.
2. May occur secondary to faulty catheterization.
3. Urine extravasation into surrounding tissues causes local pain and swelling.
4. Stranguria or anuria may result with clinical signs of fever, anorexia, and depression.

Radiographic findings

1. Survey radiographs may show loss of detail in the pelvic canal or soft tissue swelling in the ischial region.
2. Evidence of other trauma (e.g., pelvic fractures)
3. Bladder may appear well defined and intact or partially obscured.
4. If the urethra is transected, the urinary bladder may appear normal in size and shape, but may be positioned more cranial than normal.

Contrast radiographs

Retrograde urethrography

Extravasation of contrast medium from the urethral lumen into the adjacent soft tissues

Urethral Neoplasia

Clinical correlations

1. Seen in mature male and female dogs; rare in cats.
2. May be primary or metastatic.
3. In male dogs is often associated with prostatic carcinoma.
4. Differential consideration: granulomatous urethritis

Radiographic findings

1. Bladder may appear normal or distended depending on the degree of urethral obstruction.
2. If a periurethral mass is present, the rectum may be displaced dorsally.

Contrast radiographs

Retrograde urethrography (Figure 12.24 A,B)

1. Irregular urethral mucosa
2. Narrowed urethral lumen caused by stricture or periurethral mass
3. Extravasation of contrast from the urethra into the tumor, especially if necrosis or a fistula is present.

Urethrorectal Fistula

Clinical correlations

1. A persistent communication between the urethra and rectum
2. Is most often a developmental defect of the fetal cloaca but can occur as a sequel to trauma.
3. During voiding, urine is seen coming from both the urethral and anal openings.

Radiographic findings

Contrast radiography

Retrograde urethrogram

1. Demonstrates the fistula

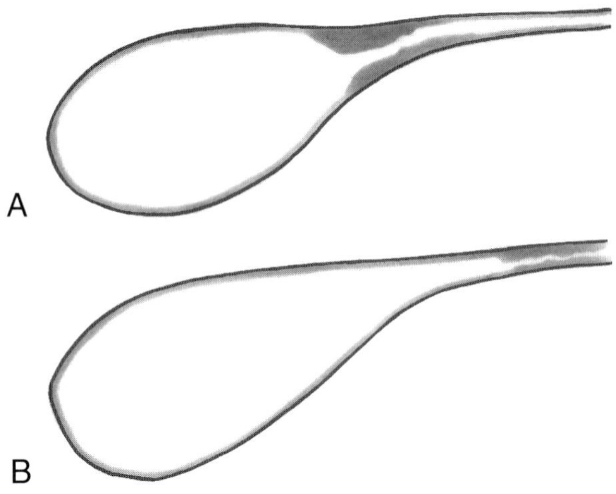

Figure 12.24. Urethral neoplasia (female): **A**) proximal urethral extending into bladder neck and **B**) distal urethra.

ADRENAL GLANDS

Radiographic Anatomy

1. The adrenal glands are located cranial and medial to the kidneys within the retroperitoneal space.
2. The left adrenal gland is bordered ventrally by the spleen, dorsally by the psoas minor muscle, laterally by the left kidney, and medially by the aorta.
3. The right adrenal gland is bordered craniolaterally by the right lateral liver lobe, laterally by the right kidney, medially by the caudal vena cava, and dorsally by the psoas minor muscle and right crus of the diaphragm.
4. The normal adrenal glands are invisible because of their small size and similar radiopacity to adjacent structures.

RADIOGRAPHIC INTERPRETATION

DISEASES/DISORDERS

Adrenal Gland Enlargement

Clinical correlations

1. Can be unilateral or bilateral.
2. Causes for enlargement include:
   a. Adenoma
   b. Adenocarcinoma
   c. Pheochromocytoma
   d. Nodular hyperplasia
3. May be hormone secreting
   a. Cortisol (e.g., hyperplasia, tumor)
   b. Catecholamines (e.g., pheochromocytoma)

Radiographic findings

1. Commonly no abnormality is seen on the survey radiographs.
2. Marked enlargement of the left adrenal gland may cause:
   a. Cranial displacement of gastric fundus
   b. Caudoventral displacement of the transverse colon
   c. Caudal displacement of the left kidney
3. Marked enlargement of the right adrenal gland may cause:
   a. Lateral displacement of the right kidney

Contrast radiographs

1. Intravenous urography
   a. The vascular phase may show adrenal circulation.
   b. Indentation of the cranial pole of the kidney may be present.
2. Pneumoperitoneography. Adrenal glands may be seen on lateral and dorsoventral projections.
3. Caudal vena cava venography. Right adrenal tumors may invade into or displace the adjacent cava.

Other imaging
1. Ultrasound
2. CT
3. MRI

Adrenal Gland Mineralization
Clinical correlations
1. May occur in neoplastic or nonneoplastic adrenal glands.
2. Seen occassionally in cats and has no known etiology or clinical significance.
3. When mineralization involves one adrenal gland, neoplasia is more likely.

Radiographic findings
1. Mineralization can be unilateral or bilateral and appear punctate, amorphous, or cystic
2. Tumors may be associated with marked enlargement of the affected adrenal gland.

Hypoadrenocorticism (Addison's Disease)
Clinical correlations
1. Is caused by decreased cortisol production from the adrenal cortex, usually associated with adrenal atrophy.
2. Common clinical signs include weakness, bradycardia, vomiting, or diarrhea. Often have electrolyte disturbance (hyperkalemia and hyponatremia).
3. The diagnosis is confirmed by cortisol analyses (e.g., ACTH stimulation).

Radiographic findings
1. Survey abdominal radiographs are usually normal.
2. Adrenal mineralization is rare.
3. Microcardia and decreased pulmonary perfusion
4. Megaesophagus

Pheochromocytoma
Clinical correlations
1. Caused by catecholamine producing tumor from the medulla of one adrenal gland.
2. May rupture causing retroperitoneal hemorrhage.
3. Tumors of the right adrenal gland may invade the caudal vena cava.
4. Clinical signs are often vague and nonspecific and can be caused by either the effect of excessive catecholamine production (systemic hypertension) or secondary to the adrenal mass and its metastasis.
5. Signs of hypertension include weakness, panting, anorexia, vomiting, and weight loss; seen in less than 50% of affected dogs.

Radiographic findings
1. Usually no radiographic abnormality seen with survey radiographs.
2. If a mass lesion of the adrenal gland is present, it may be seen in the retroperitoneal space adjacent to the kidney and may be ill-defined, especially if hemorrhage has occurred.
3. Dystrophic mineralization may be present.

Contrast radiographs
1. Intravenous urography
2. Caudal vena cava venography
3. Pneumoperitoneography

Other imaging
1. Ultrasound
2. CT
3. MRI

Hyperadrenocorticism (Cushing's syndrome)
Clinical correlations
1. Common disease in the dog; rare in the cat.
2. Caused by increased cortisol production from the adrenal cortex:
   a. Pituitary dependent disease (PDH) caused by pituitary hypersecretion and secondary bilateral adrenocortical hyperplasia is most common (80–90%).
   b. Functional adrenal tumor (adenoma or adenocarcinoma) less common (10–20%)
3. Carcinomas may metastasize to the liver, lymph nodes, kidney, and lungs.
4. Common clinical signs include: polydypsia, polyurea, polyphagia, abdominal distension, and symmetric hair loss.
5. The diagnosis is confirmed by cortisol and ACTH assays.
6. Pulmonary thromboembolism can occur as a disease complication.

Radiographic findings
1. Survey radiographs may be normal.
2. An adrenal mass may be seen.
3. Mineralization of adrenal occurs uncommonly.
4. Other radiographic findings include:
   a. Hepatomegaly
   b. Bronchointerstitial calcification
   c. Mineralization of the skin (calcinosis cutis)
   d. Osteoporosis
   e. Distended "pot bellied" appearance to ventral abdominal wall with no peritoneal effusion

Other imaging
1. Ultrasound
2. CT
3. MRI

chapter thirteen

13

Genital System

MALE

The male genital system consists of the prostate gland, the testicles and the penis (Figure 13.1).

PROSTATE GLAND

ANATOMY (Figure 13.2)

1. The prostate gland is round to ovoid and located caudal to the urinary bladder, ventral to the rectum, and dorsal to the pubis.
2. The prostatic urethra extends through the prostate gland, slightly dilated within the gland and narrowed at its caudal margin.
3. In immature or castrated dogs, the prostate gland is usually within the pelvic canal.
4. In intact males, the prostate commonly enlarges because of benign hypertrophy, and is often present cranial to the pubis within the caudal abdomen.

RADIOGRAPHIC ANATOMY

1. The prostate gland is of soft tissue opacity and its visualization depends on the presence of peripelvic or periurethral fat.
2. On the lateral projection, the cranial and ventral margins of the prostate can usually be seen because of the presence of adjacent fat.
3. The dorsal border of the prostate is usually not seen because it is silhouetted with adjacent tissues having a similar soft tissue radiopacity.
4. The prostate gland occasionally may be seen on the ventrodorsal projection, if fecal material within the rectum does not obscure it.

Radiographic findings (Figures 13.3 through 13.6)

1. Increased size of the prostate gland
   a. Benign hypertrophy and hyperplasia
   b. Prostatitis
   c. Prostatic abscess
   d. Prostatic cystic disease
   e. Paraprostatic cyst
   f. Neoplasia
2. Decreased size of the prostate gland
   a. Immature or castrated dog
   b. Chronic prostatitis with fibrosis
3. Mineralization of the prostate
   a. Prostatic calculi
   b. Chronic prostatitis
   c. Neoplasia
   d. Cyst
   e. Paraprostatic cyst

DISEASES/DISORDERS

Benign Prostatic Hypertrophy

Clinical correlations

1. Is common in intact males older than 5 years.
2. Most dogs have no clinical signs.
3. Tenesmus may be present.
4. Other prostatic disease may be present concurrently.
   a. Prostatitis
   b. Cystic disease
   c. Abscess
   d. Neoplasia

Radiographic findings (See Figure 13.3)

1. On the lateral projection, the enlarged prostate is usually seen cranial to the pubic brim of the pelvis, displacing the urinary bladder cranially and the descending colon and rectum dorsally.

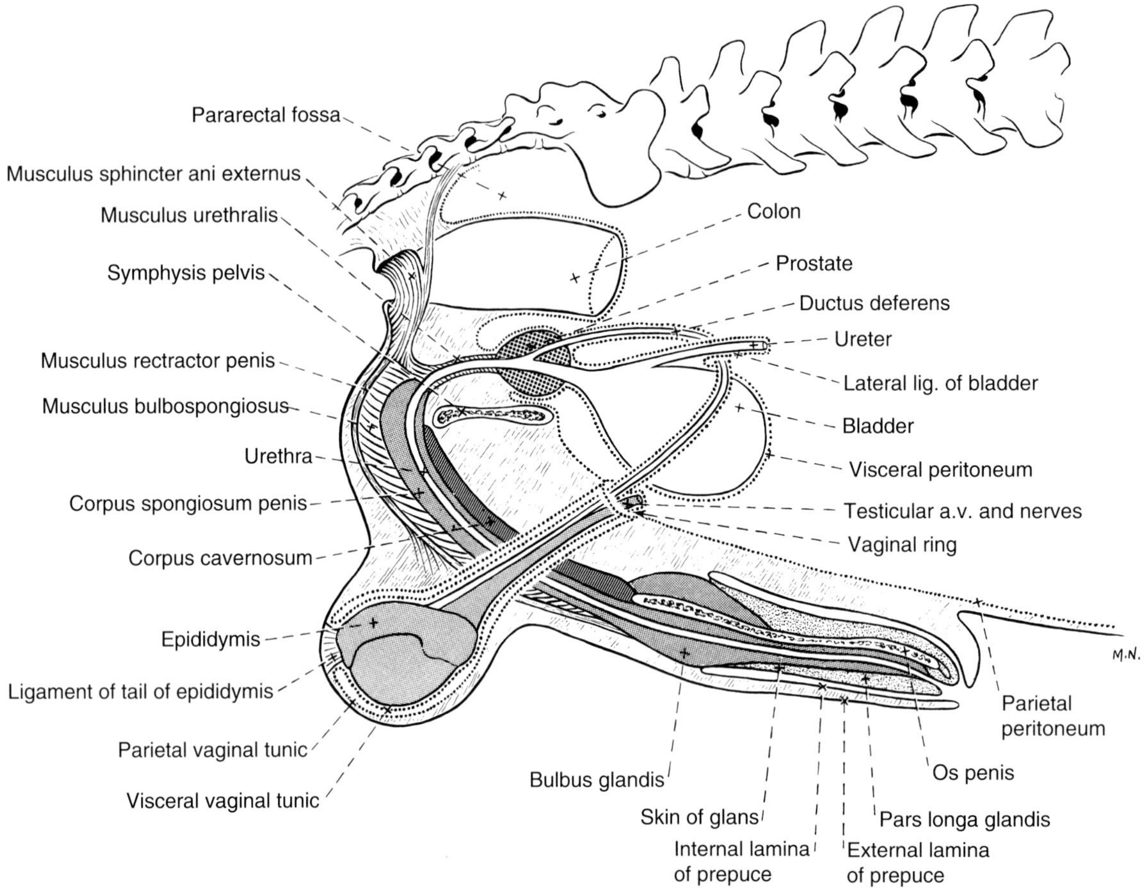

Figure 13.1. Diagram of peritoneal reflections and the male genitalia. (From Evans HE, Christensen GC. The urogenital system. In: Evans HE, ed. Miller's Anatomy of the Dog. 3rd ed. Philadelphia: W.B. Saunders; 1993:512. Courtesy of and with permission of Dr. Howard E. Evans.)

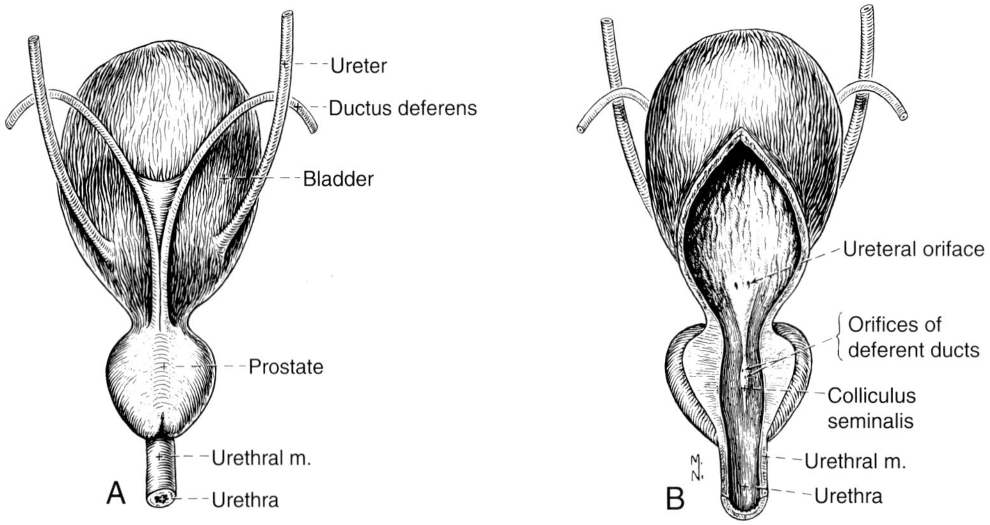

Figure 13.2. Bladder and prostate: **A**) dorsal aspect and **B**) ventral aspect, partially opened on midline. (From Evans HE, Christensen GC. The urogenital system. In: Evans HE, ed. Miller's Anatomy of the Dog. 3rd ed. Philadelphia: W.B. Saunders; 1993:501. Courtesy of and with permission of Dr. Howard E. Evans.)

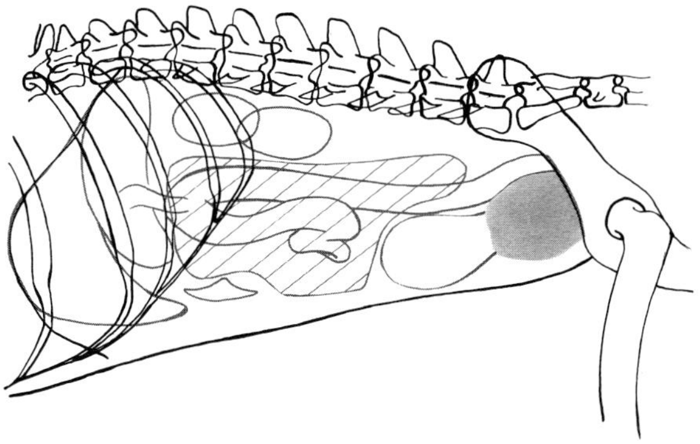

Figure 13.3. Prostatomegaly. Enlargement of the prostate gland commonly causes cranial displacement of the urinary bladder and dorsal displacement of the descending colon.

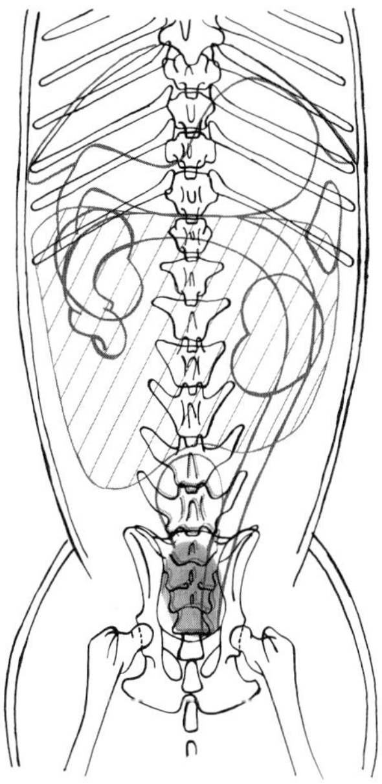

Figure 13.4. Prostatomegaly. Enlargement of the prostate gland commonly causes cranial displacement of the urinary bladder.

2. On the ventrodorsal projection, the enlarged prostate may be seen superimposed over the pubic bones on the midline.

Other imaging

1. Ultrasound
2. CT
3. MRI

Prostatitis, Prostatic Abscess

Clinical correlations

1. Is usually associated with ascending urinary tract infection.
2. Can be acute or chronic.
3. Variable enlargement of the prostate gland
4. Common clinical signs include tenesmus, dysuria, hematuria, and pyuria.

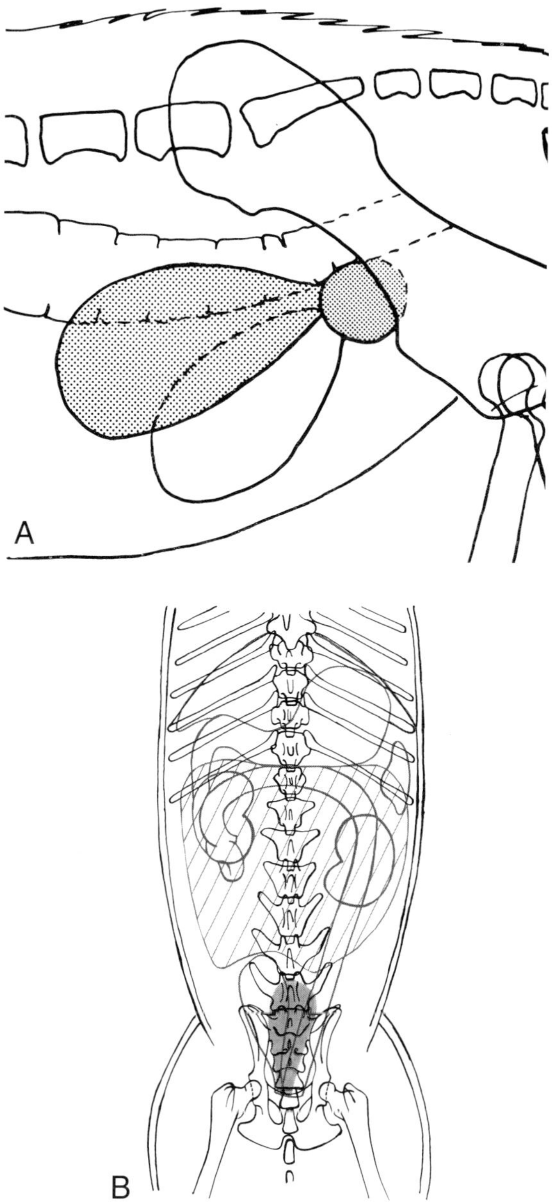

Figure 13.5 Paraprostatic cyst. **A.** A large paraprostatic cyst displaces the urinary bladder dorsally and cranially. **B.** A large paraprostatic cyst displaces the urinary bladder to the right side.

Radiographic findings

1. Prostatic enlargement with cranial displacement of the urinary bladder and often dorsal displacement of the rectum
2. The border of the prostate may be ill-defined if inflammation has extended through the capsule or if an abscess is present.
3. Severe prostatic enlargement is more suggestive of abscess or neoplasia, rather than prostatitis alone.
4. Prostatic mineralization may be present, usually as sequel to necrosis.

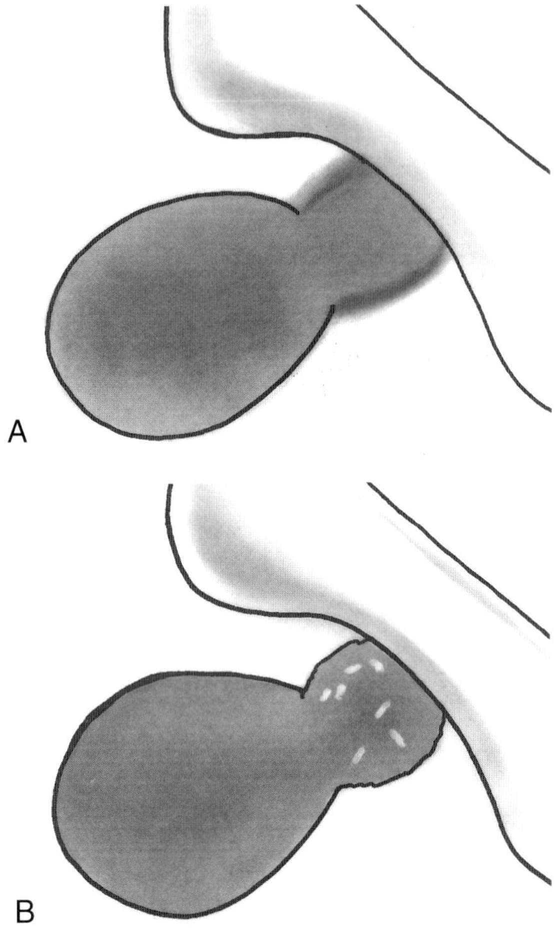

Figure 13.6 **A.** Enlarged and ill-defined enlargement of the prostate gland is most often associated with infection or neoplasia. **B.** Enlarged prostate gland with focal mineralization is most often asscociated with neoplasia, chronic inflammation, or calculi.

Contrast radiographs (cystourethrography)

1. Narrowed or enlarged prostatic urethral lumen
2. Prostatic reflux

Other imaging

1. Ultrasound

Prostatic Calculi/Prostatic Mineralization

Clinical correlations

1. Is usually associated with chronic prostatitis.
2. Calculi are usually within the prostatic ducts.
3. Mineralization may be present with neoplasia secondary to necrosis.

Radiographic findings (see Figure 13.6 B)

1. On survey radiographs, calculi are usually spherical and within the prostate gland.
2. Differentiate from dystrophic mineralization, which is usually amorphous or linear and secondary to inflammatory or neoplastic disease.

Contrast radiographs (retrograde urethrography)

1. The urethra may appear smooth or irregular.
2. Filling defects within the prostatic ducts may be visualized by seeing reflux of positive contrast into the prostatic ducts.

Other imaging

1. Ultrasound

Paraprostatic Cyst

Clinical correlations

1. Usually cccurs in older intact male dogs.
2. The paraprostatic cyst usually develops from an embryonic defect involving the persistence of the Muellerian ducts with secondary cyst formation. The cyst retains its attachment to the prostate gland.
3. Paraprostatic cysts are commonly located caudal to the bladder, but may be located cranial, ventral dorsal, or lateral to the bladder.

Radiographic findings (See Figure 13.5)

1. A caudal abdominal soft tissue mass is visible on survey radiographs.
2. Dystrophic mineralization may be present within the cyst wall.

Contrast radiographs

Retrograde urethrocystography

1. Confirms the location of the urethra and bladder relative to the paraprostatic cyst.
2. The paraprostatic cyst may be located cranial, dorsal, ventral, or lateral to the urinary bladder.
3. May contain "rim like" dystrophic mineralization.

Other imaging

1. Ultrasound

Prostatic Neoplasia

Clinical correlations

1. Occurs in mature intact or castrated dogs.
2. Is rare in the cat.
3. The most common tumor is primary adenocarcinoma.
4. Transitional cell carcinoma or leiomyosarcoma are less common.
5. Common clinical signs include tenesmus, hematuria, dysuria, tense abdomen, and a stiff gait.
6. Metastasis commonly occurs to the ileosacral lymph nodes, the lumbar spine, pelvis, and the lung.

Radiographic findings

1. The degree of prostatic enlargement seen on survey radiographs is variable.
2. The borders of the prostate may appear ill-defined if an abscess is also present or if the neoplasm has extended through capsule.

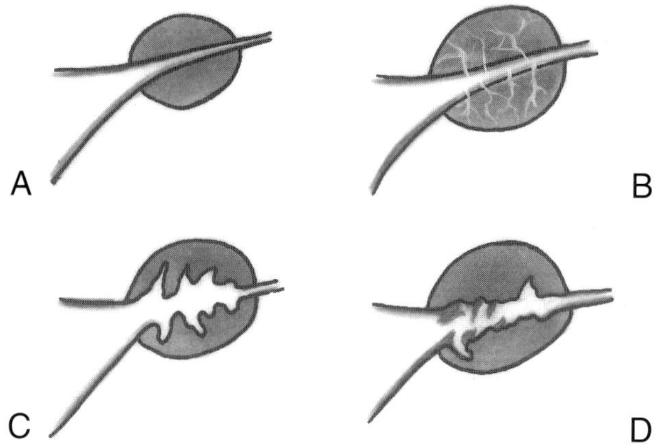

Figure 13.7. Prostatic urethra (urethrogram) with **A**) normal smooth urethra, **B**) contrast reflux into prostatic ducts, **C**) irregular cavitation into the prostate gland, and **D**) urethral neoplasia with cavitation into the prostate gland.

3. Prostatic mineralization may be present.
4. Signs of metastasis:
   a. Iliosacral lymphadenopathy with ventral displacement of the descending colon
   b. Bone metastasis is typically proliferative and most commonly involves the ventral aspects of the fourth to seventh lumbar vertebrae and may involve the pelvis, femurs, sacrum, and coccygeal vertebrae.

Contrast radiographs

Retrograde urethrocystography (Figure 13.7 A–D)

1. The prostatic urethra may be dilated, irregular, or narrowed.
2. Reflux of contrast media from the urethra into the prostate gland may occur with extravasation into the tumor.
3. Filling defects of the urethral mucosa with or without stricture may be present if the urethra is involved with neoplasia.

Other imaging

1. Ultrasound
2. CT
3. MRI

THE TESTICLE

RADIOGRAPHIC INTERPRETATION

1. Radiography is of limited value because the soft tissue opacity of the testes and epididymis and scrotum is similar.
2. Undescended testes are usually not seen on survey radiographs unless enlarged as a result of neoplasia or torsion.
3. Intraabdominal testicles when present as an abdominal mass lesion are usually in the caudoventral abdomen.
   a. May cause dorsal and lateral displacement of the small bowel.
   b. May cause indentation of the urinary bladder.

DISEASES/DISORDERS

Cryptorchidism

Clinical correlations

1. Is congenital and may be inherited.
2. The cryptorchid testicle may be located within the abdomen, the inguinal canal, or within the subcutaneous tissues of the inguinal area.
3. An abdominal testicle is more likely to have torsion or neoplasia than a scrotal testicle.
4. The most common tumor of a retained testicle is a Sertoli cell tumor, which frequently causes feminization.

Radiographic findings

1. A retained testicle is usually small and not radiographically visible.
2. If the retained testicle is neoplastic or becomes torsed, a mass lesion may be seen in the mid or caudal abdomen.
3. If the retained testicle is malignant (e.g., Sertoli cell tumor), signs of feminization (e.g., gynecomastica) or metastasis to the iliosacral lymph nodes or other sites may be present.

Other imaging

1. Ultrasound

Orchitis/Epididymitis

Clinical correlations

1. Can be secondary to trauma or infection.
2. The most common infection in the dog is due to *Brucella canis*.
3. Common clinical signs include pain, swelling, and fever.
4. Diagnosis is obtained by semen evaluation, *Brucella* titer, fine needle aspirate, or testicular biopsy.

Radiographic finding

1. Survey radiographs are not helpful in diagnosis.

Other imaging

1. Ultrasound

Testicular Torsion

Clinical correlations

1. Is a condition in which the spermatic cord undergoes rotation, leading to thrombosis or infarction of the testicle.

2. Most often occurs in retained neoplastic abdominal testicle; is rare in a scrotal testicle.
3. Common clinical signs include abdominal pain, fever, and anorexia.

Radiographic finding
1. Intraabdominal mass (if tumor involves the retained testicle), mass often is ill-defined.

Other imaging
1. Ultrasound

Testicular Neoplasia
Clinical correlations
1. Is common in the dog, rare in the cat.
2. Most common tumor is sertoli cell tumor.
3. Seminoma and interstitial cell tumor are less common.
4. More often occurs in a retained testicle.
5. Feminization may occur.
   a. Gynecomastica
   b. Pendulous prepuce
   c. Alopecia and hyperpigmentation of the skin
   d. Atrophy of the contralateral testicle

Radiographic findings
1. Intraabdominal mass, if tumor mass is present in the retained testicle.
2. Gynecomastica if feminization is present.

Other imaging
1. Ultrasound

Infections and Tumors of the Penis
Clinical correlations
1. Infections and tumors of the penis are best evaluated by physical examination.
2. Tumors may arise from urethral, adjacent soft tissues, or from the os penis bone.
3. Urethral involvement can produce clinical signs of dysuria or stranguria.

Radiographic findings
1. The soft tissues of the penile region are poorly evaluated with survey radiography.
2. If a bone tumor of the os penis is present, aggressive lytic or productive lesions may be present.

Contrast radiographs (urethrography)
1. Can evaluate urethral integrity
2. May see filling defects associated with urethritis or neoplasia

Fractures of the Os Penis Bone
Clinical correlations
1. Occasionally the os penis bone is fractured during strenuous breeding activity or other trauma.
2. Marked swelling of the penis is common; hematoma or dysuria may also be present.

Radiographic findings
1. Fracture of the os penis bone is readily identified on a survey lateral projection.
2. Differential considerations:
   a. Multiple centers of ossification of the os penis bone
   b. Urethral calculi

Contrast radiographs
Urethrogram
1. Evaluates urethral integrity at the fracture site
2. Urethral rupture or compression from adjacent hematoma

FEMALE

RADIOGRAPHIC ANATOMY (Figures 13.8 and 13.9)

1. The female reproductive tract consists of two ovaries, two uterine horns, the uterine body, the cervix, and the vagina.
2. The normal internal genitalia in a nongravid female are usually not seen on survey radiographs.
3. In some normal dogs and cats, particularly in obese individuals, the uterine body can be seen on a lateral survey radiograph between the rectum and the urinary bladder.

RADIOGRAPHIC FINDINGS

1. Generalized uterine enlargement can be caused by:
   a. Pregnancy
   b. Pyometra
   c. Hydrometra
   d. Mucometra
   e. Physometra
   f. Uterine torsion
   g. Uterine adenomatosis
2. Localized uterine enlargement
   a. Neoplasia (carcinoma, leiomyoma, leiomyosarcoma)
   b. Localized pyometra, mucometra, hydrometra, or physometra
   c. Uterine stump granuloma or abscess
3. Uterine mineralization
   a. Normal pregnancy with ossified fetal skeletons
   b. Fetal mummification
   c. Mineralized uterine cyst or tumor

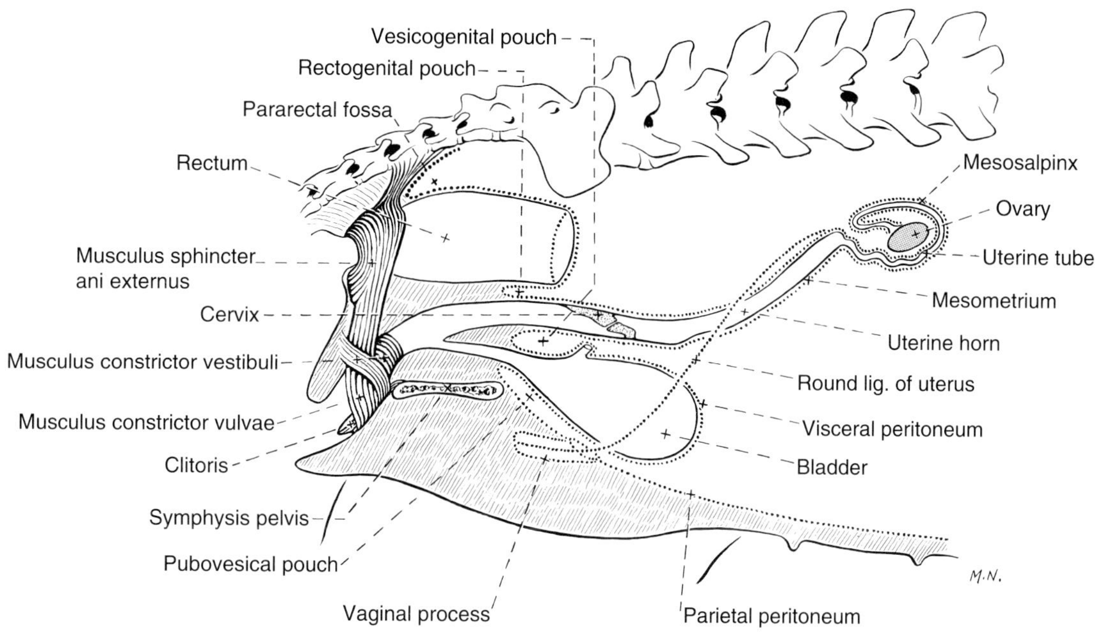

Figure 13.8. Diagram of peritoneal reflections and the female genitalia. (From Evans HE, Christensen GC. The urogenital system. In: Evans HE, ed. Miller's Anatomy of the Dog. 3rd ed. Philadelphia: W.B. Saunders; 1993:532. Courtesy of and with permission of Dr. Howard E. Evans.)

4. Uterine gas
   a. Fetal death (fetal emphysema)
   b. Uterine torsion with ischemia
   c. Physometra caused by infection with gas-forming organisms

CONTRAST RADIOGRAPHS

1. Pneumoperitoneography
2. Hysterosalpinography
3. Retrograde vaginogram, if cervix is open

Other imaging
1. Ultrasound
2. CT
3. MRI

OVARIES AND UTERUS

DISEASES/DISORDERS

Ovarian Masses

Clinical correlations
1. Types of ovarian masses include:
   a. Cyst
   b. Abscess
   c. Granulosa cell tumor
   d. Adenocarcinoma
   e. Teratoma
2. Abdominal mass may be palpable.

Radiographic findings
1. Small ovarian enlargements are undetectable radiographically.
2. Large right ovarian masses are usually located caudal to the pole of the right kidney and may cause displacement of the small intestine ventrally and the descending duodenum and ascending colon medially.
3. Large left ovarian masses are usually located caudal to the pole of the left kidney and may cause medial displacement of the descending colon.
4. Abdominal effusion may be present associated with carcinomatosis or peritonitis.

Other imaging
1. Ultrasound
2. CT
3. MRI

Uterine Masses

Clinical correlations
1. Types of masses include:
   a. Pregnancy
   b. Pyometra or endometritis
   c. Hydrometra or mucometra

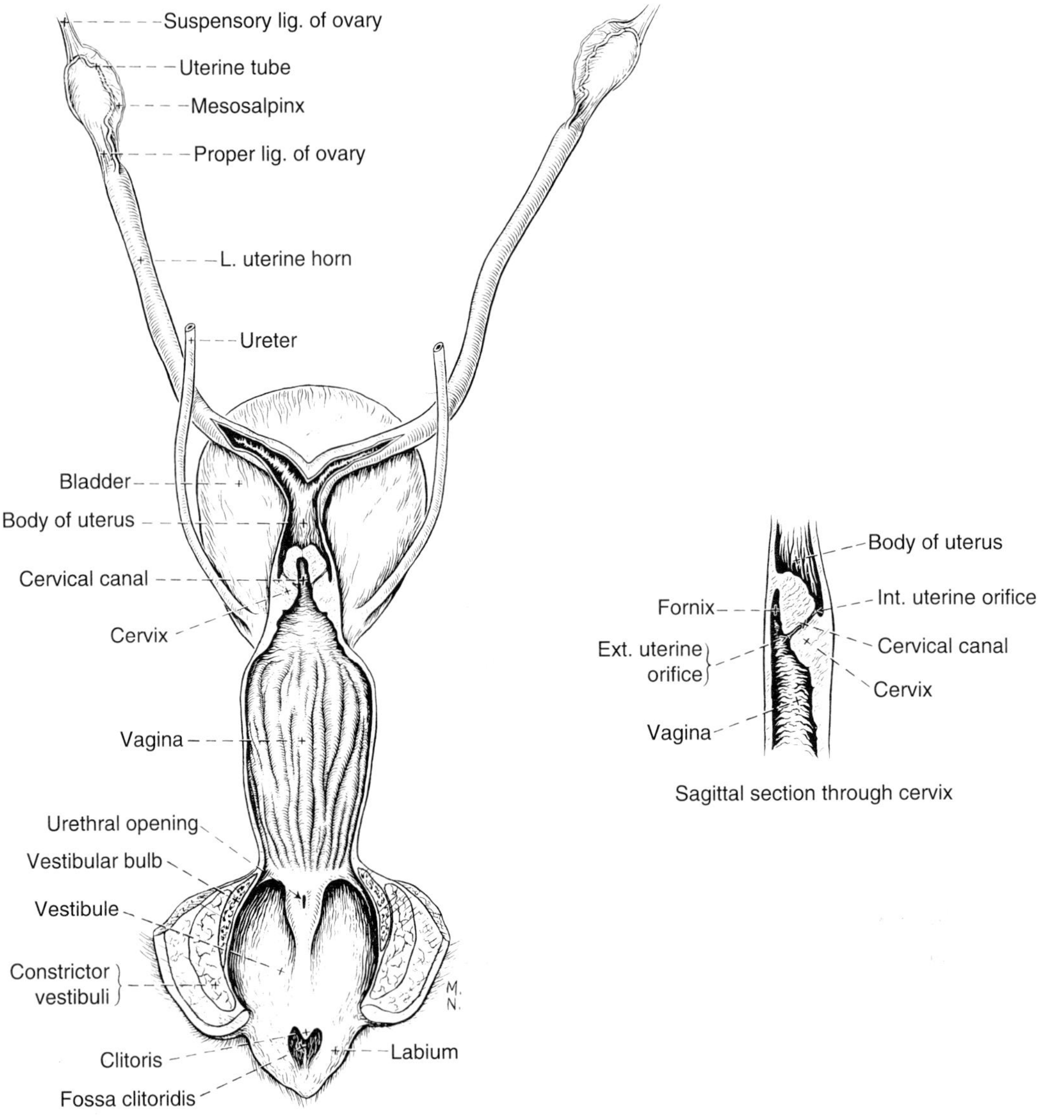

Figure 13.9. Dorsal view of the female genitalia, partially opened on the midline, smaller view shows a lateral view of a sagittal section through cervix, the fornix is ventral. (From Evans HE, Christensen GC. The urogenital system. In: Evans HE, ed. Miller's Anatomy of the Dog. 3rd ed. Philadelphia: W.B. Saunders; 1993:539. Courtesy of and with permission of Dr. Howard E. Evans.)

   d. Uterine torsion
   e. Tumor (e.g., adenocarcinoma, leiomyoma, leiomyosarcoma)
   f. Abscess of uterine body or cervix
2. Abdominal mass may be palpable.
3. Clinical signs are variable depending on type of condition present.

Radiographic findings
1. Soft tissue radiopaque mass in the caudal to midabdomen with variable displacement of adjacent bowel depending on the size of the mass.
2. Uterine stump granulomas may compress and displace the urinary bladder ventrally and may cause dorsal displacement of the descending colon and rectum.
3. Differential considerations:
   a. Bowel mass
   b. Mesenteric mass
   c. Splenic mass

Other imaging
1. Ultrasound
2. CT
3. MRI

The Gravid Uterus
Clinical correlations
1. In early pregnancy, abdominal palpation and ultrasound are more sensitive diagnostic methods than radiography for confirming uterine enlargement.

2. The fetal skeletons begin to ossify at approximately 42 to 45 days in the dog and 35 to 39 days in the cat.

Radiographic findings
1. The uterus is normally not visible before 25 to 30 days gestation.
2. When visible, the gravid uterus may be identified with soft tissue symmetrical segmentation.
3. The enlarged uterus often displaces the small bowel cranially and dorsally and may compress or be superimposed over the urinary bladder and ventral to the descending colon.
4. When the fetuses ossify, an accurate fetal count can usually be made by counting the skulls or spines of the fetuses on two radiographic projections (lateral and ventrodorsal).
5. Normal fetuses are usually of similar size and degree of ossification.

Other imaging
1. Ultrasound

Dystocia and Fetal Death
Clinical correlations
1. Dystocia may be caused by many factors, including:
   a. Prolonged gestation
   b. Maternal factors:
      1) Primary or secondary uterine inertia
      2) Uterine torsion
      3) Abdominal hernia containing uterus
      4) Vaginal or pelvic mass
      5) Narrowed pelvic canal (e.g., healed pelvic fracture)
   c. Fetal factors
      1) Oversized fetus
      2) Malpresentation
      3) Fetal anomalies
2. Common clinical signs include prolonged parturition, depression, severe pain, and hemorrhagic vaginal discharge.
3. Fetal death is usually a complication of dystocia.

Radiographic findings
1. Provides evaluation of fetal number, position and shape of individual fetuses, and estimate of fetal age.
2. Determine whether a pelvic canal deformity, stenosis, or pelvic mass is present.
3. Radiographic signs of fetal death include:
   a. Gas present within the uterus or any part of the fetus.
   b. Overlapping of the frontal and parietal bones of the skull
   c. Lysis of the fetal skeleton
   d. Abnormal angulation of the spine
   e. Mummification is characterized by contraction of the skeleton with an abnormal fetal size and shape.

Other imaging
1. Ultrasound

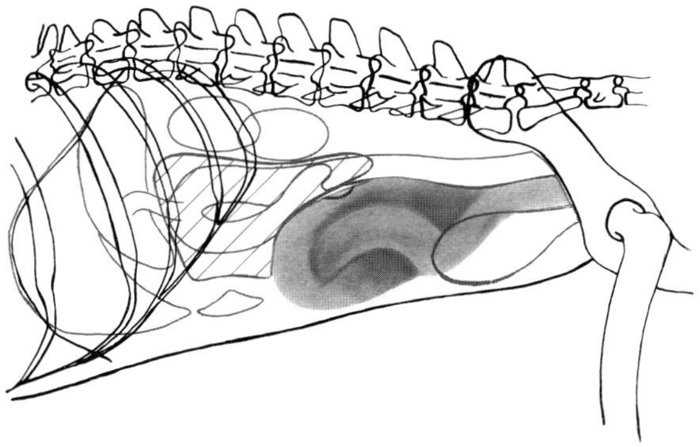

Figure 13.10. Pyometra. A tubular fluid-filled uterus is commonly superimposed over the urinary bladder and causes cranial displacement of the small intestine.

Cystic Endometrial Hyperplasia/Pyometra Complex
Clinical correlations
1. Cystic endometrial hyperplasia is commonly associated with aging and characterized by thickening of the endometrium and increased mucus within the uterine lumen. This can lead to mucometra or hydrometra.
2. Pyometra occurs secondary to bacterial infection of an abnormal uterus, often present 4 to 10 weeks after estrus.
3. Physometra is caused by uterine infection by gas-forming organisms.
4. Vaginal discharge may or may not be present depending on whether the cervix is open or closed.
5. Common clinical signs include polydypsia, polyuria, anorexia, depression, and dehydration.

Radiographic findings (Figures 13.10 and 13.11)
1. Variable enlargement of the uterus depending on the duration and severity of disease.
2. When enlarged, a tubular soft tissue mass is usually present in the caudal abdomen causing cranial and dorsal displacement of the small bowel.
3. On the lateral projection, the uterus may be seen superimposed over the urinary bladder.
4. On the ventrodorsal projection, the enlarged uterus may be seen to the left of the descending colon and in the right caudal abdomen displacing the small bowel medially.
5. Careful compression of the abdomen (i.e., radiolucent paddle) may aid in identifying the abnormal uterus between the bladder and the descending colon.

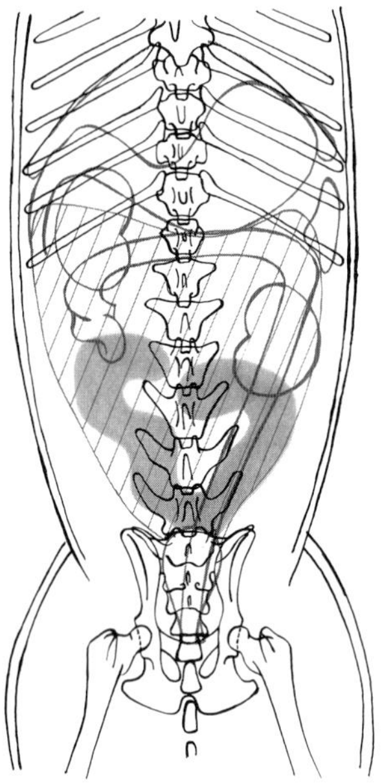

Figure 13.11. Pyometra. A tubular fluid-filled uterus is commonly seen in the caudal abdomen superimposed over or displacing the small bowel.

6. Differential considerations:
   a. Pregnancy
   b. Fluid-filled small bowel loops
   c. Uterine mass
   d. Other midabdominal mass

Other imaging
1. Ultrasound

Cervical Masses
Clinical correlations
1. Types of cervical diseases include:
   a. Tumor (e.g., carcinoma, leiomyosarcoma)
   b. Abscess
   c. Granuloma (e.g., after ovariohysterectomy)
2. Can usually be palpated rectally and abdominally.
3. May cause urinary incontinence or dysuria depending on the degree and location of the bladder compression.
4. If the mass compresses the bladder neck, bladder or ureteral obstruction may be present.
5. Hydronephrosis may occur if ureteral obstruction is severe.

Radiographic findings (Figure 13.12)
1. The normal cervix cannot be seen on survey radiographs.
2. A large cervical mass appears as a soft tissue opacity between the rectum and the neck of the urinary bladder on the lateral projection. A cervical mass may cause dorsal displacement of the rectum and ventral compression or displacement of the urinary bladder.

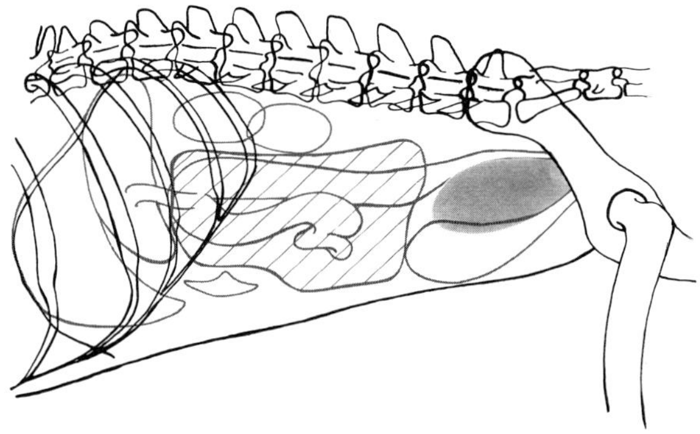

Figure 13.12. Cervical mass (lateral view). A large cervical mass may cause indentation or displacement of the urinary bladder and dorsal displacement or indentation of the descending colon.

Contrast radiographs
1. Urethrocystography
   a. Localizes the normal versus abnormal position of the urethra and bladder
   b. Can evaluate displacement or compression of the urethra or bladder
2. Vaginography
   a. Determines location of the vagina to the level of the cervix
   b. A filling defect within the vagina may be seen if the cervical mass is proliferative.
3. Pneumocolon or barium enema
   a. Determines location of rectum and colon
   b. Can evaluate displacement or compression depending on the size of the cervical mass.

Other imaging
1. Ultrasound

Diseases of the Vagina
Clinical correlations
1. Common vaginal diseases include:
   a. Vaginitis
   b. Prolapse
   c. Polyps
   d. Vaginal edema, hyperplasia, or hypertrophy
   e. Tumor (e.g., fibroma, leiomyoma, leiomyosarcoma, transmissible venereal tumor)
   f. Rectovaginal fistula
   g. Lacerations
2. Most vaginal diseases are best assessed by physical examination and endoscopy.

Radiographic findings
1. Survey radiographs are usually normal.
2. If the vagina is enlarged and a mass lesion is present, the rectum may be displaced dorsally.
3. If the urethra is compressed, the urinary bladder may be distended.

Contrast radiographs

Vaginography

1. Determine location and size of the vagina
2. Mural defects may be present.

Hermaphroditism

Clinical correlations

1. Types of hermaphrodites
   a. True hermaphrodite (rare) is presence of both ovarian and testicular tissue.
   b. Male pseudohermaphrodite has normal testes with external genitalia resembling that of a female.
   c. Female pseudohermaphrodite has normal ovaries with external genitalia resembling that of a male.
2. The most common anomaly is the female pseudohermaphrodite.
   a. Affected animals have a sheath but lack a penis and an os penis bone.
   b. No palpable prostate gland.
   c. May have an os clitoris.
   d. An internal uterus masculinus is present, which may become cystic, infected, or fluid-filled.

Radiographic findings

1. Survey radiographs (female pseudohermaphrodite) indicate no os penis bone present; may have an os clitoris.
2. If the uterus masculinus is infected, a fluid-filled mass may be seen in the caudal abdomen.

Contrast radiographs

Urethrocystography

1. Enables localization of the urethra and the urinary bladder
2. Occasionally a fluid-filled uterus masculinus will communicate with the urethra and therefore fill with contrast media during a retrograde urethrogram.

Suggested Readings

Anderson WD, Anderson BG. Atlas of canine anatomy. Philadelphia: Lea & Febiger; 1994.

Birchard SJ, Sherding RG. Saunders manual of small animal practice. Philadelphia: W.B. Saunders; 1994.

Braund KG. Clinical syndromes in veterinary neurology. St. Louis: Mosby-Year Book; 1994.

Burk RL, Ackerman N. Small animal radiology and ultrasonography. 2nd ed. Philadelphia: W.B. Saunders; 1996.

Diagnostic Imaging. Veterinary clinics of North America. Vol 23:2. Philadelphia: W.B. Saunders; 1993.

Ettinger SJ, Feldman E. Textbook of veterinary medical internal medicine. 4th ed. Philadelphia: W.B. Saunders; 1995.

Evans HE. Miller's anatomy of the dog. 3rd ed. Philadelphia: W.B. Saunders; 1993.

Farrow CS, Green R, Shively M. Radiology of the cat. St. Louis: Mosby-Year Book; 1994.

Kealy K. Diagnostic radiology of the dog and cat. 2nd ed. Philadelphia: W.B. Saunders; 1987.

Morgan J. Radiographic techniques in veterinary radiography. 5th ed. Ames: Iowa State University Press; 1993.

Morgan RV. Handbook of small animal practice. 2nd ed. NY: Churchill Livingstone; 1992.

Nelson RW, Couto CG. Essentials of small animal internal medicine. St. Louis: Mosby-Year Book; 1992.

Newton CD, Nunamaker DM. Textbook of small animal orthopedics. Philadelphia: J.B. Lippincott; 1985.

O'Brien TR. Radiographic diagnosis of abdominal disorders in the dog and cat. Philadelphia: W.B. Saunders/O'Brien, Davis; 1978.

Schebitz H, Wilkens H. Atlas of radiographic anatomy of the dog and cat. 3rd ed. Verlag Paul Parey, ed. Philadelphia: W.B. Saunders; 1978.

Suter PF, Lord PF. Thoracic radiography—A text atlas of thoracic diseases in the dog and cat. Peter F. Suter, ed. Wettswill, Switzerland; 1984.

Thrall DE. Textbook of veterinary diagnostic radiology. 3rd edition. Philadelphia: W.B. Saunders; 1998.

Ticer JW. Radiographic technique in veterinary practice. 2nd ed. Philadelphia: W.B. Saunders; 1984

Tilley LP, Smith WK. The 5 minute veterinary consult. Baltimore: Williams & Wilkins; 1997.

Veterinary Radiology & Ultrasound Journal, published by American College of Veterinary Radiology, indexes available on American College of Veterinary Radiology Web site http://www.acvr.ucdavis.edu/acvr/acvr.html and Index Medicus (MEDLINE).

Whittick WG. Canine orthopedics. 2nd ed. Philadelphia: Lea & Febiger; 1990.

Glossary

Air-bronchogram sign refers to the visualization of a bronchus because air within the bronchus stands out in contrast to surrounding parenchymal consolidation (e.g., collapsed or fluid/exudate- filled alveoli). A radiographic sign associated with an alveolar pulmonary pattern.

Alveolar pulmonary pattern a radiographic appearance when most alveoli are airless as a result of collapse of the alveoli or filling of the air spaces with fluid or cellular material.

Angiocardiography a radiographic contrast study of the heart and great vessels.

Angiography a radiographic contrast study of blood vessels.

Apophysis secondary ossification center that contributes to the overall shape of the bone and serves for attachment of tendons, but commonly does not contribute to overall bone length.

Appendicular pertaining to the legs.

Arthrography a radiographic contrast study of a joint.

Artifact a false lesion; commonly caused by technical faults (e.g. film, screens, grid, development, exposure, cassettes, x-ray table) and patient structures (e.g., debris on haircoat, superimposed cutaneous or subcutaneous lesions, nipple).

Atelectasis incomplete expansion (partial to complete collapse) of the lung usually associated with lung disease, pleural effusion, pneumothorax, or intrathoracic masses.

Avulsion fracture a fracture usually involving an apophysis or sesamoid, which involves the bony insertion of a ligament or tendon.

Axial pertains to the bones of the vertebral column, skull, hyoid, ribs, and sternum. Also may be used to describe in the direction of, or along an axis of, a structure or part.

Barium enema a radiographic contrast study of the colon.

Beak sign contrast media fills only the entrance of the lumen at the pyloric sphincter; a sign associated with pyloric stenosis.

Beam direction described in terms that indicate the entrance and exit of the x-ray beam (e.g., dorsoventral, dorsopalmar) (Refer to Figure 1.3).

Bezoar a concretion of various character commonly found in the stomach or intestine. Different types include trichobezoar (hair), phytobezoar (fruit and vegetable fibers), or trichophytobezoar (mixture of hair and fruit or vegetable fibers).

Block vertebra congenital defect caused by developmental failure of somite segmentation of the vertebral body.

Bone infarcts areas of necrosis within the medullary cavity of bones that appear as focal radiopacities.

Bone sclerosis an increase in the radiopacity of bone. Also called eburnation.

Bone spur osteophyte formation on the periarticular margins of a bone.

Brachycephalic having a short wide head.

Bronchial cuffing thickening of the peribronchial interstitial tissue sheath as a result of fluid accumulation, cellular peribronchiolar infiltration, or fibrosis. Commonly associated with the bronchial pulmonary pattern.

Bronchial pulmonary pattern a radiographic appearance when the collagenous and cartilaginous tissue and the associated mucous glands have proliferated or contain fluid to cellular infiltrates, causing the bronchial wall or lumen shape to be accentuated or altered.

Bronchiectasis abnormally shaped pulmonary airways, usually characterized by dilation of the bronchi or bronchioles with loss of normal branching and tapering.

Bronchitis inflammation of the bronchi.

Bronchography a radiographic contrast study of the major airways.

Bronchopneumonia inflammation of the lungs that usually begins in the terminal bronchioles.

Calcification deposition of calcium salts within soft tissue structures.

Calcinosis deposition of calcium salts in various tissues other than the parenchymatous viscera.

Carcinomatosis widespread distribution of cancer throughout the body; often refers to the diffuse implantation of neoplastic nodules within the peritoneal cavity.

Caudal an anatomic direction toward the tail or hind part of the body. Also used to designate the flexor side of a limb.

Caudocranial refers to a position in which the x-ray beam enters the caudal aspect of the body part first, and exits the cranial aspect of the part nearest the film (Refer to Figure 1.3).

Celiography a radiographic contrast study of the peritoneal cavity.

Central beam the imaginary x-ray photons in the center of the x-ray beam.

Cervical spondylopathy deformity of the vertebral bodies, narrowing of the vertebral canal, vertebral instability, and malarticulation with varying degrees of spinal cord compression.

Cholangiography a radiographic contrast study of the bile ducts.

Cholecystocholangiography a radiographic contrast study of the gall bladder and bile ducts.

Cholecystography a radiographic contrast study of the gall bladder.

Chondrodysplasia inherited deformities of the bony skeleton caused by abnormal cartilage development.

Coin lesion a pulmonary nodule approximately 1 cm in diameter.

Chylothorax accumulation of chyle in the pleural cavity, usually secondary to rupture of the thoracic duct.

Chylous effusion accumulation of chylous fluid in the pleural cavity usually associated with heart failure, mediastinal neoplasia, or mediastinitis.

Cineradiography the making of a cinematographic record directly from a fluorescent screen.

Comparison radiographs radiographs of the side opposite of the one in question, to aid in determining normal from abnormal.

Consolidation indicating pathology of the lung in where the alveolar air has been replaced by fluid, cells or cellular exudate, or by invasion of neoplastic cells.

Contralateral situated or pertaining to the opposite side.

Contrast media compounds or materials used to increase or decrease the radiopacity differences of an examined organ as compared with adjacent structures.

Contusion bruising.

Cranial anatomic term referring to the directional location of a body part (e.g., skull, thorax, spine, abdomen, limb). Opposed to caudal (Refer to Figure 1.3).

Craniocaudal refers to the direction in which the x-ray beam enters the cranial aspect of the part first, and exits the caudal part nearest the film (Refer to Figure 1.3).

Cretinism disproportionate dwarfism caused by arrested development of the thyroid gland, defective thyroid hormone synthesis, or iodine deficiency. Also called congenital hypothyroidism.

Cystography a radiographic contrast study of the urinary bladder.

Dacryocystorhinography a radiographic contrast study of the nasolacrimal duct.

Decubitus the animal is positioned in lateral, ventral, or dorsal recumbency, and the x-ray beam is directed horizontally.

Degenerative joint disease (DJD) degenerative arthropathy of many diverse causes (also known as osteoarthritis and osteoarthrosis).

Density radiographic density is the quantitative measure of blackening of the photographic or radiographic image.

Diaphysis a primary center of ossification of a long bone.

Diskography a radiographic study used for visualizing the central portion of an intervertebral disk.

Diskospondylitis inflammation or infection of an intervertebral disk. Also known as intradiskal osteomyelitis, diskitis.

Disseminated idiopathic skeletal hyperostosis (DISH) an ossifying condition characterized by bony hyperostosis at tendon and ligament attachments in axial and extra-axial sites.

Distal an anatomic term denoting away from the center of the body. Opposed to proximal (Refer to Figure 1.3).

Donut sign a bronchus seen end-on because of bronchial thickening, increased endobronchial secretions, or peribronchial infiltrate. A sign associated with the bronchial pulmonary pattern of disease.

Dorsoventral the x-ray beam enters the dorsal surface of the animal first, and exits the ventral surface of the animal nearest to the film.

Dolichocephalic having a long head.

Dorsal anatomic direction pertaining to the back. Opposed to ventral. Also refers to the limbs from the carpus and tarsus distally (Refer to Figure 1.3).

Dorsal recumbency animal is positioned on its back.

Dorsopalmar/plantar describes entry of the x-ray beam on the dorsum of the leg from the carpus and tarsus distally and exiting on the palmar/plantar surface of the leg (Refer to Figure 1.3).

Dorsoventral (DV) described entry of the x-ray beam dorsally and exiting ventrally on the animal (Refer to Figure 1.3).

Double contrast a contrast study using negative (e.g., gas) and positive contrast media (e.g., barium, iodinated).

Dural ossification a degenerative condition of unknown clinical significance in the dog characterized by osseous metaplasia of the dura mater.

Eburnation subchondral sclerosis.

Emphysema a swelling or inflation caused by the presence of air (e.g., mediastinal emphysema, subcutaneous emphysema, emphysematous cystitis, emphysematous cholecystitis).

Emphysema, compensatory the dilation of one part of the lung to compensate for the consolidation of another part. Also referred to as compensatory hyperinflation.

Emphysema, pulmonary increased size of the air spaces distal to the terminal bronchiole with destructive changes in their walls.

Enchondroma benign bone tumor usually located in the metaphysis of a long bone. Thought to be the result of failure of normal endochondral ossification with retention of physeal growth cartilage.

Enthesophyte a bony growth projecting outward from the bone at sites of tendinous or ligamentous attachments.

Epidurography a radiographic contrast study for assessment of the cauda equina and associated nerve roots.

Epiphysis a secondary ossification center at the proximal and distal ends of most long bones. Separated from the metaphysis by the physis during the growth of an animal.

Erect position of the animal is vertical, and the x-ray beam is directed horizontally.

Erect position animal is held upright, usually standing on its hind legs.

Esophagraphy a radiographic contrast study of the esophagus.

Excretory urography a radiographic contrast study of the kidney and ureters.

Exostosis a bony growth projecting outward from the surface of the bone.

Extension the straightening of a leg or other body part. Opposed to flexion.

Extrapleural sign term to include all lesions arising outside the parietal or mediastinal pleura. Commonly extrapleural masses originate from the wall of the thorax, diaphragm, or mediastinum.

Filling defect a space-occupying lesion or mass within a hollow organ.

Fistulography a radiographic contrast study of a fistulous tract.

Flail chest thoracic wall instability that interferes with the mechanics of ventilation. A segment of the chest wall is detached with comminuted adjacent rib fractures and the flail segment moves paradoxically, being sucked in on inspiration and thrust out on expiration.

Flexion the bending of a limb or body part. Opposed to extension.

Fluid level the horizontal interface between fluid and air. A fluid level can be demonstrated only by using a horizontal x-ray beam (e.g., standing lateral and erect ventrodorsal projections).

Gastrography a radiographic contrast study of the stomach.

Gastrointestinography a radiographic contrast study of the stomach and small intestine.

Hemivertebra congenital defect caused by developmental hemimetametric displacement of the vertebral somites resulting in only partial development of the vertebral body.

Hemothorax accumulation of blood within the pleural cavity.

Hernia protrusion of an organ or portion of an organ through an abnormal opening. True hernias have an intact serous lining. False hernias (e.g., traumatic diaphragmatic hernia) have a torn muscular portion through which viscera protrude.

Herringbone pattern the normal transverse mucosal pattern of the distal third of the feline esophagus.

Heterotopic bone formation focal bone formation within the lung, common in aged dogs. Also called pulmonary osteomas.

Hiatal a gap, cleft, or opening, usually associated with diaphragmatic lesions, e.g., hiatal hernia of the esophageal hiatus.

Horizontal beam radiographic positioning in which the x-ray beam is directed horizontally.

Hydrothorax accumulation of fluid within the pleural cavity.

Ileus abnormal dilation of the bowel, caused by mechanical or functional causes.

Infiltrate a localized or diffuse lesion visualized in an organ (e.g., lung, bone).

Interstitial pulmonary pattern a radiographic appearance when there is an increased amount of interstitial tissue or fluid, or cellular material has accumulated within the interstitial spaces.

Ipsilateral situated on or pertaining to the same side.

Lateral of or pertaining to the side. Away from the medial plane. Opposed to medial.

Lateral decubitus term describing use of the x-ray beam with a horizontal direction, directed at the dorsal or ventral aspect of the animal in lateral recumbency.

Lateral recumbency animal positioned on its side.

Lesion a detected radiographic abnormality.

Lumbosacral instability a congenital or acquired disorder characterized by narrowing of the vertebral canal or intervertebral foramina causing compression of the nerve roots that form the cauda equina in the lumbosacral region. Also called cauda equina syndrome, lumbosacral stenosis, and lumbosacral malarticulation.

Lung markings pertains to the visualization of bronchial walls and pulmonary vessels.

Lymphography a radiographic contrast study of the lymphatic vessels

Magnification (radiographic) enlargement of the radiographic image by using a small focal spot and increasing the object-film distance.

Mass lesion (pulmonary) a circumscribed solitary radiopacity larger than 4 cm in diameter.

Median being situated or occurring in the middle of the body.

Medial on the inner surface of an extremity. Opposed to lateral.

Mediastinal shift a shift of the heart or other mediastinal structures more into one hemithorax or the other, commonly caused by a mass lesion, unilateral loss or increase in lung volume, or congenital anomaly.

Meningocoele neural defect in which the meninges protrude through a dorsal spinal defect.

Meningomyelocoele neural defect in which the spinal cord, meninges, or nerve roots protrude through a dorsal spinal defect.

Metaphysis the area of the bone between the diaphysis and physis.

Microlithiasis the formation of minute concretions within an organ, usually refers to focal "sand-like" mineralization within the lung.

Miliary small in size, like a millet seed, as in miliary lung metastasis.

Mineralization addition of mineral matter to the body, often caused by calcification or ossification.

Mixed pulmonary pattern a radiographic appearance in which two or more pulmonary pattern components are visible concurrently.

Mucopolysaccharidosis a recessively inherited lysomal disease that results from metabolic defects of different glycosaminoglycans.

Myelocoele neural defect in which the spinal cord protrudes through a dorsal spinal defect.

Myelodysplastic conditions congenital malformations resulting from defective development

Myelography a radiographic contrast study of the spinal cord made possible by the injection of contrast material into the spinal subarachnoid space.

Niche a recess in the wall of a hollow organ that retains contrast. Ulcers and diverticuli are examples.

Nodular lesions (pulmonary) spherical radiopacities ranging from 2 to 40 mm in diameter.

Nodular pulmonary pattern presence of rounded pulmonary radiopacities within the terminal airspaces or interstitium. A component of interstitial pulmonary pattern of disease.

Oligocephalic a normal sized head.

Opacity property of a substance to absorb x-ray radiation. Opposed to lucency.

Ossification formation of bone or of a bony substance. Usually caused by conversion of fibrous tissue or cartilage into bone.

Osteochondroma cartilagenous exostosis. Benign bone tumor containing cartilage and bone usually affecting the metaphyses of long bones, costochondral junctions, or spinal processes. May also refer to intra-articular free bodies as seen in osteochondritis dissecans.

Osteogenesis imperfecta generalized condition caused by defect in collagen production, which causes fragile bones.

Osteolysis a localized area of bone loss caused by removal or loss of calcium

Osteomalacia softening of the bones because of faulty mineralization of available osteoid.

Osteomyelitis infection of the bones caused by a pyogenic organism (e.g., bacterial, fungal, protozoal organisms).

Osteopenia synonym for osteoporosis

Osteopetrosis increased bone opacity resulting from prenatal bone that has not converted to cancellous bone. Also called marble bone.

Osteophyte a bony growth projecting outward from the bone usually at periarticular margins. Also called bone spur.
Osteoporosis decrease in radiopacity of bone caused by reduction in bone mass or atrophy (increased porousness).
Otic canalography a radiographic contrast study to visualize the external auditory canal.
Palmar refers to the surface of the limb from the carpus distally (Refer to Figure 1.3).
Palmar-dorsal entrance of the x-ray beam on the palmar aspect of the leg and exiting on the dorsal aspect of the leg from the carpus distally.
Panosteitis self-limiting bone disorder that causes lameness as a result of an acute onset of long bone pain. Also called eosinophilic panosteitis and enostosis.
Patchy clouding (pulmonary) amorphous radiopacities with poorly defined margins, often 1 to 2 cm in diameter.
Pathologic fracture a fracture through weakened bone caused by an underlying disease or developmental defect. Often associated with bone neoplasia or secondary to metabolic bone disease.
Physis the cartilagenous growth plate located between the metaphysis and the epiphysis of a long bone.
Physis fracture a fracture through a physis occurring in immature animals. Subclassified as Salter-Harris fractures I through V according to the location of the fracture lines of the epiphysis, physis, and metaphysis.
Phytobezoar a concretion of fruit and vegetable fibers within the stomach or intestine.
Plantar refers to the surface of the limb from the tarsus distally (Refer to Figure 1.3).
Plantar-dorsal entrance of the x-ray beam on the plantar aspect of the leg and exiting on the dorsal aspect of the leg from the tarsus distally.
Pleural thickening fibrin or calcific deposits on the parietal or visceral pleura.
Pleurography a radiographic contrast study to visualize the parietal and visceral pleural surfaces.
Pneumatocoele air-filled pulmonary cyst usually secondary to pulmonary trauma.
Pneumatosis the presence of gas or air in an abnormal situation in the body. Examples include pneumatosis coli (gas in colonic wall) and pneumatosis pulmonum (pulmonary emphysema)
Pneumopericardiography a radiographic contrast study of the pericardial space to evaluate the pericardial sac, epicardial surface of the heart, and origin of the aorta and pulmonary arteries.
Pneumoperitoneography a radiographic contrast to evaluate the peritoneal cavity.
Pneumothorax presence of free air or gas within the pleural space.
Pneumothorax, open pneumothorax secondary to laceration of the chest wall
Pneumothorax, tension causes compression atelectasis of the lung through the valve or flap-like action of a tear in the visceral pleura or chest wall.
Portography a radiographic contrast study of the portal venous system.
Pronate to turn a limb inward so that the plantar or palmar surface faces downward and the dorsal or cranial surface faces upward.
Proximal anatomic term for the end of a leg or other part that is nearest the point of attachment. Opposed to distal (Refer to Figure 1.3).
Pyothorax accumulation of exudate within the pleural cavity.
Radiograph a photographic image of an object (e.g., internal structures of an animal) produced by a beam of penetrating ionizing radiation passing through the object.
Radiography the science and art of making a radiograph.
Radiologist a specialist trained in the diagnostic and therapeutic uses of x-rays, radionuclides, radiation physics, and radiation biology.
Radiology the scientific discipline of medical imaging using ionizing radiation, radionuclides, nuclear magnetic resonance, and ultrasound.
Radiolucent the characteristic of tissue or material that permits most of the x-ray photons to pass through unaffected (penetrable x-rays) and has the blacker film density when the x-ray film is processed.
Radiopaque the characteristic of tissue or material that causes it to absorb a large percentage of the x-ray beam (less penetrable x-rays) and therefore appear on the radiograph as a whiter film density.
Recumbent the animal's position is horizontal (lateral, sternal, or dorsal recumbency) and the x- ray beam is perpendicular to the long axis of the body.
Reticular shadows term to describe a fine interlacing pattern of lines. Usually part of the interstitial pulmonary pattern.
Roentgenography a synonym for radiography.
Rostral an anatomic direction toward the head, especially toward the nose. Opposed to caudal.
Sacrococcygeal dysgenesis developmental anomaly consisting of absence of one or more sacral or coccygeal vertebrae.
Sail sign a triangular "sail-like" structure representing the thymus visible on the ventrodorsal/dorsoventral projections of the thorax.
Saggital situated in the direction of the ventrodorsal plane or in a section parallel to the long axis of the body.
Scalloping alterations in the diaphragm with visibility of small muscle fascicles near their insertions on the caudal rib margins, usually seen in severe pulmonary hyperinflation.
Serial radiographs those taken in sequence during a single study (e.g., gastrointestinal series) or after longer intervals of time (e.g., days or weeks) for follow-up evaluation of a disorder.
Sialography a radiographic contrast study of the salivary ducts and glands.
Signet ring sign radiographic appearance of end-on view of a bronchus and adjacent pulmonary artery
Silhouette sign used to localize a disease process based on tenet that an intrathoracic lesion touching a border of the heart, aorta, or diaphragm will obliterate that border on the radiograph. An intrathoracic lesion not anatomically continuous with a border of these structures will not obliterate that border.
Spina bifida developmental failure of the lateral arches to fuse dorsally, causing incomplete development of the dorsal spinal processes.
Spondylitis bony reaction on a vertebral body associated with infection.
Spondylosis deformans a noninflammatory degenerative disorder associated with the intervertebral joints and characterized by osteophytes originating at the margins of the endplates.
Stress fracture a fatigue fracture caused by repetitive stress with a gradual interruption in the bone structure at a greater rate than can be offset by the reparative process.
String sign appearance of barium contrast media in the narrowed lumen through the pyloric sphincter; a sign associated with pyloric stenosis.
Supinate to turn a limb so that the plantar or palmar surface

faces upward and the dorsal or cranial surface faces downward.

Survey radiograph a standard radiographic study of a large area made without the use of contrast media, usually preceding a contrast procedure.

Synostosis union between two adjacent bones.

Table top technique radiographic technique that does not use a grid and permits positioning of the film on the top of the table just beneath the animal.

Tissue density relationship of density of the body tissues, with teeth and bone most dense and air or gas least dense.

Tit sign radiographic appearance of the pyloric antrum during a barium contrast study. There is a relatively sharp, pointed, outpouching of the pyloric antrum along the lesser curvature as a peristaltic wave pushes the contrast medium up against a mass-like or stenotic lesion around the pylorus.

Tracheoesophageal stripe sign a radiographic sign that indicates that the esophagus contains gas. The esophageal wall causes a silhouette sign with the dorsal tracheal wall and mimics a false thickening of the tracheal wall.

Tracheography a radiographic contrast study to visualize the luminal anatomy of the trachea.

Tram lines parallel opaque lines of the bronchi used to describe a bronchial pattern.

Transitional vertebra a developmental anomaly in which a vertebra has some anatomic characteristics of an adjacent vertebral region.

Trichobezoar a concretion of hair contained within the stomach or intestine.

Trichophytobezoar a concretion of hair and fruit or vegetable fibers within the stomach or intestine.

Upper gastrointestinal study a radiographic contrast study of the esophagus, stomach, and small intestine.

Urethrography a radiographic contrast study of the urethra.

Urography a radiographic contrast study of the kidneys and ureters.

Vascular pattern a radiographic pulmonary pattern in which the arteries or veins are larger or smaller than normal.

Ventral anatomic direction pertaining to the sternal and abdominal surface. Opposed to dorsal (Refer to Figure 1.3).

Ventral recumbency animal is positioned on its sternum.

Ventrodorsal the x-ray beam enters the ventral surface of the animal first, and exits the dorsum nearest the film.

Vertical beam radiographic technique in which the x-ray beam is directed vertically.

Index

Page numbers in *italics* denote figures; those followed by t denote tables.

Abdominal cavity, 217–222. (*see also specific organs*)
  anatomy, 217–219, *218–219*
  radiographic interpretation, 217
    detail, loss of, 217–219
    focal opacities, 220–221
    gas accumulation, 219–220, *219–220*
    hernias, peritoneal, 221–222
    lymph nodes, 221, *221*
Abductor pollicis longus muscle sesamoid, 28, *29*
Abscess
  diaphragm, 184
  liver, 237
  prostate, 287
  pulmonary, 164, *164*
  splenic, 238–239, *239*
Acanthomatous epulis, 123, *124*
Adamantinoma, 123, *123*
Addison's disease, 277
Adenocarcinoma
  gastric, 246
  intestinal, 254
  large bowel, 259
  pancreas, 240
  pulmonary, 169–170
  renal, 269
  urinary bladder, 274
Adrenal glands
  anatomy, 276
  enlargement, 276–277
  hyperadrenocorticism, 277
  hypoadrenocorticism, 277
  mineralization, 277
  pheochromocytoma, 277
Aeleurostrongylus abstrusus, 168
Aggressive vs. nonaggressive bone lesion patterns, 34
Air radiopacity, 10
Alveolar pattern of lung disease, 158
Ameloblastoma, 123
Anconeal process ossification, 31
Angiography, 23–24, 185
Anterior cruciate ligament injury, *93,* 93–94
Anus, imperforate, 260
Aorta, 194
  stenosis, 200, *200–201*
  thromboembolism, 213
ARDS (adult respiratory distress syndrome), 167
Arteriovenous fistula, 57
Arthritis
  erosive, 66–67
  feline polyarthritis, 67
  Greyhound polyarthritis, 67
  Reiter disease, 67
  rheumatoid, 66
  infectious, 63–64, 64t
    bacterial, 63–64
    fungal, 64
    viral, 64
  noninfectious, 64–66, 65t
    Akita heritable polyarthritis, 66
    familial renal amyloidosis, 65–66
    idiopathic polyarthritis, 65
    polyarteritis nodosa, 66
    polyarthritis/polymyositis complex, 65
    Sjogren Syndrome, 65
    systemic lupus erythematosus, 65
Arthrography, 23
Ascites, 196
Aspiration pneumonia, 162, 163–164
  contrast media, 16, 17
  laryngeal paralysis, 151
  vascular ring anomalies, 202
Asthma, feline, 156, *156*
Atelectasis, 165
  mediastinal shift, *171*
  pneumothorax, 178
Atlantoaxial subluxation, *136,* 136–137
Atrioventricular valve dysplasia, 201
Attenuation, 2
Avulsions, 45, *45*
  acromion and scapular spine, *71*
  calcaneal process, *101*
  greater humeral tubercle, *71*
  long digital extensor, 95, *95*
  popliteal muscle, 95, *96*
  scapular tuberosity, *71*
  tibial tuberosity, 97, *97*

Barium enema, 21–22
  cervical masses, 288
  double contrast, 21–22
  indications, 258
  interpretation, 258
  intussusception, 253
  large bowel disorders, 258–260
Barium sulfate, 16–17. (*see also* Contrast radiography)
  adverse reactions, 17
  small intestine, 251
Benign osseous metaplasia, 220
Biceps tendinopathy, 72–73, *73*
Blastomycosis, 168–169
Blebs, pulmonary, 165
Block vertebra, 132, *132*
Bone
  cyst, 52, *53*
  infarcts, 43, *43*
  radiopacity, 10, 34
  scintigraphy, 8
Brain scintigraphy, 8
Bronchi
  anatomy, 147–148, *148*
  asthma, feline, 156, *156*
  bronchiectasis, 155, *155*
  bronchitis, 154–155, *155*
  collapse, 154, *155*
  obstruction, 155–156, *156*
Bronchial pattern of lung disease, 159
Bronchogenic carcinoma, 169
Bronchogenic cysts, 165
Bronchography, 25
Brucella canis, 283

Calcaneon tendon injury, 101, *101*
Calcification
  bladder wall, 271
  dystrophic, 220
  metastatic, 220
  pancreas, 240
  renal, 264
Calcinosis circumscripta, 56, *57*
  spinal, 142–143
Calcinosis cutis, 220
Calcium tungstate phosphors, 2
Calculi, 220
  gall bladder, 236, *236*
  prostatic, 282, *282*
  renal, 264, 268, *268*
  salivary, 124
  ureteral, 268
  urethral, 275
  urinary bladder, 271, 272–273
Calculus, dental, 120
Carbon dioxide as contrast medium, 17, 22
Cardiogenic edema, 160–161, *161*
Cardiomegaly, 192–194, *194*
Cardiomyopathy
  Boxer, 208–209
  English Cocker Spaniel, 209
  dilated, canine, 207–208, *208*
  dilated, feline, 211, *211*
  Doberman Pincher, 208
  hyperthyroidism, 212
  hypertrophic, canine, 209
  hypertrophic, feline, 209–210, *209–210*
  indeterminate, 211
  restrictive, feline, 210
Cardiovascular contrast procedures
  angiography, 23–24
  pneumopericardiography, 24
  venous portography, 24
Caries, 120, *120*
Carpus
  anatomy, *81, 83–84*
  fractures, 81, *82*
  luxation/subluxation, 81, *81*
  physis closure, 27t, 28t
  radiographic technique, 80
  sesamoids, 28, *29, 31*
Cartilage joints (synchondroses), 59–60
Cauda equina syndrome, 137–138, *138*
Caudal cruciate ligament injury, 94
Caudal vena cava, 195
Cecal inversion, 259, *259*
Cecum, 255–257
Celiography, 22
Cervical masses, 288, *288*
Cervical spondylopathy, 137, *137*
Chemodectoma, 212
Chest wall, 179–182
  congenital anomalies, 180–181
  fractures, 181, *181*
  masses, 181–182
  pectus carinatum, 180
  pectus excavatum, 180, *180*
  soft tissue abnormalities, 179–180
  sternal dysraphism, 180
Cholecystitis, 235–236
Chondrodysplasia, 36–38, 36t
  dwarfism
    Alaskan Malamutes, 38
    Norwegian Elkhound, 38
    pituitary, 37
    Samoyed, ocular-skeletal, 38
  enchondrodystrophy, 37–38
  epiphyseal dysplasia, multiple, 37
  Great Pyrenee, 38
  hypothyroidism, congenital, 37
  Labrador Retriever skeletal-retinal dysplasia, 38
  proportionate/disproportionate, 36
  tibial metaphyseal dysplasia, 39
Chronic obstructive pulmonary disease (COPD), 165–166
Chylothorax, 26, 175
Coccidiodomycosis, 169
Codman's triangle, *33,* 34
Colitis, 258, *259*
Colon. (*see* Large bowel)
Colonic examination, positive contrast, 22
Compression fracture, 44
Compression radiography, 257
Compression/distraction radiograph, 89–90
Computed tomography (CT), 6 (*see also specific organs and areas*)
  components, *6*
  intracranial neoplasms, 114
  spine, 128
Conformational deformities, 62
Congenital diseases/disorders
  heart, 197–203
  imperforate anus, 260
  joints, 62
  megaesophagus, 230
  renal, 265–266
Congestive heart failure, 195–196
  pleural effusion, 175
Contrast radiography, 15–26
  angiography, 23–24
  arthrography, 23
  barium enema, 21–22
  bronchography, 25
  colonic techniques, 22
  cystography, 18–19, 271–274
    double contrast, 18
    indications for, 271
    interpretation of, 271–272
    pneumocystography, 19
    positive contrast, 19
  dacryocystorhinography, 25–26
  discography, 23
  echocardiography, 186
  epidurography, 22–23
  esophagography, 20
  fistulography, 24–25
  gastrography, 20–21
  gastrointestinal
    esophagus, 226–231
    large bowel, 257–260
    liver, 235
    pancreas, 240
    pharynx, 224
    small intestine, 251–254
    stomach, 244–249
  intravenous urography, 264–270
  media, 15–17, 251
    adverse reactions, 16–17
    barium sulfate, 16–17
    ionic and nonionic, 15–16
    negative, 17
  lymphography, 26
  myelography, 22
  otic canalography, 26
  patient preparation, 15
  peritoneography, 22
  pleurography, 25
  pneumopericardiography, 24
  rhinography, 26
  sialography, 25
  tracheography, 25
  upper gastrointestinal study, 21, 240, 244–249, 251–254
  urethrography, 19, 274–276
  urography, intravenous (IVU), 17–18
  vaginography, 19–20
  venous portography, 24
Cor pulmonale, 16, 153, 193
Coronoid process, medial
  fragmented, 76, 77–78
  ossification, 32
Coxofemoral joint. (*see* Hip)
Cranial cruciate ligament injury, *93,* 93–94
Cranial hyperostosis, 112–113
Craniomandibular osteopathy (CMO), *112,* 112–113
Cricopharyngeal achalasia, 224–225
Cruciate ligament injury, *93,* 93–94
Cryptococcosis, 169
Cryptorchidism, 283
CT (computed tomography). (*see* Computed tomography (CT))
Cushing's syndrome, 277
Cystic endometrial hyperplasia, 287–288
Cystine calculi, 273
Cystography, 18–19
  double contrast, 18, 272, 274
  pneumocystography, 19
  positive contrast, 19
Cystourethrography, voiding, 274
Cysts
  bone, 52, *53*
  bronchogenic, 165
  oral, *123,* 123–124
  paraprostatic, *281,* 282
  perinephric pseudocyst, 267–268, *268*
  pulmonary, 165
  renal, 267–268, *267–268*

Dacryocystorhinography, 25–26, 125
Dentigerous cyst, *123,* 124
Diagnostic radiology
  overview, 1–3
    film identification, 3
    positioning, 3
    technique, 3

Diaphragm, 182–184
abscess, 184
anatomy, 149, 182
herniation, 183, *183,* 221
peritoneopericardial hernia, 214
radiographic interpretation, 182
tumors, 183–184
Digits
anatomy, 82–83, *82–84*
fractures, 84
luxation, 84
neoplasia, 84–85
polydactyly, 36
radiographic technique, 82
sesamoids, 28, *30*
syndactyly, 36
Dirofilaria immitis. (*see* Heartworm disease)
DISH (disseminated idiopathic skeletal hyperostosis), 143
Diskography, 23, 127, 138
Diskospondylitis, 144, *144*
Distractio cubiti, 78, *78*
Distraction Index, hip, 89
Diverticuli
esophageal, *229,* 229–230
rectal, 260
Doppler echocardiography, 186
Doppler ultrasound, 5
Dorsal acetabular rim projection (DAR), 90
Dural ossification, 142
Dwarfism
Proportionate and disproportionate
Alaskan Malamute, 38
Norwegian Elkhound, 38
pituitary, 37
Samoyed, 38
Great Pyrenee, 39
Laborador Retriever, 39
hypothyroidism, 38
Dysphagia, 224–225
Dysplasia (Joints)
hip, 81–91
shoulder, 72
elbow, 74–79
tarsus, 39
Dystocia, 287
Dystrophic mineralization, 56, 220, 264

Ears
otic canalography, 26
otitis, *113,* 113–114
Echocardiography, 186
Ectrodactyly, 35, *36*
Edema
lymphedema, 57–58
pharyngeal, 223
pulmonary, 160–161, *161,* 196
Effusion
joint, 60, *61,* 93–94
pericardial, 214–215, *215*
peritoneal, 218–219, 239
Ehrlichiosis, 64
Elbow
anatomy, *74–76*
diseases/disorders
distracto cubiti, 78, *78*
dysplasia, 76, *77*
fragmented medial coronoid process, 76, 77–78
incomplete ossification of humeral condyle, 78, *79*
luxation, 79
medial epicondylar spur, 79–80, *80*
osteochondrosis/osteochondritis dissecans, 76, *77*
subluxation, 79, *80*
ununited anconeal process, 76, 77, *77*
radiographic technique, 74
sesamoids, 28, *29*
Embolism
gas, 17
pulmonary, 166–167
Emphysema, 165
abdominal, 219
gall bladder, 236
musculocutaneous, 56
subcutaneous, 116, 172
urinary bladder, 273, *273*
Emphysematous bulla, *162*
Emphysematous cystitis, 273, *273*
Empyema, 175
Enchondrodystrophy, 37–38
Enchondroma, 52
Endocardiosis, 203
Enema, barium, 21–22
Enostosis, 42
Eosinophilic panosteitis, 42
Eosinophilic pneumonia, 164, *164*
Epididymitis, 283
Epidurography, 22–23, 127, 138
Epiphysis
dysplasia, multiple, 37
growth plate injury, 63
vertebral fracture, 140, *140*
Epulis, 123, *124*
Esophagography, 20, 185, 226–231, *231*
vascular ring anomalies, *202*
Esophagus
anatomy, 225–226, *226*
contrast radiography, 226–231
diverticuli, *229,* 229–230
esophagitis, 227
foreign bodies, 227
intussusception, gastroesophageal, 230–231, *231*
megaesophagus, 230, *230–231*
neoplasia, 229
stricture, 228–229
vascular ring anomalies, 227–228, *228*
Excretory urography (EU), 17–18
Exostosis, 52, *52*
Extremities, 27–58
anatomy, 27–32
clinical and radiographic correlations, 32
diseases/disorders
bone infarcts, 43, *43*
chondrodysplasia, 36–38
ectrodactyly, 35, *36*
feline osteodystrophy, 39
growth arrest lines, 41, *41*
hemimelia, 36
hypertrophic osteodystrophy (HOD), 40, *40*
hypertrophic osteopathy, 41, *42*
lead poisoning, 43
mucopolysaccharidosis, 39
osteogenesis imperfecta, 39–40
osteopetrosis, 35
osteoporosis, 34, 35, *35*
panosteitis, 42, *42*
polydactyly, 36
retained enchondral cartilage, 40, *41*
rickets, 41
syndactyly, 36
fractures
complications, 47–52
delayed union, 47–48, *48*
malunion, 48, *48*
nonunion, 48, *48*
osteomyelitis, 50–52
physeal closure, premature, 48–50, *49–50*
pseudoarthrosis, 48
healing, 46–47, 46t
type classification, 43–46, 43t, *44–46*
interpretation, radiographic, 33–35
definitions, 34–35, 34t
musculocutaneous diseases, 55–58
neoplasia, 52–55
ossification, 27–32, 27t–28t, *29–32,* 32t
sesamoids, 28, *29–31*
technique, radiographic, 33

Fat
opacity, 10
radiographic contrast, 217
saponification, 240
Feline
asthma, 156, *156*
cardiomyopathy, 209–211
congenital heart disorders, 198t
hypervitaminosis A, 135
mucopolysaccharidosis, 135–136, *136*
osteochondromatosis, 52
perirenal cysts, 267–268, *268*
polyarthritis, 67
Feline infectious peritonitis (FIP), 175, 214, 262–263
Feminization, 283, 284
Femur
head/neck fractures, 87, *87*
ischemic necrosis of head, *87,* 87–88
physis closure, 27t, 28t
Fetus
death, 287
ossified, 220–221
Fibrocartilage joints, 60
Fibrous joints (synarthroses), 59
Fibula, physis closure of, 27t, 28t
Filaroides osleri, 154

Film, x-ray, 2–3
identification, 3
object-film distance, 10
FIP (feline infectious peritonitis), 175, 214, 262–263
Fistula
arteriovenous, 57
fistulography, 24–25
salivary duct, 124
Fluoroscopy, 4
dysphagia, 225
esophagography, 20
gastric emptying, 244
gastrography, 20–21
pyloric outflow obstruction, 249
Focal spot
oral radiographs, 120
x-ray tube, 10
Foramen magnum, *107*
Foreign bodies
diskospondylitis, 144
esophageal, 227
gastric, 247, *247*
linear, 253, *253*
nasal, 117
small intestine, *252–253*, 253
soft tissue, 58
tracheal, 154
Fractures. (*see also* Avulsions)
carpus, 81, *82*
central tarsal bone, *100*
complications, 47–52
delayed union, 47–48, *48*
malunion, 48, *48*
nonunion, 48, *48*
osteomyelitis, 50–52
physeal closure, premature, 48–50, *49–50*
pseudoarthrosis, 48
digits, 84
femoral head/neck, 87, *87*
healing, 46–47, 46t
os penis, 284
patella, *98*
pelvis, 86, *86*
rib, 181, *181*
shoulder, 71, *71*
skull, 109, *111*, 111–112, 116
tooth, 122, *122*
type classification, 43–46, 43t, *44–46*
vertebral, 139–140, *139–140*
Fragmented medial coronoid process (FMCP), 76, 77–78
Frontal sinuses, *106*
Fungal infections
arthritis, 64
rhinitis, 117, *117*

Gall bladder
anatomy, *232*, 235, *235*
cholecystitis, 235–236, *236*
cholelithiasis, 236, *236*
parasitic disease, 236
Gas opacity, 10
Gastric dilation and volvulus (GDV), 247–248, *248*
Gastrocnemius tendon rupture, *96*
Gastrography, 20–21
Gastrointestinal system
contrast procedures, 20–22
barium enema, 21–22
colonic examination, 22
gastrography, 20–21
upper GI study, 21
esophagus
anatomy, 225–226, *226*
contrast radiography, 226–231
diverticuli, *229*, 229–230
esophagitis, 227
foreign bodies, 227
intussusception, gastroesophageal, 230–231, *231*
megaesophagus, 230, *230–231*
neoplasia, 229
stricture, 228–229
vascular ring anomalies, 227–228, *228*
gall bladder
anatomy, *232*, 235, *235*
cholecystitis, 235–236, *236*
cholelithiasis, 236, *236*
parasitic disease, 236
large bowel
anatomy, 255, *256–257*
cecal inversion, 259, *259*
colitis, 258, *259*
contrast radiographs, 257–260
diverticuli, 260
hernia, 260
imperforate anus, 260
neoplasia, 259–260, *260*
radiographic interpretation, 255–258
liver
anatomy, 231–233, *232*
hepatomegaly, 233–234, *233–234*
small, 234–235, *235*
pharynx/larynx, 223–225
anatomy, 223, *224*
dysphagia, 224–225
inflammation, 223
masses, 223–224, 225, *226*
small intestine
anatomy, 243, 249–250
enteritis, 251
inflammatory bowel disease (IBD), 251
intussusception, *252–253*, 253–254
mesenteric thrombosis, 254–255
mesenteric volvulus, 254
neoplasia, 254, *254*
obstruction, 251–252, *252*
perforation, 255
radiographic interpretaion, 250
spleen
abscessation, 238–239, *239*
anatomy, 237
neoplasia, 238, *238–239*
rupture, 239
splenomegaly, *237*, 237–238
torsion, 238, *238*
stomach
anatomy, 240–242, *241–243*
dilation and volvulus (GDV), 247–248, *248*
emptying, 244
enlargement, 242
foreign bodies, 247, *247*
gastritis, 245, *245*
neoplasia, *246*, 246–247
pyloric outflow obstruction, 248–249, *249*
radiographic interpretation, 241–242, *242*
ulceration, 245–246
wall anomalies, 244
Genital system, 279–289
female
anatomy, 284, *285–286*
cystic endometrial hyperplasia, 287–288
dystocia/fetal death, 287
hermaphroditism, 289
masses
cervical, 288, *288*
ovarian, 285
uterine, 285–286
pregnancy, 287
pyometra, 285, 287–288, *287–288*
vaginal, 288
male
anatomy, 279–280, *280*
penis disorders, 284
prostate gland
abscess, 281–282
anatomy, 279, *280*
benign hypertrophy, 279–281, *281*
calculi/mineralization, 282
cyst, paraprostatic, *281*, 282
neoplasm, 282–283
prostatitis, 281–282
testicles
cryptorchidism, 283
neoplasia, 283, 284
orchitis/epididymitis, 283
torsion, 283–284
Geometry of radiographic images, 10–11
Glucagon, 20
Growth arrest lines, 41, *41*
Gynecomastica, 283, 284

Heart
anatomy, radiographic
dorsoventral projection, *187–188*, 188–189, *192*
lateral projection, 186–188, *187*, *192*
diseases/disorders
acquired
endocardiosis, 203
endocarditis, infectious, 205
heartworm disease, 205–207, *206*
mitral valve insufficiency, 203, *204*

tricuspid valve insufficiency, 204–205, *205*
cardiomyopathy
Boxer, 208–209
dilated, canine, 207–208, *208*
dilated, feline, 211, *211*
Doberman Pincher, 208
English Cocker Spaniel, 209
hyperthyroidism, 212
hypertrophic, canine, 209
hypertrophic, feline, 209–210, *209–210*
indeterminate, 211
restrictive, feline, 210
congenital, 197–203
aortic stenosis, 200, *200–201*
AV valve dysplasia, 201
in cats, 198t
in dogs, 197t–198t
PDA (patent ductus arteriosus), 198–199, *199*
pulmonic stenosis, 199–200, *200*
situs inversus, 202–203
Tetralogy of Fallot, 201
vascular ring anomalies, *202*, 202
VSD (ventricular septal defect), 201
congestive heart failure, 195–196
hypertension, systemic, 212
microcardia, 196–197, *197*
neoplasia, 212–213, *213*
pericardial, 213–216
constrictive pericarditis, 215–216
cysts, 214
effusion, 214–215, *215*
hernia, 214
masses, 216
thromboembolism, aortic, 213
interpretation, radiographic, 189
radiographic technique, 185–186
contrast procedures, 185–186
echocardiography, 186
size and shape, 186–187, 189–194
cardiomegaly, 192–194, *194*
left atrial enlargement, 193
left ventricular enlargement, 193
microcardia, 196–197, *197*
normal, 189–192
right atrial enlargement, 192–193
right ventricular enlargement, 193
variables, *190–191*, 190–192
vessel evaluation
aorta/aortic arch, 194
caudal vena cava, 195
hypervascularity, 195
hypovascularity, 195
pulmonary artery segment, 194–195
Heart base tumors, 212–213, *213*
Heartworm disease, 193, 205–207, *206*
canine, 206
eosinophilic pneumonia, 164
feline, 206–207
hypervascularity, 199199
thromboembolism, 166
Heel effect, 10–11
Hemimelia, 36
Hemivertebra, 132–133, *133*
Hemothorax, 175
Hepatomegaly, 233–234, 241
Hermaphroditism, 289
Hernias
common locations, *222*
congenital, 221
contrast radiography, 222
diaphragmatic, 183, *183*, 214
inguinal, 221
perineal, 260
peritoneal, 221–222
peritoneopericardial diaphragmatic, 214
Hip
anatomy, 85–86, *85–86, 88*
diseases/disorders
dysplasia, 88–91, *90*
accuracy of radiographic diagnosis, 90
control programs, 90–91
radiographic techniques, 88–90
femoral head/neck fractures, 87, *87*
ischemic necrosis of femoral head, *87*, 87–88
luxation, 86, *86*
pelvic fractures, 86, *86*
ossification, *31*
radiographic technique, 85, 88–90
Histiocytic colitis, 258
Histoplasmosis, 168, *168*
Horizontal beam radiography, 147, 165
peritoneal gas, 220
pleural effusion, 176
Humerus, physis closure of, 27t, 28t
Hyaline cartilage, 59–60
Hydrocephalus, 110, *111*
Hydronephrosis, 268–269, *269*
Hyperadrenocorticism, 277
Hyoid bones, 152
Hyperparathyroidism, *123*
Hypertension, systemic, 212
Hyperthyroid myocardial disease, 212
Hypertrophic cardiomyopathy, 209–210, *209–210*
Hypertrophic osteodystrophy (HOD), 40, *40*
Hypertrophic osteopathy (HO), 41, *42*
Hypertrophic pulmonary osteoarthropathy (HPOA), 41, *42*
Hypervitaminosis A, 135
Hypoadrenocorticism, 196, 277
Hypothyroidism, congenital, 37
Hypovolemic shock, 196

Idiopathic polyarthritis, 65
Iliopsoas muscle sesamoid, *31*
Imaging procedures
computed tomography, 6
diagnostic radiology, 1–3
fluoroscopy, 4
magnetic resonance imaging (MRI), 6–8
nuclear imaging, 8
ultrasound, 4–6
Imperforate anus, 260
Infarcts, bone, 43, *43*
Inflammatory bowel disease (IBD), 251, 258
Infraspinatus muscle
sesamoid, *30, 73*
tendinopathy, 73, *73*
Inguinal hernia, 221
Institute for Genetic Disease Control in Animals (GDC), 91
Insulinoma, 240
International Elbow Working Group (IEWG), 76
Interpretation of radiographs
principles, 9–13
Interstitial pattern of lung disease, 159
Interstitial pneumonia, 163, *163*
Intervertebral disk disease, 140–142, *141*
myelography, 129–131
Intestinal obstruction, 251–252, *252*
Intravenous urography (IVU), 17–18, 264–270
indications, 264
interpretation, 264–265
Intussusception
gastroesophageal, 230–231, *231*
gastrointestinal, 251–252, *252–253*
Iodinated contrast media, 15–16. (*see also* Contrast radiography)
excretion, 16
gastric emptying, 244
gastric lesions, 244
side effects, 16
small intestine, 251
Ischemic necrosis of femoral head, *87*, 87–88

Joints, 59–103
arthrography, 23
carpus, 80–82
clinical and radiographic correlations, 61
digit, 82–85
diseases/disorders
arthritis
erosive, 66–67
infections, 63–64, 64t
noninfectious, 64–66, 65t
classifications of, 61t
conformational/deformities, 62
congenital malformations, 62
neoplasia, 67–68
metastatic, 68
primary bone sarcoma, 67
synovial cell sarcoma, 67
osteochondrosis/osteochondritis dissecans, 62
synovial osteochondromatosis, 68, *68*
trauma, 63
villonodular synovitis, 68
effusion, 60, *61*, 93–94
elbow, 74–80
hip, 85–91

Joints–*Continued*
  interpretation, radiographic, 60–61
  shoulder, 68–74
  stifle, 91–98
  tarsus, 99–103
  technique, radiographic, 60
  types, 59–60

Kartagener's syndrome, 202
Kidneys. (*see also* Urinary system)
  anatomy, 261–262, *262*
  contrast radiography, 264–270
    indications, 264
    interpretation, 264–265
  diseases/disorders
    calculi, 268, *268*
    congenital, 265–266
    cysts, 267–268, *267–268*
    hydronephrosis, 268–269, *269*
    neoplasia, 269
    nephritis/pyelonephritis, 266–267
    rupture, 269–270
  radiographic interpretation, 262–264, *263–264*
Kyphosis, 134

Labrador Retriever retinal dysplasia, 38
Large bowel
  anatomy, 255, *256–257*
  cecal inversion, 259, *259*
  colitis, 258, *259*
  contrast radiographs, 257–260
  diverticuli, 260
  hernia, 260
  imperforate anus, 260
  neoplasia, 259–260, *260*
  radiographic interpretation, 255–258
Larynx, 223–224
  anatomy, *151*
  hypoplasia, 151
  laryngeal paralysis, 151
  mineralization, 150–151
  neoplasia, 151–152
  radiographic interpretation, 150–151
Lead poisoning (plumbism), 43
Linear foreign bodies, 253, *253*
Liver
  anatomy, 231–233, *232*
  hepatomegaly, 233–234, *233–234*
  small, 234–235, *235*
Liver fluke, 241
Long digital extensor avulsion, 95, *95*
Lordosis, 134
Lumbosacral instability, 137–138, *138*
Lungs
  anatomy, 149
  diseases/disorders
    abscessation, 164, *164*
    ARDS (adult respiratory distress syndrome), 167
    atelectasis, 165
    cavitary lesions, 165
    chronic obstructive pulmonary disease (COPD), 165–166
    emphysema, 165
    hematoma, 162
    hemorrhage, 162
    neoplasia, 169–170, *170*
    pneumonia, 162–164
      aspiration, 163–164
      eosinophilic, 164, *164*
      interstitial, 163, *163*
      mycotic, *168,* 168–169
      parasitic, 167–168, *167–168*
    pulmonary edema, 160–161, *161*
    radiopacity and differential diagnosis, 157t–158t
    thrombosis/thromboembolism, 166–167
    torsion, 166
  radiographic interpretation
    patterns of disease, 158–160
      alveolar, 158
      bronchial, 159
      interstitial, 159
      vascular, 159–160
    radiopacity
      increased, 157t–158t
      mineralization/calcification, 158t
      multiple focal, 157t
      multiple ill-defined, 157t
      solitary lesions, 157t
Luxation
  carpus, 81
  coxofemoral, 86, *86*
  digits, 84
  elbow, 79
  patella, 95, 97–98, *98*
  shoulder, 70–71, *71*
  stifle, 95
  tarsus, *100,* 100–101
  temporomandibular, *111,* 112
Lymph nodes, retropharyngeal, 224
Lymphadenopathy, 57
Lymphangectasia, 26, 175
Lymphedema, 57–58
Lymphography, 26
Lymphosarcoma
  gastric, 246
  intestinal, 254
  larynx, 151
  myocardial, 212
  pleural effusion, 175
  pulmonary, 169–170
  renal, 269

Magnetic resonance imaging (MRI), 6–8
  components, *7*
  intracranial neoplasms, 114
  spine, 128
Mandible
  periostitis, *112,* 112–113
  radiographic technique, *107*
Manx cat spina bifida, 132
Marie's disease, 41, *42*
Maxilla, radiographic technique for, *107*
Medial epicondylar spur, 80, *80*
Mediastinum, 171–174
  anatomy, 149, 171
  enlargement, 173–174, *174*
  esophageal foreign bodies, 227
  masses, 172–173, *173*
  pneumomediastinum, 172, *172*
  shift, *171,* 171–172
Megacolon, 255
Megaesophagus, 152, 230, *230–231*
Meningioma, 114, *116*
Meningitis/polyarthritis syndrome, 65
Mesentery
  hernia, 221–222
  thrombosis, 254–255
Metacarpus physis closure, 27t, 28t
Metatarsal physis closure, 27t, 28t
Metaphyseal tibial dysplasia, 39
Microcardia, 196–197, *197*
Mineralization
  abdominal cavity, 220
  adrenal gland, 277
  dystrophic, 264
  intervertebral disc, *141*
  laryngeal cartilages, 150–151
  lung disease, 158t
  prostate, 281–282
Mitral valve insufficiency, 193, 203, *204*
Monteggia fracture, 79
Motion artifact, 3
MRI. (*see* Magnetic resonance imaging [MRI])
Mucometra, 287
Mucopolysaccharidosis, 39, 135–136, *136*
Multiple myeloma, 114, *115*
Musculocutaneous soft-tissue disease, 55–58
  emphysema, 56
  fistula, 57
  foreign bodies, 57
  lymphadenopathy, 57
  lymphedema, 57–58
  masses, 55
  mineralization, 56, 56t
  swelling, 55
Mycoplasma species, 64, 67
Mycotic infections
  osteomyelitis, 50–52, *51*
  pneumonia, 162, *168,* 168–169
Myelography
  indications and technique, 22
  lumbosacral instability, 138
  nonionic contrast media, 15
  spinal neoplasms, 146
Myelosclerosis, 35
Myositis ossificans, 56

Nasal cavity
  anatomy, 116, *116*
  nasopharyngeal polyps, 113, *114*
  neoplasia, 117–118, *118*
  radiographic technique, *106, 107*
  rhinitis/sinusitis, 116–117, *117*
  rhinography, 26
Nasolacrimal duct
  abnormalities, 125
  dacryocystorhinography, 25–26
Nasopharyngeal polyps, 113, *114,* 224, *225*
Nephritis, 266–267
Nephrocalcinosis, 264

Nitrous oxide as contrast medium, 17, 22
Nocardiosis, 169
Norberg angle, 88, *89*
Nuclear imaging. (*see* Scintigraphy)

Occipital dysplasia, 111, *111*
OCD. (*see* Osteochondrosis/osteochondritis dissecans)
Odontoid process, 136
Omphlophlebitis, 64
Opacity, 9–10
  bone, 10, 34
  fat, 10
  gas, 10
  interpretation
    decreased, 13t
    increased, 12t
  soft-tissue, 10
Oral cavity. (*see also* Teeth)
  neoplasia, *123,* 123–124
Orchitis, 283
Orthopedic Foundation for Animals (OFA), 90–91
Os coxae physis closure, 27t
Os penis
  fracture, 284
  ossification, 32
Ossicles
  dorsal acetabular rim, *31*
  glenoid, *30*
  table of, 32t
Ossification, *30–31,* 32t
  accessory centers, 28–32, 32t
  DISH (disseminated idiopathic skeletal hyperostosis), 143
  dura mater, 142
  incomplete of humeral condyle, 78, *79*
  intraarticular, 97
  physis closure
    canine, 27t
    feline, 28t
  sesamoids, 28, *29–31*
  soft tissue, 56, 56t
  tendonitis, ossifying, 56
  vertebrae, 127, *128*
Osteochondroma, 52–53, *53*
Osteochondromatosis, spinal, 144–145, *145*
Osteochondrosis/osteochondritis dissecans
  clinical correlations, 62
  elbow, 76, *77*
  shoulder, 72, *72*
  spine, 138, *139*
  stifle, *94,* 94–95
  tarsus, 102, *102*
Osteogenesis imperfecta, 39
Osteolysis, 34
Osteoma, 52, 114, *115*
Osteomalacia, 34–35
Osteomyelitis, 50–52
Osteopetrosis, 35, *35*
Osteophytes and spondylosis deformans, 143
Osteoporosis, 35, *35*
  defined, 34
  differential diagnosis, 135t
  spinal, 134–135
Osteosclerosis, 35
Otic canalography, 26
Otitis, *113,* 113–114
Ovarian masses, 285

Pancreas, 239–240, *240*
Panosteitis, 42
Paragonimus kellicotti, 167, *168*
Paraprostatic cysts, *281,* 282
Parasitic disease
  gall bladder, 236
  pneumonia, 167–168, *167–168*
Patella, 28
  fracture, *98*
  luxation/subluxation, 95, 97–98, *98*
  tendon rupture, 98, *98*
PDA (patent ductus arteriosus), 198–199, *199*
Pectus carinatum, 180
Pectus excavatum, 180, *180*
Pelvis
  fractures, 86, *86*
  sacroiliac luxation, 87
PennHIP, 89, *89,* 90–91
Pericardial sac
  constrictive pericarditis, 215–216
  cysts, 214
  effusion, 214–215, *215*
  hernia, 214
  masses, 216
  pneumopericardiography, 24
Perineal hernia, 260
Perinephric pseudocyst, 267–268, *268*
Periodontal disease, 121, *121*
Periosteal reactions
  hypertrophic osteopathy (HO), *42*
  types, *33,* 33–34
Peritoneal cavity
  anatomy, 217–219
  radiographic interpretation
    detail, loss of, 217–219
    gas accumulation, 219–220
    hernias, 221–222
    lymph nodes, 221
Peritoneography, 22
Peritoneopericardial diaphragmatic hernia, 214
Peritonitis, 218, 253
Persistent right aortic arch (PRAA), 227, *228*
Phalanx physis closure, 27t, 28t
Pharynx, 223–225
  anatomy, 223
  dysphagia, 224–225
  inflammation, 223
  masses, 223–224, *225*
Pheochromocytoma, 277
Philosophy of imaging, 1
Physis
  closure, premature, 48–50, *49–50*
  epiphyseal growth plate injury, 63
  fracture, 45, *46*
Pituitary dwarfism, 37
Platynosomum concinnum, 236
Pleura, 174–179
  anatomy, 149–150, 174
  effusion, 175–176, *175–176*
  masses, *176,* 178
  pleurography, 25
  pneumothorax, 178–179, *179*
  thickening, 176–177, *177*
Pleural effusion, 175–176, *175–176*
Pneumatocoeles, 162, 165
Pneumocolon, 22, 257
Pneumocystis carinii, 169
Pneumocystography, 19, 219
Pneumomediastinum, 172, *172,* 219
Pneumonia, 162–164
  aspiration, 16, 17, 151, 162, 163–164, 202, 228
  eosinophilic, 164, *164*
  interstitial, 163, *163*
  mycotic, *168,* 168–169
  parasitic, 167–168, *167–168*
Pneumopericardiography, 24, 186
Pneumoperitoneography, 219, 276–277
Pneumothorax, 172, 178–179, *179*
Pneumocystography and gas embolism, 17
Polyarteritis nodosa, 66
Polyarthritis/meningitis syndrome, 65
Polyarthritis/polymyositis complex, 65
Polycythemia, 199
Polydactyly, 36
Popliteal fabella, 28
Popliteal muscle avulsion, 95, *96*
Portosystemic vascular shunts, 8, 234
Positioning, 3
Pregnancy
  dystocia/fetal death, 287
  radiographic findings, 287
Prostate gland
  abscess, 281–282
  anatomy, 279, *280*
  benign hypertrophy, 279–281, *281*
  calculi/mineralization, 282
  cyst, paraprostatic, *281,* 282
  neoplasm, 282–283
  prostatitis, 281–282
Protozoan osteomyelitis, 52
Pseudoarthrosis, 48
Pseudodiverticulum, *229*
Pulmonary artery segment enlargement, 194–195
Pulmonary edema, 160–161, *161,* 196
  laryngeal paralysis, 151
Pulmonary hemorrhage, 162
Pulmonary infiltrates with eosinophilia (PIE), 164, *164*
Pulmonary thromboembolism, 166–167
Pulmonary vasculature, 159–160
  anatomy, 148–149, *149*
  hypervascularity, 195
  hypovascularity, 195
  radiographic anatomy, 188
Pulmonic stenosis, 199–200, *200*
Pyelonephritis, 266–267
Pyloric outflow obstruction, 242, 248–249, *249*
Pyometra, 287–288, *287–288*
Pyothorax, 175

Radiograph identification, 3
Radionuclides, 8
Radiopacity. (*see* Opacity)
Radius
  physis closure, 27t, 28t
  premature physeal closure, 49–50, *49–50*
Rare earth phosphors, 2
Reactions, adverse, 16–17t
  barium sulfate, 17
  iodinated contrast media, 16
  negative contrast media, 17
Rectum. (*see also* Large bowel)
  diverticuli, 260
  urethrorectal fistula, 276
Reiter disease, 67
Resorption, tooth, 120, *121*
Respiratory system. (*see* Thorax; *specific organs*)
Retrograde urethrogram and ectopic ureters, 266
Retroperitoneal space
  anatomy, 217
  gas accumulation, 219–220
  lymph node enlargement, 221, *221*
Rheumatoid arthritis, 66, 66t
Rhinography, 26
Ribs, 180–181
Rickets, 41
Rickettsial arthritis, 64

Sacrococcygeal dysgenesis, 134, *134*
Sacroiliac luxation, 87
Salivary glands
  anatomy, 124, *125*
  calculi, 124
  fistula, salivary duct, 124
  nasolacrimal duct disorders, 125
  neoplasia, 124–125
  sialoceole, 124
Salter Harris Classification, 45, *46*
Sarcoma
  primary bone, 67
  synovial cell, 67
Scapula
  avulsions, *71*
  physis closure, 27t, 28t
Schmorl's nodes, 142, *142*
Scintigraphy, 8
  gastric emptying, 244
  pulmonary thromboembolism, 167
  uses, 8
Scoliosis, 134, *135*
Scottish fold feline osteodystrophy, 39
Screens, intensifying, 2
Scrotal hernia, 221
Sertoli cell tumor, 283, 284
Sesamoids, 28
  carpus, 28, 29, *31*
  digits, 28, *30*, *83–84*, 84
  elbow, 28, *29*
  fractures, 84
  physis closure, 28t
  shoulders, 73
  stifle, 28
  tarsus, 28, *29*
Shoulder
  anatomy, *69–70*
  diseases/disorders
    biceps tendinopathy, 72–73, *73*
    dysplasia, 73
    fracture, 71, *71*
    luxation, 70–71, *71*
    osteoarthritis, 73–74
    osteochondrosis/osteochondritis dissecans, 72, *72*
  glenoid ossicles, *30*
  radiographic technique, 68–70
  sesamoids, 27t, 28t, *30*
Sialocoele, 124
Sialography, 25, 124
Silhouette sign, 217
Situs inversus, 202–203
Sjogren Syndrome, 65
Skull, 105–125
  anatomy, 108, *108–110*
    calvarium, *108–110*, 110
    dental, 118–119, *118–119*, 119t
    nasal cavity, 116, *116*
    salivary gland, 124, *125*
  diseases/disorders
    craniomandibular osteopathy (CMO), *112*, 112–113
    dental
      abscessation, 121–122, *122*
      anomalies, 120
      calculus, 120
      caries, 120, *120*
      fracture of tooth, 122, *122*
      metabolic disease, 122–123, *123*
      neoplasia, *123*, 123–124
      periodontal disease, 121, *121*
      resorption, 120, *121*
    ear lesions, *113*, 113–114
    fractures, *111*, 111–112, 116, 122, *122*
    hydrocephalus, 110, *111*
    neoplasia, 114–116, *114–116*
    occipital dysplasia, 111, *111*
    osteomyelitis, 112
    rhinitis/sinusitis, 116–117, *117*
    salivary gland, 124–125
    temporomandibular luxation, *111*, 112
  imaging modalities, 108
  interpretations, radiographic, 110
  technique, radiographic, 105–108
    dental examination, *107*, 120
    projections, 105t, *106–107*
Small intestine
  anatomy, 243, 249–250
  enteritis, 251
  inflammatory bowel disease (IBD), 251
  intussusception, *252–253*, 253–254
  mesenteric thrombosis, 254–255
  mesenteric volvulus, 254
  neoplasia, 254, *254*
  obstruction, 251–252, *252*
  perforation, 255
  radiographic interpretaion, 250
Soft tissue
  emphysema, 56
  fistula, 57
  foreign bodies, 57
  lymphadenopathy, 57
  lymphedema, 57–58
  masses, 55
  mineralization, 56, 56t
  opacity, 10
  swelling, 55
Spina bifida, 131–132, *132*
Spine
  anatomy, 127, *128*
  development, vertebral, 127, *128*
  diseases/disorders
    atlantoaxial subluxation, *136*, 136–137
    block vertebra, 132, *132*
    calcinosis circumscripta, 138–139
    cervical spondylopathy (wobblers), 137, *137*
    curvature deformities, 134, *135*
    DISH (disseminated idiopathic skeletal hyperostosis), 143
    diskospondylitis, 144, *144*
    dural ossification, 142
    hemivertebra, 132–133, *133*
    hypervitaminosis A, 135
    intervertebral disc disease, 140–142, *141*
    lumbosacral instability, 137–138, *138*
    mucopolysaccharidosis, 135–136, *136*
    neoplasia, 145–146
    osteoarthritis, 143
    osteochondromatosis, 144–145, *145*
    osteochondrosis, 138, *139*
    osteoporosis, 134–135, *135*
    sacrococcygeal dysgenesis, 134, *134*
    Schmorl's nodes, 142, *142*
    spina bifida, 131–132, *132*
    spondylitis, *143*, 143–144
    spondylosis deformans, 142, *142–144*
    transitional vertebrae, *133*, 133–134
    trauma, 139–140, *139–140*
  interpretation, radiographic, 128–129, 129–131
  intramedullary lesions, 130–131, *130–131*
  myelography, 127, 129–131
    extradural lesions, 130, *130*
    intradural lesions, 130, *130–131*
    technique, 129
  technique, radiographic, 127
Spiricerca lupi, 229
Spirochetal arthritis, 64
Spleen
  abscessation, 238–239, *239*
  anatomy, 237
  neoplasia, 238, *238–239*
  rupture, 239

splenomegaly, *237,* 237–238
torsion, 238, *238*
Splenoportography, 24
Spondylitis, *143,* 143–144
Spondylosis deformans, 142, *142–143*
Sternal dysraphism, 180
Stifle
anatomy, *91–93*
disease/disorders, 93–98
avulsions, 95–97, *95–97*
caudal cruciate ligament injury, 94
cranial cruciate ligament injury, *93,* 93–94
luxation, 95
ossification, intraarticular, 95
osteochondrosis/osteochondritis dissecans, *94,* 94–95
patellar luxation/subluxation, 95, 97–98, *98*
patellar tendon rupture, 98, *98*
joint effusion, *61*
radiographic technique, 91–93
sesamoids, 28
Stomach
anatomy, 240–242, *241–243*
dilation and volvulus (GDV), 247–248, *248*
emptying, 244
enlargement, 242
foreign bodies, 247, *247*
gastritis, 245, *245*
neoplasia, *246,* 246–247
pyloric outflow obstruction, 248–249, *249*
radiographic interpretation, 241–242, *242*
ulceration, 245–246
wall anomalies, 244
Stress fracture, 45
Stress radiograph for lumbosacral instability, 138
Subluxation
atlantoaxial, *136,* 136–137
carpus, 81, *81*
elbow, 79
patella, 97–98
tarsus, 100–101
Supinator muscle sesamoids, 28, *29*
Supraspinatus muscle
sesamoid, *30, 73*
tendinopathy, 73, *73*
Syndactyly, 36
Synovial joints (diarthroses), 59, *60*
Synovial osteochondromatosis, 68, *68*
Systemic lupus erythematosus (SLE), 65

Tarsus
anatomy, 99–100
diseases/disorders, 100–102
calcaneon tendon injury, 101, *101*
luxation/subluxation, *100,* 100–101
osteochondrosis/osteochondritis dissecans, 102, *102*
physis closure, 27t, 28t
radiographic technique, 99–100, 103
sesamoids, 27, *31*
Tc-99m, 8
Technique charts, 3
Teeth
age and, 119, *119*
anatomy, 118–119, *118–119,* 119t
diseases/disorders
abscess, 121–122, *122*
anomalies, 120
calculus, 120
caries, 120, *120*
fracture of tooth, 122, *122*
metabolic disease, 122–123, *123*
neoplasia, *123,* 123–124
periodontal disease, 121, *121*
resorption, 120, *121*
formulae, 119t
technique, radiographs, *107,* 120
Temporomandibular joint
luxation, *111,* 112
osteodystrophy, 112–113
radiographic technique, *106*
Tendinopathy
biceps, 72–73, *73*
supraspinatus/infraspinatus, 73, *73*
Tendonitis, ossifying, 56
Tension pneumothorax, 178, 197
Testicles, 283–284
Tetralogy of Fallot, 201
Thorax. (*see specific structures*)
Thromboembolism
aortic, 213
heartworm disease, 206
Thrombosis, mesenteric, 254–255
Thymus, 171, *174*
Thyroid scintigraphy, 8
Tibia
physis closure, 27t, 28t
tuberosity avulsion, 97, *97*
metaphyseal dysplasia, 39
Torsion
lung, 166
splenic, 238, *238*
testicular, 283–284
Toxoplasmosis, 167
Trachea
anatomy, 147
diseases/disorders
collapse, 153, *153*
foreign body, 154
hypoplasia, 153, *153*
masses, endotracheal, 153–154
rupture, 154
stenosis, 153, *153*
tracheitis, 154
radiographic interpretation, 152
Tracheography, 25
Transitional vertebrae, 132–134, *133*
Trauma, joint, 63
Tricuspid valve insufficiency, 204–205, *205*
Tympanic bullae
craniomandibular osteopathy (CMO), 113
otitis, 113, *113–114*
radiographic technique, *106*
tumor, *114*

Ulceration, gastric, 244, 245–246
Ulna
physis closure, 27t, 28t
premature physeal closure, *49,* 49–50
retained enchondrial cartilage, 40, *41*
Ultrasound. (*see also specific organs and areas*) 4–6
echocardiography, 186
Umbilical hernia, 221
Ununited anconeal process, 31, *31,* 76, 77, *77*
Upper gastrointestinal study (UGI), 21
Ureters
anatomy, 262
calculi, 268
contrast radiography, 265, 266
ectopic, 266, *266*
rupture, 269–270
Urethra
anatomy, 274
calculi, 275
contrast radiography, 274–275
neoplasia, 275
radiographic interpretation, 274–275
rupture, 275
urethritis, 275
urethrorectal fistula, 276
Urethrography, 19, *283*
retrograde, 274–276, 282
Urinary bladder
anatomy, 270, *270*
calculi, 272–273
contrast radiography, 271–274
cystitis, 272
emphysema, 219
emphysematous cystitis, 273, *273*
neoplasia, 273–274, *274*
radiographic interpretation, 270–271, *271*
rupture, 273
Urinary system. (*see also specific structures*)
contrast procedures, 17–19
cystography, 18–19
intravenous urography, 17–18
urethrography, 19
Urinary tract infection and prostatitis, 281
Urography and nonionic contrast media, 15
Uterus
masses, 285–286
physometra, 219
pyometra, 285, 287–288
stump granulomas, 286

Vaginography, 19–20, 289
cervical masses, 288
ectopic ureters, 266
Vascular calcification, 220

Vascular ring anomalies, 202, *202,* 227–228
Vasculature, pulmonary, 159–160
  anatomy, 148–149, *149*
Venography, caudal vena cava, 276
Venous portography, 24
Ventricular septal defect (VSD), 201
Vertebra. (*see* Spine)
Vertebral Heart Sum (VHS), 190
Villonodular synovitis, 68
Volvulus
  gastric, 247–248, *248*
  mesenteric, 254
Ventricular Septal Defect (VSD), 201
Wobbler syndrome, 137, *137*

X-rays. (*see also* Computed tomography (CT); Fluoroscopy)
  attenuation, 2
  film, 3
  focal spot, 10
  overview, 2–3, 9